NATIONAL ACADEMIES Sciences Engineering Medicine

NATIONAL ACADEMIES PRESS
Washington, DC

Launching Lifelong Health by Improving Health Care for Children, Youth, and Families

---

Tina L. Cheng and James M. Perrin,
Editors

Committee on Improving the Health and Wellbeing of Children and Youth through Health Care System Transformation

Board on Children, Youth, and Families

Division of Behavioral and Social Sciences and Education

Board on Health Care Services

Health and Medicine Division

Consensus Study Report

NATIONAL ACADEMIES PRESS 500 Fifth Street, NW Washington, DC 20001

This activity was supported by contracts between the National Academy of Sciences and the American Board of Pediatrics (18452-81001), the Health Resources and Services Administration and the Agency for Healthcare Research and Quality (75R60221D00002/75R60222F34004), the Robert Wood Foundation (79272), and The David and Lucile Packard Foundation (2022-73646), and was supported by the American Academy of Pediatrics, Academic Pediatric Association, Children's Hospital Association, and Silicon Valley Community Foundation. Any opinions, findings, conclusions, or recommendations expressed in this publication do not necessarily reflect the views of any organization or agency that provided support for the project.

International Standard Book Number-13: 978-0-309-72194-3
International Standard Book Number-10: 0-309- 72194-6
Digital Object Identifier: https://doi.org/10.17226/27835
Library of Congress Control Number: 2024948442

This publication is available from the National Academies Press, 500 Fifth Street, NW, Keck 360, Washington, DC 20001; (800) 624-6242; http://www.nap.edu.

Printed in the United States of America.

Suggested citation: National Academies of Sciences, Engineering, and Medicine. 2024. *Launching Lifelong Health by Improving Health Care for Children, Youth, and Families*. Washington, DC: National Academies Press. https://doi.org/10.17226/27835.

The **National Academy of Sciences** was established in 1863 by an Act of Congress, signed by President Lincoln, as a private, nongovernmental institution to advise the nation on issues related to science and technology. Members are elected by their peers for outstanding contributions to research. Dr. Marcia McNutt is president.

The **National Academy of Engineering** was established in 1964 under the charter of the National Academy of Sciences to bring the practices of engineering to advising the nation. Members are elected by their peers for extraordinary contributions to engineering. Dr. John L. Anderson is president.

The **National Academy of Medicine** (formerly the Institute of Medicine) was established in 1970 under the charter of the National Academy of Sciences to advise the nation on medical and health issues. Members are elected by their peers for distinguished contributions to medicine and health. Dr. Victor J. Dzau is president.

The three Academies work together as the **National Academies of Sciences, Engineering, and Medicine** to provide independent, objective analysis and advice to the nation and conduct other activities to solve complex problems and inform public policy decisions. The National Academies also encourage education and research, recognize outstanding contributions to knowledge, and increase public understanding in matters of science, engineering, and medicine.

Learn more about the National Academies of Sciences, Engineering, and Medicine at **www.nationalacademies.org**.

Consensus Study Reports published by the National Academies of Sciences, Engineering, and Medicine document the evidence-based consensus on the study's statement of task by an authoring committee of experts. Reports typically include findings, conclusions, and recommendations based on information gathered by the committee and the committee's deliberations. Each report has been subjected to a rigorous and independent peer-review process and it represents the position of the National Academies on the statement of task.

Proceedings published by the National Academies of Sciences, Engineering, and Medicine chronicle the presentations and discussions at a workshop, symposium, or other event convened by the National Academies. The statements and opinions contained in proceedings are those of the participants and are not endorsed by other participants, the planning committee, or the National Academies.

Rapid Expert Consultations published by the National Academies of Sciences, Engineering, and Medicine are authored by subject-matter experts on narrowly focused topics that can be supported by a body of evidence. The discussions contained in rapid expert consultations are considered those of the authors and do not contain policy recommendations. Rapid expert consultations are reviewed by the institution before release.

For information about other products and activities of the National Academies, please visit www.nationalacademies.org/about/whatwedo.

COMMITTEE ON IMPROVING THE HEALTH AND WELLBEING OF CHILDREN AND YOUTH THROUGH HEALTH CARE SYSTEM TRANSFORMATION

TINA L. CHENG (*Co-Chair*), Cincinnati Children's Hospital Medical Center; University of Cincinnati College of Medicine
JAMES M. PERRIN (*Co-Chair*), Harvard Medical School; Massachusetts General Hospital for Children
LOUIS P. APPEL, People's Community Clinic
CHRISTINA BETHELL, Johns Hopkins Bloomberg School of Public Health
ASHLEIGH F. BOWMAN, University of South Alabama, College of Nursing; USA Health Children's & Women's Hospital
NATHAN T. CHOMILO, Minnesota Department of Human Services; University of Minnesota Medical School
ASHLEIGH D. COSER, Cherokee Nation
ALISON E. CUELLAR, George Mason University; National Bureau of Economic Research
HALA H. DURRAH, Independent Patient Family Engagement Consultant
CAROLE R. GRESENZ, Georgetown University
KELLY J. KELLEHER, Nationwide Children's Hospital; The Ohio State University
WILLIAM MARTINEZ, University of California, San Francisco; Zuckerberg San Francisco General Hospital
PHILIP O. OZUAH, Montefiore Einstein Medicine; Albert Einstein College of Medicine
SARAH A. STODDARD, University of Michigan School of Nursing and School of Public Health
LEQUISHA S. TURNER, University of Nebraska Medical Center Munroe Meyer Institute
JENNIFER R. WALTON, University of Miami Miller School of Medicine

Study Staff

JULIE ANNE SCHUCK, Study Director
ABIGAIL ALLEN, Associate Program Officer (from August 2023)
SUNIA YOUNG, Senior Program Assistant (until February 2024)
EMMA MOORE, Senior Program Assistant (from January 2024)
SHAAKIRA PARKER, Associate Program Officer (until August 2023)
EMILY P. BACKES, Deputy Board Director, Board on Child, Youth, and Families

FOPEFOLUWA ATANDA, Intern (Summer 2023)
ALLISSA MASSE, Intern (Summer 2023)

National Academy of Medicine Fellow in Global Health Leadership

KAI CHEONG, Hong Kong Children's Hospital,
University of Hong Kong

BOARD ON CHILDREN, YOUTH, AND FAMILIES

BOARD ON HEALTH CARE SERVICES

Reviewers

This Consensus Study Report was reviewed in draft form by individuals chosen for their diverse perspectives and technical expertise. The purpose of this independent review is to provide candid and critical comments that will assist the National Academies of Sciences, Engineering, and Medicine (National Academies) in making each published report as sound as possible and to ensure that it meets the institutional standards for quality, objectivity, evidence, and responsiveness to the study charge. The review comments and draft manuscript remain confidential to protect the integrity of the deliberative process.

We thank the following individuals for their review of this report:

CHARLES BRUNER, Director, Child Equity
PAUL CHUNG, Department of Health Systems Science, Kaiser Permanente Bernard J. Tyson School of Medicine
TUMAINI R. COKER, General Pediatrics, Seattle Children's Hospital
CHRISTOPHER B. FORREST, Department of Pediatrics at Children's Hospital of Philadelphia, and Director, Applied Clinical Research Center
KIMBERLY E. HOAGWOOD, Department of Child and Adolescent Psychiatry, New York University
BRUCE LESLEY, President, First Focus on Children
MICHAEL C. LU, School of Public Health, University of California, Berkeley
PAULA MAGEE, Department of Anesthesiology and Critical Care Medicine at Children's Hospital of Philadelphia

CINDY MANN, Partner, Manatt, Phelps & Phillips, LLP
LINDA MENDONCA, Community/Public Health Nursing, Zvart Onanian School of Nursing, Rhode Island College
LISA A. PROSSER, Department of Pediatrics and Department of Health Management and Policy, University of Michigan
COLLEEN REULAND, Director, Oregon Pediatric Improvement Partnership, Department of Pediatrics, Doernbecher Children's Hospital, Oregon Health & Sciences University
ZIRUI SONG, Department of Health Care Policy, Harvard Medical School and Department of Medicine, Massachusetts General Hospital
JOSHUA TRAYLOR, Executive Director, Center for Health and Research Transformation
DAVID W. WILLIS, Senior Fellow, Center for the Study of Social Policy

Although the reviewers listed above provided many constructive comments and suggestions, they were not asked to endorse the conclusions or recommendations of this report, nor did they see the final draft before its release. The review of this report was overseen by **ROSEMARY A. CHALK,** Independent Consultant, and **SUSAN J. CURRY,** Department of Health Management and Policy, The University of Iowa, emeritus. They are responsible for making certain that an independent examination of this report was carried out in accordance with the standards of the National Academies and that all review comments were carefully considered. Responsibility for the final content rests entirely with the authoring committee and the National Academies.

Acknowledgments

The committee thanks the sponsors of this study for their support: the American Board of Pediatrics, the Health Resources and Services Administration and the Agency for Healthcare Research and Quality, the Robert Wood Johnson Foundation, The David & Lucile Packard Foundation, the American Academy of Pediatrics, the Academic Pediatric Association, the Children's Hospital Association, and Pediatrics Supporting Parents through the Silicon Valley Community Foundation.

This report would not have been possible without the contributions of many people. Special thanks go to the members of the committee, who dedicated extensive time, expertise, knowledge, and energy to the preparing of the report. The committee also thanks the members of the staff of the National Academies for their significant contributions to the report: Julie Schuck, Abigail Allen, Emma Moore, Shaakira Parker, and Sunia Young, as well as Kai Cheong, National Academy of Medicine Fellow, and summer interns Fopefoluwa Atanda and Allissa Masse.

In addition to its own research and deliberations, the committee received input from numerous outside sources, whose perspectives and experiences were fundamental to the committee's effort. We thank Mary Applegate, Ohio Department of Medicaid; Prameela Boorada, Mental Health America, Youth Mental Health Leadership Council; Renée Boynton-Jarrett, Boston University, Vital Village Community Engage ment Network; Jacey Cooper, California Department of Health Care Services; Sneha Dave, Generation Patient; Doug Eby, Southcentral Foundation; David Erickson, Federal Reserve Bank of New York; Sherry Glied, New York University; Christopher Greeley, Baylor College of Medicine, Texas Children's Hospital; Neal

Halfon, University of California, Los Angeles; Dana Hargunani, Oregon Health Authority; Kay Johnson, Johnson Group Consulting, Inc.; Nat Kendall-Taylor, FrameWorks Institute; Stephen Kingsmore, Rady Children's Hospital; Elizabeth Koschmann, University of Michigan, TRAILS to Wellness; Daniel Kraft, NextMed Health; Bruce Lesley, First Focus on Children; Cindy Mann, Manatt Health; Kenny McDonald, The Columbus Partnership; Eneida Mendonça, Cincinnati Children's Hospital; Tamela Milan-Alexander, EverThrive; Nikki Montgomery, Family Voices; Carley Riley, Cincinnati Children's Hospital, All Children Thrive; Tim Robinson, Nationwide Children's; Sara Rosenbaum, The George Washington University; Edward Schor, health care system consultant; Jim Taylor, Google; Sara Watson, Watson Strategies, LLC; and Paul Wise, Stanford University. The committee also gathered information through commissioned papers. We thank Irene Papanicolas, Brown University, London School of Economics, Harvard University, and Mark Stabile, INSEAD, University of Toronto, for their papers.

The committee is also grateful to National Academies staff Pamella Atayi and Javed Khan for their administrative and financial assistance on this project. From the Office of Reports and Communication of the Division of Behavioral and Social Sciences and Education (DBASSE), Kirsten Sampson Snyder, Douglas Sprunger, and Kimberly Halperin shepherded the report through the review and the production process and assisted with its communication and dissemination. Hannah Fuller of the Office of News and Public Information and Sandra McDermin of the Office of the Congressional and Government Affairs were instrumental in the release and promotion of the report. The committee also thanks Clair Woolley of the National Academies Press and Bea Porter of DBASSE for their assistance with the production of the final report. We also thank Health and Medicine Division staff member Marc Meisnere and consultants Eli Cahan and Megan Snair for their writing and editing contributions; editors Rona Briere and Allie Boman provided skillful editing of the report manuscript.

Throughout the project, Natacha Blain and Emily Backes, director and deputy director of the Board on Children, Youth, and Families, and Carlotta Arthur and Patti Simon, executive director and associate executive director of DBASSE, provided valuable oversight and guidance.

Contents

Boxes, Figures, and Tables

BOXES

FIGURES

TABLES

Preface

The true measure of a nation's standing is how well it attends to its children—their health and safety, their material security, their education and socialization, and their sense of being loved, valued, and included in the families and societies into which they are born.

—*United Nations Children's Fund*

The foundation and promise of lifelong health start in childhood. Children are the workforce of tomorrow and the human capital that will drive our nation forward. That future, however, is threatened by the precarious state of child health and wellbeing in America today. The United States significantly lags in child health status among the world's industrialized countries. Our nation's enduring health disparities deprive too many children of the care, support, and opportunity they need to thrive.

If we fail to address these circumstances, our nation faces grave economic, social, and health-related risks. A strong economy relies on a highly skilled workforce, but the business community increasingly warns that the United States is losing ground. No fewer than three branches of the military failed to meet their recruitment goals last year, with 77% of young people ineligible for reasons of health. The growing population of older adults will rely on an undersized youth cohort and a declining U.S. birth rate.

Good evidence supports national and local strategies for changing the trajectories for young Americans. There are many well-studied innovations on health care for children and youth that, if brought to scale, can strengthen young peoples' health, wellbeing, and development. The path forward accelerates the move to team care in communities, inclusion of mental and behavioral health and community health workers, and major improvements in the science and organization of pediatric subspecialty care. Greater inclusion of families in all aspects of their health care—using their voice and experience to improve care—builds trust, capacity, and solutions. Schools can increase their efforts in prevention and providing health services that keep children active, alert, and engaged in their education. Many critical public health efforts—from nutrition, to surveillance and prevention, to delivery to particularly vulnerable groups, to ensuring the health of the nation's children and parents—merit focus, collaboration, and more support.

It will take consistent, sustained, and permanent national leadership and strong state and local engagement to institute and maintain the changes needed. Many previous efforts have led to important progress in programs for children's health, but the lack of a sustained vision and focus has limited those gains. Attention to children's health needs in times of national crisis often comes too little and too late. The nation needs to pay more, and more wisely, for change and to support the future health care system that can be built from the strong evidence this report offers. Critically, public insurance (mainly Medicaid and the Children's Health Insurance Program) support health care for half of U.S. children. Reform of these programs, along with the investment needed to prevent discrimination based on insurance provider, can form the basis of a high-quality universal health care system for all children who lack other insurance. Ensuring the full implementation of key Medicaid benefits, especially the Early and Periodic Screening, Diagnosis, and Treatment statute, will strengthen that progress. Payment reform in general, both commercial and public, can greatly enhance the transformation of care and help bring to scale the many innovations available in pediatric care and wisely implement the many scientific advances in prevention, diagnosis, and treatment of childhood conditions.

This project benefited from the support of a diverse group of public and private sponsors. We very much appreciate their support and the questions they provided us early in the study. Our committee included an array of members with varied experiences, backgrounds, and disciplines, who engaged actively in this work. Their talents helped us build a vigorous and well-rounded approach to a complex and important set of questions.

Nelson Mandela noted that "our children are our greatest treasure." However, America's young lack voice in decision making and are often an afterthought in policy and innovation. Changing this situation requires "the wisdom, the will, and the wallet," as co-chair Cheng puts it. This report relays the wisdom: the committee documents the substantial knowledge base regarding child health and wellbeing, identifying essential levers for change, and underscoring the essential role of families and communities in creating necessary progress. The enduring oversight structure and investment strategy recommended in this report are a blueprint for ensuring the health and wellbeing of America's most valuable asset: all our children. Investing in their future is the key to a healthy community, a stable and prosperous nation, and the next generation of adults that realizes its full human potential.

Tina L. Cheng and James M. Perrin, *Co-Chairs*
Committee on Improving the Health and
Wellbeing of Children and Youth through
Health Care System Transformation

Acronyms and Abbreviations

AACAP	American Academy of Child and Adolescent Psychiatry
AAFP	American Academy of Family Physicians
AANP	American Association of Nurse Practitioners
AAP	American Academy of Pediatrics
ACA	Patient Protection and Affordable Care Act
ACF	Administration for Children and Families
ACGME	Accreditation Council for Graduate Medical Education
ACO	accountable care organization
ACOG	American College of Obstetricians and Gynecologists
ACP	American College of Physicians
ACS	American Community Survey
ADDM	Autism and Developmental Disabilities Monitoring (Network)
ADHD	attention deficit hyperactivity disorder
AHA	American Hospital Association
AHEAD	Accelerating All-Payer Health Equity and Development
AHRQ	Agency for Healthcare Research and Quality
AI	artificial intelligence
AI/AN	American Indian/Alaska Native
ASPE	Office of the Assistant Secretary for Planning and Evaluation
ASQ	Ages and States Questionnaire
ASTHO	Association of State and Tribal Health Officials
BLS	Bureau of Labor Statistics
BMI	body mass index

BPCA	Best Pharmaceuticals for Children Act
BSCA	Bipartisan Safer Communities Act
CACFP	Child and Adult Care Food Program
CAHMI	Child and Adolescent Health Measurement Initiative
CAP	child and adolescent psychiatrist
CARES	Coronavirus Aid, Relief, and Economic Security
CAY	Center for the Advancement of Youth
CBO	Congressional Budget Office
CBT	cognitive-behavioral therapy
CCBHC	certified community behavioral health clinic
CCDF	Child Care and Development Fund
CDC	U.S. Centers for Disease Control and Prevention
CHCS	Center for Health Care Strategies
CHIP	Children's Health Insurance Program
CHW	community health worker
CLS	child life specialist
CMMI	Center for Medicare and Medicaid Innovation
CMS	Centers for Medicare & Medicaid Services
CNMI	Commonwealth of the Northern Mariana Islands
CNS	Clinical Nurse Specialist
COI	Child Opportunity Index
CPEHN	California Pan-Ethnic Health Network
CPSTF	Community Preventive Services Task Force
CRA	Community Reinvestment Act
CSSP	Center for the Study of Social Policy
CTC	Child Tax Credit
CW	Child Welfare (Administration for Children and Families)
CYBHI	Children and Youth Behavioral Initiative
DBP	developmental-behavioral pediatrician
DoD	Department of Defense
DSH	Disproportionate Share Hospital (program)
DULCE	Developmental Understanding and Legal Collaboration
EBT	electronic benefit transfer
ECHO	(Project) Extension for Community Healthcare Outcomes
ED	U.S. Department of Education
EHR	electronic health record
EI	Early Intervention (U.S. Department of Education)
EIP	economic impact payment
EnAct!	Engagement in Action (framework)

EPA U.S. Environmental Protection Agency
EPSDT Early and Periodic Screening, Diagnosis, and Treatment
ERS Economic Research Service

FCFS Federal Interagency Forum on Child and Family Statistics
FDA Food and Drug Administration
FMAP Federal Medical Assistance Percentage
FNS Food and Nutrition Service
FPL federal poverty level
FQHC federally qualified health center
FY fiscal year

GAO Government Accountability Office
GDP gross domestic product
GDP2 Global Developmental Potential
GHWIC Good Health and Wellness in Indian Country
GRPA Government Performance and Results Act

HDHP/SO high-deductible health plan/savings option
HEDIS Healthcare Effectiveness Data and Information Set (managed care organization measures; National Committee for Quality Assurance)
HHS U.S. Department of Health and Human Services
HMG Help Me Grow
HMO health maintenance organization
HNHF Healthy Neighborhoods Healthy Families
HomVEE Home Visiting Evidence of Effectiveness (project)
HRSA Health Resources and Services Administration
HV Maternal, Infant, and Early Childhood Home Visiting (Health Resources and Services Administration)

IDEA Individuals with Disabilities Education Act
IECMH Infant Early Childhood Mental Health
IECMHC Infant and Early Childhood Mental Health Consultation
IEP individualized education program
IFSP individualized family service plan
IHS Indian Health Service
IIHS Insurance Institute for Highway Safety
IMPACT Integrated Model for Parents and Children Together
InCK Integrated Care for Kids (model)
IOM Institute of Medicine
IPFCC Institute for Patient- and Family-Centered Care
IRS Internal Revenue Service

KIDs	Kids Inpatient Database
LAUNCH	Linking Actions for Unmet Needs in Children's Health
MACPAC	Medicaid and CHIP Payment and Access Commission
MCD	Medicaid and CHIP (Centers for Medicare & Medicaid Services)
MCH MRN	Maternal and Child Health Measurement Research Network
MCHB	Maternal and Child Health Bureau
MCO	managed care organization
MFP	medical-financial partnership
MIECHV	Maternal, Infant, and Early Child Home Visiting (program)
MLP	medical–legal partnership
MLR	medical loss ratio
NACHC	National Association of Community Health Centers
NAM	National Academy of Medicine
NASN	National Association of School Nurses
NASW	National Association of Social Workers
NCBDDD	National Center on Birth Defects and Developmental Disabilities
NCCPA	National Commission on the Certification of Physician Assistants
NCHWA	National Center for Health Workforce Analysis
NCTSN	National Child Traumatic Stress Network
NCUIH	National Council of Urban Indian Health
NHGRI	National Human Genome Research Institute
NHIS	National Health Interview Survey
NHOPI	Native Hawaiian or Other Pacific Islander
NHQDR	National Healthcare Quality and Disparities Report
NICHD	National Institute of Child Health and Human Development
NICWA	National Indian Child Welfare Association
NIH	National Institutes of Health
NP	nurse practitioner
NPC-QIC	National Pediatric Cardiology for Everyone Improvement Collaborative
NRC	National Research Council
NRHA	National Rural Health Association
NSCH	National Survey of Children's Health
NSLP	National School Lunch Program
ODM	Ohio Department of Medicaid
ODPHP	Office of Disease Prevention and Health Promotion

OECD	Organisation for Economic Co-operation and Development
OMB	Office of Management and Budget
ONC	Office of the National Coordinator for Health Information Technology
OSG	Office of the U.S. Surgeon General
PA	physician assistant
PARENT	Parent-focused Redesign for Encounters, Newborns to Toddlers
PEDS	Parent's Evaluation of Developmental Status
PHHS	Preventive Health and Health Services
PNCB	Pediatric Nursing Certification Board
POS	point of service
PPO	preferred provider organization
PTSD	post-traumatic stress disorder
R3	Ready! Resilient! Rising!
REACH	Racial and Ethnic Approaches to Community Health
RMTS	Random Moment Time Study
RN	registered nurse
ROI	return on investment
RUC	Relative Value Scale Update Committee
SAMHSA	Substance Abuse and Mental Health Services Administration
SBHA	School-Based Health Alliance
SBHC	school-based health center
SBP	School Breakfast Program
SCF	Southcentral Foundation
SDOH	social determinants of health
SEEK	Safe Environment for Every Kid
SFSP	Summer Food Service Program
SNAP	Supplemental Nutrition Assistance Program
SPP	Solutions for Pediatric Psychology
SPS	Solutions for Patient Safety
SSA	U.S. Social Security Administration
SSI	Supplemental Security Income
SWYK	Survey of Well-Being of Young Children
TANF	Temporary Assistance for Needy Families
TFICC	Transnational Forum on Integrated Community Care
TRAILS	Transforming Research into Action to Improve the Lives of Students
TV	Title V (Health Resources and Services Administration)

UNICEF	United Nations Children's Fund
USDA	U.S. Department of Agriculture
USVI	U.S. Virgin Islands
VA	U.S. Department of Veterans Affairs
VFC	Vaccines for Children
VIP	Video Interaction Project
WHO	World Health Organization
WIC	Special Supplemental Nutrition Program for Women, Infants, and Children
WSCC	Whole School, Whole Community, Whole Child
WVP	Well-Visit Planner

Key Terms

Adolescent	An individual in the transitional period between childhood and adulthood, which has been viewed as spanning ages 10–19 (World Health Organization [WHO], n.d.a) or 10–24 (Sawyer et al., 2018). The term "youth" is used interchangeably.
Adult	An individual who has reached full physical growth and maturity (Arain et al., 2013; Arnett, 2000; Sawyer et al., 2018; WHO, n.d.a). A legal adult is seen as age 18 or older. Older adults are viewed to be age 65 or older.
Adverse Childhood Experiences	Potentially traumatic events that occur in childhood, including (among other forms) physical, emotional, or sexual abuse; neglect; and household dysfunction. (Centers for Disease Control and Prevention [CDC], 2019b).
Child	An individual in a period of rapid growth and development from birth to adulthood, encompassing infancy, childhood, and adolescence (Food and Drug Administration [FDA], 2022; Williams et al., 2012).

Child Health	This term is used broadly to include preconception, maternal, prenatal, child, adolescent, family, and community health and wellbeing. A multigenerational and life course perspective considers that all health and developmental stages build on each other and are inextricably linked.
Children and Youth with Special Health Care Needs	Individuals with existing or heightened vulnerability to chronic physical, developmental, behavioral, or emotional conditions. These children need health care and associated services beyond the typical requirements for children in general (McPherson et al., 1998).
Co-Creation and/or Co-Design	Active collaboration among stakeholders in designing solutions to a prespecified problem. Co-creation and co-design emphasize involving diverse stakeholders in all parts of a process, beginning with determining and defining the problem through the final stages of a project. These concepts promote citizen participation when formulating or addressing specific concerns (Vargas et al., 2022).
Community	Any configuration of individuals, families, and groups whose values, characteristics, interests, geography, and/or social relations unite them in some way (National Academies of Sciences, Engineering, and Medicine [National Academies], 2017a).
Community Engagement	The process of working collaboratively with and through groups of people affiliated by geographic proximity, special interest, or similar situations to address issues affecting the wellbeing of those people (CDC, 1997).
Community Health Centers	Community-based and patient-directed organizations that provide affordable, accessible, high-quality primary health care services to individuals and families, including people experiencing homelessness, agricultural workers, residents of public housing, and veterans (Health Resources and Services Administration [HRSA], 2023e).

Community Health Worker	A frontline public health worker who is a trusted member or has a particularly good understanding of the community served. Serves as a liaison between health and social services and the community to facilitate access to services and improve the quality and cultural competence of service delivery (American Public Health Association, n.d.; CDC, 1997).
Cross-Sector Collaboration	A process in which various community organizations come together to focus their expertise and resources collectively on a complex issue of importance to a community they serve. The fields of community development and public health are interconnected, and the partnership models they use jointly can inform how sectors come together to foster health and wellbeing (Towe et al., 2016). For child health, other sectors of particular import include child welfare, education, juvenile justice, and social services.
Family	A group of two or more persons related by birth, marriage, or adoption who live together; all such related persons are considered members of one family. For purposes of this report, "family" is extended to include "functional family," which encompasses caregivers and support systems for children, as well as "cultural family," which determines beliefs and reasons for behavior; these extended concepts of family can inform the negotiation of treatment and care (HRSA, 2023d; Medalie & Cole-Kelly, 2002).
Family-Centered (Community-Centered)	A partnership approach to health care decision making between the family (or community) and health care provider (Kuo et al., 2012).
Federally Qualified Health Centers	Federally funded nonprofit health centers or clinics that serve medically underserved areas and populations. Provide primary care services regardless of ability to pay.[1]

[1]https://www.healthcare.gov/glossary/federally-qualified-health-center-fqhc/

Flourishing	A state of positive wellbeing. Typically focuses on parents' or other adults' reports of observable attributes, such as whether children show interest and curiosity in learning new things, are able to regulate emotions and behaviors in challenging situations, and can focus and persist to achieve goals (Bethell, Gombojav, & Whitaker 2019).
Health	Encompasses the extent to which individuals are able or enabled to (a) develop and realize their potential; (b) satisfy their needs; and (c) develop the capacities that allow them to interact successfully with their biological, physical, and social environments (Institute of Medicine [IOM], 2004).
Health Disparities	Differences among specific population groups in the attainment of full health potential. Can be measured by differences in incidence, prevalence, mortality, burden of disease, and other adverse health conditions (National Academies, 2017a).
Health Equity	The state in which everyone is able to achieve their optimal health and wellbeing, with no systemic disparities in health outcomes between groups with different levels of underlying social advantage or disadvantage (Braveman et al., 2018; National Academies, 2017a, 2021b).
Historically Marginalized Populations	Groups and communities that have been poorly served by the health care system, have faced systemic oppression and denial of access to quality care, and have experienced disproportionate impacts from discrimination (National Academies, 2017a, 2020b).
Institutional Racism	Policies and practices within institutions that, intentionally or not, produce outcomes that chronically favor White individuals and put individuals from historically marginalized racial and ethnic groups at a disadvantage (National Academies, 2023b).

Life Course Theory	The life course health and development framework addresses the developmental origins of health across life stages, the role of biological and behavioral plasticity in facilitating different levels of adaptation, and how mismatches between biological propensity and environmental context interact to produce breakdowns in health, known as disease (Halfon et al., 2018).
Maternal Health	Health during pregnancy, childbirth, and the postnatal period (WHO, n.d.b).
Medical Home	An approach to delivering comprehensive and high-quality primary care that goes beyond a physical location. Emphasizes accessibility, family-centered care, continuity, comprehensiveness, compassion, and cultural effectiveness, as well as coordination and partnership among clinicians, families, and community resources (American Academy of Pediatrics [AAP], 2022). High-performing medical homes are practices that provide comprehensive well-child visits and preventive services based on Bright Futures and Early and Periodic Screening, Diagnosis, and Treatment standards, emphasizing care coordination tailored to children's and families' needs (InCK Marks, 2018).
Positive Childhood Experiences	Includes positive interpersonal experiences with family, friends, and in school or the community. Current theory identifies seven types (e.g., felt safe and protected by an adult in their home, felt sense of belonging in school; Bethell et al., 2019).
Public Health	The science and pursuit of promoting and protecting the health of all people in a community. Dimensions include a focus on primary prevention, population health, and diverse public and private collaborators (IOM, 2012c).

Relational Health	The capacity to develop and maintain safe, stable, nurturing relationships with others; relational health is an important predictor of wellness across the lifespan (Garner & Yogman, 2021a).
School-Based Health Centers	Located on or near primary and secondary school campuses; provide primary and preventive medical care, behavioral health services, diagnostic care such as routine screenings, and/or dental preventive care (Medicaid and CHIP Payment and Access Commission, 2018b).
Social Determinants of Health	The conditions in the environments in which people live, learn, work, play, worship, and age that affect a wide range of health, functioning, and quality-of-life outcomes and risks (National Academies, 2017a; Office of Disease Prevention and Health Promotion, n.d.a).
Structural Racism	The totality of ways in which a society fosters racial and ethnic inequity and subjugation through mutually reinforcing systems, including housing, education, employment, earnings, benefits, credit, media, health care, and the criminal legal system. These structural factors organize the distribution of power and resources (i.e., the social determinants of health) differentially among racial, ethnic, and socioeconomic groups, perpetuating racial and ethnic health inequities. The key difference between institutional and structural racism is that structural racism happens across institutions, while institutional racism happens within institutions. "Systemic racism" is a synonym (National Academies, 2024b).

Team-Based Care	Two or more health care professionals working collaboratively with patients and their caregivers to accomplish shared goals. Potentially involving a wide range of team members in various settings, a health care team strives to meet patient needs and preferences by actively engaging patients and families as full participants in their care, while encouraging all health care professionals to function to the full extent of their education, certification, and experience. Members may include physicians, nurses, pharmacists, social workers, community health workers, and others identified as persons necessary to help achieve shared goals (Smith et al., 2020).
Telemedicine and Telehealth	"Telemedicine" refers to the use of telecommunications technologies to facilitate the provision of various medical, diagnostic, and treatment services, typically by physicians. Encompasses activities such as conducting diagnostic tests, closely monitoring a patient's progress post-treatment or therapy, and facilitating access to specialists not located in the same geographic area as the patient. "Telehealth" is similar but encompasses a broader range of remote health care services extending beyond the doctor–patient relationship; frequently involves services provided by nurses, pharmacists, or social workers, supporting patient health education, social assistance, medication adherence, and addressing health concerns for patients and their caregivers (Federal Communications Commission, n.d.).
Whole Child and Family Health Care	A child, family, community-centered, integrated approach to health care that focuses on health promotion and disease prevention early in the life course and addresses family health and the social conditions in which children and families live (National Academies, 2023a).

Abstract

Launching lifelong health for the country's children has never been more important. It is time to reverse troubling trends in the health and wellbeing of child, adolescent, and young adult populations. This report documents increases in the incidence of chronic diseases, growing concerns with children's mental, emotional, and behavioral health, and significant disparities among population subgroups. Rising rates of mortality and disability among youth and working-age Americans also reflect the long-term consequences of not providing the care that children need.

Even with expanded insurance coverage, many children lack access to adequate preventive care. Furthermore, models of health care payment, usually relying on fee-for-service structures or value-based arrangements focused on lowering expenditures for high-cost adult patients, do not provide child health clinicians the flexibility or incentives to work with families and partner with communities to address their health and developmental needs.

In response to rising concerns about the adequacy of pediatric health care to meet evolving challenges and societal needs, the Committee on Improving the Health and Wellbeing of Children and Youth through Health Care System Transformation was assembled to identify key levers of change for improving the health care system for children and youth. The focus of this report and its recommendations is on the health care sector, defined broadly to include clinical and community care, along with public health investments in child and family health and school-based efforts in health care. This report is not the first assessment of opportunities for transformative pediatric care; it builds on an ever-expanding body of research on health care for children, families, and communities.

Robust science on the importance of early life experiences, relationship-based care, genetics and epigenetics, and developmental origins of health and disease demonstrates potential for enhancing society through a focus on prevention and health promotion. A substantial research base shows that efforts to promote positive childhood experiences that provide safe, stable, and nurturing relationships and environments in early life can reduce adult physical, mental, social, and relational health problems.

Health care systems in the future will need to engage in broader, cross-sector collaborations that build on community strengths and address family and community health needs. With the proper infrastructure and financing, many recent, well-evidenced advances in health care can continue to support change and the progress needed in the next 10 years. These advances include better and earlier diagnosis and treatment, innovations in team-based primary and subspecialty care, integration of mental and behavioral health services with care, effective strategies for child and family engagement in care and co-design of care, and improved screening and co-ordination of care with other community services. The health care financing system for children, with support from Medicaid and the Children's Health Insurance Program, insures almost 95% of U.S. children, but current incentives inhibit critical innovations. Key strategies exist to reform payment and transform care.

The committee identified five implementation goals to set the country on a path toward improved health care and better health and wellbeing of children and youth. Each goal includes a set of recommendations aimed at critical federal, state, and community-level actions.

1. Elevate the importance of child and adolescent health for the nation through continuous public focus on children and youth.
2. Finance health care systems for all children, emphasizing prevention and health promotion.
3. Strengthen community-level health promotion and disease prevention.
4. Ensure co-creation and co-design of programs and structures with youth, family, and community voices and leadership.
5. Implement measurement and accountability to ensure equitable achievement of these goals.

The report's recommendations call for sustained and coordinated leadership at the federal level to maintain focus on children and youth and their health care and better assess the child health impact of public policies. The report identifies four key levers of change: (1) health care financing reform with incentives for preventive care; (2) increased investment in public health efforts, school-based health care, and activities designed to address community health needs; (3) inclusion of children and families and especially historically marginalized communities in all aspects of program and policy improvement; and (4) development of measurement strategies for population health outcomes. (See the Summary and Chapter 10 for fuller description and discussion of the recommendations.)

Investing in the health and wellbeing of children and youth not only helps young people and their families now but has longer-term social and economic benefits for the next generation of productive and healthy adults and healthy children. At a population level, child health is the foundation of a thriving nation.

Summary

Ensuring that every child is on an optimal trajectory to a healthy and productive adulthood is imperative for the nation's future. Investment in children and families improves not only child health but also population health, health equity, education outcomes, workforce productivity, and cost-effectiveness in public spending. The foundations of lifelong health are established early in the life course. Longitudinal studies show clearly that major causes of adult morbidity and mortality and aging have their roots in childhood. Emerging scientific and technological advances in genomics, artificial intelligence, relational health, and social determinants highlight the promise of early identification, health promotion, and prevention to optimize the health of children, adults, and society.

Innovations in health care delivery have been implemented over the past few decades in various locations to expand the reach of pediatric primary care and enhance disease prevention and health promotion through strengthened connections with other community resources. In addition, scientific advancements and quality improvement approaches have increased life expectancy for children and youth with special health care needs. The health care system is positioned to play a fundamental role in advancing these innovations and promoting the early and lifelong wellbeing of children and youth. Yet, the main sources of financing for health care have not transformed to support broad implementation of key innovations.

Meanwhile, in the context of this tremendous advancement and opportunity, the birth rate is declining and children's health, wellbeing, and survival rates have all worsened. The nation faces the consequences of this poor state of health in rising mortality, chronic disease, and mental health problems among working-age adults, a less capable workforce, and too few healthy young people to ensure military preparedness and economic stability.

Despite calls to improve the child and adolescent health care system that have been made for more than 20 years, the nation today faces a crisis with serious consequences for the coming decade. Without change, the next 10 years will see larger numbers of young people enter adulthood with chronic illness and disability and worse mental health, leaving fewer adults capable of productive work. This report underscores earlier calls to action on the need to advance health equity, strengthen accountability, promote cost-effectiveness, ensure quality, and engage patients and families through health care transformation. National progress on improving long-term outcomes for all Americans will come only from a dedicated and ongoing commitment to improving the wellbeing of children, youth, and families.

THE STUDY CONTEXT AND CHARGE

In response to rising concerns about the adequacy of pediatric health care to meet evolving challenges and societal needs, the National Academies of Sciences, Engineering, and Medicine (National Academies) assembled the Committee on Improving the Health and Wellbeing of Children and Youth through Health Care System Transformation to provide advice on key levers of change to facilitate health promotion, resilience, disease prevention, and equitable treatment. Committee members included physicians, nurses, hospital system leaders, Medicaid experts, youth and family advocates, community health center providers, economists and health care financing experts, and experts in mental health and school-based health care.

In its charge, the committee was tasked with addressing six questions. The first question asked the committee to identify key levers of change to guide innovation and transformation within the child and adolescent health care system. The second asked for promising policies and programs for achieving transformation. Other questions focused on systemic inequities and disparities, and the gaps and barriers in current payment models. The committee was also asked to examine ways to improve family engagement and community-centered care; team-based care; and integration of major programs serving children and adolescents.

The focus of this report is on the health care sector, defined broadly to include public health investments in child and family health and school-based efforts in health care. However, the committee recognizes the many other important policies and programs that influence child and family health, especially those around poverty and income support, housing, labor markets and employment, community wellbeing, family leave and child care support, juvenile justice, education, and financing of these.

"Child health," as described in this report, includes preconception, maternal, prenatal, child, adolescent, family, and community health and wellbeing. Throughout the report, the committee takes a multigenerational and life course perspective because research has shown that all health and developmental stages are inextricably linked. To develop a plan to address its charge, the committee ascribed to a set of principles to guide its work and the development of program and policy recommendations: (1) employ a life course perspective; (2) partner with families and communities, which are central to child health and wellbeing; (3) prioritize and drive equitable outcomes through resources and accountability; and (4) make it sustainable over time. The committee views the present time as a clear opportunity for the nation to transform child and adolescent health care, making the United States a place for children to grow and thrive, and building a lasting, effective, diverse, and creative workforce.

OVERARCHING CONCLUSIONS

Based on the background and findings presented in the chapters of this report and in the extensive literature on the state of children's health and health care delivery in the United States, the committee makes these overarching conclusions:

1. The United States faces a major crisis with the poor and worsening health and wellbeing of children and youth and the impact on the workforce of the future. Despite many advances, the United States currently ranks at the bottom among wealthy nations on the mental wellbeing, physical health, and academic and social skills of children. Children living in poverty, from historically marginalized groups, in foster care, or involved with the juvenile justice system all face poorer health and higher rates of mental health conditions. The incidence of several chronic diseases among children has increased over the past half century, along with growing concerns with children's mental, emotional, and behavioral health. Many of these conditions are preventable or can be well managed with little disability. Further, working-age adults in the United States have experienced substantial increases in mortality and morbidity, with high rates of mental health conditions, obesity and associated cardiovascular and pulmonary disease, and substance use. These increases make the U.S. workforce less prepared for the needs of business and industry and diminish military preparedness. At a time when the U.S. birth rate has also decreased, increasing numbers of older people have rising support needs but fewer workers to assist.

2. The committee examined the evidence of what works to improve child health and health care and to advance health equity. Social and relational experiences and environments shape the health and wellbeing and development of children and youth in positive and negative ways. Major advances in early childhood science show that health early in the life course sets the foundation for health throughout childhood, adolescence, young adulthood, and beyond. Many adult chronic illnesses have early antecedents that are discernable in childhood. Scientific and technological advances in epigenetics, advanced treatments, and new prediction by artificial intelligence help identify conditions earlier and provide strategies for prevention and early treatment. Health care has seen growth in innovations applying this knowledge to clinical care, with positive outcomes in both primary and subspecialty care.
3. Previous efforts have led to real progress in some communities, but the lack of an ongoing focus on children, youth, and families has hampered continuing progress. Broader health care discussions and policy, program, and funding in the United States have paid limited attention to the health care delivery needs of children and youth. Most health care investment and reform have been directed toward the adult care delivery systems.
4. Families and communities are experts in their own health needs and have expressed desires to be informed and part of the process of improving health care. Their engagement in broad aspects of health care decisions has led to real changes in some communities and improvements in the organization and delivery of services and their impact on the populations engaged.
5. The current child health care system has made major gains in broadening primary care content and building teams in primary and subspecialty care, with many strong programs presenting clear evidence for their impact. Multidisciplinary teams often involve nurses, mental/behavioral health providers, community health workers, and others. Recent innovations include providing family supports and building capacity to address mental and behavioral health and school issues, as well as linking the health care team to other sectors and community services that support child and family wellbeing and development. Nonetheless, current health care financing arrangements have made it difficult to bring innovations to scale.
6. Community health centers have had leading roles in providing high-quality and comprehensive services to many low-income children. Hospital and subspecialty care have changed in recent years,

with fewer hospitalizations; more concentration in urban centers; and greater capacity in subspecialty care, coordinated with the primary care community. However, access to quality health care continues to be problematic for many individuals and communities, including those with certain health conditions (e.g., mental health conditions, where health care delivery and financing are often siloed), children with special health care needs, low-income and historically marginalized populations, and those in certain geographic areas.

7. Schools have been a central partner in child health through health education, socioemotional learning, nursing services, counseling, and the provision of nutritious meals and other wellbeing supports. They provide important services, and their growth offers opportunities to strengthen the health of young people. In many communities, school-based health clinics have increased access to clinical care and improved outcomes for children.
8. Children benefit from many public health activities, including those to improve the health of communities as well as many programs directed to maternal and child health, including vaccine programs, various preventive efforts (e.g., car seats, toxin exposures, climate preparedness), and efforts to support families during early childhood (e.g., Head Start, several nutrition programs), among many others. Key federal agencies engaged in public health efforts include the Health Resources and Services Administration (and its bureaus of Primary Care and Maternal and Child Health), Centers for Disease Control and Prevention, Indian Health Services, and U.S. Department of Agriculture.
9. The current health care financing for children and youth has major strengths but also numerous weaknesses that need correction. Current health insurance coverage for children is high—around 95% have some insurance. About half of U.S. children and youth depend on public health insurance through Medicaid and the Children's Health Insurance Program (CHIP), two critical programs that provide a major safety net for large numbers of children who would otherwise lack any health insurance. However, major fluctuations in Medicaid and CHIP administration can change coverage levels significantly and contribute to racial and geographic inequities. Current payment mechanisms, funding, and financial incentives within both public and commercial insurance programs tend to emphasize diagnosis and treatments rather than prevention and health promotion—and limit opportunities to implement health care innovations widely.

10. Medicaid and CHIP have characteristics that make them strong supports for children, including the requirement that states enroll all eligible children who apply and the major Early and Periodic Screening, Diagnosis, and Treatment statute that requires states to provide a wide range of health care services to younger populations. Major state variations, while allowing states to experiment with services and payment strategies focused on their own population needs, have also meant that children have access to very different services and providers in different states, even to the degree that a child would be eligible for Medicaid in one state but not in a neighboring one. Opportunities exist to standardize key characteristics of public insurance across states, including eligibility, enrollment, scope of services, payment, and quality, and to make payment levels high enough to assure equal access to needed services.
11. Most efforts at payment reform have focused on older populations. Although many of these advances could have value for child health as well, payment reform for children must recognize the limited short-term financial return on investment and the need to value longer-term outcomes, often in sectors other than health care. Managed care organizations currently cover the large majority of children in Medicaid and CHIP, and most still pay providers using some form of fee for service. Experimentation and improvement in payment through managed care could enhance progress in health care transformation.
12. The committee found good evidence that transformation of health care for children can take place. The growth in innovations, new science, evidence from family engagement, recognition of how to center health, and opportunities for reformed financing provide the basis for transformation.

THE VISION FOR IMPROVED HEALTH CARE

Prevention has been a cornerstone of child and adolescent health care, and the current state of child health calls for even greater investment in prevention, given the strong evidence of major poor health outcomes downstream. Critically, preventive gains cannot be achieved without greater equity in access and receipt of quality care. Sustained progress in transforming child and adolescent health care requires a coordinated and ongoing focus from federal, state, and local governments on children, youth, and families in all relevant programs and policies, and it requires strong and predictable financing. Moving toward health equity requires an intentional focus on communities that have long endured underinvestment and structural disadvantage. With these aims, the committee identified five implementation goals:

1. Elevate the importance of child and adolescent health for the nation through continuous public focus on children and youth.
2. Finance health care systems for all children, emphasizing prevention and health promotion.
3. Strengthen community-level health promotion and disease prevention.
4. Ensure co-creation and co-design of programs and structures with youth, family, and community voices and leadership.
5. Implement measurement and accountability to ensure equitable achievement of these goals.

The following sections articulate the importance of each goal and how it relates to the issues in the committee's charge, along with key recommendations. Further details on the implementation goals and recommendations can be found in Chapter 10.

Goal 1: Elevate the Importance of Child and Adolescent Health for the Nation through Continuous Public Focus on Children and Youth

Without dedicated and sustained policy and funding prioritization of children at federal, state, and local levels, the nation will continue to lag behind other industrialized countries in most indicators of child, adolescent, and adult health and wellbeing. Limited and late concern for children during the COVID-19 pandemic and other social crises exemplifies the major lapses that occur without sustained federal leadership around the central needs of children. Coordination and communication among agencies serving children and a child-health-in-all-policies lens will be important and will necessitate aligning strategies and funding plans and maintaining a robust process for collecting and disseminating actionable data on the health and wellbeing of all children across federal agencies. The locus of leadership and coordination will need to be at the highest levels of the federal government, but clear participation and shared accountability across key government agencies, states, and the private sector will also be needed. Additionally, similar structures will be needed at the state level.

Recommendation 1-1: Federal policy makers should convene an expert panel of key stakeholders, families, community partners, and state and federal agencies to develop a framework for promoting health and well-being for all children and adolescents and an enduring implementation plan. The framework should strive to integrate health programs among

health care, education, labor, child welfare, and justice systems and foster shared goals of improving health and wellbeing throughout the life course and advancing health equity. The framework should present options for (1) financing enhanced services, (2) monitoring coordination over time, and (3) designating key leaders and agency structures that can focus attention on the health care needs of children, youth and families.

Recommendation 1-2: Federal policy makers should enact child health and health equity impact statements that include impact and cost/benefit over longer time horizons for (1) Office of Management and Budget regulations in the federal register; (2) Congressional Budget Office (CBO) scoring of legislation; and (3) all major federal programmatic and research actions involving the U.S. Departments of Health and Human Services, Education, Housing and Urban Development, Agriculture, Labor, and Justice. The CBO should expand its scoring of health programs to address longer-term outcomes (including Medicare and other public health expenditures) and impacts on federal sectors beyond health care. The president's annual budget line items should also report on inclusion of children and child health and health equity impact.

Recommendation 1-3: State legislatures and agencies should implement scoring of legislation and major programmatic initiatives to inform decisions based on their impact on the health and wellbeing of children and families and on health equity.

Recommendation 1-4: Foundations and child and youth wellbeing advocacy organizations should fund and implement a long-term, multifaceted public awareness campaign that highlights issues of child and adolescent health and describes the importance of children and adolescents for the nation's future wellbeing and economic and national security.

Recommendation 1-5: The U.S. Department of Health and Human Services—through the Agency for Healthcare Research and Quality, the Advanced Research Projects Agency for Health, the National Institutes of Health, and other research and technology funders and developers—should continue and accelerate investment in research on whole child and family health, including mothers, children, adolescents, and families. Key elements of this research follow:

- Inclusion of children, as well as child health and equity impact evaluations, in major research and technology initiatives
- Longitudinal research early and throughout the life course, assessing long-term return on investment in health and developmental/educational outcomes and across sectors

- Research that includes individuals' family and community context.
- Research on developmental transitions and care, such as from the prenatal period to infancy and from adolescence to adulthood.
- Clinical trials and dissemination and implementation research, especially related to incorporating scientific and technological advances in practice and policy.
- Engagement of youth, families, and community in the co-creation and co-design of research.

Goal 2: Finance Health Care Systems for All Children, Emphasizing Prevention and Health Promotion

The committee was tasked with considering the gaps and barriers in current payment models for both public and commercial insurance, and with suggesting potential solutions for addressing them. Goal 2 and its recommendations focus on reform of Medicaid and the CHIP and on changing payment incentives to transform the pediatric health care system so that it provides more prevention and health promotion services. Although the current child health care system promotes wellbeing and prevention, it is hampered by being modeled after an adult system focused on disease identification and treatment and reinforced by fee-for-service payment models. These models do not allow clinicians the flexibility to work with families and communities to address health and developmental goals for children. Instead, payment models are needed that can support team and cross-sector care, including mental and behavioral health integration and other innovations that support the development of safe, stable, and nurturing relationships between caregivers and children; improve health equity; and build community health.

Medicaid and CHIP, the payers for health care for about half of children and youth, ensure a major safety net for large numbers of American children who would otherwise have no insurance. Yet, state variation in implementation of federal Medicaid law creates barriers to enrollment and differences in program eligibility and accessibility that have widened gaps between groups in insurance coverage and access to care. On the other hand, state variation can have positive impacts, especially in allowing innovations and rewarding improvements in accessibility, quality, and costs. Barriers to care affect historically marginalized populations disproportionately, contributing to place-based racial and ethnic health inequities.

Because of their prominence in the lives of most children and families, schools offer unique opportunities to advance child health. The number of school-based health centers that provide primary and preventive medical care to children is growing, serving more than 6 million children in communities that face barriers to health care access. Expansion of school-based health centers is a promising strategy for improving equitable access to high-quality care for children; however, state variation on Medicaid payments currently makes broad expansion challenging.

Recommendation 2-1: Federal and state policy makers and the Centers for Medicare & Medicaid Services (CMS) should reform Medicaid and the Children's Health Insurance Program (CHIP) to ensure coverage and services for every child and parent under age 65 who lacks other insurance. Specific actions to ensure insurance coverage include

- Providing presumptive continuous eligibility for all children through their 6th birthday and universal access to Medicaid for all those under age 26 years who lack other health insurance.
- Enrolling all newborns at birth in Medicaid/CHIP if not covered by another plan.
- Allowing undocumented children and their parents access to Medicaid/CHIP, the Health Insurance Marketplace, and other federally funded health care services.
- Ensuring continuous Medicaid coverage for low-income parents.
- Aligning the financing of child coverage in the territories with that of states through Medicaid and CHIP.

Specific actions to improve benefits and payment include

- Reducing state and territory variability in eligibility, enrollment, quality, and payment by raising minimum federal standards.
- Ensuring a national base of high-quality services by modernizing Early and Periodic Screening, Diagnosis, and Treatment (EPSDT) benefits and rules. CMS and Congress should update EPSDT regulations, and CMS and the states should implement ongoing strategies for ensuring statutory compliance.
- Enforcing managed care organization contracts and implementation to ensure meeting all Medicaid/CHIP standards and requirements. States should ensure transparency in managed care organization contracts and public accountability.
- Designing and requiring integration of Medicaid and CHIP into a single program, making CHIP permanent, establishing the same provisions as Medicaid, and eliminating differences in eligibility and benefits.
- Increasing transparency in provider payment rates and direct provider subsidies and raising provider payments to levels that ensure that children and adolescents have equitable access to

comprehensive, team-based primary and specialty care without discrimination based on payer.

- CMS and the Medicaid and CHIP Payment and Access Commission should collect and analyze data that speak to the adequacy of payment for child health care services.
- CMS should implement a Medicaid Beneficiary Survey, modeled after the Medicare Current Beneficiary Survey, that captures beneficiaries' health and functioning; satisfaction with health care; usual source of care; and access to care, including primary care and specialty care for new and established patients.

Recommendation 2-2: Public and commercial payers should transition from relying predominantly on fee-for-service arrangements and explore payment incentives that emphasize prevention and health promotion services, team-based and cross-sector care, health equity, health outcomes, and longer-term return on investment. While enhancements in fee-for-service models can support needed change, related payment strategies, including direct incentives, various withholding mechanisms, and alternative payment methods, should support this transition. The Centers for Medicare & Medicaid Services (CMS) and commercial payers should use payment methods that provide direct incentives toward population health, health equity, and the health of communities. Strategies for incentivizing practice change could include tiered payments that reward high-performing pediatric care. Current payment innovations, including numerous state efforts such as per member per month or population payments, serve as key experimental steps for covering health care services for children, youth, and families.

- CMS and commercial payers should test and implement episodic and bundled payment models that are designed for the service needs of children, youth, and families, especially those with more complex conditions.
- CMS, through its Center for Medicare and Medicaid Innovation (CMMI), should innovate in pediatric payment strategies and assure inclusion of children in their programs. For example, as CMMI implements state total-cost-of-care models in the States Advancing All-Payer Health Equity Approaches and Development Model, children should be included and child health and health equity impact statements addressed.
- Payment should support team-based and cross-sector care, including high-performing medical homes, mental and behavioral health integration, and other innovations that support development of safe, stable, and nurturing relationships between caregivers and children; improve health equity; and build community health.

Recommendation 2-3: State legislatures and Medicaid programs should adopt and enforce policies that promote equitable payment for services delivered in school-based health centers (SBHCs) and by other school providers. Policies that have been effective in several states include those that (1) define SBHCs as a specific provider type; (2) waive prior approval or authorization from primary care providers for all SBHC billing; (3) allow Medicaid managed care organization payment for "self-referred" children seen in SBHCs; and (4) incorporate clarification of laws related to data sharing, including the Health Insurance Portability and Accountability Act and the Family Educational Rights and Privacy Act. Such policies should be implemented with intent to prioritize communities that face the largest health inequities, including gaps in access to pediatric health care services, and to encourage school-based programs to leverage, support, and enhance collaborations between schools and community health centers and health care systems.

Goal 3: Strengthen Community-Level Health Promotion and Disease Prevention

The committee was tasked with examining the interaction and integration of the child and adolescent health care system with key services that heavily influence the health and wellbeing of children and adolescents and with identifying ways to strengthen those connections. In the United States, far more of the investment in health flows through the health care system for medical care rather than to public health services for primary prevention. Given that a defining feature of public health is its focus on community-level actions to promote health and prevent disease, and given that children have the most to gain from a focus on primary prevention, the nation's underinvestment in public health represents a missed opportunity to benefit child health and protect the nation from future high costs of health care and other services attributable to preventable poor health conditions. The committee views the expansion and intensification of the nation's investment in public health as essential for strengthening population-level health promotion and disease prevention and launching lifelong health for children. Child- and family-focused programs with proven benefits merit substantial new investments. Moreover, because public health spending is highly uneven across communities, the committee calls for assessing and strengthening local health departments to ensure that each has a minimum standard of core, foundational capabilities.

Schools provide a central focus and experience for children and youth—unlike any similar set of institutions for older populations. Schools already provide substantial amounts of preventive health and treatment services, and their health care role should be continued and expanded to reach more children and families that need assistance, including early care and health education programs.

> Recommendation 3-1: Federal policy makers and agencies should expand funding for population-level whole child and family health promotion and disease prevention resource investments in ways that (1) provide greater and equitable support for children and families in need; (2) integrate community-level resources with child health care systems; and (3) ensure that all eligible children and families receive the highest-quality services in current public health programs. Federal programs that have particular relevance to younger populations and should be expanded to build core services for communities include
>
> - The Administration for Children and Families Head Start and Early Head Start programs.
> - The U.S. Department of Agriculture Special Supplemental Nutrition Program for Women, Infants, and Children and the Supplemental Nutrition Assistance Program.
> - The Prevention and Public Health Fund, administered through the Centers for Disease Control and Prevention, with elevated focus on younger populations.
> - Investments in early childhood health and prevention administered through the Health Resources and Services Administration (HRSA) and the Substance Abuse and Mental Health Services Administration. Within HRSA, the Maternal and Child Health Bureau Title V block grant and targeted funding for maternal health, child health, and child development particularly merit expansion.
>
> Recommendation 3-2: Federal, state, and local agencies should reduce inequities in local public health department capacity and improve execution of current evidence-based support programs aimed at children to reap long-term benefits of improving child health and wellbeing.
>
> - Federal policy makers should create a permanent Public Health Infrastructure Fund to ensure that each local health department has basic, core capabilities and technology support and to ameliorate existing inequities in public health resource availability.
> - State and local agencies should evaluate existing public health capacity across communities and support coordination with other local health departments and health care systems.

- Federal and state agencies should evaluate how competitive grant-in-aid mechanisms may exacerbate resource inequities across local health departments and test alternative approaches to allocating limited resources.
- Federal and state agencies should coordinate and streamline processes and systems for ensuring strong execution of current evidence-based programs that support child health, in order to reach all who are eligible for services, using multiple points of access.

Recommendation 3-3: Federal, state, and local policy makers and agencies—in collaboration with health care systems, schools, foundations, employers, and other community partners—should expand investment, through blended and braided funding, to support the infrastructure and resources to enhance school-based health promotion and disease prevention. Key actions include

- Funding expansion of the Centers for Disease Control and Prevention Healthy Schools program to meet community needs.
- Expanding resources to meet community needs and provide nutritious meals to all eligible students through the National School Lunch Program and the School Breakfast Program.
- Expanding the School-Based Mental Health Services Grant Program distributed through the Bipartisan Safer Communities Act to improve the ability of communities and schools to reach all children in need.

Recommendation 3-4: To expand investment in community-based prevention and health promotion for children, federal agencies should strengthen existing community benefit requirements and accounting mechanisms to support and incentivize health care system initiatives to advance community health.

- The Internal Revenue Service (IRS) should strengthen community benefit requirements for tax-exempt hospitals and create similar requirements for tax-exempt health plans. Reporting under the IRS Community Benefit Standards should require that nonprofit hospitals and health plans (1) use best-practice community needs assessment and improvement protocols and coordinate with existing community partnerships—or establish such partnerships—to create and implement action plans for addressing findings of community health needs assessments; (2) ensure community representation, accountability measures, and enforcement mechanisms in action plans; and (3) publicly report on progress for community-defined, cross-sector outcomes and measures for child and community health.

- The Centers for Medicare & Medicaid Services should reclassify community-based prevention programs as an allowable service, as part of the medical loss ratio.

Recommendation 3-5: State legislatures should mandate investment in community health from for-profit health care providers and managed care organizations. Such mandates should ensure that for-profit providers employ best practices for assessing community needs, engaging community representation, developing initiatives, and publicly reporting on progress for community-defined, cross-sector outcomes and measures for child and community health and health equity.

Goal 4: Ensure Co-Creation and Co-Design of Programs and Structures with Youth, Family, and Community Voices and Leadership

The committee was tasked with considering promising policies and practices that incorporate the lived experiences of underserved children, adolescents, parents, and caregivers and build needed trust, partnerships, and long-term relationships with health care systems. It was also tasked with looking at workforce development in regard to team-based care and more community-based, culturally and linguistically competent workers. The impact of family and community voices on system change has not yet been fully realized. Health disparities and structural racism remain and are prominent concerns, and for many families and communities in the United States, the health care system is still untrustworthy. Engaging youth, families, and community members in the design of health care systems provides an opportunity to improve trust and the delivery of care.

Recommendation 4-1: Health care systems should partner with community members and leaders from historically marginalized backgrounds to co-design policies and build programs that support a more child-, family-, and community-centered health care system, supporting quality improvement, patient safety, and health equity initiatives. Such partnerships should

- **Ensure the active involvement of patients, youth, and families in the development and implementation of new science and technologies (e.g., genome sequencing, prediction models that use artificial intelligence) and models of care.**
- **Strengthen the role and diversity of patient and youth family advisory councils that reflect the communities served and address community needs.**

- Provide education and training opportunities as well as compensation to patient, youth, and family advisors that engage in child health care system transformation initiatives and efforts.
- Create pathways with local community programs to involve high school and college students from marginalized communities in early mentorship and job programs, in order to promote community engagement and develop a sustained and diverse health care workforce.
- Provide and encourage training and volunteer opportunities for health care system employees to partner with the community to co-design, build, implement, and evaluate programs, in order to achieve excellent and equitable child health outcomes.

Recommendation 4-2: Federal research agencies, state governments, and foundations should eliminate barriers that make it challenging for health care entities to financially compensate patients and families for their participation in efforts to improve services or programs; they should also eliminate barriers that limit collaboration among health care, child health–related public health programs, and family- and community-based services.

Recommendation 4-3: Accrediting and certifying bodies for the training and certification of physicians, nurses, nurse practitioners, physician assistants, mental and dental health providers, and other health care workers should require training to ensure that the health care workforce is competent, diverse, team oriented, and antiracist, and able to promote relational health.

Recommendation 4-4: Hospital or health care system accrediting bodies (e.g., The Joint Commission) and recognition programs (e.g., *U.S. News & World Report* Hospital Rankings, American Nurses Association Magnet Recognition Program) should continue efforts to assess and recognize activities related to patient and family experience; diversity, equity, and inclusion; and achievement of excellent and equitable health outcomes.

Recommendation 4-5: Federal and state agencies should mandate and utilize the expertise of youth, families, and communities by generating and sustaining community representation and advisory practices that are integrated with accountability measures and enforcement mechanisms.

- Federal agencies should incorporate requirements in grants to states and territories for greater youth, family, and community engagement, including those from historically marginalized communities.

- State agencies should instruct community advisory boards to make proceedings and minutes of meetings public to ensure strong engagement.
- Federal and state agencies should support quality improvement efforts and learning health networks—with a specific focus on co-design with patients, children, youth, families, and communities—to improve outcomes tied to decreasing health disparities and quality measures that align with communities' needs.
- The Centers for Medicare & Medicaid Services should reinvigorate its Partnership for Patients program by funding capacity and capability building for children, youth, families, and community leaders to fully engage and co-lead quality improvement efforts within hospital and community innovation networks and quality improvement organizations.

Recommendation 4-6: Federal and state agencies, foundations, and other funders should provide financial support for youth-led services in local communities. This support could include

- Research funding directed at strengthening scientific understanding of the efficacy, effectiveness, and implementation of youth-led services.
- Funding of youth-led services, through AmeriCorps' Healthy Futures focus area, to include training and credentialing, which should be deployed locally. The proposed expansion of funding for this program should target young people in delivering peer-led services, to massively expand their access to health promotion and mental health supports.
- Funding to co-create and co-design a national credential for peer-support specialists with youth-led organizations, graduate student–led national organizations, and the credentialing bodies for allied health care professionals, to expand the workforce of youth leaders. This is pivotal to providing consistency in delivery of youth-led services and to sustaining the development of the future health care workforce.

Goal 5: Implement Measurement and Accountability to Ensure Equitable Achievement of These Goals

The committee was tasked with considering levers for establishing integration within health care and with other systems and with identifying promising mechanisms and policies for enhancing collaboration among and integration of data systems for health care, mental health, public health, welfare, education, and other agencies. The committee concluded that a transformed health care system will emphasize accountability for equitable, whole child, family, and community population health outcomes among the health care system and public–private partners. Ongoing innovations in measurement, payment, and cross-sector service integration suggest that a child health care system that is accountable for improved child wellbeing outcomes is possible. These recommendations build on a renewed commitment to greater accountability for child and adolescent health and call on federal agencies to support expansion of evolved accountability systems to all communities and health care systems.

Recommendation 5-1: The Centers for Medicare & Medicaid Services, in collaboration with other federal agencies, should support health care systems' implementation of new and evolved accountability measurement systems that minimize overall measurement burden, have meaning for families and communities, and highlight equity. Measures should address population health, disparities, and the functioning of children, and they should promote integrated, cross-sector child health care systems of care. Key efforts include

- Providing technical support for state demonstrations on the application of an outcome-based, shared, cross-system measurement and accountability framework focused on a narrowed and integrated set of measures aimed at population health and equity using a whole child and family health approach. Such support could be coordinated with the Administration for Children and Families, the Health Resources and Services Administration, and the U.S. Department of Education.
- Partnering with other federal agencies to support state and local child health accountability-related programs, and working with the Interagency Working Group on Youth Programs and private-sector partners and experts, to develop a toolkit for best practices in engaging families, youth, and communities in the co-design and effective use of accountability measurement systems.

Recommendation 5-2: Federal research agencies tasked with improving the health and wellbeing of children and youth should continue to advance the data resources and research necessary to evolve accountability measurement systems in ways that produce robust state and local area estimates from national surveys and existing federal data systems, support digital tools for local data collection and reporting to allow for comparable health care, public health, and policy studies, and

fill key knowledge gaps in the practice of designing and using population health measures aligned with communities' needs for better health outcomes for children.

Recommendation 5-3: Federal and state governments should coordinate cross-agency efforts to monitor system performance and eliminate barriers to shared accountability across child health programs, in areas such as health care, education, child welfare, home- and community-based services, and juvenile justice. These efforts should support the development of interoperable cross-sector portals, including patient- and family-facing portals.

Recommendation 5-4: The Office of the National Coordinator for Health Information Technology should partner with the Centers for Medicare & Medicaid Services and a national committee comprising both public- and private-sector members, in order to develop a transparent reporting protocol for data submission that all payers and child-serving health care systems can use to monitor a small set of agreed-upon measures amenable to real-time (daily, weekly, monthly) electronic record submissions that include family- or patient-reported outcomes data.

CONCLUDING REMARKS

This report comes at a point of national crisis in the health and wellbeing of U.S. children and youth—and the graphic evidence of the effects of this crisis on the U.S. workforce, military preparedness, and burgeoning costs of adult ill health. Transforming child and adolescent health care requires an ambitious agenda. This report reviews the opportunities and challenges in several areas, including the science of early childhood, innovations in health care delivery, scientific advances and developing technology (e.g., epigenetics, predictive technologies, telehealth and other communication methods, new treatments), health care financing, advancement of health equity, public health, engagement of families and youth in their health care programs, and measurement of health outcomes. This work provides a guide and framework for needed transformation and seeks to establish the national imperative for change, to reverse troubling trends in the health of America's children and in the current and future workforce and to promote wellbeing proactively.

Previous studies from the National Academies and elsewhere have highlighted many of the advances and opportunities documented in this report. Few have had broad impact, in part because of the lack of a coordinated, sustained focus on improving the health of all children, youth, families, and communities.

The report recommendations include strategies for strengthening the nation's commitment and focus on children and youth and their health care, including better assessment of the child health and health equity impact of public policies, ways to reform health care financing for children, strategies for improving public health and school health, methods of including children and families and historically marginalized communities in all aspects of program and policy, and ways to measure and ensure accountability for change and outcomes.

Such changes will require strong leadership and incentives at the federal and state levels. The need for sustained and focused attention on children, youth, and families is painfully clear, and lack of this effort will burden U.S. society with tremendous costs in the near future and for generations to come.

1

Child Health and Health Care: Uniqueness, Societal Importance, and Vision for the Future

Invest in children's health for lifelong, intergenerational, and economic benefits. The evidence is clear: early investments in children's health, education, and development have benefits that compound throughout the child's lifetime, for their future children, and society as a whole.

WHO–UNICEF–*Lancet* Commission, 2020[1]

The United States is rebounding from the COVID-19 pandemic at a time of tremendous growth in science, medicine, innovation, and technology. Continued progress in these areas will require the efforts of creative and productive young people. Fortunately, the connection between health and wellbeing for children and the nation's capabilities and capacity has never been clearer. Advances in genomics, new technology, and community-based health promotion offer incredible opportunities to improve child health and prevent adult chronic diseases by intervening early in the life course.

Robust science on the importance of early life experiences, relationship-based care, genetics, and developmental origins of health and disease demonstrates potential for enhancing society through a focus on prevention and health promotion in maternal, preconception, prenatal, child, adolescent, family, and community health and wellbeing. A substantial research base shows that efforts to promote positive childhood experiences in early life can reduce adult physical, mental, social, and relational health problems, again highlighting the need for preventive strategies (Bethell et al., 2019; Bethell,

[1]Clark et al., 2020, p. 605.

Gombojav, & Whitaker, 2019; Braveman & Barclay, 2009; Bruner & Johnson, 2018; Gluckman et al., 2008; Halfon et al., 2018; National Academies of Sciences, Engineering, and Medicine [National Academies], 2019b). The major causes of adult morbidity and mortality have their roots in childhood (Simmonds et al., 2016). For instance, obesity and diabetes often start in childhood, as do most cases of mental, emotional, behavioral, and substance use disorders (National Academies, 2019b,d). Major diseases of older populations, such as atherosclerosis and Parkinson's disease, can also trace their roots to childhood. Adverse childhood experiences are associated with adult physical and mental health disorders, as well as lower education and productivity in adulthood (Felitti et al., 1998). Emphasizing early intervention and preventive care, such as health education, vaccinations, and regular screenings, can reduce the long-term need for more intensive services (AbdulRaheem, 2023; Fowler et al., 2020; Schor & Bergman, 2021).

Achievements in pediatric research in the past 40 years have driven solutions that have dramatically reduced childhood morbidity and mortality (Cheng et al., 2016). However, this progress is now under threat as evidenced by rising morbidity and mortality rates (Ely & Driscoll, 2022). Many see persistent inequities in child health, high rates of adverse childhood experiences (Camacho & Clark Henderson, 2022), and rising rates of mental and behavioral health conditions and obesity as contributing to this threat (see Chapters 2, 3, and 4). The pandemic made clear that the United States is at a crisis point regarding poor physical and mental health among the nation's children and youth (Bauer, Chriqui, et al., 2021; Cheng, Moon, & Artman, 2020; National Academies, 2023b; Parolin & Wimer, 2020). High rates of childhood poverty; racism in health care and outcomes; and growing health problems and mortality among working-age adults have major implications for the nation's economic productivity and prosperity. Rising rates of mortality and disability among youth and working-age Americans reflect outcomes of not providing the care that children and youth need. The U.S. military has raised concerns about the eligibility of young Americans for military service, with the largest increase in reasons for disqualification for mental health and overweight conditions (Department of Defense [DoD], 2020). The contrast between the opportunities presented by scientific and health knowledge and the clearly worsening health of young Americans shows the urgency of addressing child and adolescent health care transformation now.

Many organizations and partnerships, across both public and private sectors, are experimenting with bold place-based initiatives, new online services, artificial intelligence, and other innovations to help children and families in their communities. Innovative businesses are exploring new ways to care for their employees and families; others are investing in public–private partnerships to improve child and community health (Johns & Rosenthal, 2022). The foundation of many of these efforts is the moral imperative for addressing child health. Investing in healthy children is the right thing to do because children are the least able to care for themselves and are the most dependent members of society. Yet, as detailed below and understood by some business leaders (Johns & Rosenthal, 2022), this investment also helps parents and their role in the workforce immediately, and the future workforce and healthier communities in the longer term.

Pediatric health care has evolved with many innovations to address salient present-day challenges to child and adolescent health. Pediatric health care has long championed prevention and health promotion from the earliest work of the Children's Bureau and the development of the medical home in the 1960s. Over the ensuing decades, much progress has occurred, broadening the content of pediatric primary care and including programs that support healthy development (e.g., HealthySteps, Reach Out and Read), integrate mental and behavioral health with primary care, and strengthen coordination and collaboration with community resources (e.g., community health workers, Help Me Grow; see Chapters 3 and 5). Many of these advances have had extensive evaluation and testing, although bringing them to scale and building universal comprehensive advanced primary care have not occurred. Main barriers include lack of financial incentives and support for the complex process of transformation and lack of a trained workforce, especially among community health workers and co-located mental health providers. Successful programs have relied in large part on philanthropy and grants rather than the main financing structure from public and commercial health insurance.

CHARGE TO THE COMMITTEE

With the support of a broad coalition of sponsors (see Box 1-1), the National Academies assembled the Committee on Improving the Health and Wellbeing of Children and Youth through Health Care System Transformation to examine ways to improve policies, practices, and norms, and to enable child and adolescent health care systems to embrace the scientific evidence for health promotion, disease prevention, and early intervention. The committee was also tasked with investigating how financing approaches can be updated to incentivize these changes. Committee members included physicians, nurses, hospital system leaders, Medicaid experts, youth and family advocates, community health center providers, economists and health care financing experts, and experts in mental health and school-based health care. Appendix A presents brief biographies of the committee members, fellow, and staff. The committee was charged with addressing a series of questions that would set forth a vision for a health care system that would improve the health and wellbeing of children, youth, and families (see Box 1-2).

BOX 1-1
Study Sponsors

- Academic Pediatric Association
- Agency for Healthcare Research and Quality
- American Academy of Pediatrics
- American Board of Pediatrics
- Children's Hospital Association
- Health Resources and Services Administration
- Robert Wood Johnson Foundation
- Silicon Valley Community Foundation/Pediatrics Supporting Parents
- The David & Lucile Packard Foundation

The committee's work and approach to addressing the questions in its charge focused on mechanisms at the system level, with attention to levers, policies, and engagements that will support necessary changes to establish equitable health care. Chapters 1–5 provide background for the reader to understand the importance of child health for society, recent advances in medicine and health care, the current state of child health and health disparities, and the structure and innovations of the existing health care system. Throughout this material, the committee examines both opportunities and challenges for health care. Chapters 6–9 discuss the key levers identified by the committee for transformation within the child and adolescent health care system: financing through insurance for health care services, public health investment, leveraging school settings, and measuring population health outcomes. Chapter 10 sets out important goals and recommendations for improving the health and wellbeing of children and youth.

The committee's focus is on the health care sector, defined broadly to include clinical care, public health investments in child and family health, and school efforts in health care. The committee recognized the many other important influences on child and family health, especially poverty and income support, housing, labor markets and employment, community wellbeing, family leave and child care support, juvenile justice reform, and educational reform and financing, but focused its efforts on the health care system. Other recent National Academies consensus studies provide strong evidence of the impact of these nonhealth sector influences on children and families (see Appendix B). This report emphasizes how the health care sector—its structure, components, incentives, governance, and financing—can transform to improve the health and wellbeing of the nation's children and youth.

Throughout the report, the committee uses the term "child health" broadly to include preconception, maternal, prenatal, child, adolescent, family, and community health and wellbeing. The report takes a multigenerational and

BOX 1-2
Committee's Charge

The National Academies will appoint an ad hoc panel of experts to examine what innovations can be made to the child and adolescent health care system to improve the health and wellbeing of children, youth, and families. The study will address the following questions:

1. What are key levers of change to guide innovation and transformation within the child and adolescent health care system to facilitate health promotion, resiliency, disease prevention, and appropriate treatments and interventions for all children, youth and families?
2. What are promising policies and practices that incorporate the lived experiences of underserved children, adolescents, parents, and caregivers, and build the needed trust, partnerships, and long-term relationships to promote family-centered engagement, promote protective factors, and help address systemic inequities and disparities in access to and use of high-quality child and adolescent health care?
3. What are the gaps and barriers in current payment models, for both public and commercial insurance, and what are potential solutions to overcome them?
4. How can innovation in workforce development within the health care system facilitate team-based care and produce more community-based, culturally and linguistically competent workers? What strategies can stabilize the workforce to enable the formation of long-term relationships within the community?
5. What are promising levers available within the health care system to enhance interaction and integration of the child and adolescent health care system with major programs that support education, child and youth development, public health, child welfare, juvenile justice, and other key services that heavily influence the health and wellbeing of children and adolescents?
6. What are promising mechanisms and policies to enhance collaboration among and integration of data systems for health care, mental health, public health, welfare, education, and other agencies at the community, state, and federal levels for improved individual and population health?

life course perspective because research has shown that all health and developmental stages build on each other and are inextricably linked. Substantial evidence demonstrates that health early in the life course sets the foundation for health through childhood, adolescence, young adulthood, and tomorrow's workforce and parents (see Chapter 2).

The committee also recognized deep concerns around systemic inequities and disparities in access to and use of high-quality child and adolescent health care, and it sought solutions to address these concerns. Such inequities are often viewed through the lens of race and ethnicity. However, health disparities exist across a broad range of dimensions, including socioeconomic status, age, geography, language, gender, disability status, citizenship status, and sexual identity and orientation. Such dimensions are not mutually exclusive and often intersect in important ways (Ndugga & Artiga, 2023). Furthermore, there is much heterogeneity within population groups. In this report, the committee uses the term "historically marginalized" to reference groups and communities that have been and are served poorly by the health care system, have faced and continue to face systemic oppression and denial of access to high-quality care, and experience disproportionate impacts from discrimination (National Academies, 2017a, 2020c). Where possible, the text refers to specific populations (e.g., low-income families; immigrants; Black, Hispanic, Indigenous communities) to be intentional about the particular barriers and lived experiences of these groups.

In undertaking its study, the committee recognized that families and communities have varied goals for healthy living and expectations of the health care system. The committee took steps to ensure that a range of perspectives was considered, including listening to community voices through multiple formats, including invited speakers at committee meetings (see Appendix C), online collection of public comments, and review of community murals and children's drawings that illustrate concerns and visions for healthy communities (see, e.g., Figure 1-1).

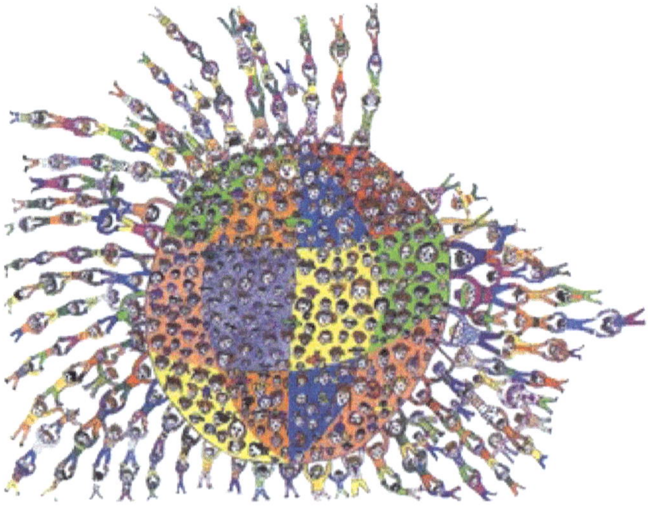

FIGURE 1-1 Children unite for a healthy world.
SOURCE: Wang Schuchi, age 7, China; © Peace Child International, used with permission.

STUDY APPROACH

The committee held five two-day hybrid meetings and a set of virtual calls between February 2023 and February 2024 to gather information, deliberate on findings, and develop this report. At its first meeting, representatives from the nine sponsors of the study participated and provided guidance and expectations for the committee's work. At four of the meetings, outside speakers were invited to public sessions to inform the committee's deliberations. The speakers provided valuable perspectives on a broad range of topics, including the rise of diversity among U.S. populations of children and youth; ways to engage families and communities in health care; chronic health needs of youth and young adults; current gaps and barriers in payment models; innovative collaborative care models in Alaska, Texas, Ohio, and Michigan; partnerships with the business sector; scientific advancements for health care delivery; the purpose of transformation; and levers of change. Agendas from the committee's public sessions can be found in Appendix C.

Through the study's website, the committee solicited input from patients, families, health care providers, researchers, and the general public to raise awareness of broader concerns and ideas. While public comments addressed several topics, mental and behavioral health care was mentioned consistently. Commenters called attention to the need for changes in the health care system and emphasized prevention initiatives, early health promotion, and greater support and inclusion of community and social services to address the social determinants of health. Comments also highlighted multiple insurance barriers and challenges with developing, implementing, and validating performance measures.

The committee also reviewed the existing literature, including peer-reviewed scientific literature and publications by private and public organizations and governmental agencies. Topics relevant to this report are broad: healthy development at all ages and across the generations, health and wellbeing measures, societal and community conditions and social determinants of health, health care system characteristics and innovations, public and private financing mechanisms, federal programs and resources, school-based services, family and community needs, and scientific and technological advances related to the delivery of health care. The committee commissioned two papers to review information and findings on international policies and programs for preventive care and mental health care (Niksch & Papanicolas, 2023; Stabile, 2023). The interdisciplinary nature of the committee's membership meant that various scientific traditions of understanding, methodology, and ways of knowing were present.

Building on the growing field of community-based participatory research, the committee also carefully considered the important evidence provided by patient, family, and community voices, reflecting its belief that transformation of health care must be done in partnership. The perspectives of children, youth, and families engaged in the health care system have often been omitted from the process of research question development, study execution, and data analysis and dissemination. Children, youth, and families engaged in the health care system are closest to the issue at hand, and consulting and learning from these communities improves the scientific process and has the potential to create more impactful solutions. Centering research on those with lived experience adds crucial insight into what works and what does not, helps researchers better understand the full context of an issue and the full implications of research findings, creates opportunities for meaningful work for those with direct experience, and may build trust in communities where generations of neglect and harmful actions have built a foundation of earned distrust (Israel et al., 1998; National Academies, 2021c, 2022b, 2023h).

As will be discussed in depth in later chapters, the committee strongly believes that the experiential knowledge and expertise of children, youth, families, and communities engaged in the health care system need to inform the design and implementation of health care system transformation. With this in mind, the committee modeled an "inclusive research frame" in its work and was intentional about involving people who are experts—by way of training, education, and/or lived experience—on the topic under study.

TRANSFORMING CHILD AND ADOLESCENT HEALTH CARE

For decades, numerous calls to improve the child and adolescent health care system have highlighted improving health equity, accountability, cost-effectiveness and quality, and patient and family engagement. The evidence cited by most of these calls supports emphases on preventive care, including community-based prevention and health promotion; direct attention to inequities and population health; new financing and metrics to assess progress; and new models of care.

This report is by no means the first assessment of opportunities for transformative pediatric care; it builds on an ever-expanding body of research targeting children, families, and communities (Perrin, Duncan, et al., 2020). The importance of person-centered, community-oriented care has been recognized for decades, coupled with calls for new conceptualizations and models of care that reform public health approaches and primary care delivery (Bruner & Hayes, 2023; National Academies, 2021b; Perrin, Duncan, et al., 2020; Shortell et al., 2023; Whole Child Health Alliance, 2023), as well as large-scale efforts to transform health care delivery and payment systems. Despite these calls for action, populations face unequal access to care, driven by economic, mental health, and social health disparities, which disproportionately impact historically marginalized communities. The United States has not taken full advantage of substantial evidence supporting pediatric health care reforms, leaving many of the nation's children, parents, and communities disadvantaged across the life course. The committee's work and this report leverage findings and conclusions from a number of prior National Academies reports relevant to this topic (see Appendix B). This body of work represents decades of accumulating knowledge on the importance of health and wellbeing across the life course, beginning with preconception conditions and including supports and positive environments at each stage of life to ensure a healthy and productive society.

In discussing how to guide and implement effective change in the health care system, the committee considered successes and limitations of these prior efforts to innovate health care, as well as key evidence, all of which emphasized the potential and value of earlier identification of disease and prevention, correcting health inequities, and the importance of implementing changes to the child and adolescent health care system in the next 10 years. This review of previous efforts also clarified the need for a sustained focus rather than short-term changes or policies.

Prevention and Health Promotion

While prevention and health promotion have long been a cornerstone of child and adolescent health care, the current national situation, given the evidence of poor health outcomes downstream, calls for even greater investment in these efforts. Prevention can save money as well as lives and health. For example, vaccines save both costs in medicine and millions of lives (National Academies, 2024c). Routine immunization of children born from 1994 to 2023 has been projected to prevent nearly 1.6 million early deaths, 508 million illnesses, and 32 million hospitalizations, and to save nearly $2.9 trillion in total societal costs—more than $5,000 for each American (Andre et al., 2008; Centers for Disease Control and Prevention [CDC], 2024j,p; Stack et al., 2011; Zhou et al., 2014). For example, the incremental lifetime medical cost of an obese 10-year-old child relative to a child who maintains a healthy weight through adulthood is $19,000. Multiplying this by the number of obese 10-year-olds yields a total direct medical cost of obesity of $14 billion for this age alone (Finkelstein, Graham, & Malhotra, 2014). Oral health care for children is another crucial component of preventive care. Regular preventive dental visits improve oral health and reduce later costs, particularly for children at high risk of dental disease (Downing et al., 2022; National Institutes of Child Health and Human Development, 2021; Rowan-Legg, 2013). Fluoride treatments, increasingly given in primary care, significantly decrease dental caries in children (Downing et al., 2022; National Institutes of Child Health and Human Development, 2021; Rowan-Legg, 2013). Economic studies show that adverse childhood experiences are associated with trillions of dollars of costs from adult physical, mental, and behavioral health problems and loss in quality of life. Preventing and mitigating the impact of adverse childhood experiences can likely decrease these long-term costs

(CDC, 2019b,d; Peterson et al., 2023). Regarding mental health, universal and targeted school-based cognitive behavioral therapy programs reduce depression and anxiety symptoms in children (Werner-Seidler et al., 2021). Exciting scientific advancements in developmental origins of health and disease, genomics, and predictive artificial intelligence all emphasize the potential of early intervention, prevention, and health promotion.

Addressing Inequities

However, many children lack access to adequate preventive care. Disparities in access to and quality of care for the nation's poorest children continue in the current system. The United States is one of a few countries in the world that does not entitle all young children and pregnant persons to health care and has some of the lowest rates of access to preventive care and routine services among resource-rich countries. Notably, many U.S. cities and states report high rates of inequities in infant mortality, preventable disease outbreaks, and higher costs of care for many specialty conditions. As the following paragraphs show, the main health financing systems cover racial and ethnic groups differentially, with historically marginalized populations having higher public insurance coverage and lower commercial coverage.

Financing

Current mechanisms of financing health care are struggling to keep up with changing demographics; environmental influences on health; new clinical strategies; and technological advances, such as increased use of telehealth. Models of health care payment—usually relying on traditional fee-for-service structures or value-based arrangements focused on lowering costs for high-cost adult patients—do not provide child health clinicians the flexibility or incentives to work with families and partner with communities to address their health and developmental needs (Counts, Mistry, & Wong, 2021; Counts, Roiland, & Halfon, 2021). Instead, current models incentivize billable encounters and procedures or lowering costs, rather than measures to address the health of communities. Payment models limit the ability of clinicians to work across sectors to address the social and family challenges that underlie many child health concerns (Johnson, Willis, & Doyle, 2020).

The main public insurance programs for children and youth (Medicaid and the Children's Health Insurance Program [CHIP]) cover almost half of all U.S. children and youth and have benefited young populations by assuring eligibility with little or no cost-sharing and a broad set of benefits, including the Early and Periodic Screening, Diagnosis, and Treatment statute that requires an exceptionally strong service base for the health care needs of children. A large majority of covered children would have had no insurance without Medicaid and CHIP. Furthermore, the high rate of managed care for children in these programs (~85%) offers real opportunities to test new payment models and incentives. Nonetheless, Medicaid and CHIP also reinforce structural racism in health care, in part because they disproportionately insure children of color and have low payment rates (Perrin, Kenney, & Rosenbaum, 2020).

Despite many well-documented advances in pediatric care, including primary and specialty care, payment for care has kept much care delivery based in a model of acute pediatric visits, originally focused on short-term illness care by office-based clinicians with less attention to chronic conditions (which were less common 50 years ago). Pediatric care has expanded its commitment to well-child care, incorporating immunizations and screening for various health conditions and providing guidance to families about upcoming growth and development milestones. However, child health settings often experience challenges in providing coordinated, longitudinal care for chronic illnesses and comprehensive care that addresses social determinants of health and relational health, in part because of limited financial incentives. Children, families, and communities often report that the child health care system does not meet their needs (see Chapter 3).

Innovations in Health Care

Many innovations have effectively improved preventive care, health promotion, long-term care coordination, specialty care, and health equity. Federal agencies and states are investing in efforts to integrate early child health care systems to drive comprehensive, high-quality well care (Health Resources and Services Administration, 2021). Schools and community settings in some locales offer prevention services in partnership with large health care systems (Boudreaux, Chu, & Lipton, 2023). And some health care systems serving children and youth have begun to use innovative financing models. For example, through accountable care organizations, participating systems receive global payments for a population (Center for Evidence-Based Policy, 2022), although few focus on younger populations (Perrin et al., 2017). Several state Medicaid programs now support team-based care models, integrating mental and behavioral health and including community health workers as part of the care team (Haldar & Hinton, 2023). Some communities have integrated health care practices with a variety of community resources, including health and social services, home visiting and family supports, educational resources, and housing programs (Garner & Yogman, 2021a; National Academies, 2019d). Additionally, health care organizations are implementing new models of community investment, which can have upstream impacts on child health and cascading benefits for both the investor and the community (Hacke & Deane, 2017).

These many innovations have documented improvements in health status, equity, care coordination, and child behavior and development. Promising payment reforms have lessened the incentives to produce visits and procedures, and have increased support for long-term outcomes and population health. The task now is to transform the larger health care system in ways that decrease chronic conditions, decrease disparities, shift payment and spending, and enhance wellbeing.

UNIQUENESS OF HEALTH CARE SERVICES FOR CHILDREN: THE 5 Ds

The health care system for children is often modeled after the adult health care system, yet several fundamental characteristics of children and youth differ from those of adults. The committee presents here current and enduring differences between pediatric and adult care (the 5 Ds) and the need for attention to these differences in all policies and programs with special approaches to child health. Consideration of and investment that recognizes these unique developmental needs result in population health over the life course. The 5 Ds are developmental change, disease/differential epidemiology, dependence, demographics, and dollars (Cheng & Mistry, 2019, 2023; Forrest, Simpson, & Clancy, 1997; Stille et al., 2010).

Developmental Change

While health care for adults focuses on health maintenance, remediation, and rehabilitation, children's health care attends to unique developmental needs and stages of children as they develop competencies and basic skills for their own self-care. Child and adolescent development is characterized by continuous new skills, growth, and transition, setting a trajectory for health across the life course (Halfon & Hochstein, 2002; see Chapter 2). Health care must focus on prevention, health promotion, and enhancing developmental progress to ensure that children are healthy and learning. Over the life course, a child meets experiences that can support or hinder growth and development, and the effects of these experiences accumulate through their lifetime. Health conditions manifest differently at different stages of life, respond differently to prevention and treatment, and lead to different consequences as a result of development (Halfon & Hochstein, 2002). Health and illness for an 18-month-old are very different from that of an 18-year-old. Useful health metrics address these differences across an individual's entire life course, including the preconception and prenatal health of mothers and their children, and consider a broader range of indicators over time, such as wellbeing, life chances, opportunity, risk and resilience, health potential, educational outcomes, and quality of life, in addition to the traditional focus on disease status and health care provision (Horn et al., 2009; National Research Council [NRC] & Institute of Medicine [IOM], 2004).

Disease/Differential Epidemiology

Child health conditions have differential epidemiology compared with adults and require different solutions. A growing proportion of children have complex physical, mental, and social conditions, although this proportion is still far lower than that of older populations. Some of the growth in chronic conditions among children and youth reflects advances in medical and surgical care, although a greater proportion of the growth is associated with adversity and environmental risks in early childhood, especially asthma, obesity, developmental problems, oral health problems, and mental and behavioral conditions (CDC, 2021e,f, 2024b,f,g). The number of children with mental and behavioral health conditions is epidemic, and this growth in large part reflects earlier life experiences and community and environmental exposures. Many other childhood conditions (e.g., cancers, heart disease, spina bifida, arthritis, cystic fibrosis), occur in relatively small to very small numbers (Bai et al., 2017; Perrin, Bloom, & Gortmaker, 2007).

The preconception and prenatal health of parents influences child health. Chronic child health problems such as obesity, cognitive disability, and neurodevelopmental disorders are often related to preventable maternal conditions (Capra et al., 2013; Johnson et al., 2023). Maternal and child exposures to psychosocial (e.g., maternal stress, adverse childhood experiences) and environmental threats (e.g., toxins) may manifest differently and accumulate over time in utero and during childhood. (See further discussion of the influences on child health and trajectory into adulthood in Chapter 2.)

Dependence

The wellbeing and support of caretakers and families help determine the health of children. Family capacities include physical and mental health and wellbeing, financial resources, time, and human capital (education and employment opportunities; Mistry et al., 2012; National Academies, 2019d). Families in turn depend on resources in their neighborhoods and communities (Minh et al., 2017). Optimal functioning of the family unit requires assessment and investment in family health, income supports and services, and community collaboration (National Academies, 2019d). Children rely directly on adults in child care, schools, and social services, in ways that differ markedly from family relationships among adults. This dependence requires that health care systems support healthy families and communities and partner across sectors of health, schools, child care, social services, juvenile justice, and child welfare.

Demographics

American children are more likely to live in poverty than are adults and older individuals. The highest rate of poverty of any age group is children under age 5 (Children's Defense Fund, 2023). In 2024, households with incomes below the federal poverty level (FPL) have annual incomes under $30,000 for a family of four, for example, or $14,580 for an individual. About 15% of Americans reside in households with incomes at or below 125% of the FPL, encompassing approximately 50 million low-income individuals, including around 15.2 million children under age 18 (Creamer et al., 2022). As of 2022, nearly two out of every five children lived in low-income families, defined as being at or below 200% of the FPL (Kids Count Data Center, 2023a). Children of color experience disproportionately high poverty rates—27.1% of Black children and 29.1% of American Indian/Alaska Native children lived in poverty in 2021, compared with just 8.8% of White children (Children's Defense Fund, 2023). Additionally, young children under age 5 face the highest poverty rates, at 16.3%. With the pandemic child tax credit, child poverty dropped to 5.2% in 2021, but since the ending of pandemic emergency supports in 2022, poverty rates and associated racial/ethnic disparities have increased to over 12% (Shrider & Creamer, 2023). Historically, economic downturns have affected children the most, with longer-lasting consequences in adulthood than those who were already adults during the downturn (Golberstein, Gonzales, & Meara, 2019; Kalil, 2013).

The number of children experiencing social adversities—including poverty, death, and incarceration or illness of a parent—is unacceptably high. Exposures to poverty, hunger, homelessness, and environmental threats (e.g., toxins) for children are higher than among adults, and require different and intentional primary and secondary prevention strategies. Epidemiologic research has demonstrated a strong dose–response relationship between adverse childhood experiences and child health, adult physical and mental health, and workforce outcomes (Ely & Driscoll, 2022; Felitti et al., 1998).

Children and youth are more diverse than the rest of the U.S. population (see illustration in Figure 1-2). In 2020, fewer than half of children were non-Hispanic White, and births of non-White babies have surpassed births of White babies since 2011 (Census Bureau, 2023a). This diversity is associated with disparities in child health and education by race, ethnicity, and socioeconomic status.

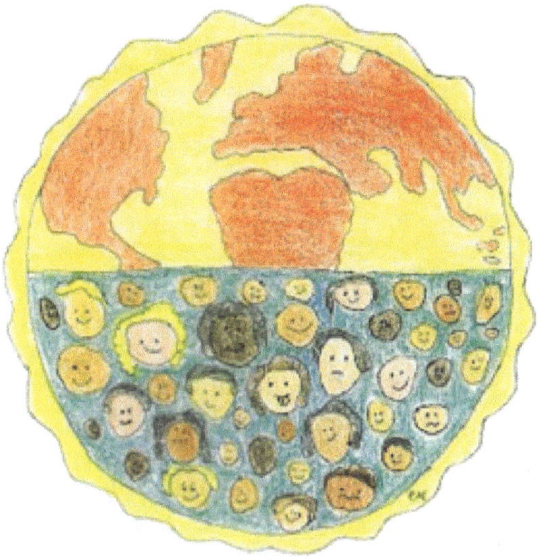

FIGURE 1-2 Child population.
SOURCE: Anonymous child artist; © Peace Child International, used with permission.

Dollars

For their health care, children depend on (1) family income, wealth, and supports; (2) educational attainment; (3) public health and education spending; and (4) commercial insurance, Medicaid, and CHIP. Half of all American children ages 0–18 are insured by public sources (e.g., Medicaid, CHIP, other), and 5% are uninsured (Centers for Medicare & Medicaid Service [CMS], 2023f,g). Black, Latino, and American Indian/Alaska Native children are disproportionately uninsured (Assistant Secretary for Planning and Evaluation, 2023a) or from low-income households (Keisler-Starkey & Bunch, 2022). A quarter of women who delivered a child were uninsured in the month prior to pregnancy, over half of whom had less than 12 years of education (Wherry, 2018). No other age group—other than older populations with Medicare—depend so much on public investment for their health care. However, Medicaid low payment rates (about two-thirds of rates paid by Medicare for the same services) threaten families' access to primary and subspecialty care, providing insufficient margins for many clinicians to participate in Medicaid (Galbraith et al., 2023; Perrin et al., 2020).

In 2020, children ages 0–18 accounted for about 10% of total health spending but represented 23% of the population (CMS, 2023f). Directing the majority of health care dollars to expensive hospital-based adult care fails to consider the short- and long-term value of child health. Return on investment (ROI) in child health occurs not only in the health care sector, but also in education, social services, and juvenile justice (Flanagan, Tigue, & Perrin, 2020). However, most ROI for child health programs accrues over a longer period of time as children develop. The long-term trajectory for ROI calls for different incentives for payers, hospitals, and legislators than short-term cost savings.

SOCIETAL GAINS FROM INVESTING IN CHILD HEALTH

The U.S. health care system today consumes about 20% of the nation's gross domestic product (GDP)—far more than any other country; yet the nation sustains generally poor health status and outcomes, including for children and youth (Keehan et al., 2023; National Academies, 2021b). Growing costs have engendered many calls for change and financing reforms to contain costs (Perrin, Cheng et al., 2023; Perrin, Flanagan et al., 2023), although the low expenditures for populations under age 21 offer few opportunities for savings in the short run. Adult health expenditures represent an enormous share of health care costs, yet poor health outcomes remain (McGough et al., 2024).

Invest in Child Health for Savings and Benefits to the Nation

Importantly, growing evidence spotlights opportunities to address the early conditions that cause individuals to become high-cost and high-need patients in the first place (IOM, 2010; McGough et al., 2024; National Academies, 2019d). The path to becoming a high-risk, high-need, high-cost adult patient starts as early as before conception, in utero, and infancy; conditions and experiences during childhood greatly affect individual health trajectories across the entire life course (Halfon & Hotchstein, 2002; Perrin, Cheng, et al., 2023; Perrin, Flanagan et al., 2023). These opportunities can have a major impact on bending the cost curve and improving health outcomes, but doing so demands that health care efforts focus on upstream factors and prevention, payment reform, and eliminating racial/ethnic and socioeconomic disparities. Demographic shifts in the U.S. population have led to a growing population of individuals over age 65, along with a declining birth rate and relative scarcity of working-age adults able to support and take care of older populations (see details below). Ensuring the best growth and development of each child has become vitally important for the future.

There are numerous urgent reasons to invest in children and families. Strong evidence suggests that Medicaid for children, investments to reduce child poverty, and investments in healthy development have significant financial payoffs (Ash et al., 2023; Hendren & Sprung-Keyser, 2020; Lou et al., 2023; Maag et al., 2023). Nobel laureate James Heckman has demonstrated that early investment in the wellbeing and skill formation of disadvantaged children pays off economically and is just and equitable (Heckman & Masterov, 2007). His research and economic modeling show that parental influences are primary in developing children's cognitive, social, emotional, and learning skills, and that quality of early childhood development heavily influences health, economic, and social outcomes for individuals and society at large. Heckman and Masterov (2007) concluded that there are great economic gains to be had by investing in families and early childhood development. Other studies show that eliminating racial/ethnic disparities dramatically reduces medical care costs and indirect costs of excess morbidity and mortality (LaVeist, Gaskin, & Richard, 2011; Thornton et al., 2016). Investments in child health also have positive effects on parental health and parental productivity, as well as the child's future health as they become an adult, with societal return on investment bridging multiple sectors (e.g., health, education, social services; Cheng & Solomon, 2014). Hendren and Sprung-Keyser (2020) reviewed 133 social policies to determine which improved social wellbeing the most and yielded the largest marginal value of public funds. They found that direct investments in the health and education of low-income children offered the highest returns.

Public Health Investment Benefits Child Health

Short-term, public spending benefits children and families directly. These benefits include access to health care and education; reduced poverty and food insecurity (especially for infants and toddlers who have particularly high poverty rates; Lou et al., 2023); better nutrition; lower family stress; healthier relationships; and conditions that allow children to be healthy, ready to learn, and on an optimal trajectory to adulthood. Long term, the benefits accrue to children and families and to society broadly. These payoffs include greater adult productivity resulting from having a more educated, healthier, and more skilled labor force—and the associated tax revenues (Ash et al., 2023; Maag et al., 2023; McLaughlin & Rank, 2018). Public investments in children also save societal and governmental expenditures on criminal justice, health care for chronic diseases (both public and private spending, including Medicare), and social services and public programs for adults (Maag et al., 2023).

Societal return on any single government investment is difficult to measure because children are affected by a constellation of programs and influences; however, research suggests that some programs have returns reaching $10 or more per dollar invested (Garfinkel et al., 2022; Hendren & Sprung-Keyser, 2020). Payoffs are particularly high from investments in

Medicaid; a Congressional Budget Office (CBO) study found that "long term fiscal effects of Medicaid spending on children could offset half or more of the program's initial outlays" (Ash et al., 2023, para. 1). Such investments reduce child poverty (McLaughlin & Rank, 2018) and promote healthy development and skills (Heckman & Masterov, 2007).

Investment in Child Health Benefits Children Now

The cost of *not* investing in child wellbeing must also be considered. Economists estimate that child poverty costs the United States between $800 billion and $1.1 trillion annually, 4.0–5.4% of the GDP, with the largest cost from reduced productivity later in life (Maag et al., 2023; National Academies, 2019a). Children growing up in poverty are more likely to have poorer health, earn less, pay less in taxes, and require more public supports in adulthood.

Historically, investment in child health has occurred during times of technologic change and health crisis. With emergence of new technology, rising child morbidity and mortality, and declaration of a national emergency in child and adolescent mental health, the time is ripe for change (American Academy of Pediatrics [AAP], 2021a). In U.S. history, categorical arguments to elevate health equity for vulnerable groups have included moral, performance or outcomes, economic or workforce, and national security arguments (Dawes, 2020, p. 72).

Realizing opportunities for improved population health and lower societal costs over time requires a sustained investment and a long-term commitment. This report addresses ways to achieve better health outcomes and health equity for children and provides a roadmap for doing so. The benefits of improving child health are both immediate and lasting. American identity and national values lie in providing opportunity for all and nurturing the young. The societal gains that result from investing in the health and wellbeing of children and youth are summarized below and in Figure 1-3 and Table 1-1. These echo the influential National Academies report *From Neurons to Neighborhoods*, which called for "a new national dialogue focused on rethinking the meaning of both shared responsibility for children and strategic investment in their future. The time has come to stop blaming parents, communities, business, and government, and to shape a shared agenda to ensure both a rewarding childhood and a promising future for all children" (NRC & IOM, 2000, p. 414). Health in childhood is insurance for healthier adulthood and is essential for a productive and healthy society.

Ensuring that every child is healthy, ready to learn, and on their optimal trajectory to productive adulthood is imperative for the nation.

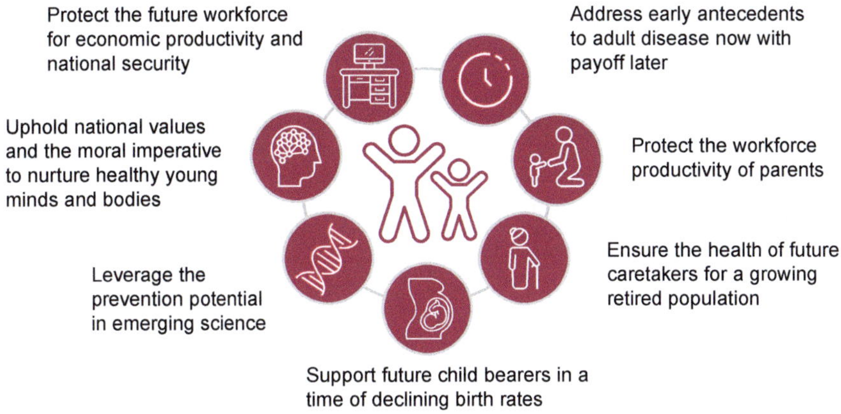

FIGURE 1-3 Societal gains in investing in children.
SOURCE: Generated by the committee.

This imperative arises from the inherent value of child health, their future health as adults, parent and societal health, and intergenerational health. It also comes from understanding the multigenerational antecedents of child growth and development, as well as the impact of child health and wellbeing on other generations. The committee notes below how these ideas affect Generation 0 (grandparents), Generation 1 (parents), Generation 2 (children), and Generation 3 (children's future children). Research underscores these value propositions described below and summarized in Table 1-1.

Societal Gain 1: It is a national value and moral imperative to give all children a healthy start in life. The future depends on nurturing young minds and bodies (Gen 2).

Research demonstrates that investment in children and families improves health and education outcomes and health equity, and reduces short- and long-term costs in the childhood years and adulthood (Ash et al., 2023; Chorniy, Currie, & Sonchak, 2018; Heckman, 2006; Hendren & Sprung-Keyser, 2020; Miller & Wherry, 2019). Health in childhood benefits children directly by improving daily lives and progress through childhood tasks. High childhood poverty rates and racial inequities lead to inequities in children's opportunity to thrive. Community, family, and individual quality of life are enhanced when children are healthy and active. Children have inherent worth beyond economic calculations, and ensuring that all children can thrive affirms values as a society.

TABLE 1-1 Societal Gains from Investing in Child Health

	Societal Gains	Selected Supporting Research
1. 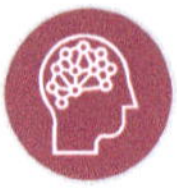	**It is a national value and moral imperative to give all children a healthy start in life. The future depends on nurturing young minds and bodies (Gen 2).**	• Investment in the health and wellbeing of children and families improves health and education outcomes and health equity, and reduces short- and long-term costs (Ash et al., 2023; Bailey et al., 2020; Bellis et al., 2019; Gaudette, Pauley, & Zissimopoulos, 2016; Qureshi & Gangopadhyaya, 2021). • Children are the poorest and most racially and ethnically diverse age group in America; the opportunity and imperative to close these equity gaps are great. • Early investment produces the greatest returns in human capital (Heckman et al., 2010).
2. 	**Child health and wellbeing support the nation's tax base, workforce, economic prosperity, and sustain a high standard of living (UNICEF, 2005). The current young adult workforce does not meet national economic and security needs (Gen 2).**	• From 2000 to 2015, the number of children under age 18 increased by only 1.9%, while the rest of the population grew by 18.5%—nine times faster (Myers, 2017). • Demographic shifts—including aging of the population, the large-scale retirement of older workers from the workforce, and declines in international migration—threaten the U.S. workforce. • Today, 77% of adolescents and young adults are not eligible for military service because of poor physical and mental health (Council for a Strong America, 2022) and for the first time the U.S. Army, Navy, and Air Force all missed their active-duty recruiting goals in fiscal year 2023, with a combined shortfall of more than 20,000 enlistees (Council for a Strong America, 2023a,b). • Poverty and poor child physical and mental health are associated with reduced work productivity in adulthood (Alaie et al., 2022, 2023; Felitti et al., 1998; Roth et al., 2024). • Investment in child health and wellbeing leads to greater adult productivity (Ash et al., 2023; Gaudette, Pauley, & Zissimopoulos, 2016; Qureshi & Gangopadhyaya, 2021).

TABLE 1-1 Continued

	Societal Gains	Selected Supporting Research
3.	**Children who are sick prevent parents from working, playing, resting, and being their full selves. Parent health, happiness, and productivity depend on child health and wellbeing.**	• Parents cannot work if children are not healthy or not in school. • Healthy children and healthy families are linked: child health affects family health and family health affects child health (Shafer, 2024). • Chronic illness in children often leads to a parent dropping out of the workforce and can weaken parent health (Cohn et al., 2020; Foster et al., 2021). • Interventions for improving child health also protect adults and older populations from illness (e.g., pertussis or Respiratory syncytial virus [RSV] vaccines).
4.	**Child health and wellbeing are essential because children are future caretakers of a growing older population (Gen 0, 1). Maximizing the capabilities of a shrinking population of children is a societal need.**	• By 2030, the ratio of seniors to working-age adults will have doubled the 20th-century ratio (Myers, 2017). • A demographic flip is occurring: the 1970 ratio of three children aged 10–14 for every senior aged 65–69 is projected to be one child per senior by 2030 (Hamilton, Martin, & Osterman, 2023; Myers, 2017; The Pew Charitable Trusts, 2022). • The growing number of retired people will rely on an undersized working-age population.
5.	**Child health is the foundation for adult health. Most adult health problems, including heart disease, diabetes, and mental health, have origins in childhood, and the most effective prevention starts early in life (Gen 2).**	• Research has established clear early antecedents to adult chronic disease and the pace of aging (Belsky et al., 2017; Braveman & Barclay, 2009; Halfon et al., 2018). • Poor child health is associated with worse adult physical and mental health (CDC, 2019b; Felitti et al., 1998; Merrick et al., 2019). • Investment in child health and wellbeing improves health and wellbeing in adulthood and saves money in health care, education, social services, and criminal justice (Campbell et al., 2014; Flanagan, Tigue, & Perrin, 2019; Heckman et al., 2010; Hughes et al., 2021; Perrin, Cheng et al., 2023; Perrin, Flanagan et al., 2023).

(*continued*)

TABLE 1-1 Continued

	Societal Gains	Selected Supporting Research
6. 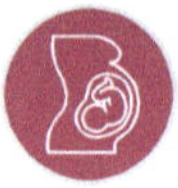	**Child health and wellbeing are essential, as children are the next generation of child bearers at a time of declining fertility rates and rising maternal mortality (Gen 3). Healthy reproduction and parenting are essential for the next generation.**	• Healthy childhood is essential for healthy pregnancies, childbirth, and parenting (Kang et al., 2023). • Research demonstrates the importance of preconception and prenatal health for healthy babies (Braveman & Barclay, 2009; Halfon et al., 2018; Johnson et al., 2006). • There has been a historic decline in U.S. fertility rates, and some states are already feeling the effects in lower school enrollment, threatening future tax revenues (Hamilton, Martin, & Osterman, 2023). • The combination of rising U.S. maternal mortality associated with racial disparities and declining birth rates threatens health and economic outcomes and accentuates the importance of optimal health in every pregnancy and birth (Hoyert, 2021).
7. 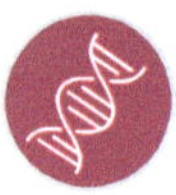	**Scientific and technologic advancement point to the promise of earlier identification and prevention of disease to improve societal health (e.g., genomics, artificial intelligence prediction) (Gen 2). Identification, prevention, and health promotion in the preconception, prenatal, childhood, and adolescent stages pay off.**	• The genomic revolution offers the promise of prediction, preemption, and precision medicine, enabling disease identification and intervention earlier in the life course (Cheng, Cohn, & Dover, 2008). • Scientific advancements on several fronts—prediction by artificial intelligence, understanding of social determinants of health, health services research, population health research and interventions, and health care financing—all emphasize the potential of earlier identification, prevention, and health promotion to improve societal health.

NOTE: Generation indicators refer to the following: Gen 0 = grandparents; Gen 1 = parents; Gen 2 = children; Gen 3 = children's future children.
SOURCE: Generated by the committee.

Societal Gain 2: Child health and wellbeing support the nation's tax base, workforce, economic prosperity, and sustain a high standard of living (UNICEF, 2005). The current young adult workforce does not meet national economic and security needs (Gen 2).

At a time of U.S. labor shortages, a healthy and prepared workforce is essential. However, the rising youth and young adult mortality rates and the child mental and behavioral health crisis threaten this workforce. In early 2023, the U.S. military reported that 77% of American youth ages 17–24 would not qualify for military services, an increase from 71% in 2017, because of health issues including obesity and behavioral health conditions and because of lack of necessary academic requirements. For the first time, the U.S. Army fell 15,000 recruits short of its annual goal (Council for a Strong America, 2022, 2023a,b). The Navy and Air Force also fell short of their goals.

The United States is also experiencing a historic decline in fertility, with all states but one reporting lower 2020 birth rates compared with averages over the decade ending in 2010 (The Pew Charitable Trusts, 2022). While lower birth rates may save education and health costs, they portend resource challenges related to a smaller pool of workers, which will likely suppress income, sales, and other tax revenues. Several factors influence the declining birth rate in the United States, including high child care costs, economic instability, and changing societal norms regarding family planning and women's roles in the workforce (Annie E. Casey Foundation, 2023a; CDC, 2024o). However, healthy and thriving children are necessary to grow the nation's economy, improve public safety, and strengthen national security. Adverse childhood experiences and mental health disorders impact lifelong health and opportunity, as well as productivity in adulthood (CDC, 2019b; Felitti et al., 1998; Jones, Merrick, & Houry, 2020a).

There is also strong evidence that investing in the health of children can improve workforce outcomes. A recent CBO working paper found that Medicaid enrollment during childhood has been shown to increase earnings in adulthood, supporting earlier research on the benefits of Medicaid (Currie & Chorniy, 2021; Hakim, Boben, & Bonney, 2000). The report went on to find that long-term fiscal effects of Medicaid spending on children could offset half or more of the program's initial outlays (Ash et al., 2023).

Societal Gain 3: Children who are sick prevent parents from working, playing, resting, and being their full selves. Parent health, happiness, and productivity depend on child health and wellbeing.

The COVID-19 pandemic starkly demonstrated that parents cannot work and experience heightened levels of stress if children are not healthy or not in school (Alonzo, Popescu, & Zubaroglu Ioannides, 2022). In addition, because children can be vectors of illness to caretakers, child health interventions can protect the health of adults. For instance, pertussis vaccination of children protects adults from illness (Choi et al., 2022). Child and family health are intertwined: child health affects family health and family health affects child health.

Societal Gain 4: Child health and wellbeing are essential because children are future caretakers of a growing older population (Gen 0, 1). Maximizing the capabilities of a shrinking population of children is a societal need.

At a time of low birth rates, an increasing proportion of the U.S. population is over age 60, which will leave a large retired population relying on an undersized group of working-age people. Demographers have suggested that this shortage of children will significantly impact a critical balance of workers and taxpayers with nonworkers (Myers, 2017). The best hope is to invest in and maximize capabilities of all children, thus strengthening the workforce supporting and caring for older people. It is the right thing to do for children, and it benefits older populations as well (Myers, 2017).

Societal Gain 5: Child health is the foundation for adult health. Most adult health problems, including heart disease, diabetes, and mental health, have origins in childhood, and the most effective prevention starts early in life (Gen 2).

The greatest threats to the health of Americans today—such as heart disease, diabetes, and mental health—have their origins in childhood, as do key morbidities of aging populations (e.g., atherosclerosis, metabolic conditions, cancer, neurodegenerative diseases such as Alzheimer and Parkinson's disease; Chung, Krenek, & Magge, 2023; Koskinen et al., 2023; Reuben, 2018; Wehrle et al., 2020). Life course research has demonstrated early antecedents to adult disease and developmental origins of health and disease (Carmeli et al., 2020; Hajat, Nurius, & Song, 2020; Lynch & Smith, 2005). Longitudinal studies have identified childhood antecedents to the pace of aging (Belsky et al., 2017; Colich et al., 2020; Wehrle et al., 2020). Inequities affect health early and may accumulate across the life course. Therefore, prevention and health promotion early in the life course offer opportunity to improve the nation's long-term health and longevity. Interventions in childhood have both health and economic payoffs in adulthood (Ash et al., 2023; Olds et al., 1986). Health and educational interventions have the highest return on investment when they are focused early in the life course (Heckman, 2006).

Societal Gain 6: Child health and wellbeing are essential, as children are the next generation of child bearers at a time of declining fertility rates and rising maternal mortality (Gen 3). Healthy reproduction and parenting are essential for the next generation.

Today's children are the child bearers of the next generation, and their health and wellbeing are essential for healthy reproduction, optimal parenting, and healthy offspring. Currently, the United States faces a declining fertility rate and increasing maternal mortality with wide racial disparity. CDC reports that four in five pregnancy-related deaths in the United States are preventable with adequate patient-centered care (Trost et al., 2022). Research demonstrates the importance of preconception and prenatal health and culturally competent care in birth outcomes (National Academies, 2019d).

Societal Gain 7: Scientific and technologic advancement point to the promise of earlier identification and prevention of disease to improve societal health (e.g., genomics, artificial intelligence prediction; Gen 2). Identification, prevention, and health promotion in the preconception, prenatal, childhood, and adolescent stages pay off.

Advancing science in genetics, prediction by artificial intelligence, understanding of social determinants of health, health services research, population health research and interventions, and health care financing innovations all emphasize the potential of earlier identification of health conditions, prevention, and health promotion (see Chapters 3, 4, and 5). The capability to ascertain the whole genome sequence of a fetus in utero is available. Health care providers will increasingly predict and preempt diseases that may manifest later in life. With these advances and appropriate ethical and legal safeguards, health care can shift to treating diseases earlier in the life course and minimizing or eliminating health consequences for individuals and society. This shift both improves quality of life and reduces the financial burden on health care systems, particularly in the senior years, when the costs of adult entitlements are most significant (Musich et al., 2016; Seow et al., 2022).

DECLINING INVESTMENT IN CHILD WELLBEING DESPITE DEMONSTRATED BENEFIT

The previous section lays out the importance and value of investing in children for the nation's future. U.S. public spending on children and families as a percentage of GDP is lower than in other industrialized countries, and such spending is correlated with child health outcomes (National Academies, 2019a). The Urban Institute's 2022 *Kids Share* report shows that outlays for children under age 18 were the focus of only 9.8% of the federal budget (Lou et al., 2023). Figure 1-4 depicts how this share is projected to decline to 6.2% over the next decade (a 37% decline), based on laws in place as of March 30, 2023. It is estimated that in 2023, the federal government spent more on interest payments on debt than it spent on children. And by 2033, the federal government is projected to spend far more on adult entitlement programs than on children, as depicted in Figure 1-5 (Lou et al., 2023). These expenditures include adult Social Security,

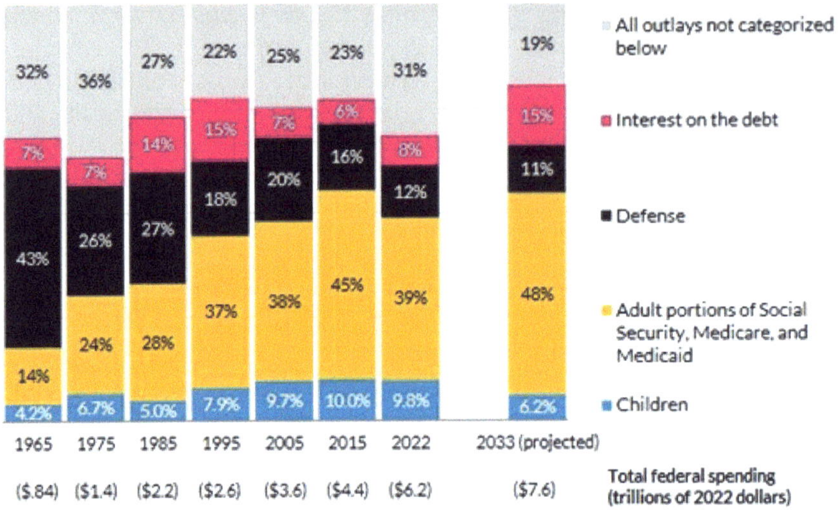

FIGURE 1-4 Share of federal budget outlays spent on children and other items, selected years, 1965–2033.
NOTE: Numbers may not sum to totals because of rounding.
SOURCES: Lou et al., 2023. Authors' estimates based primarily on Congressional Budget Office, 2023a, Office of Management and Budget, 2023, and past years' release of these reports.

Medicare, and Medicaid spending, which in recent years has reached approximately 40% of total federal outlays. Even after including state and local spending that covers high child educational costs, total public spending benefiting seniors is still about twice the amount spent on children each year (Lou et al., 2023). While children under age 18 made up 40% of Medicaid enrollees in 2019, they consumed only 17% of total Medicaid spending (KFF, 2019). With adults imposing the largest costs in the health care system, many population health efforts have focused on adults with high health care costs and the Medicare population, with less attention to prevention and child health.

COVID-19 relief bills benefited children and families, but other budget priorities grew even more. During the pandemic, it is estimated that total federal outlays grew from 20% of the GDP to a post–World War II high of more than 30%, then fell to 25% of the GDP in 2022. In contrast, spending on children grew from around 2% of the GDP prepandemic to 2.8% in 2021, and declined to 2.4% in 2022 (Lou et al., 2023).

Many pandemic benefits for children and families were short lived, despite evidence of the deleterious long-term effects of the COVID-19 pandemic on child socioemotional, educational, and mental and physical

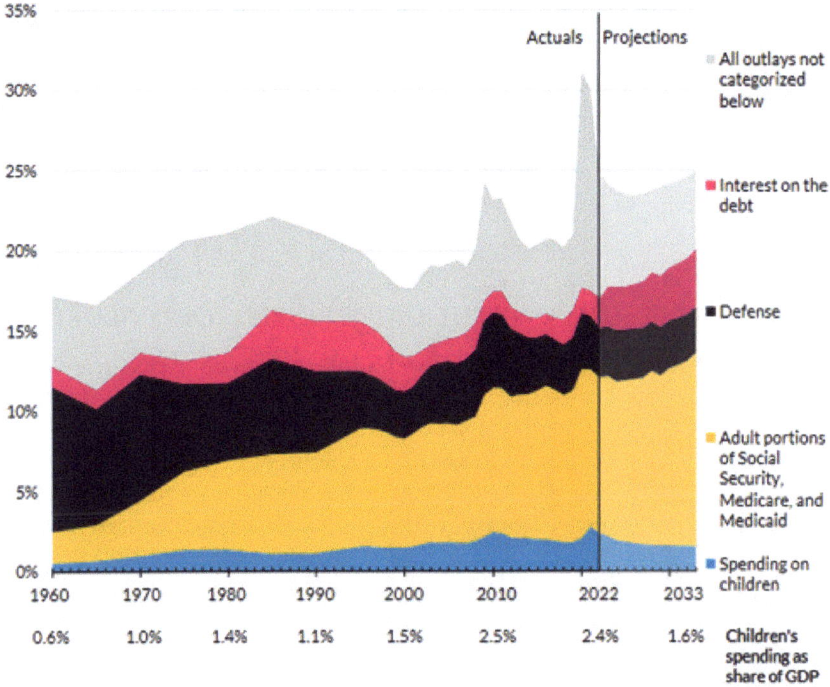

FIGURE 1-5 Federal outlays on children and other major budget items as a share of gross domestic product (GDP), 1960–2033.
NOTE: Totals shown along the horizontal axis are the share of GDP spent on children in the corresponding year.
SOURCE: Lou et al., 2023. Authors' estimates based primarily on Congressional Budget Office, 2023a, Office of Management and Budget, 2023, and past years' release of these reports.

health outcomes, especially among those from low-income and historically marginalized communities (National Academies, 2023c). Three rounds of economic impact payments were made; the child tax credit, the Supplemental Nutrition Assistance Program, and federal Medicaid funding were all increased; and the Education Stabilization Fund expanded child care funding. The pandemic child tax credit reduced poverty in 2021 (Burns & Fox, 2022; as had been demonstrated historically; National Academies, 2019a), decreased child abuse and neglect reports (Bullinger & Boy, 2023), and alleviated food insecurity (Bovell-Ammon et al., 2022; Shafer et al., 2022). As COVID-19 emergency funds were spent down and the pandemic child tax credit expired, child poverty more than doubled in 2022—from 5.2% in 2021 to 12.4% according to the supplemental poverty measure (Shrider

& Creamer, 2023)—and child abuse and neglect reports have again risen (Department of Health and Human Services, 2024). The pandemic highlighted racial, ethnic, and socioeconomic inequity; structural racism; slow response; and long-lasting negative impact on children, pregnant women, and families (National Academies, 2023c). Nonetheless, it is projected that by 2033 all categories of expenditures on children as a share of GDP will decline below current levels and most will decline below prepandemic levels (Lou et al., 2023).

LACK OF ATTENTION TO THE UNIQUE NEEDS OF CHILDREN

The differences between pediatric and adult care noted above (the 5 Ds) lead to differences in health care delivery and research needs. Most of health care innovation occurs in adult delivery systems, given the higher expenses for older groups. This approach often leaves out the needs of children, especially those with rare conditions, and innovations in adult health care may have unintended negative consequences for children. A few examples are discussed below.

Pediatric Health Care and Pediatric Clinicians

Pediatric health care and maternity care require specialized medications, diagnostics, therapeutics, equipment, and staff. Pediatric health care relies on Medicaid/CHIP, covering almost half of U.S. children, yet lower payment makes access to primary care and subspecialty care difficult for many children with public insurance. Pediatric inpatient beds are less profitable than adult beds, contributing to the closure of pediatric units and maternity wards, which has resulted in further access challenges (Cushing et al., 2021; Shachar, Gruppuso, & Adashi, 2023). More than half of U.S. rural hospitals no longer offer birthing services (Anderer, 2024; Center for Healthcare Quality and Payment Reform, n.d.). A retrospective study of 4,720 U.S. hospitals using the 2008–2018 American Hospital Association survey found that pediatric inpatient units decreased by 19.1% and pediatric inpatient unit beds decreased by 11.8%, with rural areas seeing the largest decreases (Cushing et al., 2021). It was estimated that one-quarter of U.S. children experienced an increase in distance to their nearest pediatric inpatient unit. While some evidence has found increased care quality associated with regionalization of medical services, there is also evidence of poor outcomes related to distance and transportation barriers.

Additionally, pediatricians remain the lowest-paid specialty in medicine (Ickes, 2023; USAFacts, 2023); other child-focused professionals, including nurses, mental health providers, teachers, and child care workers, also have low salaries. The lifetime earning potential for adult physicians averaged 25% more ($1.2 million higher) than for pediatric physicians across all comparable areas of both general and subspecialty academic practice (Catenaccio, Rochlin, & Simon, 2021). With many medical students graduating with high debt, the percentage of U.S. medical school graduates entering pediatrics has been in decline, with earning potential cited as a factor (Azok et al., 2024; Vinci, 2021). The National Academies (2023e) report *The Future Pediatric Subspecialty Physician Workforce* also detailed the growing shortages of many pediatric subspecialists. The lowest-paid specialties have the greatest shortages in fellowship program fill rates (e.g., pediatric nephrology, child abuse pediatrics, pediatric infectious disease, pediatric rheumatology, developmental-behavioral pediatrics, pediatric endocrinology).

Pediatric Drug Development and Diagnostic Testing

Diagnostic tools, devices, and treatments developed for adults do not immediately or easily translate to pediatrics, and some disorders present only in childhood. The economic environment for drug discovery and development strongly favors a focus on therapeutics for common adult conditions over conditions affecting children or rare diseases. As a result, off-label drug use and drug shortages are more frequent and even commonplace in pediatric care, despite some evidence that off-label use is associated with higher rates of adverse effects in children (Turner et al., 1999). High rates of off-label prescribing outside of an approved age, indication, weight, dose, formulation, or route of administration occurs in inpatient settings (36–92%) and especially neonatal and pediatric intensive care units (80–97%; Cuzzolin, Atzei, & Fanos, 2006; Pandolfini & Bonati, 2005; Turner et al., 1999). In the ambulatory setting, nearly 1 in 5 pediatric visits resulted in the ordering of one or more off-label drugs; 45–60% of pediatric visits when drugs were prescribed included off-label orders (Bazzano et al., 2009; Hoon et al., 2019). Off-label use has risen in recent years, most notably for antihistamines and psychotropic drugs, including antidepressants (Hoon et al., 2019). Testing of pharmaceuticals is especially limited in pediatric oncology—at the time of first approval of adult oncology drugs, only 5.1% have pediatric labeling information (Bicer et al., 2023; Hwang et al., 2020). In a study using a ClinicalTrials.gov review of pediatric-relevant cancer drugs that were starting efficacy testing in adults, only 34% of the 185 drugs were evaluated in minors (Bicer et al., 2023).

Laws and policies have attempted to incentivize or mandate pediatric clinical trials to reduce off-label use. The Best Pharmaceuticals for Children Act (BPCA, 2002), Pediatric Research Equity Act (2003), and European Pediatric Regulation (2007) have helped increase pediatric studies, and BPCA provides a voluntary incentive. However, drug companies still often fail to include children, with off-label pediatric drug use increasing.

Finally, shortages of essential drugs, including chemotherapy drugs, have been increasing in the United States and Europe (Huss et al., 2023), disproportionately and negatively impacting care of pediatric patients (Butterfield, Cash, & Pham, 2015). Pediatric patients may be at particular risk of harm because of a comparative increase in the use of impacted medications (e.g., parenteral nutrition) and the relative lack of quality pediatric data (or Food and Drug Administration–approved indications for pediatric use) to guide the selection of alternative medications (Butterfield, Cash, & Pham, 2015). Children are a vulnerable group with very limited pharmaceutical treatment options. Strengthened protections are needed.

The development, safety, and effectiveness of laboratory tests is another area requiring unique consideration for children. Diagnostic tools developed for adult populations may not translate to pediatrics and require validation study. Again, the economics of developing diagnostic tests for a relatively small population are a challenge. Reference ranges for children may vary significantly by age, gender, and other factors, requiring additional effort. Laboratory-developed tests by children's hospitals and pediatric academic medical centers fill a critical gap in developing and validating diagnostic tests.

Health Care Innovations and Pediatrics

With continual innovation in health care, addressing the unique needs of children and impacts on children and low-income and minoritized communities must be considered and addressed early. Three examples of health care innovations are discussed: one results in delays in realizing the benefits of technology for children; another results in children suffering unintended consequences of innovation focused on adults; in the third, children have not been included.

While electronic health records (EHRs) and related innovations now function in almost all pediatric health care settings, initial design was for adult care, and use of pediatric customization and functionality continue to lag. While EHR adoption has increased significantly in pediatric practices since 2005, when only 21.3% of pediatric primary care practices had EHRs (Kemper, Uren, & Clark, 2006), challenges persist in implementing pediatric-specific functionalities. The Children's Electronic Health Record Format, developed by the Agency for Healthcare Research and Quality (AHRQ) and CMS, outlines critical functionalities and data elements specific to pediatric EHRs, highlighting the need for specialized features (Dufendach et al., 2015). Yet, over 80% of pediatric clinicians use EHRs lacking optimal functionality for pediatric care, leading to potential errors in clinical decisions, misdiagnosis, and medication dosage miscalculations (Temple et al., 2019), and many EHR systems lack essential pediatric features such as specialized growth charts, vaccine management tools, and age-appropriate developmental screening templates (AHRQ, 2014; Dufendach et al., 2015; Lehmann et al., 2014). These ongoing challenges suggest that while progress has been made, EHRs and related innovations continue to fall short in fully addressing the unique needs of pediatric care, and progress has still fallen behind progress for older populations (Nakamura et al., 2013; Weinberg et al., 2021).

Another example of health care innovation that left out or had unintended negative consequences for children has involved the move to alternative payment models and value-based care. The majority of these experiments have occurred with adults and Medicare recipients. In fact, the Center for Medicare and Medicaid Innovation was directed to address the likelihood of cost savings within an unspecified period of time, typically defined as 18–36 months (Badger, 2022; CBO, 2023a). This short time frame for return on investment is particularly difficult to demonstrate for innovations for children, and the cost-saving directive has stymied effort in payment reform to support prevention and health promotion early in the life course.

Experiments with alternative payment models can deprioritize focus on children and primary prevention. One example is in the state of Maryland, which has a unique all-payer rate-setting system for hospital services (Cheng, 2023). The model approved in January 2014 was developed by the state and CMS to shift from volume-based reimbursement to a global budget revenue system in an effort to align hospital incentives with community and primary care efforts and to decrease health care costs. Since children contribute only a small portion of the total cost in the health care system, this population health effort focused on Medicare patients and other adults.

Initial areas of priority in Maryland's initiative were diabetes, opioid use, and establishment of the Maryland Primary Care Program. Despite clear roots of many health conditions in childhood, primary prevention efforts in childhood would not show needed short-term cost savings, resulting in exclusion of children in these initiatives with a focus on secondary and tertiary prevention with adults. The Maryland Primary Care Program offered prospective payments for advanced primary care, but eligibility was based on a minimum number of Medicare beneficiaries. Very few in the maternal and child health population are insured by Medicare, and thus maternal and child health practices were not included. Health care delivery systems followed the state's lead in their investments. Because pediatrics and obstetrics fall under global budgets for large health care delivery systems, the focus was on the majority adult population and Medicare metrics. As CMS expands new voluntary, state total-cost-of-care models, attention to prevention and inclusion of children are needed.

Finally, the current National Institutes of Health initiative to develop a database of 1 million Americans, an example of precision public health, has been an exciting opportunity for understanding developmental origins of health and disease starting early in the life course. However, after over 6 years of recruiting nearly 800,000 adults and publication of the monograph *Opportunities Enabled Through the Enrollment of Children in the* All of Us *Research Program* in 2018, child enrollment has just begun (All of Us Research Program Investigators, 2019; Kaiser, 2024).

Inclusion of children, consideration of their unique needs, and addressing health equity are prerequisites for policy initiatives, legislation, and innovation.

VISION FOR IMPROVING THE HEALTH AND WELLBEING OF CHILDREN AND YOUTH

Early in its deliberations, drawing on the expansive literature discussed above and the growing consensus within the health care field on principles and attributes of health care, the committee crafted a vision for improving the health and wellbeing of children and youth. We envision a child and adolescent health care system a decade from now built on traditional knowledge and the evidence regarding early life experiences, human development, and disease prevention (see Chapter 2) to provide comprehensive, family-engaged, community-integrated, and equitable care focused on optimizing the healthy development and lifelong wellbeing of all children, youth, and their families. This health care system will exist in a broader, cross-sector system, especially including the work of schools, which equitably promotes flourishing, builds on community strengths, and addresses family and community needs to create the safe, stable, and nurturing relationships and environments that all children need to thrive. The major causes of child and adolescent morbidity and mortality and the lived knowledge and expressed needs of children, youth, and families will guide the priorities for how the health care system allocates its resources to achieve this vision (see Chapter 3). Figure 1-6 illustrates how the characteristics of care would change.

Ensuring that the lived knowledge and expressed needs of children, youth, and families set the priorities for the health care system is a critical component of a future transformed system. Existing endeavors to advance health care transformation often fail to include people with lived experience in their development and evaluation. Many local health care systems have sought ways to incorporate such experiences into the design and improvements of policies and services.

Several key advances in health and health care already support change and progress expected in the next 10 years, including better and earlier diagnosis and treatment of medical conditions, innovations in team-based care, integrated mental and behavioral health, inclusion of the family and child

Pediatric Care Now and Future

	OLD MODEL		FUTURE MODEL
WHO	Primarily doctors and nurse practitioners	➡	Interdisciplinary teams, community health workers, co-production with families, communities, virtual
WHAT	Individual patient-oriented, 1:1	➡	Individual patient, family, and public health-oriented, 1:many
	Clinical treatment	➡	Whole child and family health, prevention, outreach
WHEN	Health maintenance and acute care	➡	Visits with other team members, group visits, self management, virtual
WHERE	Clinic and hospital-focused	➡	Community-based and community-integrated, networks, virtual
HOW	Continuity through visits and phone	➡	Continuity through visits, phone and other information technology
	Reactive, episodic	➡	Proactive, outreach, education/empowerment, coordination/navigation
	Funded through insurance	➡	Insurance, block grants, braided and blended funding across sectors
	Lesson plan	➡	Listen plan, co-design and co-creation with youth, families, communities
	Focus on medical conditions	➡	Longer time frames, investment in lifelong health and prevention

FIGURE 1-6 Present and future pediatric care models.
SOURCE: Generated by the committee, adapted from Cheng, 2004.

voice, and improved coordination of care with community services that address social determinants of health. The growth of artificial intelligence and genomics will support and expand these advances. The major mental health crisis—combined with the effects of the COVID-19 pandemic on schooling with clear inequities between different population groups among America's children and youth—has highlighted needs and led to efforts to expand mental and behavioral health services, especially in primary care and schools but indeed across the spectrum of child and adolescent health services (National Academies, 2023b). Going forward, mental and behavioral health will have a prominent place in health care, which will necessitate expanding prevention and early identification of conditions affecting mental and behavioral health and integrating treatment (see Chapter 5).

Recognizing that the major causes of child and adolescent morbidity and mortality involve injury, violence, and social determinants of health, primary care involvement in addressing family and community challenges and needs will be important for improving child health. Furthermore, as medicine has advanced and more children survive previously fatal conditions, the larger proportion of children with chronic and complex conditions will challenge the health care system to design new models of care, including remote patient monitoring and intensive home care.

What will the child health care system of the future look like? Healthy children entering adulthood will have histories without major family or community adversity and will have healthy behaviors and mental and behavioral wellness, along with educational skills and resilience. Any chronic condition and identified risk conditions will be well managed, and their health will support them as they enter the workforce and childbearing ages. To achieve these outcomes, we expect that the clinical workforce will transform even more into coordinated team-based care—with physicians and nurses working alongside integrated mental and behavioral health workers and community health workers or navigators (Brykman, Jacobs, & Casau, 2024; Katkin et al., 2017; Shalaby & Agyapong, 2020). Inclusion of families—and children, in developmentally appropriate ways—in care teams will expand, building in part on new communication strategies. Teams may be housed in offices but also will be based in communities (e.g., schools, community centers) and virtual settings. Families will experience teams as trusted partners for easy access to the complex variety of services that promote children's healthy development and family and community wellbeing. Teams will ensure that families receive (1) preventive and health-promoting services, especially focused on social and relational health and positive childhood experiences, and including immunizations and early identification and treatment for growth and developmental problems; (2) assessment and management of common acute illnesses; (3) integrated mental and behavioral care providing prevention, early identification, short-term management, and referral as needed; and (4) access to community resources in areas such as housing, nutrition, education, and income support. Many aspects of a child's life—including those outside the realm of clinical care—impact growth, development, socioemotional health, and education; therefore, more effective links are needed between clinical care and the wide variety of other community services and programs that affect the health and wellbeing of children and youth.

Hospitals will increasingly limit their work to necessary acute or interventional services, such as needed surgery and follow-up, care for acutely ill individuals, and specialized evaluations. Pediatrics will continue to be important in birthing hospitals with well-baby and neonatal intensive care units. The pediatric health care system will experience greater regionalization of centralized high-technology and specialized services. Subspecialty care, too, will use new technologies for remote monitoring of many acute and chronic conditions and maximize new communication and support strategies to help families care for their children at home. Children and families will have less need to travel to hospitals for checkups and follow-up care.

New communication modalities will increase, especially in rural communities, although local community-based primary care will also expand. These communication methods will allow earlier identification of needs with increased use of artificial intelligence, genomics, and monitoring of growth and development and health conditions, especially for children and families facing threats to healthy development and for children with chronic health conditions and other special needs. Convenient retail clinics will provide increasing amounts of acute care, although most of the developmental,

mental and behavioral, and chronic condition care likely will come from community teams and virtual care. The diverse ways that households interact with team members will encourage personal relationships with the team, ensuring that families and youth have team members they trust and partner with across time.

Schools will build on their already extensive provision of health care to children and youth, especially mental and behavioral health services, with greater collaboration between early care and education, providing a continuum through childhood, adolescence, and young adult life. Digital tools will strengthen communication and collaboration between schools and health providers.

Integrating children who have more complex conditions with the community-based system will help ensure that care is close to home when possible and also provide needed attention to mental and behavioral conditions and social and relational health risks, which occur at higher rates among children and youth with chronic conditions and special needs. Policies will ensure that children with complex conditions have access to essential services, including preventive and health-promoting supports, impacting their quality of life and wellbeing.

Investing in the child and adolescent health care system will diversify, with recognition that all of society has reasons and sees value to provide equal opportunity and to invest in children and youth. Cross-sector collaboration in meeting the health and developmental needs of children and young people will become routine, eliminating silos across public health, education, social services, and health care (Wong, Houry, & Cohen, 2024). Current health insurance investments from Medicaid, CHIP, and commercial insurance will continue with changing incentives for providers based largely on promoting the service transformation outlined above and on improving population health, while continuing to finance necessary medical and health-promoting services. Payment will support key team members and schools. Payment mechanisms will diversify, providing strategies other than insurance models to implement comprehensive prevention and health promotion programs. Coordinated child health and wellbeing investments will come from a diverse range of public and private sources committed to building a successful and effective young adult population. Cross-sector and braided funding will support a broad and coordinated tapestry of services for children, youth, and families.

GUIDING PRINCIPLES

To develop a plan to achieve its vision and address its charge, the committee ascribed to a set of principles to guide its work and the development of program and policy recommendations: (1) employ a life course perspective; (2) partner with families and communities, which are central to child health and wellbeing; (3) prioritize and drive equitable outcomes through resources and accountability; and (4) make it sustainable over time. We view the present as a clear priority for the nation to transform child and adolescent health care, making the United States a place for children to grow and thrive, and building a lasting, effective, and creative workforce.

Principle 1: Employ a Life Course Perspective

A transformed health care system must be rooted in the science underlying the healthy development of children and youth, especially recognizing the early and lifelong influences impacting healthy development at every stage of childhood, adolescence, and young adult life. Science has shown the importance of early life experiences for later health and wellbeing and the cumulative effects of such experiences throughout development, translating to the health and capacity of working-age adults in both positive and negative ways. A life course approach requires a system-wide focus on prevention and promotion from preconception to adulthood, emphasizing upstream prevention of many health problems and promotion of healthy experiences. Major threats to thriving among children include early adversity, relational risks, persistent hunger, and unstable housing. Strong communities and families help to mitigate these threats by providing supports for anatomic, physiological, and psychological needs and building trusting relationships that support children. The outcomes of a life course perspective with continuing commitment to strengthen positive experiences over the early years and build strong and effective relationships include an effective, engaged, and skilled workforce for the nation and a healthier population as it ages.

Principle 2: Partner with Families and Communities, Which Are Central to Child Health and Wellbeing

Unhealthy families facing adversity cannot raise healthy children. As noted in the "5 Ds" above, children have distinct health care needs given their unique developmental stages, anatomic and physiological differences, and emotional and psychological characteristics that differ from adults. These distinct needs make clear the case for different design and incentives in the child and adolescent health care system. Moreover, children depend on adults, and children's needs must be viewed in the context of family and community. Principles of family-centered care recognize the importance of collaboration with families and communities in decision making (American Institutes for Research, 2017; Gears et al., 2021). The American Academy of Pediatrics calls children and families "essential partners," working together with health care providers and other team members (Katkin et al., 2017). Community partners (e.g., schools, pharmacies, home care, and state agencies) coordinate with teams to help ensure preventive care, health promotion, and health maintenance for all children for lifelong health and wellbeing (Katkin et al., 2017). Screening for health-related community, social, economic, and environmental risks to health (e.g., food insecurity, housing instability, lack of transportation), with subsequent integration with and provision of cross-sector resources, is critical for addressing health disparities (Buitron de la Vega et al., 2019).

Principle 3: Prioritize and Drive Equitable Outcomes through Resources and Accountability

The emergence of health disparities starts early in the life course. To address upstream causes of health disparities appropriately, a framework for change must include a cultural shift toward systems and care that understand and address racism as a root cause of health inequities (Trent, Dooley, & Dougé, 2019). As racism drives inequities across every identity that individuals and communities share, addressing structural, institutional, and interpersonal racism is critical to achieving health equity (Jones, 2000; National Academies, 2023c). Moving toward health equity, or "everyone [having] a fair and just opportunity to be as healthy as possible" (Braveman et al., 2018, p. 2), requires an intentional redistribution of focus to communities that have long endured underinvestment and structural disadvantage. While this could be viewed as describing all children, Black, Native American, Hispanic, and other children of color; those who live with disabilities; and those who identify as LGBTQ+ have borne the brunt of health inequities.

Centering historically oppressed and underserved communities requires collaborating across the health care field to disaggregate and standardize the data used to assess health disparities and allocate resources; integrating measurement that drives change defined by children, youth, families, and the communities that support them; and defining success not by how well the average child does but by true child health equity. The path forward includes existing ideas and models for pediatric care—such as addressing social determinants of health and adversity, focused team-based care efforts on the needs of children and families, interventions that mitigate the "negative early experiences and exposures" through community collaborations and provision of resources, and incentivization of these efforts (Perrin, Lu et al., 2020c, p. 2). A health equity approach also encourages and implements ideas that appear unconventional and finds ways to elevate traditional and Indigenous knowledge (White House Council on Environmental Quality & Office of Science and Technology Policy, 2022). It challenges the notion that only evidence produced by systems that have currently and historically upheld a racist, inequitable status quo are worthy of investment and action. Achieving health equity requires not only redistributing focus but also confronting the imbalance of power within current pediatric health care systems. If one defines "power" as "the capacity to influence social and structural conditions" (Rosino, 2016, p. 340), then along every step of this new framework must exist a checkpoint where current power imbalances are interrogated, and steps taken with communities most disadvantaged to remediate and rectify historical and current injustices (Iton, Ross, & Tamber, 2022). A framework for health care transformation that centers health equity therefore ensures along every step that transformation is not worsening inequity and is in fact achieving health equity.

Principle 4: Make It Sustainable over Time

Sustained progress in child and adolescent health care transformation will require strong and predictable financing by strengthening public and commercial health insurance and by strengthening the financial base of the nation's public health and school health structures. Children's health progress has suffered from a lack of sustained public attention and commitment to the issues driving child, adolescent, and young adult health and wellbeing. Sustaining it will require ongoing governmental focus centered on the needs of children, youth, and families in all relevant programs and policies. Successful children's health care system transformation relies on leaders; partners; payers; and activated communities, families, and youth that establish agreements that incentivize and track performance on shared goals, ensuring transparency and open exploration of performance in partnership with health care systems and families and the communities they serve. Infrastructure to support the real-time and sustained identification and promotion of success factors is critical, as are financing approaches that pay for the efforts and changes needed to achieve transformative improvements. Essential to these goals is the specification and routine tracking and actionable reporting of measures of positive health and equity-based quality of care and individual and population-based outcomes that are agreed upon by key partners and payers of care.

ORGANIZATION OF THE REPORT

The committee divided the report into 10 chapters. Chapters 2–9 provide background that serves as the basis for the committee's recommendations and implementation plan (Chapter 10). Chapter 2 discusses social influences affecting the delivery of health care, including scientific and technological advances in medicine and medical and personal tools, and the familial and environmental influences that affect health trajectories. It captures a set of frameworks for thinking about optimal health, health care delivery, and the health care system. Chapter 3 examines child and family health needs and expectations of the health care system. It draws on lived experiences to identify the current challenges that families and communities face in receiving appropriate health care. It also takes stock of different models of family and child engagement. Chapter 4 provides context for changing demographics and needs in the United States and captures the current state of child and adolescent health and wellbeing. The chapter makes comparisons with other countries on certain health indicators. It considers social trends that have an impact on health care as well as the health and wellbeing of children and youth. Chapter 5 overviews the organization, features, and new initiatives of the current health care system in the United States. It also examines the changing nature of and challenges for the health care workforce. Chapter 6 details current financing mechanisms and their opportunities, barriers, and challenges. It discusses the role that redirecting funding streams can play in supporting preventive care practices. Chapter 7 discusses current public health programs and the opportunities for federal programs and resources aimed at supporting and improving the health and wellbeing of children, families, and communities. Chapter 8 discusses how schools currently provide a significant proportion of health and mental health care and the opportunities in expanding health and health care in school settings. Chapter 9 identifies levers and strategies for promoting accountability for child and youth wellbeing and monitoring quality with metrics. Chapter 10 presents the committee's recommended actions that comprise its implementation plan. In addition to the core content, there are four appendixes. Appendix A presents the biographies of the committee members, fellow, and staff. Appendix B lists the numerous National Academies consensus study reports and National Academy of Medicine publications of relevance to this study and documents the accumulating evidence for large-scale reform of the health care system. Appendix C provides the agendas from the committee's public sessions. Appendix D summarizes performance measurement topics used across seven child health programs involving federal funding.

CONCLUSION

Although most U.S. children and youth are healthy, significant increases in rates of chronic conditions, especially mental and behavioral health conditions, along with worsening indicators of the state of child health, call for major redirection of the way the health care system influences child health and wellbeing. The results of worsening child health and wellbeing now affect the working-age population, which also experiences higher rates of disease and disability (e.g., mental and behavioral health problems, obesity, pulmonary, and cardiovascular disease) than seen in previous generations. This poor state of health of working adults combined with the prospects of falling birth rates and rising numbers of retired individuals create a workforce crisis.

This chapter has introduced the committee's task of identifying key levers of change within the child health care system and highlighted findings from prior reports of the accumulating knowledge on the importance of child health for health across the life course. This review indicates the importance of prevention and health promotion in early childhood, as well as the need to address disparate health outcomes and inequities in access to quality health care. Growing evidence points both to the challenges of current financing mechanisms to support broad changes to health care and to the opportunities of innovations that have tested different models for payment, care coordination, and family and community supports. Subsequent chapters discuss this background and literature in greater detail.

This chapter has focused on defining what investment in child health means to children, families, communities, and the nation and has articulated seven societal gains demonstrated by research. It has called attention to declining investment in child health despite these demonstrated gains. Given this assessment of trends, the committee concludes that a health care system that focuses predominantly on adults deprioritizes children's health and threatens long-term societal health. The distinct needs of younger populations often get little attention in new delivery models, in development of diagnostics and therapeutics, and during public health crises. Effective transformation of child and adolescent health care to meet life course needs of children and greater family and community needs and to build a resilient future for the nation will require ongoing commitment and leadership within the health care system to address whole child and family health care, engage families and communities in improvements, and foster partnerships across diverse agencies and sectors for a thriving future for all.

Building on this expansive literature and committee members' experiences in health care, the committee set forth a vision for improving health care for children and youth and developed four principles to guide its deliberations and recommendations (see Chapter 10). These principles include (1) employ a life course perspective; (2) partner with families and communities, which are central to child health and wellbeing; (3) prioritize and drive equitable outcomes through resources and accountability; and (4) make it sustainable over time.

2

Science and Frameworks to Guide Health Care Transformation

The first mandate [...] is to ensure that our decision-making is guided by consideration of the welfare and well being of the seventh generation to come.

—Bemidji Statement on Seventh Generation Guardianship

Development of children and youth is characterized by continuous skills attainment, growth, and transition, thereby setting a trajectory upon which adult health builds. Such health, wellbeing, and developmental trajectories are shaped by consequential influences across social, environmental, and relational contexts. This chapter discusses the science of healthy child and youth development as the base for a life course perspective on improving child and family health and clarifying the importance of relational health throughout the life course. To describe the dynamic nature of child health and development, the chapter provides an overview of critical stages in development. It describes the scientific bases and important advances in science and technology that guide efforts to improve child health and well-being, and it outlines social and environmental factors—at individual and community levels, as well as at the broader population level—that influence the life course. The chapter concludes with a discussion of the implications of these scientific streams—the science of child and youth development, key scientific and technological advances, and the social determinants of health—to guide health care transformation.

LIFE COURSE AND MULTIGENERATIONAL PERSPECTIVE

Childhood is a time of wonder, with developmental stages progressing from conception and infancy to childhood, adolescence, and adulthood. Growing research demonstrates many early antecedents to adult health and disease and aging (Braveman & Barclay, 2009; Horvath & Raj, 2018; Joseph & Kramer, 1996; National Academies of Sciences, Engineering, and Medicine [National Academies], 2019b,c,d; Raffington, 2024; Wehrle et al., 2020). Multiple factors affect life course developmental stages, including structural inequities and racism; social determinants of health; environmental exposures; and individual behavioral, social, and biological mechanisms. A previous report by the National Academies, *Children's Health, The Nation's Wealth,* provides a model of children's health and its influences across life stages (see Figure 2-1; National Research Council [NRC] & Institute of Medicine [IOM], 2004). The model illustrates multiple influences—including biology, behavior, and physical and social environments—that interact over time to create children's health. Programs, services, and policies affect how these influences operate in a child's life. The relative weight of these

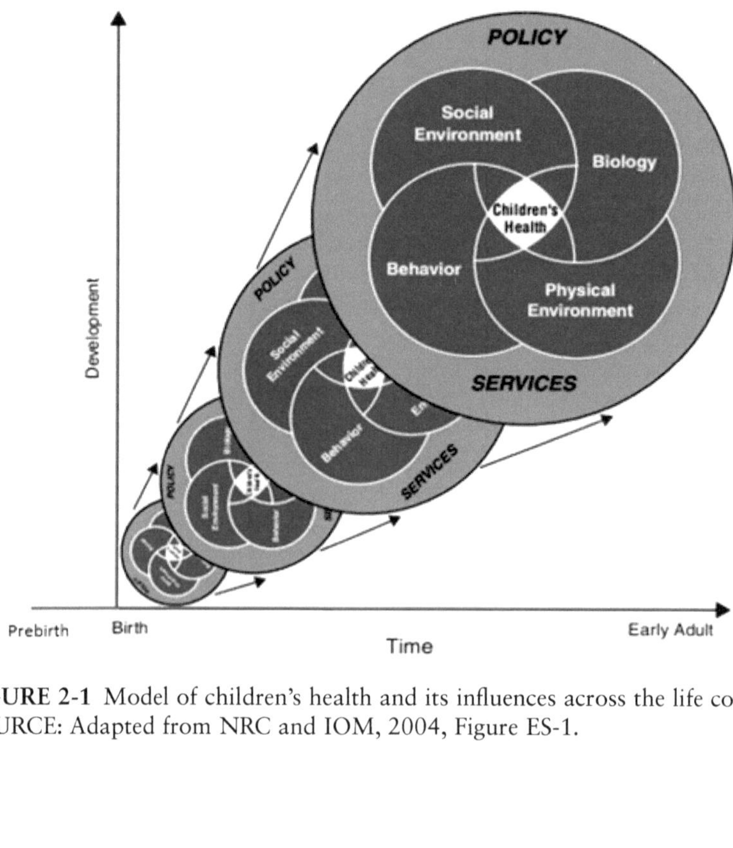

FIGURE 2-1 Model of children's health and its influences across the life course.
SOURCE: Adapted from NRC and IOM, 2004, Figure ES-1.

influences and interactions varies in different developmental stages; previous stages influence later development. Changes in a child's health resemble a kaleidoscope of glass pieces representing various influences that create different patterns of health over time from birth to adulthood.

An addition to this model was the extension of the x-axis to include prebirth. Research demonstrates the importance of fetal health and parents' preconception health on a child's health (National Academies, 2019d; Schrott, Song, & Ladd-Acosta, 2022). Ensuring child wellbeing requires considering conditions prior to birth, as well as the health of the family unit across the life course. Understanding how to support healthy developmental trajectories will be important for transformation at the practice, policy, and systems levels to ensure that all children and families have the opportunity to realize positive trajectories.

Pediatric practice has long adopted a two-generation approach to care, with focus on both children and parents. With recognition of genetic, epigenetic, and environmental factors affecting health risks for the next generation, a longer view is needed (Cheng, Johnson, & Goodman, 2016; Hanson & Gluckman, 2014). A growing body of literature documents the intergenerational transmission of health and disease and transgenerational effects of social and environmental exposures and epigenetics on health (Benincasa, Napoli, & DeMeo, 2024; Breton et al., 2021; Kioumourtzoglou et al., 2018; Scorza et al., 2019; Tan et al., 2024). In addition, beyond the importance of their health today, as future adults, children and youth are also the child bearers for the next generation. A three-generation approach considers the health of children, the adults they will become, and the new families they will create (see Figures 2-2 and 2-3). This proactive prevention approach for the next generation emphasizes child and family health, child educational success, family planning, and parenting education starting before childbearing (Cheng, Johnson, & Goodman, 2016).

Modern understanding of the origins of health confirms long-understood traditional and Indigenous knowledge. Many Indigenous communities have followed the principle of Seven Generations, which understands that present actions will affect the next seven generations (Loew, 2014). Based on ancient Haudenosaunee (Iroquois) philosophy, this principle emphasizes present decision making that considers potential effects on descendants seven generations in the future (Haley, 2021). These Indigenous principles do not focus solely on the intergenerational impact of trauma; instead, they center a strengths-based approach that understands, among many things, the value of relational health, intergenerational healing, and collective wisdom in realizing communal health and wellness (Fish et al., 2023; O'Keefe, Fish et al., 2022; O'Keefe, Maudrie et al., 2023). This report is guided by a life course and multigenerational framework for health care transformation.

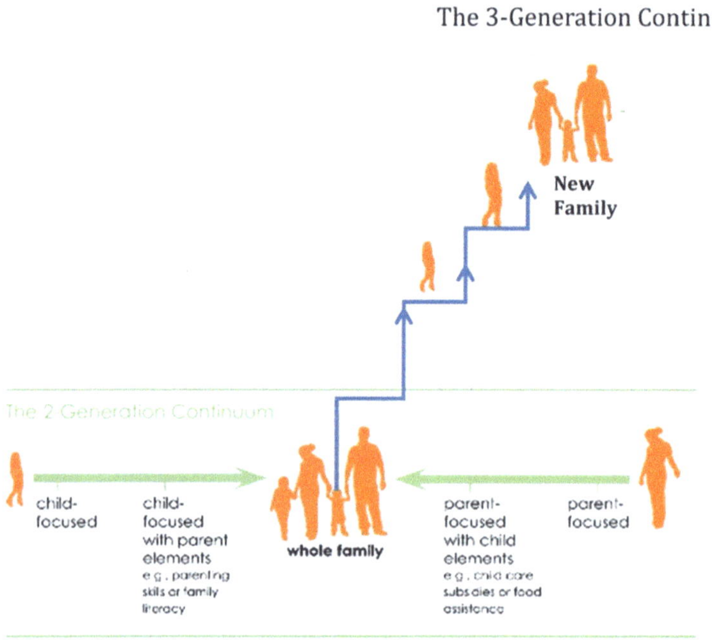

FIGURE 2-2 The three-generation continuum.
SOURCE: Cheng, Johnson, & Goodman, 2016a.

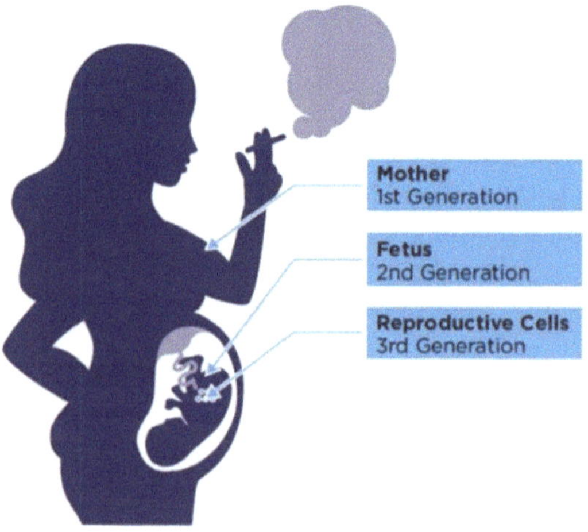

FIGURE 2-3 Multigenerational transmission of health effects from environmental exposures.
SOURCE: Child Enrollment Scientific Vision Working Group, 2017.

CRITICAL PERIODS IN DEVELOPMENT: OPPORTUNITIES FOR HEALTH CARE TRANSFORMATION

Life course theory highlights critical and sensitive periods in development. These concepts have been part of developmental science recognizing periods when certain experiences, exposures, or conditions exert disproportionate influence or malleability over long-term outcomes (Colombo, Gustafson, & Carlson, 2019). "Sensitive periods" are limited developmental time windows during which experiences have great effect; "critical periods" are subsets of sensitive periods in which normal development is impaired without appropriate nurturing and stimulation (Knudsen, 2004; Voss, 2013).

For example, the National Academies report *Addressing the Long-Term Effects of the COVID-19 Pandemic on Children and Families* noted that the pandemic was an adverse childhood experience for many and that the effects on child development and outcomes differ depending on child age and developmental stage (National Academies, 2023b). Further examples include pregnancy and childbirth, which usher in excitement for opportunities from the start and hope for the future. Infancy, childhood, and adolescence celebrate the wonders of child growth and development in the domains of social, emotional, physical, cognitive, and language development. Late adolescence and young adulthood mark the transition to adulthood—becoming independent; developing one's identity; handling more complex relationships; and taking on new roles and responsibilities in education, employment, and family formation.

Understanding and optimizing these developmental periods and ensuring that the health care system provides developmentally appropriate care across these life stages are necessary for children to thrive. The following sections summarize these developmental periods and give examples of health care opportunities to strengthen these stages and transitions.

Preconception and Prenatal Women's Health

Considerable evidence demonstrates the impact of baseline maternal health (e.g., diabetes, obesity, hypercholesterolemia, hypertension, depression) and behaviors (e.g., smoking, drug use, physical activity, nutrition) on offspring outcomes in childhood and adulthood (Castro & Avina, 2002; Kleinman et al., 1988; Orr & Miller, 1997; Ryder, 2018; Walford et al., 2011; Xiong et al., 2006; Zuckerman et al., 1989). These associations indicate the need for early prevention in mothers before or during pregnancy (Ryder, 2018). The story of folic acid supplementation is a powerful example of how a preconception intervention influences child health. The educational campaign and fortification of grains led to a 26% drop in the rate of neural tube defects (De-Regil et al., 2010; Howse, 2008). Recent evidence suggests that women should start taking folic acid supplements at least 3 months before conception for optimal effectiveness, as neural tube defects occur during the first 28 days of pregnancy (Kim et al., 2017; Viswanathan et al., 2023). In a multisite cluster-randomized trial, a maternal health screener and brief interconception intervention in pediatric primary care were found to be feasible and effective in increasing daily folic acid use and decreasing smoking (Upadhya et al., 2020). With growing scientific recognition that early antecedents of child and adult health start prenatally and even preconceptionally, women's health is key (American College of Obstetricians and Gynecologists [ACOG], 2019).

Family health affects child health. Thus, family health care access and intended family size may have large influence on a child's health. Pediatric health care providers have the opportunity to address the health of children, their mothers and fathers, adolescents and young adults who will be future child bearers. Preconception and interconception health affect future generations; improving population health must embrace the entire life course and the origins of disease.

Early Childhood and Family Health

The National Academies report *From Neurons to Neighborhoods* emphasized the rapid brain development that occurs from birth to age 5 years, with children rapidly developing foundational capabilities on which subsequent development builds (NRC & IOM, 2000). Early experiences influence brain development, and the prenatal and early childhood years are particularly sensitive periods in development. Additionally, parental well-being is an important determinant of children's health and developmental outcomes: what happens to parents before, during, and after pregnancy has major implications for their children (Center on the Developing Child, 2009; Goodman & Garber, 2017; National Academies, 2019b,c).

Promoting health and resilience requires—beyond reducing exposure to adversity—increasing relational health and forming and maintaining safe, stable, and nurturing relationships (National Scientific Council on the Developing Child, 2020). Strong relationships not only help downregulate the stress response in a child but also help build skills, such as self-regulation and executive function, that assist children in managing future adversity (National Academies, 2019b,c; National Scientific Council on the Developing Child, 2020).

There is evidence that not only are the brains of infants primed to interact socially and emotionally with adult caregivers but that the brains of parents of a newborn infant also enter a critical period such that they are primed to interact with their child (Garner & Yogman, 2021a,b). Responsive interactions between children and engaged adults appear to be of fundamental importance to establishing healthy brain architecture and the health-promoting body system responses that go along with it (Garner & Yogman, 2021a,b). Healthy caregiver–child relationships develop a dyadic synchrony that can include synchronized autonomic function, hormone release, and brain-to-brain synchrony with coordinated oscillation in brain wave types between caregiver and child (Garner & Yogman, 2021a,b).

School-Age Children

The years children are in school ("school age" generally refers to ages 5–12 years) is a period of rapid acquisition of physical, cognitive, language, and socioemotional skills. Children move from playing alone to having multiple friendships and social groups. They develop independence and take on more responsibility for their activities, schoolwork, health, and safety. School occupies much of their time. The Community Preventive Services Task Force (CPSTF), an independent, nonfederal panel that provides evidence-based recommendations to improve population health, recommends the implementation and maintenance of school-based health centers (SBHCs) in low-income communities to improve educational and health outcomes. Research demonstrates that SBHCs improve educational outcomes—including school performance, grade promotion, and high school completion—and health outcomes—including the delivery of vaccinations and other recommended preventive services, as well as decreases in asthma morbidity and emergency department and hospital admission rates (CPSTF, 2015). Schools also offer an effective and opportune place for addressing health and chronic disease management, and potentially preventing, identifying, and managing mental health conditions among school-age children and adolescents (Office of the Surgeon General [OSG], 2021; see also Chapter 8 in this report).

Adolescents and Young Adults

Adolescence (ages 13–25) is another time of significant social, emotional, physical, and cognitive development (National Academies, 2019c). Puberty triggers not only visible growth and changes in physical characteristics, including primary and secondary sex characteristics, but also neurobiological and cognitive changes. These changes enable youth to engage in more complex thinking and heighten sensitivity to rewards; willingness to take risks (sensation seeking); identity development; reorientation of attention and motivation (toward peers, social evaluation, status and prestige, and sexual and romantic interests); and changes in social contexts, roles, and responsibilities. In emerging adulthood (approximately age 19 through the mid- to late twenties), young people become even more independent and begin exploring various life possibilities. The process of identity formation (in the realms of relationships, education, and work) that began during adolescence continues to materialize during these emerging adult years.

Parents and other adult caregivers are no less important for adolescents than they are for young children: both young children and adolescents need secure attachment with parents or other important adults as a foundation for healthy development and strong relationships (National Academies, 2019c). There is evidence that strong parent or other adult relationships, involvement, and connectedness are associated with better adolescent health and reduced problem behavior (National Academies, 2020d). In a study that looked at flourishing for children ages 6–17 years, a measure of family resilience and connection was strongly associated with a greater percentage of children flourishing, regardless of the number of adverse childhood experiences reported for the children (Bethell, Gombojav, & Whitaker, 2019).

Health-related behaviors during adolescence and emerging adulthood are strongly associated with health status in adulthood (National Academies, 2020b). Engaging in unhealthy (unhealthy diet, lack of exercise) and/or risky behaviors (alcohol and other substance use, tobacco use and vaping, sexual behavior, violence, dangerous driving) can have a long-term impact on both physical and mental health in adulthood (National Academies, 2020b). A growing body of research examines associations between social media use and mental and behavioral outcomes, of key concern for adolescents and youth who increasingly spend time on such platforms. A recent National Academies report, *Social Media and Adolescent Health*, did not support the conclusion that social media causes changes in adolescent health at the population level but pointed out potential harms and benefits and needed actions to protect young people (National Academies, 2023g).

Adolescents are also more sensitive than children or adults to the presence of peers (Casey et al., 2010). By middle to late adolescence, youth report relying more on either best friends or romantic partners than on parents for emotional support (Farley & Kim-Spoon, 2014). Although these interpersonal relationships can increase stressors and negative emotions, they can also, when of high quality, protect against the negative effects of stressful experiences (Farley & Kim-Spoon, 2014; Yeung, Thompson, & Leadbeater, 2013). Social isolation, peer rejection, and bullying are associated with numerous unhealthy risk behaviors and adverse health outcomes, such as increased delinquency, depression, numbers of suicide attempts, and low self-esteem (Smokowski & Evans, 2019). Notably, evidence consistently shows a reduction in risky sexual behaviors and substance abuse among U.S. adolescents over the past 20–25 years; however, experiences of violence are increasing in some cases and poor mental and suicidal thoughts and behaviors are increasing for nearly all groups of youth (Borodovsky et al., 2020; Centers for Disease Control and Prevention [CDC], 2023i; National Academies, 2020d). Positive peer modeling and awareness of peer norms have been found to be protective against violence, substance misuse, and unhealthy sexual risk (Viner et al., 2012). A network of supportive relationships with parents, peers, and other caring adults can set the foundation for lifelong health and development.

SCIENTIFIC BASES FOR HEALTH CARE TRANSFORMATION: DEVELOPMENTAL ORIGINS OF HEALTH AND DISEASE

The interplay among life experiences, genes, age, and the environments in which children live lays the foundation for early childhood development and health later in life (National Academies, 2019c,d; National Scientific Council on the Developing Child, 2020). Animal studies and epidemiological observations have demonstrated that environmental influences early in development affect the risk of later pathophysiological processes associated with chronic disease. These interconnected factors are known as the developmental origins of health and disease (Hanson & Gluckman, 2014).

Large bodies of evidence make clear how health and development reflect the interplay among genes and the environment, with major effects of the environment especially early in life. As summarized in a recent National Academies report, *Vibrant and Healthy Kids*, "New research has clarified that altered nutrition, exposure to environmental chemicals, and chronic stress during specific times of development can lead to functional biological changes that predispose individuals to manifest diseases and experience altered physical, socio-emotional, and cognitive functions later in life" (National Academies, 2019d, p. 6). *Vibrant and Healthy Kids* provides evidence about the importance of intervening early, especially in light of U.S. problems with infant mortality, low birth weight, childhood chronic disease and mental and behavioral conditions, early life adversity, poverty, lapses in health insurance, and inequities in care. While the environment influences individuals throughout life, early months and years carry the most import for changes in many human systems, from brain development to immune function to endocrine responses to physical development. Early life experiences, both positive and negative, tremendously influence how a child grows, thrives, interacts, learns.

The body's "fight or flight" stress response system, and inflammation related to activation of that system, plays a central role in mediating these effects. When a stressor occurs, the body's autonomic nervous system, immune system, metabolic systems, and neuroendocrine system all interact with the brain and each other to respond (National Scientific Council on the Developing Child, 2020). If the stress response is short lived because of either the nature of the stressor or the mitigating effect of supportive relationships (e.g., a child's first day at school), the body systems return to a baseline state and the experience can promote development for the child. If the stress response activation is prolonged, severe, or frequent—for example in the context of ongoing physical abuse, exposure to community violence, or discrimination—in the absence of supportive relationships, the body systems responses that are adaptive and helpful in dealing with the stressor can lead to allostatic overload or wear and tear on the brain and body, resulting in negative long-term health outcomes. Chronic inflammation—associated with unmitigated chronic stress activation—is associated with increased risk for a number of chronic conditions, including heart disease, diabetes, depression, arthritis, gastrointestinal disorders, autoimmune disorders, multiple types of cancer, dementia, and asthma (National Scientific Council on the Developing Child, 2020).

"Genes," heritable units of genetic material composed of DNA, provide the molecular instructions that determine specific traits (National Human Genome Research Institute [NHGRI], 2024b). "Epigenetics" refers to chemical modifications in DNA that alter the degree to which genes are turned on or off without modifying the underlying genetic code itself (NHGRI, 2024a). The interaction of experiences and genes in the context of relationships affects brain architecture and the regulation of the autonomic nervous system, the immune system, metabolic systems, and the neuroendocrine system (National Scientific Council on the Developing Child, 2020). In addition to known genetic predispositions to specific chronic diseases, variations in genes and gene expression are associated with a person's physiologic response to stressors, which can result in an increase or a decrease in the negative consequences of exposure to adversity (Boyce et al., 2021; National Academies, 2019b). There is evidence that some children are more sensitive to their social environment than others, such that more sensitive children have more positive outcomes in supportive environments and more negative outcomes in unsupportive environments, with genes and gene expression underlying the differences in sensitivity (Boyce, 2016; Boyce et al., 2021). There are many examples of links between health risks and outcomes and specific genes or specific epigenetic modifications in gene regulation (Boyce et al., 2021).

A life course view of health risk (Figure 2-4) outlines the opportunity for early intervention. During windows of plasticity, brain architecture is most sensitive to the effects of experience (Boyce et al., 2021). Sensitive and critical periods are specific windows during development when the brain is particularly receptive to certain environmental stimuli, which significantly shape neural circuits and subsequent behavior.[1] These periods are crucial for the development of various functions, including sensory processing,

[1]Different neural circuits have distinct sensitive and critical periods for different functions. For example, during sensory development, the visual and auditory systems have critical periods early in life when exposure to visual and auditory stimuli is essential for normal development (Zeanah & Fox, 2019). Sensitive periods for emotional regulation and cognitive functions extend beyond early childhood into adolescence. During these periods, experiences such as caregiving quality and educational opportunities significantly shape the brain's emotional and cognitive circuits (Cisneros-Franco et al., 2020; Zeanah & Fox, 2019).

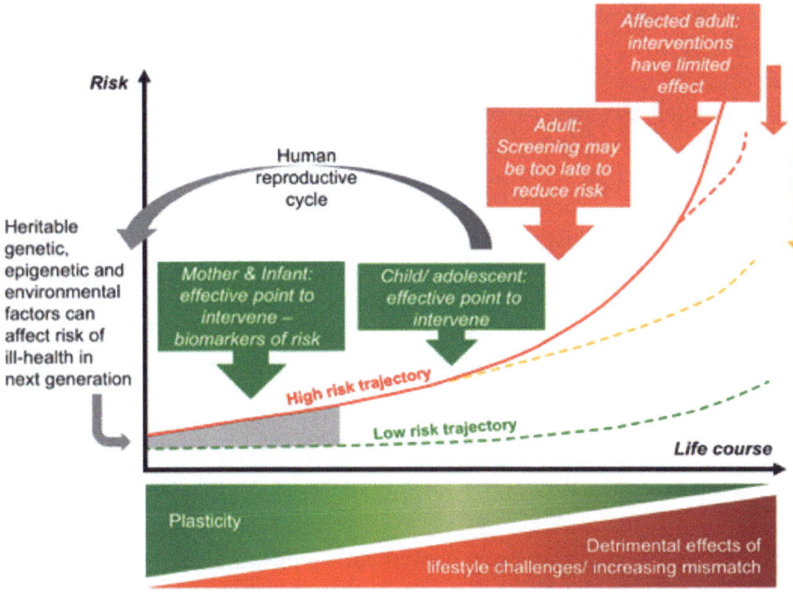

FIGURE 2-4 A life course view of health risk.
SOURCE: Hanson & Gluckman, 2014.

emotional regulation, and cognition (Boyce et al., 2021; Heun-Johnson & Levitt, 2018; Morishita et al., 2015; Nelson, Lau, & Jarcho, 2014). Because of rapid development during the prenatal period and early childhood (from birth through age 8 years), brain architecture is notably responsive to both positive and adverse experiences, making them particularly important periods for the promotion of health and wellbeing (NRC & IOM, 2015). There is also evidence for adolescence being another critical period, specifically for the development of neural circuits in the prefrontal cortex, which is responsible for functions, such as executive function (Larsen & Luna, 2018).

The goal is to diminish the risks to health on this trajectory. Opportunities to do so decrease with age as neuroplasticity declines. Life challenges in earlier stages may lead to cumulative damage in later ones. For adults, who are already on the steeper part of the risk trajectory, screening may be too late to reduce substantial risk.[2] Conversely, interventions in childhood, adolescence, and young adulthood offer major opportunities to effectively

[2]It is important to note that research has shown that experiences outside of critical periods can still change outcomes, although more intensity of effort is required. Interventions to promote healthy development of the brain and other body systems can be achieved at all ages (NRC & IOM, 2015).

and cost-effectively influence health later in the life course and in the next generation.

Experiences over the life course have lasting effects. Positive childhood experiences, including the presence of safe, stable, and nurturing relationships, are associated with positive outcomes later in life (Bethell, Gombojav, & Whitaker, 2019; Bethell, Jones et al., 2019; Garner & Yogman, 2021a,b; National Scientific Council on the Developing Child, 2020). Negative experiences, on the other hand, increase the likelihood of poor health in childhood, lower educational achievement, adolescent mental health conditions, adverse risk taking and substance use, incarceration (NRC & IOM, 2015). What is more, negative experiences over the life course lead to higher rates of several chronic health conditions in adulthood, including diabetes, substance use, obesity, mental health conditions, and early death (NRC & IOM, 2015). Adversities in childhood at the population level link to negative health outcomes in adulthood with the risk of negative health outcomes increasing as the number of adversities increases (Felitti et al., 1998). A significant portion of cases of conditions such as depression, asthma, kidney disease, coronary heart disease, and diabetes in the United States have been associated with adverse childhood experiences (Merrick et al., 2019).

As childhood adversity activates chronic stress and the associated, intertwined cascade of brain and body system responses, it also increases the risk of negative health outcomes in childhood and adulthood and helps explain the development of important chronic health conditions.

SCIENTIFIC AND TECHNOLOGICAL ADVANCES

The science of maternal child health and development, coupled with scientific advances in medicine, charts a path forward to applying the tools of precision medicine and precision population health to health promotion, starting early in the life course. Precision medicine seeks to use patient-level phenotypic and genotypic data to tailor care recommendations to improve individual health outcomes (Costain, Cohn, & Malkin, 2020), while precision population and public health addresses social, behavioral, and environmental influences (Bayer & Galea, 2015; Lyles et al., 2018). Both precision medicine and precision public health, combined with technological advances, allow earlier identification of and intervention on health problems at the individual or population level to ensure optimal conditions for health and wellbeing from the start. Including children in these advances is essential for them to realize their potential. Lyles and colleagues (2018) give the All of Us Program—an effort by the National Institutes of Health (NIH) to develop a database of 1 million Americans—as an example of precision public health; however, recruitment of children to All of Us just started after more than 6 years of recruiting nearly 800,000 adults (All of Us Research Program Investigators, 2019), with continued funding to recruit children uncertain. This section discusses examples of exciting new science and technology that has and will continue to transform health care and health, with particular promise early in the life course.

Genetics, Epigenetics, and Gene Therapy

The sequencing of the human genome was completed in 2003, and technological advances have led to an explosion of discoveries in matching genotypes to phenotypes (Hamosh et al., 2021). However, no single genome can fully represent the diversity of the human species; recently, a first draft of a human "pangenome" reference was published that includes both sets of chromosomes from 47 individuals with diverse ancestral backgrounds (Liao et al., 2021). This pangenome will contribute to further equitable and fundamental insights (Frazer & Schork, 2023).

With the genetics revolution, former NIH director Elias Zerhouni (2006) suggested a paradigm shift for medicine, characterized by four "Ps": predictive, preemptive, participatory, and personalized care. It has been suggested that the fifth and sixth Ps should be pediatrics and prenatal, as it is early in the life course when molecular evidence is knowable and when opportunity for intervention will be possible and potentially more effective (Cheng, Cohn, & Dover, 2008). Future health care will likely center around these six Ps, seizing the opportunity to predict the emergence of future health conditions and prevent, preempt, and buffer the anticipated health trajectory. Prenatal care and pediatrics are at the leading edge.

Genome sequencing has become a standard of care for a growing number of medical conditions and has high diagnostic yield in many conditions, including pediatric rare diseases (Wright et al., 2023). For instance, a recent systematic review and meta-analysis on exome sequencing in cerebral palsy supported the recommendation of exome sequencing in the diagnostic evaluation of individuals with neurodevelopmental disorders (Gonzalez-Mantilla et al., 2023). A recent issue of the *Journal of Pediatrics* included three articles reporting high yields of genetic testing in children with congenital heart disease, liver dysfunction, and neonatal encephalopathy (Durbin et al., 2023; Lenahan et al., 2023; Stewart et al., 2023). Postmortem study of infant deaths found undiagnosed genetic diseases that would have reclassified infant mortality data (Owen et al., 2023). Polygenic prediction of weight and obesity trajectories across the life course has also been described, with new opportunities for mechanistic assessment and clinical prediction (Khera et al., 2019). The interaction of experiences and genes in the context of relationships brings in epigenetic changes that affect brain architecture and the regulation of the autonomic nervous system, the immune system, metabolic systems, and the neuroendocrine system (National Academies, 2019d; National Scientific Council on the Developing Child, 2020). Epigenetic mechanisms are responsible for the incredible developmental plasticity in childhood and are exciting areas of research.

Diagnostic yield for genomic sequencing is higher than targeted neonatal gene sequencing, although time to return of results was slower (Maron et al., 2023). As technology for sequencing has become more accurate and rapid, many neonatal intensive care units are expanding use of whole genome and exome sequencing in sick neonates, with studies demonstrating high diagnostic yield (Kingsmore & Cole, 2022). Studies in children's hospitals have demonstrated improved clinical outcomes and cost savings (Dimmock et al., 2021). In addition, wider use of genome sequencing in utero and as part of newborn screening are imminent. Fetal genome sequencing could become as routine as the fetal ultrasound.

Finally, pharmacogenomics to personalize therapeutics, as well as gene therapy and gene editing to treat, prevent, or cure a disease or medical disorder, are making rapid progress. Gene therapy may involve replacing a disease-causing gene with a healthy copy of the gene, inactivating a disease-causing gene that is not functioning properly, or introducing a new or modified gene into the body to help treat a disease. The promise of gene editing approaches, including CRISPR/Cas9 gene editing—discovered in 2020 by Nobel prize winners Emmanuelle Charpentier and Jennifer Doudna—opened the possibility of cure for many genetic disorders (Park & Bao, 2021). Gene therapy is being used in a growing number of inherited genetic conditions (e.g., hemophilia, thalassemia, sickle cell disease) and acquired diseases (e.g., leukemia). It has also opened a myriad of access, implementation, and ethical questions to be addressed.

NHGRI has outlined a strategic vision for improving human health, with bold predictions that by 2030, generating and analyzing a complete human genome sequence will be routine for any research laboratory; the biological function of every human gene will be known; features of the epigenetic landscape and transcriptional output will be routinely incorporated into predictive models; genome testing will be routine, with an individual's complete genome sequence accessible on their smartphone; and curative gene therapies will be available to all for dozens of genetic diseases (Green et al., 2020).

The six Ps paradigm shift is occurring now, with opportunities for predictive, preemptive, and preventive care greatest early in the life course; this requires engagement and inclusion of obstetrics and pediatrics. Understanding adolescent, family, and community perspectives on how genetic data should be used (Cakici et al., 2020) and coproducing strategies will be essential for addressing acceptance and ethical and equity issues.

Cancer Identification and Treatment

Cancer treatment has also been a success story in pediatrics. Forty years ago, acute lymphoblastic leukemia in a child was a death sentence for most. Today, over 90% are cured. Chemotherapy and radiation therapy have been the mainstays of treatment (Rathore & Kadin, 2010). Immunotherapy, which uses the cells of the immune system to eliminate cancer, has revolutionized treatment of many pediatric and adult cancers. These therapies include tumor-infiltrating lymphocyte therapy, engineered T cell receptor therapy, chimeric antigen receptor T cell therapy, and natural killer cell therapy (Cancer Research Institute, n.d.). Finally, many gene therapies for cancer are on the horizon (Arjmand et al., 2020; Mulcrone, Herzog, & Xiao, 2022).

Cancer treatment is moving to a precision model of care, where treatment decisions are optimized to a patient's tumor molecular profile (Tsimberidou et al., 2020). As the next generation of pediatric precision trials is ushered in, needs include attention to the unique factors influencing pediatric drug development and precision oncology trials for pediatric cancers (DuBois et al., 2019).

Radiation therapy has also advanced with proton beam therapy. Compared with traditional radiation therapy, proton beam therapy more precisely delivers a beam of protons to disrupt and destroy tumor cells, sparing damage to surrounding tissue, which is especially important for children. Proton therapy has been found to have fewer side effects than traditional radiation therapy (Baumann et al., 2020). A systematic review and meta-analysis found that neurocognitive outcomes were improved in pediatric brain tumor patients after treatment with proton versus photon radiation (Lassaletta et al., 2023). Ultra-high-dose millisecond FLASH proton therapy and combining proton therapy with immunotherapy are areas of active research (Mascia et al., 2023; Zhang et al., 2021).

While advancements in therapy have been tremendous, advancements in diagnosis have also been exciting. Genetic technology has allowed earlier identification of risk and diagnosis of cancer cells in the bloodstream before clinical symptoms (Armakolas, Kotsari, & Koskinas, 2023). Liquid biopsies are already being used routinely to monitor cancer recurrence. As the field advances, recurrence, secondary cancers, and survivorship are growing areas of focus for pediatric and adult oncology.

While prevention is a key focus in pediatrics, preventing childhood cancer presents unique challenges. Unlike many adult cancers, most childhood cancers are not strongly linked to modifiable lifestyle or environmental factors (World Health Organization, 2021). The vast majority of childhood cancers do not have a known cause, making prevention strategies difficult to implement. However, some preventive measures can be taken, such as vaccinations against certain infections and avoiding exposure to known carcinogens like ionizing radiation (American Cancer Society, 2024). For children with genetic predispositions, which account for approximately 10% of cases, early screening may be beneficial (American Cancer Society, 2024). Currently, the most effective approach to reducing the burden of childhood cancer focuses on early diagnosis and prompt treatment, as these factors significantly improve outcomes and survival rates (Pan American Health Organization, n.d.).

Stem Cells, Organoids, and Regenerative Medicine

Regenerative medicine engineers biologically functional tissues or organs for therapeutic testing or tissue replacement (Elisseeff, Badylak, & Boeke, 2021; Shi et al., 2017; Trounson, Boyd, & Boyd, 2019). It is now possible to take one's blood, isolate pluripotent stem cells, and grow these cells in a petri dish into complex organoid tissue of stomach, intestine, retina, or neural tissue. This is another area of precision medicine featuring personalized cell therapy and the creation of essential platforms for targeted drug development. Enabled by Nobel prize scientist Shinya Yamanaka, a small number of genes within the genome of mice were identified that allowed a mature or specialized cell to return to an immature state, which, in turn, could grow into different types of cells within the body. This discovery of a renewable cell source of adult and induced pluripotent stem cells, which could potentially avoid immunologic rejection, has accelerated research on the creation of new organoids, microtissues, and body-on-a-chip systems in the context of immunoengineering and regenerative immunology, for basic biology discovery and clinical application. The possibility of using pluripotent stem cells to correct conditions identified in the fetus is another area of active research (Bergh, Buskmiller, & Johnson, 2021).

Advances in Vaccines and Monoclonal Antibody Development

Routine childhood immunization has been a success story in averting death and disability from disease. A recent study found that routine immunizations have led to reductions in incidence of all vaccine-targeted diseases, ranging from 17% for influenza to nearly 100% for diphtheria, *Haemophilus influenzae* type B, measles, mumps, polio, and rubella—equating to more than 24 million cases averted in the United States in 2019 (Talbird et al., 2022).

The continued development of vaccines will influence health care needs in the future as well. The rapid development of an effective COVID-19 vaccine was a public health success story. Many more vaccines are on the horizon that will have far-reaching impact on health and health care. RSV infection is the leading cause of pneumonia and bronchiolitis in young children globally and is the most common cause of hospitalization among American infants (CDC, 2024i; Karron, 2023). Approved in 1998, palivizumab (Synagis), a monoclonal antibody product has protected high-risk young children from severe RSV infection. A second monoclonal antibody, nirsevimab (Beyfortus), has been recently approved for infants and offers easier administration (Hammitt et al., 2022). A new bivalent RSV vaccine has shown great promise in older adults and in infants born to women who received the vaccine (Kampmann et al., 2023; Walsh et al., 2023).

Recovering from pandemic-related childhood vaccine disruptions and addressing vaccine hesitancy will need to be priorities to maintain and further progress. For example, low vaccination rates and vaccine hesitancy have led to polio outbreaks in the past 2 years, with cases of paralysis from polio in the United States and London (Census Bureau, 2024), and measles outbreaks are becoming more common. Improving science communication is an important topic in need of further research (National Academies, 2017c). CDC estimates that vaccination of children in the United States born between 1994 and 2021 will prevent 472 million illnesses (29.8 million hospitalizations), help avoid 1,052,000 deaths, and save nearly $2.2 trillion in total societal costs (Whitney et al., 2014). Vaccines save lives and are cost-effective (see an illustration of such protection in Figure 2-5). New vaccines and monoclonal antibodies addressing current and emerging diseases will continue to transform child, youth, and societal health and health care into the future.

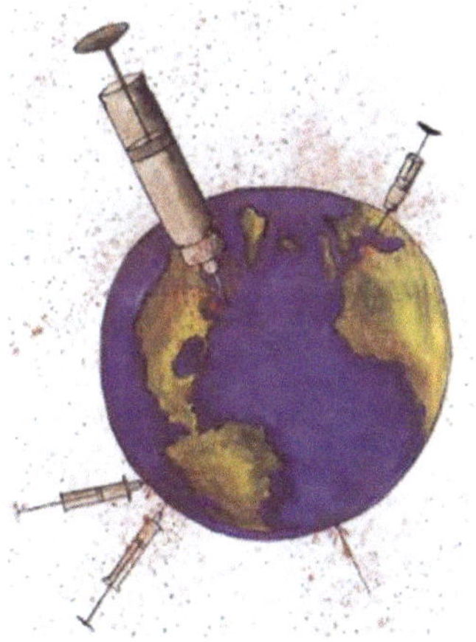

FIGURE 2-5 Human world, protected by vaccines.
SOURCE: Ekaterina Kotova, age 15, Russia; © Peace Child International, used with permission.

Maternal–Fetal Health

Women's health in preconception and prenatal health are major determinants of child health. The specialty of maternal–fetal medicine has seen profound and rapid growth and progress since its emergence in the 1960s. This field, which covers the science of the effects of women's health on fetal health and diagnosis and treatment of maternal and fetal complications, progressed from fetal movement and heart rate monitoring to amniocentesis to ultrasound to the complex fetal medical and surgical interventions of today.

Medical or surgical fetal intervention has become standard of care for certain conditions, including the administration of maternal glucocorticoids to speed lung maturation in premature fetuses at risk for respiratory distress syndrome and in utero surgery for certain neural tube defects (ACOG, 2013; Bergh, Buskmiller, & Johnson, 2021; Committee on Obstetric Practice, 2017). Mostly under research protocols, additional interventions are being offered for fetal diseases, including structural abnormalities (e.g., myelomeningocele, renal or urologic abnormalities, congenital diaphragmatic hernia, hypoplastic left heart syndrome), cardiac arrhythmias, fetal metabolic diseases, and abnormalities of the placental vessels or membranes. While many of these diseases would be lethal without treatment, some receive in utero treatment to improve child outcomes. While a beneficence-based motivation (i.e., to improve fetal and neonatal outcomes, do good, and to ameliorate suffering) guides this treatment, it raises many ethical issues surrounding maternal autonomy and decision making, child outcomes, resource utilization, and innovation versus research (ACOG, 2011).

Many areas of research discovery enhance knowledge about maternal–fetal health and disease, with the goal of optimizing pregnancy and perinatal outcomes extending to improved child and adult health outcomes (CDC, 2024l). Some of these areas are maternal–fetal immunology and the recent approval of an RSV vaccine for use in pregnant women to protect their infants, additional genetic screening and intervention, new fetal surgery targets, and the possibility of using pluripotent stem cells to correct conditions identified in the fetus (Bergh, Buskmiller, & Johnson, 2021).

Artificial Intelligence (AI) and Digital Health

As in many sectors, the convergence of a number of rapidly developing technologies—such as apps, robotics, virtual reality, AI, 3D printing, and networks, among others—has the potential to revolutionize health and medicine for children and youth. Such technologies could transform the health care system from one that is predominantly a "sick care" system based on episodic, in-person, one-size-fits-all care that relies on human cognition to a system based on continuous, virtual, personalized, and AI-enhanced care (Kraft, 2023). These technologies can enhance diagnostic accuracy, improve training and skill acquisition, support mental health, and provide continuous health monitoring (Hasan et al., 2023; Laspro et al., 2023; Pinto-Coelho, 2023; Sousa, Ferrinho, & Travassos, 2023). For example, AI-based technology systems have been used in analyzing medical images, detecting drug interactions, identifying high-risk patients, and coding medical notes (Lee, Bubeck, & Petro, 2023; Pinto-Coelho, 2023; Whitehead et al., 2024). In these examples, digital health tools and systems remove some of the "friction" in health care delivery, making certain processes more efficient and potentially freeing up providers' time for other tasks. Augmented, extended, and virtual reality technologies are also being used for surgical navigation systems through small, wearable displays such as headsets or glasses and for engaging children to reduce anxiety and pain during medical procedures and recovery (Antonovics, Boitsios, & Saliba, 2024; Food and Drug Administration, 2023).

Wearables for patients have shifted the health landscape; individuals can not only track their blood pressure and perform urinalysis at home, but detect genetic abnormalities, and use smart pacifiers to monitor infants' electrolyte levels in real time (Gurovich et al., 2019; Kraft, 2023). In addition, some technologies may allow for prescribing through an app health intervention instead of a traditional pharmaceutical intervention (Children's Bureau, n.d.). For instance, apps are now available for youth mental health interventions and prescription video games can treat young people with attention deficit hyperactivity disorder (ADHD; Children's Bureau, n.d.). While evidence supports the effectiveness of these technologies, continued research and development are necessary to fully realize their potential and address challenges such as user engagement and device reliability.

Technologies also have the potential to enhance patient and provider partnerships, especially for chronic conditions. In a study of an electronic health record–linked mHealth platform that supports patient and clinician collaboration through real-time, bidirectional data sharing, Opipari-Arrigan and colleagues (2020) found that participants using the platform reported improvement in self-efficacy and positive impacts on care, including improved visit quality, collaboration, and preparation. The authors concluded that "use of an mHealth tool to support closed feedback loops through real-time data sharing and patient-clinician collaboration is feasible and shows indications of acceptability and promise as a strategy for improving pediatric chronic illness management" (Opipari-Arrigan et al., 2020, p. 1).

The health care system could enhance care delivery for children and families by leveraging advances in AI and other digital tools, such as AI-driven applications to screen for rare genetic conditions and personalize treatment plans, thereby improving diagnostic accuracy and access to specialized care (Children's National Hospital, 2023a). However, it is crucial to develop and implement these technologies with a focus on equity and inclusivity, ensuring that AI algorithms and digital health solutions are designed to serve diverse populations effectively (Kan Yeung et al., 2023; Mennella et al., 2024; see also Chapter 3).

The use of telehealth has also expanded significantly in recent years, particularly in response to the COVID-19 pandemic. Virtual technologies—such as remote patient monitoring, telehealth for high-risk or technology-dependent patients, preprocedural evaluation, and postprocedural follow-up care—can increase practices' quality, efficiency, and capacity (Ashwood et al., 2017; CDC, n.d.e; Ong et al., 2016). Providing asynchronous care by telehealth can improve the pediatric clinician's time management and efficiency, reduce the need for ancillary office staff to handle real-time interaction, improve documentation of encounters, improve compensation for remote services, and meet the needs of families who are increasingly demanding care on nontraditional schedules (Curfman et al., 2022).

Telehealth may offer opportunities to transform adolescent health care specifically, as young people are spending increasing amounts of time on digital platforms. Telehealth enables adolescent care to be offered through secure chats, asynchronous visits, video visits with peripherals, and digital therapeutics, and to increase adolescents' engagement in their health care. North (2023) posited:

> Telehealth may allow an ongoing, adaptive conversation focused on adolescent wellness. For example, periodic risk behavior and mental health screening could be conducted with short, chat-based questions delivered at regular intervals. The provision of care in this manner would allow access to a private space and increase confidentiality. Responses would trigger timely, developmentally appropriate, and culturally sensitive anticipatory guidance through a secure app or an immediate video visit with a medical team member for an acute crisis. Additionally, when appropriate, parent-focused health information could be delivered immediately. (p. 3)

Research on telehealth has found positive outcomes regarding patient, parent, and provider satisfaction; feasibility; and equivalence of telehealth encounters to in-person encounters (see, e.g., Curfman, Hackell et al., 2021; Curfman, McSwain et al., 2021a; Curfman, McSwain et al., 2021b; Fleischman et al., 2016; Milne Wenderlich & Herendeen, 2021; Myers et al., 2015; Shah & Badawy, 2021). School-based telehealth programs have been shown to increase opportunities for both acute and chronic care for children and adolescents (Bian et al., 2019; Holland et al., 2021; Knopf, 2013; McConnochie et al., 2015; Reynolds & Maughan, 2015; Ronis et al., 2017), and to provide an early means of evaluation and intervention for acutely ill patients, as well as address developmental, behavioral, and educational issues (Curfman et al., 2022; Halterman et al., 2018).

Integrating digital health tools such as telehealth platforms and mobile health apps can facilitate continuous and person-centered care, ensuring timely interventions and better health outcomes for pediatric patients (Granström et al., 2020; Oh, 2023). However, adoption and implementation of these technologies raise questions of equity, bias, and quality. Algorithmic bias is a significant concern, as combining data from adults and children can lead to age-related biases, compromising the generalizability and effectiveness of AI and machine learning models for pediatric populations (Muralidharan et al., 2023). Additionally, racial and socioeconomic disparities can be perpetuated if the data used to train these algorithms reflect historical inequities, leading to differential treatment and outcomes for minority children (Nong, 2023). The lack of digital health literacy and access among underserved populations further exacerbates these inequities, as seen in regions with high poverty and low educational attainment, where families struggle to utilize digital health tools effectively (Shimamoto, 2023). Equitable implementation of telehealth services will require inclusion of children and specific attention to under-resourced populations, appropriate training for providers and health care professionals, support for the expansion of broadband infrastructure, attention to digital literacy, and financial support to ensure all patients have equitable access to care (Curfman et al., 2022).

Precision Population and Public Health

Beyond individual precision medicine "omics" (e.g., genomics, proteomics, metabolomics), precision population and public health have advanced in identifying and addressing particular social, structural, behavioral, and environmental factors influencing health and ensuring that all benefit (Lyles et al., 2018). This includes precisely identifying specific communities and populations for focus and specific social or structural determinants to address, and using population approaches to improve health and wellbeing. Precision approaches to population health build on the science and public health interventions over the last century, which have led to an increase of 20 years in the American life expectancy at birth.

An example of a visible and successful population approach includes universal newborn metabolic screening to identify serious and treatable inherited conditions (Green et al., 2020; National Academies, 2023j). Incorporating more genetic tests and conditions into this screening will further precision population health, as will AI and big data algorithms predicting risk and response. Adolescent, family, and community engagement will address health needs and health equity more precisely. Utilizing quality improvement methods to standardize processes; implementing structures to reduce system variation; and establishing collaborative-learning health networks to enable patients, families, clinicians, researchers, and communities to improve together offer the opportunity to achieve population outcomes at scale. This requires a shift from treating individuals with acute and chronic illnesses to also focusing on detailed and focused population management of disease and primary and secondary prevention. The potential impact of both individual precision medicine science and precision population health starting early in the life course is powerful.

The following sections further describe the science on the social, structural, and environmental influences on health; the importance of including patients, families, and communities in co-creation and co-design of solutions; and the importance of implementation and dissemination research to ensure excellent and equitable benefit (National Academies, 2023e,g,i).

Implications of Scientific and Technological Advancement for Transformation

The scientific advances outlined in this chapter reflect major successes in understanding the causes of health and wellbeing and the role of major medical advances on the prevention, elimination, and treatment of diseases. The pace of discovery is rapid as research is being translated to clinical care and public health. These discoveries have many implications for health care and health care transformation.

As change occurs, it is vital to consider proactively how to fairly distribute the benefits and risks associated with these advancements and to ensure equity and community co-design and co-creation. The evidence regarding persistent racism and inequities in child and adolescent health care call for vigilance and repair in association with the applications of the innovations noted above into practice and daily life. For example, while the possible uses of AI offer hope of efficiency and improvement, potential unintended consequences need focused attention. AI models using existing data can perpetuate inherent biases. Studies have found that AI chatbots' responses to clinical vignettes differed based on a patient's gender, race and ethnicity, and socioeconomic status (Kim et al., 2023).

Adolescent, family, and community perspectives must be at the center of change with partnership in translation of science to practice. This is especially important in a time of rampant health misinformation, vaccine hesitancy, and questioning of science. Co-production and careful messaging are imperative. For example, many parent-led disease-based organizations have been influential advocates in scientific advancements and are essential partners.

In addition to equity and access issues, ethical issues abound, especially as children are a vulnerable population and controversy remains on when life begins. For children, ethical considerations are complex, as they often lack the capacity to provide informed consent for medical procedures or research participation (Banerjee, 2020). Additional safeguards are required when conducting research with children, including assessing risks carefully and obtaining permission from parents or guardians (Canadian Pediatric Society, 2008). Furthermore, debates around the beginning of life have significant implications for issues affecting children, such as access to reproductive health services for minors and protections for pregnant adolescents (Ziegler, as cited in Simmons-Duffin, 2022) and in the conduct of maternal–fetal medicine interventions. Also, the cost of new therapies is significant, raising societal concerns on who might benefit and how to pay. The National Academies report *Toward Equitable Innovation in Health and Medicine* provides guidance on managing the risks, benefits, and ethical and societal implications of new technologies in health and medicine (National Academies, 2023j). Attention to the coordinated, cross-sector governance framework and recommendations in the report is vital for an innovation system that is more equitable, community engaged, and responsive to inequities as they arise, and mindful of the myriad ethical issues.

New science and technology are bound to change health care delivery in process, structure, and outcomes. **A shift to more outpatient care, virtual care, and home care** is likely. Children hospitalized today have greater acuity, severity, and complexity of illness compared with previous decades. Cancer therapy, which used to involve long inpatient stays, now has shifted to more outpatient care. New discoveries may facilitate additional shifts to outpatient care (e.g., FLASH proton therapy eliminating multiple radiation therapy visits, liquid biopsy enabling earlier identification of cancer), virtual care (e.g., counseling on genetic risks, mental health), and home care. This shift will likely be accompanied by **a shift to multidisciplinary teams to address and preempt health risks.** With great focus on health risks and attention to social determinants of health, interventions will require the assistance of social workers, genetic counselors, developmentalists, nutritionists, mental and behavioral health counselors, and community services.

It is likely that there will also be **a shift to more predictive and personalized care.** With earlier identification of health risks, counseling and early intervention will be important health care services. Primary and specialty care will increasingly incorporate more screening and AI-based digital prediction tools. Genomic and digital prediction tools will facilitate more personalized care, including pharmacogenomic tailoring of therapeutics and risk assessment based on multisource data specific to an individual child or family.

Maternal–child health is at the forefront of many exciting advances. Subsequent chapters discuss considerations of these areas of progress on health transformation.

The transformed child health care system will need to address several key ethical and equity issues arising from scientific advances, to avoid perpetuating or exacerbating existing disparities. These include algorithmic bias in AI and machine learning systems, differential access to expensive new therapies, privacy concerns with increased data collection, and potential misuse of genetic technologies, among others (Abràmoff et al., 2024; Jeyaraman et al., 2023; Ndugga, Pillai, & Artiga, 2024). To mitigate these risks, safeguards—such as rigorous testing of algorithms for bias, innovative financing models to improve access to high-cost treatments, and robust data privacy protections—are needed, as are ethical frameworks to guide the responsible development and use of new technologies (Chin et al., 2023; Tilala et al., 2024; Turner Lee, Resnick, & Barton, 2019). Additionally, the system needs to actively work to ensure that scientific advances benefit all children equitably by engaging diverse stakeholders, addressing social determinants of health, and improving diversity in the health care workforce (National Academies, 2023e). Ongoing collaboration between health care providers, researchers, policy makers, ethicists, and communities will be crucial to navigate the complex ethical terrain as technologies continue to evolve.

SOCIAL AND ENVIRONMENTAL INFLUENCES ON CHILD HEALTH AT COMMUNITY AND INDIVIDUAL LEVELS

The U.S. Department of Health and Human Services's Office of Disease Prevention and Health Promotion (ODPHP, n.d.a) defines the "social determinants of health" as "the conditions in the environments where people are born, live, learn, work, play, worship, and age that affect a wide range of health, functioning, and quality-of-life outcomes and risks" (para. 1). These are grouped into five domains: economic stability, education access and quality, health care access and quality, neighborhood and built environment, and social and community context (ODPHP, n.d.b). The importance of these domains for child health is well established. For instance, poor living conditions and housing instability affect children's health detrimentally and increase mortality, even after controlling for socioeconomic status (Anderst et al., 2022).

Experiences across environmental contexts play a significant role in child and youth development. *Vibrant and Healthy Kids* provides a conceptual model and environmental context for understanding development across life stages (see Figure 2-6; National Academies, 2019d). The diagram's nested circles illustrate the complex sociocultural environment that shapes development at the individual level. Individual social and biological mechanisms and culture operate and interact within and across the three levels.

Structural inequities operate at the outermost level of socioeconomic and political drivers. As summarized in *Vibrant and Healthy Kids,* "Structural

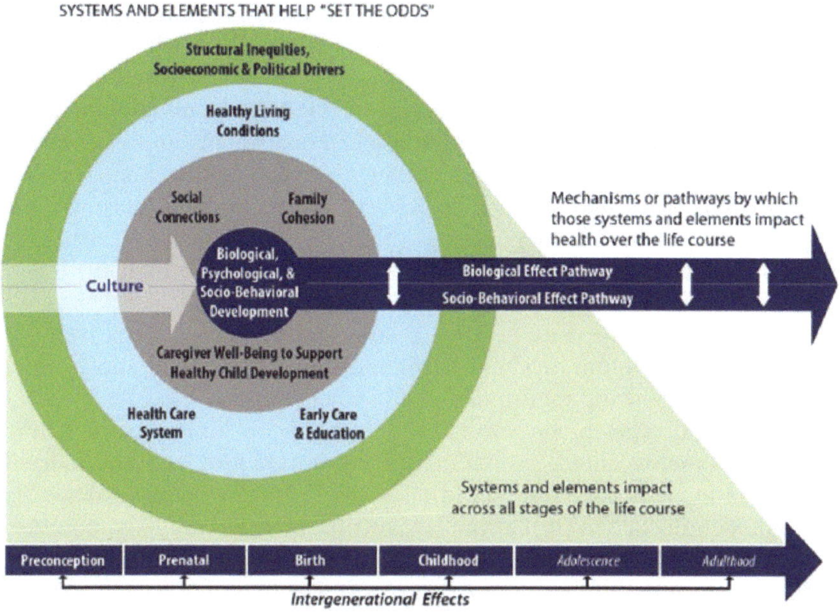

FIGURE 2-6 Socioecological model of development across the life course.
SOURCE: National Academies, 2019d.

inequities are deeply embedded in policies, laws, governance, and culture; they result in the differential distribution of power and resources across individual and group characteristics (including race, ethnicity, sex, gender identity, class, sexual orientation, and gender expression)" (National Academies, 2019d, p. 57). The next level, second from the outermost circle, represents social, economic, cultural, and environmental states (i.e., the social determinants of health). The third level represents the factors that most directly and proximally shape children's daily experiences, routine patterns, and access to resources: family cohesion, social connections, and caregiver wellbeing. Both developmental risk and protective factors can be transferred intergenerationally. In sum, long-term psychological, behavioral, and physical health is shaped by biological and environmental factors and social context, and their interactions, before conception and throughout the life course.

Structural Inequities and Racism

The various forms of racism so prevalent in the United States have profound effects on child and adolescent health care outcomes. Racism is a system of exclusion and oppression based largely on physical appearances.

Jones (2000) described it as the application of power against a group for the advantage of the oppressor group (see also Jones et al., 2009). Elsewhere, it has been equated with an American caste system, whether manifested as slavery, Jim Crow laws, or mass incarceration. "Race," the underpinning for racism, is not a biological construct but a social one, and its implementation varies widely within and across countries (Wilkerson, 2020). Race was not derived from genetics or biology but for social and political reasons, and racism has led to significant inequities (National Academies, 2023d). Racism was foundational to the formation of the U.S. economy and contributed to American economic growth and expansion over the centuries through the exploitation of inexpensive labor. It continues to have a pervasive hold over many U.S. communities with large numbers of children, adolescents, and adults experiencing racism daily.

The several types of racism include (but are not limited to) systemic or structural racism, interpersonal racism, cultural racism, and internalized racism (National Academies, 2023d). "Systemic" or "structural racism" is oppression embedded in regulation, law, institutions, and even communities over time that limit opportunities or punish certain marginalized persons disproportionately. "Institutional racism," a concept within systemic racism, arises when the system provides inconsistent access to opportunities and services, based on race and where groups differ in their power and influence, via policies that have been normalized and legalized (Jones, 2000), marginalizing groups and providing different access to housing, education, employment, and health care. "Interpersonal racism" includes direct forms of aggression or oppression between individuals. Sometimes referred to as personally mediated racisms, interpersonal racism is discrimination and prejudice, or what most people consider when the term "racism" is mentioned (Jones, 2000). Concepts within interpersonal racism include microaggressions and cyber-racism. "Cultural racism" is the broad acceptance of cultural attributes as more attractive or desirous in media, communications, and public spaces (Cogburn, 2019). "Internalized racism" refers to when individuals from historically marginalized groups accept the negative message that they are inferior, substandard, or lack potential, or otherwise underestimate their worth and value (Jones, 2000).

Racism appears to act as a chronic stressor that increases allostatic load at key developmental stages, including prior to and during the prenatal periods, such that effects are seen as early as birth and worsen over time. Allostatic load maintains a high state of stress and hypervigilance in the body and mind. Although it is adaptive in some environments, when confronted with frequent challenges, stress system activation becomes chronic, resulting in ongoing inflammation, increased chronic illnesses, and premature mortality. Because of its chronic nature, racism can have a "weathering effect" (Forde et al., 2019; Geronimus, 1996), increasing biological age faster than chronological age as measured by telomere shortening, methylation, and related assays, and likely increasing susceptibility to chronic diseases such as cancer and heart disease.

More than two decades ago, the landmark IOM (2003b) report *Unequal Treatment: Confronting Racial and Ethnic Disparities in Health Care* raised awareness of and reviewed the literature on the health effects of racism. Of the 103 studies reviewed in *Unequal Treatment*, only five focused on disparities for children, even though it is known that that disparities early in life can have lifelong impact (Cheng & Jenkins, 2009).

More than 20 years after *Unequal Treatment* was published, disparities remain persistent and pervasive, as seen recently during the COVID-19 pandemic, when some racial groups experienced higher rates of infection, hospitalization, and death than others. Today there is much literature on maternal, child, and adolescent health inequities, including a sentinel review by the American Academy of Pediatrics, *The Impact of Racism on Child and Adolescent Health* (Trent, Dooley, & Dougé, 2019). Racism continues to have devastating effects on child and adolescent health, especially for conditions that have substantial associations with social and economic influences, such as prematurity, emotional and behavioral disorders, asthma, and obesity (Trent, Dooley, & Dougé, 2019). These conditions all show marked gradients in outcomes among diverse groups of children, with consistently poorer outcomes for historically marginalized youth. For example, institutional racism is associated with infant morbidity and mortality, as well as asthma mortality, specifically in the Black population (Fanta, Ladzekpo, & Unaka, 2021).

Residential racial segregation is a fundamental cause of racial and ethnic health disparities (Williams & Collins, 2001). Babies born to mothers who lived in very segregated areas are shown to have higher rates of intraventricular hemorrhage (Murosko, Passerella, & Lorch, 2020). Pabayo and colleagues (2019) measured proportions of Black versus White individuals in each state around employment, criminal justice, and voting and legislative representation as indicators of racism. These disparities were associated with infant mortality—Black infants had increased odds of mortality compared with White infants in states with increased levels of racism (Pabayo et al., 2019). A review of California Census tract data showed that children with asthma living in communities severely affected by historical redlining were predominantly non-Hispanic Black and Hispanic, living in poverty, and living in neighborhoods with higher diesel exhaust particle emissions (Nardone et al., 2020). These children also had higher rates of emergency department visits due to asthma exacerbations (Nardone et al., 2020).

Racism affects pediatric health care institutions, often exacerbating child and adolescent experiences of racism in other contexts. Health care institutions expose patients and families to interpersonal and structural racism throughout the care process, resulting in more expensive care and poorer patient outcomes. Racism affects which patients are accepted for appointments (as shown in secret shopper studies) or how long it takes to get appointments, the location of specialty resources in pediatrics, the types of diagnoses that are offered, and the types of treatments provided (National Academies, 2023d; Rankin et al., 2022). For example, in behavioral health, specialists are less likely to accept racially or ethnically marginalized children and adolescents as patients; racially or ethnically marginalized children wait longer to get appointments, have different rates of diagnoses such as externalizing disorders, and are more likely than their White peers to be prescribed antipsychotics rather than antidepressants (Hoffmann et al., 2022; Substance Abuse and Mental Health Services Administration, 2015). Similarly, Black children with appendicitis presenting to the emergency department with moderate pain were less likely than White children to receive pain medication. With severe pain, Black children were less likely than White children to receive opioid medication (Goyal et al., 2015). In a study by Wakefield and colleagues (2018), all Black youth with sickle cell disease reported experiencing bias in a community setting, and some also in a medical or health setting. A study of fifth-grade children documented an association between discrimination and developing symptoms of depression, ADHD, oppositional defiant disorder, and conduct disorder (Coker et al., 2009). In short, the process of receiving health care can worsen existing racial disparities for children and adolescents.

Internalized racism may also impact child and family health. Children as young as age 3 years can recognize racial differences and begin categorizing people by race (Hilario et al., 2023). For example, in a study, Black and White children as young as age 3 years assigned different characteristics to a White doll and a Black doll, preferring to play with the White doll, while assigning negative characteristics to the Black doll and preferring not to play with it. Black children became "emotionally upset at having to identify with the doll that they had rejected" (Jordan & Hernandez-Reif, 2009, video interview, timestamp 5:55; see also Clark & Clark, 1939). Subsequent research explains that children's racial awareness emerges early in their lifetimes. By ages 4–5, many children have already developed racial biases and stereotypes influenced by their environment and experiences (Hilario et al., 2023). This early racial awareness means children of color may internalize negative stereotypes and racism from a young age, impacting their self-esteem and mental health (Byrd et al., 2017; Hilario et al., 2023; Pachter & García Coll, 2009; Sullivan, Wilton, & Apfelbaum, 2020).

The inequities around identifying and managing autism in Black children provide one example of racism in pediatric health. Black children have an average age of autism diagnosis of 64.9 months, more than 3 years on average after parents stated their initial concerns (Constantino et al., 2020).

This study called for increasing participation of non-White children in research, especially in efforts to address the adverse impact of racism in autism care—namely, policies that adversely affect access to evaluations and interventions, including suboptimal payment and the lack of a diverse and culturally humble workforce conducting the evaluations, potentially exacerbating the bias clinicians have and discrimination families experience (Broder-Fingert, Mateo, & Zuckerman, 2020):

> Finally, any study of racial inequity warrants discussion of racism and racial injustice in the United States, including the long-standing, complex system of oppression and exclusion that allocates and concentrates unfair advantage to white communities and disadvantages to multiracial communities (para. 6).

Hispanic children face significant health care disparities compared with their White, non-Hispanic counterparts in various aspects of medical care. Hispanic children are less likely to have health insurance coverage and a usual source of care, which can lead to reduced access to preventive services and regular checkups (Escarce & Kapur, 2006; Funk & Lopez, 2022). They also experience longer wait times in emergency rooms and are less likely to receive adequate pain management for conditions such as broken bones, appendicitis, and migraines (Samuelson, 2024). Hispanic children with special health care needs receive fewer specialist services than their White peers, and they are less likely to be diagnosed with developmental disabilities before preschool or kindergarten (Samuelson, 2024). In end-of-life care, Hispanic children are more likely to die in the hospital and receive medically intense care during their final days compared with White children (Samuelson, 2024).

Changes to well-child visits present a unique opportunity to better address racism, poverty, and nutritional and environmental influences on child health. Examples include the implementation of an antiracist framework with comprehensive screening for social determinants of health and implicit bias training for health care providers (Pachter & García Coll, 2009; Pyone et al., 2021). Systematic screening for financial strain, food insecurity, and housing instability could be incorporated, along with referrals to community resources and social services (Garg et al., 2023). Additionally, detailed assessments of nutritional status and environmental exposures could be conducted, with pediatric clinicians advocating for policies to improve neighborhood conditions and collaborating with local organizations to provide families with resources. These changes have the potential to foster trust, mitigate health care disparities, alleviate poverty-related stressors, and ensure children grow up in environments conducive to their overall health and wellbeing (Pachter & García Coll, 2009; Pyone et al., 2021).

Childhood Poverty

Childhood poverty remains the strongest predictor of child health, wellbeing, and poor health outcomes (Council on Community Pediatrics et al., 2016). Children whose families live in poverty experience worse health early in life than children growing up in higher-income families, and this disparity worsens as they age (National Academies, 2023c,g). Childhood poverty significantly impacts life course health and wellbeing by increasing the risk of chronic health conditions, such as obesity, diabetes, and cardiovascular diseases, which can persist into adulthood (National Academies, 2019a). The stress and deprivation experienced in an impoverished childhood can lead to long-term psychological and emotional challenges, influencing mental health outcomes throughout life. Additionally, limited access to quality health care, nutritious food, and educational opportunities further exacerbates the cycle of poverty and its detrimental effects on overall wellbeing across the lifespan.

The intersectionality of poverty and racism creates compounded challenges for minoritized children in accessing and receiving quality health care. Research shows that children from racial and ethnic minority groups are more likely to live in poverty, and this combination of factors leads to worse health outcomes and disparities in care (National Academies, 2019a, 2023g). Poverty limits access to resources, nutritious food, safe housing, and quality education—all social determinants that impact health (National Academies, 2019a, 2023g). At the same time, systemic racism in health care and other institutions creates additional barriers through discrimination, implicit bias, and unequal treatment (Beech et al., 2021; Castro-Ramirez et al., 2021; Cheng, Goodman, & Committee on Pediatric Research, 2015). For minoritized children, this intersection means they are more likely to lack health insurance, receive lower-quality care when they do access services, and experience the cumulative health effects of chronic stress from both poverty and racism (National Academies, 2017a; Slopen et al., 2024). The cognitive burden of dealing with resource scarcity and racial discrimination also takes a toll, leaving families with less bandwidth to navigate complex health care systems (National Academies, 2017a; Paradies et al., 2015; Slopen et al., 2024). Ultimately, this intersectionality perpetuates a cycle where poverty and racism reinforce each other, leading to persistent health disparities for minoritized children that can have lifelong impacts (Beech et al., 2021; Castro-Ramirez et al., 2021).

Two recent National Academies reports (2019a, 2023g) identified ways to reduce childhood poverty in the United States and to decrease intergenerational poverty among U.S. households. The latter report, *Reducing Intergenerational Poverty* (National Academies, 2023g), specified the value of health insurance coverage—through Medicaid—as one factor that can diminish poverty. The committee recognizes the fundamental importance of addressing childhood poverty to improve the health and wellbeing of U.S. children and youth, and supports the recommendations of those two key reports.

Healthy Living Conditions

A strong causal link has been established between child health and exposure to pollution, particularly in utero, based on both epidemiological and quasi-experimental methods (Currie, Ray, & Neidell, 2011). More recently, this research has been extended to show causal impacts of childhood exposure to pollution on adult outcomes and even the health of the next generation (Colmer, Voorheis, & Williams, 2022; Isen, Rossin-Slater, & Walker, 2017). Major stationary pollution sources include power plants, refineries, and industrial facilities; mobile sources include cars, buses, and planes, which pollute areas near major roadways; additionally, residual lead and other toxins remain in the environment. Families with low income and from racially and ethnically marginalized groups have historically been (and continue to be) exposed disproportionately to pollution, because of the high degree of residential segregation by income and race in the United States and the concentration of polluting sources in neighborhoods where these families live (Alexander & Currie, 2017; Teye et al., 2021). For example, children living in more racially segregated cities are exposed to twice the pollution, as measured by fine particulate matter ($PM_{2.5}$), compared with those in less segregated cities, and this difference increases to tenfold when one considers exposure to toxic metals (Kodros et al., 2022).

Housing instability also has large impacts on children and families, and addressing the issue improves parents' stress, promotes family preservation, and improves families' ability to engage in health care (Marcal, 2018). Studies have shown that evictions increase the odds of losing Medicaid coverage, with subsequent disruptions in health care access (Schwartz et al., 2022). They have also found that exposure to evictions in utero is associated with higher rates of preterm birth and low birth weight among infants (Khadka et al., 2020), and that greater neighborhood-level eviction rates are associated with higher rates of child maltreatment, particularly among older children (Bullinger & Fong, 2020). Families that are already vulnerable—for example, because of a child with special health needs—are more likely to be evicted (Schwartz et al., 2021). Homelessness also poses severe challenges, with an estimated 2.5 million children experiencing homelessness annually in the United States (De Sousa et al., 2022). The physical environment has a notable impact on the health and wellbeing of children, as well-maintained sidewalks, parks, and green spaces promote physical activity and social interaction (Bole, Bernstein, & White, 2024). Racial segregation remains a persistent issue, with studies showing that Black children living in highly segregated neighborhoods are at higher risk of elevated blood lead levels, even when controlling for socioeconomic status (Miranda et al., 2023; Wang et al., 2022). This highlights how structural racism can create enduring health impacts (Beck et al., 2020; Wallerich et al., 2023). Additionally, the built environment, including access to grocery stores and safe outdoor spaces, significantly influences children's health outcomes, particularly in minoritized communities and those experiencing poverty (Wallerich et al., 2023).

Adequate nutrition during infancy and early childhood is also essential for growth, health, and development for children to reach their fullest potential as adults (Schwarzenberg & Georgieff, 2018). Low-income communities and individuals from racially and ethnically marginalized groups are more likely than others to experience "food insecurity" (i.e., inadequate access to affordable, high-quality, nutritious food; Coleman-Jensen et al., 2022). Food insecurity during childhood is associated with worse physical health (Gundersen & Kreider, 2009; Thomas, Miller, & Morrissey, 2019) and mental health (McIntyre et al., 2013), and lower academic achievement in childhood (Jyoti, Frongillo, & Jones, 2005), as well as worse psychological distress and physical health during adulthood (Fertig, 2019). Food access is a significant concern, with approximately 19 million people living in food deserts, areas characterized by limited access to affordable and nutritious food (Key et al., 2023). This affects low-income and minority communities disproportionately, contributing to health disparities. Addressing these interconnected factors is essential for promoting equitable health outcomes and ensuring that all children have the opportunity to thrive.

SOCIETAL INFLUENCES ON CHILD HEALTH AT THE POPULATION LEVEL

In addition to the socioenvironmental influences detailed above, other broad societal and cultural externalities influence the wellbeing of children markedly. This section discusses three key societal influences on the health and wellbeing of children and families: gun violence, global infectious pandemics, and the climate crisis. The co-occurrence of each of these threats contributes to the feelings of dread and hopelessness that many persons, including some children and adolescents, experience. Some have argued that this "syndemic" of civilization-threatening events may be the leading cause of the marked increase in depression and anxiety among adolescents and young adults (Marazziti et al., 2021). The constant exposure to news, social media, misinformation, and politicization pertaining to each of these threats adds to worsening mental health symptoms and interferes with functioning for children and adolescents. Each is associated with ongoing loss of life and danger, each is prominent in the news and media, and each has become part of the culture wars that further alienate young people.

Gun Violence

Firearm-related injury has risen significantly over time and is now the primary cause of death among children in the United States, surpassing motor vehicle injuries and accounting for 20% of all child deaths, with significant disparities by income and race. Youth in counties with the highest poverty rates had nearly five times higher rates of firearm-related mortality than those living in counties with the lowest poverty rates (Barrett et al., 2022). Black children experienced nearly six times higher rates of firearm-related deaths (12 per 100,000) than White children and three times higher than Native American children in 2021 (Panchal, 2022).

Evidence shows that even indirect exposure to neighborhood or family violence (i.e., witnessing or knowing victims of violence) can result in significant long-term harm related to physical and mental health, problem behaviors, and poor academic performance and educational attainment (for reviews, see Osofsky, 1999; Rivara et al., 2019; Sharkey, 2018; see also Bor et al., 2018). Perhaps the best evidence of causal impact of exposure to gun violence on children's long-term outcomes is the work linking school shootings to short-term mental health outcomes and long-term economic outcomes. That research addresses confounding in exposure to violence by examining the timing of school shootings and comparing children living closest to the affected schools, and therefore exposed, with those living slightly further away and therefore similar but not exposed themselves (Cabral et al., 2021; Rossin-Slater & Wüst, 2020).

Additional evidence highlights that child and adolescent survivors of gun violence face a 68% increase in psychiatric disorders and a 144% increase in substance use disorders, with health care spending rising by $34,884 within a year postinjury, mostly covered by insurers or employers (Song et al., 2023). Parents of survivors experience a 30–31% increase in psychiatric disorders, with mothers having 75% more mental health visits and reductions in routine medical care for mothers and siblings, while family members of deceased children face even larger increases in psychiatric disorders and mental health visits (Song et al., 2023).

Notably, the U.S. Surgeon General's Advisory on Firearm Violence, issued in 2024, qualifies firearm violence as a public health crisis in America (OSG, 2024). This advisory highlights the profound impact of gun violence on children, families, and communities. The pervasive threat of gun violence contributes to widespread trauma and fear, exacerbating the nation's mental health crisis. Children are particularly vulnerable to unintentional firearm deaths at home, and there has been a notable increase in firearm-related suicides among young people. Families, especially in communities of color and marginalized groups, face disproportionate risks and long-term psychological trauma from gun violence.

To address this public health crisis, the advisory recommends several interventions. These include regulatory measures such as banning automatic rifles and implementing universal background checks, as well as mandating safe firearm storage and promoting education on gun safety. The advisory also emphasizes the importance of increasing access to mental health services, investing in community-based programs to address root causes of violence, and implementing hospital-based violence intervention programs. Additionally, it calls for enhanced research efforts to better understand and develop evidence-based solutions to firearm violence. The Surgeon General urges a collective, public health approach to combat gun violence and protect the wellbeing of all Americans. Gun violence is a uniquely American problem with tremendous impact on child health. Prevention is possible and will require multilevel interventions beyond the scope of this report.

Infectious Pandemics

The COVID-19 pandemic changed the world, killing millions and causing economic disruption that has further punished families and young people. The effects of the pandemic on children and adolescents were thought to be minimal at first because older adults seemed to be most vulnerable. However, children and adolescents suffered from both direct and indirect effects of the pandemic, often exacerbated by existing societal inequities (National Academies, 2023b).

During the pandemic, attention to maternal and child health issues was slow. Vaccines and therapeutics for children were seriously delayed (Permar, 2022). Attention to children's issues in the pandemic most commonly arose from their parental or workforce needs, with focus on children and their wellbeing coming significantly later. While COVID relief efforts did help children and families, many of these interventions were short lived, with ensuing increases in child poverty rates and further declines in child investment projected (see Chapter 1).

More than 5 million children have been infected directly with the COVID-19 virus in confirmed cases, and more than 1,000 U.S. children have died from infection, a number that is likely underestimated, given the increase in overall child mortality. At its peak, the pandemic resulted in hospitalization rates of 1,500 children per week, and 15% of all documented cases nationally (Howard-Jones et al., 2022). Children and youth who have underlying medical concerns, including obesity, diabetes, and asthma, are at increased risk of infection and hospitalization due to COVID-19 (CDC, 2023d; Kompaniyets et al., 2021; Vicetti Miguel et al., 2022; White, Liburd, & Coronado, 2021).

These disparate outcomes persist into 2024 (CDC, 2024r). The pandemic worsened family stress, child hunger, and poverty, and exacerbated preexisting epidemics in child mental health, childhood obesity, educational disparities, and maternal morbidity and mortality (Bauer, Chriqui et al., 2021; National Academies, 2023b; Parolin & Wimer, 2020). Disparities in the rates of COVID-19 infection, hospitalization, and death across communities highlighted deep-seated health inequities, structural racism, and the failures of safety nets for children and families.

The indirect effects of COVID-19 on children are equally compelling. Recently labeled the "shadow effects" of COVID-19, dramatic increases in depression and anxiety, increases in obesity, marked educational loss, continued school absenteeism and social isolation, and other effects are presenting overwhelmed health care systems with pandemic effects for which they are poorly prepared (Harrison et al., 2022; Howard-Jones et al., 2022). In addition, the pandemic impacted the number of children who lost a parent or caregiver—more than 140,000 children from April 1, 2020, to June 30, 2021—with alarming disparities by race and ethnicity (National Academies, 2023b). American Indian/Alaska Native children were 4.5 times, Black children 2.4 times, Hispanic children 1.8 times, and Asian children 1.1 times more likely than White children to lose a parent or caregiver during that time period (Hillis et al., 2021). These indirect effects of the pandemic will have consequences well into adulthood, with reduced workforce participation, lower educational achievement, greater requirement for social programs, and increased chronic disease.

The COVID-19 pandemic is only the latest infectious disease to result in loss of life and economic devastation (Alqahtani et al., 2022; Arnold, 2002; Carlson et al., 2021, George Washington University School of Business, 2020; Rehman et al., 2021). Influenza epidemics with significant mortality and economic consequences have occurred four times in the past 100 years. Other emerging infectious diseases are increasing, even after controlling for reporting bias, because of increased animal–human interaction, greater connectivity of transportation systems, increasing poverty, and the lack of surveillance in areas most likely to be the source of emerging infectious diseases. More than 60% of these are zoonoses, with most originating in wildlife; and almost all are strongly related to ecological and economic factors (Rahman et al., 2020).

Importantly, numerous tools have emerged for improving surveillance and capabilities to confront these emerging infections. These new tools include large-scale testing capacities such as sewage and water system monitoring, RNA vaccine development, broad-scale telemedicine capacity, and AI for early threat detection and tracking in large datasets (CDC, 2024c). Unfortunately, most of these systems are deployed in developed economies with low likelihood of emerging infections rather than countries where substantial risk of new agents is concentrated (Campbell, 2022; Carabin, 2021; Haldane et al., 2021; United Nations International Children's Emergency Fund, n.d.).

The committee supports the implementation of the recommendations in the National Academies report *Addressing the Long-Term Effects of the COVID-19 Pandemic on Children and Families*, which discusses the health, education, and socioemotional effects of the pandemic and recommends prioritizing prevention measures to protect children in future pandemics (National Academies, 2023b).

Climate Change

Climate change threatens the health and wellbeing of children, adolescents, and their families with current and ongoing consequences. To date, climate change is associated with worsening of storms, hurricanes, monsoons, and other specific weather events (Ebi et al., 2021). Climate change also worsens air pollution, fires and smoke exposure, crop failure, and increased exposures to pests and invasive plants and animals in populated areas, all of which influence children more than adults. Similarly, rapid climate change and news about it is associated with increased anxiety and depression, especially among young adults (see Figure 2-7; Cianconi et al., 2023; Clayton & Karazsia, 2020; Schwartz et al., 2022; Taylor, 2020).

The physical and mental consequences of climate change–related catastrophes on children and adults have been less well studied, but new work suggests that the effects will be most dramatic among the youngest citizens (Hickman et al., 2021a,b; Ramadan & Ataallah, 2021). First, children and adolescents typically lack the resources to prepare independently for severe

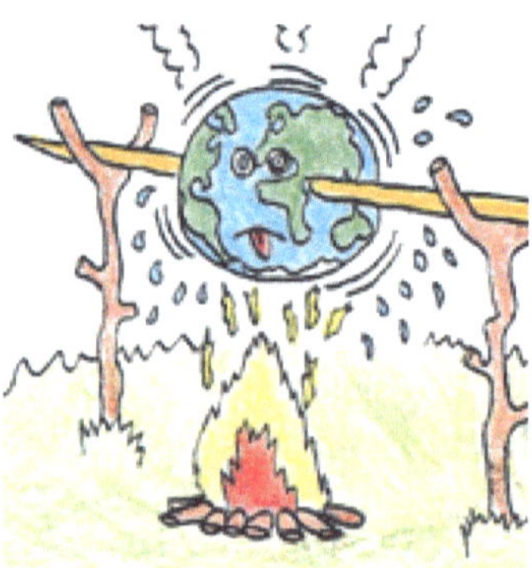

FIGURE 2-7 Climate change and anxiety.
SOURCE: Anonymous child artist; © Peace Child International, used with permission.

and inclement weather (Arpin et al., 2021). Secondly, they live disproportionately in climate-vulnerable communities with poor housing stock that is vulnerable to severe weather (Bezgrebelna et al., 2021). Within cities, children and adolescents in communities of color are most likely to live in the neighborhoods most often affected by extreme heat (Benz & Burney, 2021). Finally, the youngest children may also be the least able to tolerate extremes of weather outside of the older adult population, and damage from environmental exposures may accumulate across the lifespan (Bennett & Friel, 2014).

Along with many physical and mental health consequences, climate change also has profound effects on the health care delivery system and services to children and adolescents, as it increases admissions and visits because of the health effects of extreme weather conditions (Bennett & Friel, 2014). It also leads to increases in asthma and respiratory admissions, infections with vector-borne diseases, and heat-related conditions—especially among those least able to pay for care (Rossati, 2017). Severe weather events have also been associated with hospital closures, disruptions in supply chains for health care facilities, and disruption in staffing due to emergency medical needs for disaster relief efforts (Melnychuk, Sallade, & Kraus, 2022).

The United States remains the top emitter of health care greenhouse gas emissions globally, accounting for 27% of Earth's total health care emissions (Christrup et al., 2023). Like most industries, the health care sector contributes to the worsening climate crisis. By some estimates, health care contributes 8.5% of all U.S.-generated greenhouse gas emissions; any serious national effort to decarbonize the economy must include health care, as it is the largest industry in the United States (Centers for Medicare & Medicaid Services, 2024j). Several general recommendations have been put forward for transforming the health care industry from a contributor to the global crisis that harms children and adolescents, to a leader in the decarbonized future (Harrison, Haley, & Shattuck, 2023). In addition to these interventions, further research is needed on the impact of climate change on children and its legacy in their lives.

HEALTH CARE TRANSFORMATION TOWARD WHOLE CHILD AND FAMILY HEALTH

As detailed above, child health depends on family health and wellbeing. This relationship is also generational. Given this understanding, this report discusses strategies to assess, scale, and spread a whole family approach to health. "Whole health" is defined as "the physical, behavioral, spiritual, and socioeconomic well-being as defined by individuals, families, and communities. *Whole health care* is an interprofessional, team-based approach

TABLE 2-1 Principles of Whole Child and Family Health Care

Principles of Whole Person, Whole Population Health Care (National Academies, 2024b)	**Principles Applied to Whole Child and Family Health Care (this report)**
1. Personal health services oriented toward health promotion and prevention, in addition to treatment;	Health promotion and prevention are salient early in the life course, when there is best opportunity for prediction and preemption.
2. Ability to equitably enhance the health and wellbeing of an entire community or population;	Health equity starts early in the life course, and health care must address the social conditions in which children live in partnership with the community.
	Population and cross-sector approaches are essential for equitable child health, requiring collaboration with schools, child welfare, juvenile justice, and community organizations.
3. Person-centered rather than provider-centered;	Care must be centered around the child and the family. Family health is necessary for optimal child and adolescent development.
4. Relationship-based rather than transactional;	Relationships form the foundation for trust on the individual and community levels and must be a focus in system design.
5. Holistic, integrative, and continuous rather than fragmented and episodic; and	Whole child and family health addresses physical and psychosocial health of children and families over time.
6. Utilize measures that matter most to people, families, and populations, and support continuous learning and improvement in processes and structures that deliver better health, higher quality care, lower costs, and optimal individual and clinician experience.	Child- and family-produced measures; aligning incentives for child, family, and community outcomes; and accountability and governance are necessary for successful transformation.
Unique Considerations for Children	Children are not little adults. Child health forms the foundation for adult health. Whole child and family health care must be designed to address the unique needs of children, adolescents, and families.
	Transforming health care for children requires collaboration across multiple sectors, including providers, health care system leaders, payers, education leaders, child welfare, community members, and policy makers.

SOURCE: Adapted from National Academies, 2024b.

anchored in trusted relationships to promote well-being, prevent disease, and restore health. It aligns with a person's life mission, aspiration, and purpose" (National Academies, 2023a, p. 356). It shifts the focus from a reactive, disease-oriented medical care system to one that prioritizes disease prevention, health, and wellbeing. It changes the health care conversation from "What's wrong with you?" to "What matters to you?"

In this framing, health and wellbeing are understood to be interchangeable with whole person and whole population health. For this report, the committee adapted the principles of whole person, whole population health care, as outlined in the National Academies report *Valuing America's Health: Aligning Financing to Reward Better Health and Well-Being* (see Table 2-1; National Academy of Medicine, 2024). Concepts the committee added include the fact that children are not little adults—so they require unique consideration in health and health care—and that improving child health requires collaboration across multiple sectors, including providers, health care system leaders, payers, education leaders, child welfare, community members, and policy makers.

CONCLUSION

This chapter provides an overview of the science underlying child health and wellbeing and life course trajectories. It also outlines new science and technology that is likely to shape the future of health care. It provides background on environmental threats to child health, such as poverty and housing instability, as well as broader societal threats (gun violence, pandemics, and climate change). The committee kept this background and knowledge in mind as it examined the characteristics and opportunities of a future health care system.

A large body of evidence demonstrates that children's and youth's health and wellbeing and positive development are shaped by their experiences and environments. Because childhood and adolescence are sensitive periods impacting life course health trajectories, there is great opportunity to build a strong foundation for long-term health. Positive experiences cultivate capable, well-functioning, and healthy children into adulthood. Conversely, childhood and adolescence can be a period of unique vulnerability. Negative experiences increase the probability of adverse effects, such as poor health during childhood, lower educational attainment, elevated rates of mental health issues, substance abuse and criminal activity, and a heightened likelihood of developing chronic health conditions in adulthood. Optimizing health and wellbeing developmental trajectories is the foundation necessary for children, youth, families, and society to thrive.

Drawing from the science of development, the committee summarizes core concepts that are critical for transforming the health care system:

- The interaction of the brain, biology, behavior, and environments shapes child and youth development and health with implications for adult and intergenerational health.
- The early caregiving environment, exposure to trauma, stress, racism, and access to resources significantly influence long-term health and development.
- Adolescents are active participants in their own development. Their developing competencies in flexible problem solving, awareness of and concern for others, and openness to exploration and novelty make adolescence a particularly opportune time for supporting agency and engagement in health promotion.

These core concepts point to the need for a transformed health care system that is attuned to achieving whole child and family health. Both the life course and multigenerational frameworks of development recognize the complex interactions between individuals and their environments, emphasizing the need to consider broader societal and familial contexts when supporting child development and facilitating health care transformation. New science about genes and gene regulation and environment and experiences over time offers the opportunity to strengthen the foundation of health formed early in the life course and guide health care transformation.

3

The Role of Children, Youth, Families, and Communities in Achieving Health Care System Transformation

Getting health care should not require resilience. Health care should be prepared to deal with all families.

—Nikki Montgomery, Family Voice

As discussed in Chapter 2, clear scientific evidence demonstrates that safe, stable, and nurturing relationships are critical for healthy development and can buffer mechanisms of adversity and support positive trajectories for both children and youth. Children, youth, families, and the communities in which they live are therefore important partners across all facets of pediatric care, as they are experts in their health and health needs. They are also experts in how health care is currently delivered and have reported on the many challenges they encounter when seeking care. Disturbing trends in child health have prompted calls for the health care system, often characterized as industry centric and provider centric, to become child, family, and community centered (Neuwirth, 2019; see also Chapters 1, 2, and 4).

It is essential to understand the perspectives of children, youth, families, and communities on their health and health care needs. Their lived experiences and insights can provide valuable guidance for reimagining a more responsive health care system, and overlooking these perspectives, as illustrated in Figure 3-1, has led to the inefficiencies and distrust discussed in this chapter.

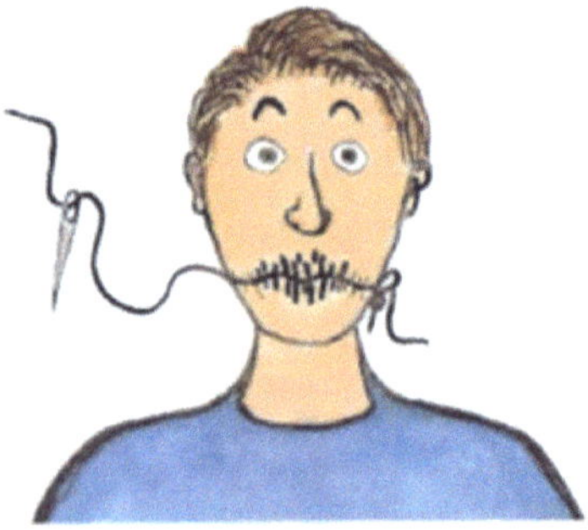

FIGURE 3-1 Youth gagged.
SOURCE: Anonymous child artist © Peace Child International, used with permission.

This chapter summarizes findings on common priorities for health care. It covers perspectives on the trustworthiness of the health care system and access to health care. It offers examples of how children, youth, families, and communities are currently engaged in decision making within the health care system. The committee acknowledges that children, youth, families, and communities are not monolithic entities. It is critical to recognize the diverse and intersecting identities that shape individual, familial, and communal experiences and health outcomes. While the chapter provides broadly applicable insights into health care system transformation, it underscores that effective and transformative actions must be tailored to address the unique needs and contexts of different groups.

CHILD- AND FAMILY-CENTERED HEALTH CARE

Patient experience has become an increasingly important focus in health care, with movement to encompass the overall quality of care from the patient's perspective instead of just tracking clinical outcomes (Bastemeijer et al., 2019; National Academy of Medicine [NAM], 2023). The concept of patient- and family-centered care has emerged as a holistic approach to health care that emphasizes the importance of partnerships between health care providers, patients, and their families (Clay & Parsh, 2016; Hsu et al., 2019; Institute for Patient- and Family-Centered Care [IPFCC], n.d.). This model is particularly salient in pediatric health care, where the family plays a crucial role in children's wellbeing (Meert, Clark, & Eggly, 2013; Seniwati et al., 2023). The goals of this approach are to improve health outcomes, enhance patient and family satisfaction, and ensure that care is respectful, responsive, and inclusive of the family's needs and values (Clay & Parsh, 2016; IPFCC, n.d.; Hsu et al., 2019).

In this model, patients and families have the autonomy to define who constitutes their "family" and decide their level of involvement in care and decision-making processes (Hsu et al., 2019). Each child and family are recognized as unique, with specific needs and preferences (Clay & Parsh, 2016; IPFCC, n.d.; Hsu et al., 2019). Multiple studies have uncovered that patients want care that responds to their unique needs and actively involves them in care plans. These include studies on adolescents (Daley, Polifroni, & Sadler, 2017; see also Diaz et al., 2004; Fox, McManus, & Yurkiewicz, 2010; Ginsburg, Menapace, & Slap, 1997; Ginsburg et al., 2002; McIntyre, 2002; Rosen et al., 1997; Sadler & Daley, 2002; Tylee et al., 2007), pregnant people (Adalia et al., 2021; Jenkins et al., 2014; Petit-Steeghs et al., 2019), and families of children with special health care needs (Coker, Rodriguez, & Flores, 2010; Kuhlthau et al., 2011). For example, during interactions with health care professionals, adolescents desire to be treated as individuals and to engage in respectful communication with providers that helps them to better understand their health and treatment options (Hardin et al., 2021; Larcher, 2005). This includes accounting for concerns around sensitive health topics, including gender and sexual identity, drugs, sex, and mental health (Brown & Wissow, 2009; National Academies of Sciences, Engineering, and Medicine [National Academies], 2023i).

COMMUNITY-CENTERED CARE

This report refers to communities as any configuration of individuals, families, and groups whose values, characteristics, interests, geography, and/or social relations unite them in some way (National Academies, 2017a). Community engagement in care or community-centered care is seen as the process of working collaboratively with and through groups of people affiliated by geographic proximity, special interest, or similar situations to address issues affecting their wellbeing (CDC, 1997). While communities are not a monolith, they generally expect pediatric health care system transformation to move beyond traditional medical models to more comprehensive, equitable, family-centered approaches that address the holistic needs of children and families in their communities (Center for Health Care Strategies, 2019a). In this vein, community engagement is a foundational aspect of developing effective health policies and programs (Aguilar-Gaxiola et al., 2022). The community mural in Figure 3-2 is an expression of the holistic health needs of families in a community.

"Community-defined" (or "practice-based") evidence refers to the knowledge, experiences, and information generated and validated by a particular community to address its unique needs, challenges, and aspirations (California

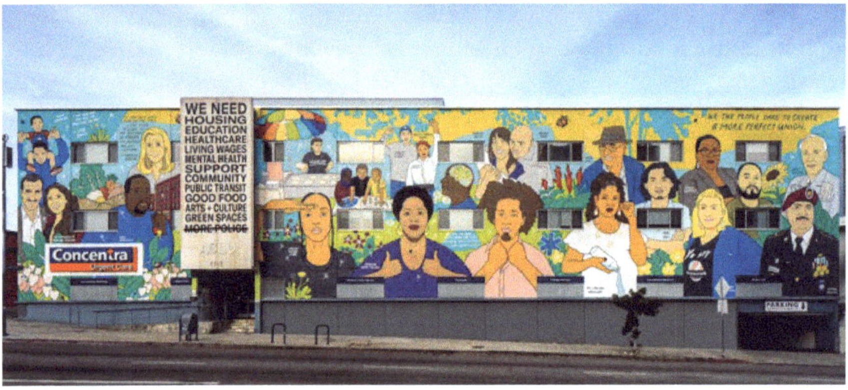
WE NEED
HOUSING
EDUCATION
HEALTHCARE
LIVING WAGES
MENTAL HEALTH
SUPPORT
COMMUNITY
PUBLIC TRANSIT
GOOD FOOD
ARTS + CULTURE
GREEN SPACES
MORE POLICE
Concentra

FIGURE 3-2 *The Care We Create*: A community mural.
NOTES: *The Care We Create* is a mural on the façade of the Westlake building of the American Civil Liberties Union (ACLU) in Los Angeles, California. The piece is a tribute to the enduring efforts of activists, organizers, and advocates across Southern California who have steadfastly fought and continue to fight for justice. Derived from the People's Budget LA coalition, encompassing organizations such as Black Lives Matter—Los Angeles, People's City Council, Ktown For All, and the TransLatin@ Coalition, the mural passionately advocates for diverting funds toward community care instead of policing. Collaborating closely with ACLU SoCal staff, coalition organizers generously contributed to the selection of portraits appearing in the mural. The individuals portrayed symbolize various issues such as racial justice in policing and legal matters, immigrants' rights, LGBTQ+ rights, economic justice and housing, and First Amendment rights, as well as students and their rights.
SOURCE: Audrey Chan, *The Care We Create*, 2020. Painted mural and vinyl facade of the Los Angeles offices of the ACLU of Southern California (1313 West 8th Street, Los Angeles, CA 90017). Fabrication by the Los Angeles Art Collective and Wilson Cetina Group. Photo by Elon Schoenholz. Courtesy of the artist.

Pan-Ethnic Health Network, 2018; Isaacs et al., 2005). Box 3-1 details the California Reducing Disparities Project, an example of a community-defined evidence initiative. It encompasses a diverse range of locally relevant data, perspectives, and practices that may not fit traditional scientific or academic criteria but hold immense value within specific cultural, social, or geographic contexts (Bauer, Churchill et al., 2021). This type of evidence emphasizes the importance of community engagement, participation, and empowerment in defining, generating, and utilizing knowledge to inform decision making and problem solving. While evidence-based practices take a "top-down" approach (i.e., evidence is generated by researchers and then, with or without the partnership of communities, is implemented in target communities), community-defined evidence takes a more grassroots, "bottom-up," approach, in which needs and practices are defined by communities, and then communities work to build evidence for these practices.

BOX 3-1
California Reducing Disparities Project

The California Reducing Disparities Project, a state-led initiative, has incorporated community-defined evidence to improve behavioral health outcomes across historically marginalized populations (California Pan-Ethnic Health Network [CPEHN], 2018). In 2009, a statewide policy initiative was launched that focused on prevention and intervention efforts for behavioral health conditions, with five priority populations: Latinxs, African American, LGBTQ, Native Americans/American Indians, and Asians and Pacific Islanders. The first phase of the project developed a strategic plan to transform the public mental health care system in California; the second phase focused on funding and evaluating these promising practices.

In 2022, the Children and Youth Behavioral Initiative (CYBHI) was established as part of a multiyear, public-sector investment of $4.7 billion in the behavioral health of children and adolescents in California. CYBHI was informed by community-defined practices in a report by CPEHN. It is currently scaling evidence-based practices, as well as promising community-defined practices, across several rounds of grant funding. In July 2023, the first round awarded over $30 million to 63 programs across California, with an emphasis on improving parenting support and practices. One example of a community-defined practice funded in the first round is the phidin ya' ja' (Celebrating Families Through Wellness) program that was awarded to the Sherwood Valley Band of Pomo Indians (n.d.). The program brings Native American families together to discuss issues related to boundary setting, healthy nutrition, drug and alcohol use, communication, and other skills to improve parenting practices.

As part of its deliberative process, the committee sought the input of a diverse group of individuals whose lived experiences and community engagement work intersects with the pediatric and maternal health care systems. Key takeaways from these information-gathering sessions[1] included the need to welcome diverse forms of wisdom, including intergenerational and cross-cultural perspectives, the need to adopt practices of inviting and maintaining the presence of family leadership, the need to focus on language and communication exchanges for families and communities where literacy or access to information might be an issue, and the need to form partnerships with community entities to address holistic health needs. An important point was recognizing that members of a community are not necessarily hard to reach, as often believed, but engagement can be difficult if trust is not established (further discussion follows).

[1]See Appendix C for agendas of public sessions. Further information on and archived recordings of these information-gathering sessions can be found at the project website: https://www.nationalacademies.org/our-work/improving-the-health-and-wellbeing-of-children-and-youth-through-health-care-system-transformation

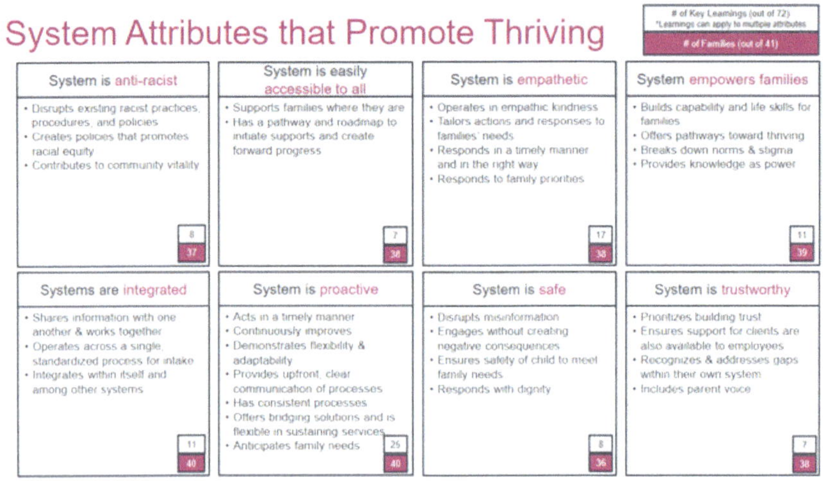

FIGURE 3-3 Family perspectives on system attributes that promote thriving.
SOURCE: Riley, 2023. Presentation to the Committee on Improving the Health and Wellbeing of Children and Youth through Health Care System Transformation.

At one of these information-gathering sessions (June 15, 2023), Carley Riley spoke about Cincinnati Children's Hospital's increased commitment to and capacity for community-engaged co-production, in collaboration with All Children Thrive Learning Network Cincinnati. This initiative created a process to identify family-prioritized systems and policy changes to address their needs and hopes around equitable child and youth thriving.[2] Eight ideal system attributes were determined to promote thriving: antiracist, accessible to all, empathetic, empowering to families, integrated, proactive, safe, and trustworthy (Riley, 2023; Figure 3-3).

The eight ideal system attributes for health care systems transformation promote a holistic approach to improving health outcomes and experiences for all individuals, families, and communities (Riley, 2023).

1. The first attribute is being antiracist. An antiracist system actively works to dismantle systemic racism and promote equity in health care delivery and outcomes (Hassen et al., 2021). An antiracist health care system acknowledges the historical and ongoing impacts of racism and takes deliberate action to create racial equity (NAM, 2023).

[2]This initiative included a recruitment period from November 2020 to May 2023, during which 44 families referred from school, community, and health care settings engaged for a median of 4 months in a multidisciplinary, cross-sector community–academic team process that co-developed a family-centered learning process.

2. The second attribute is being accessible to all. This ensures that health care services and resources are readily available and easily obtainable for all individuals, regardless of their socioeconomic status, geographic location, or other potential barriers (Levesque, Harris, & Russell, 2013; Qi et al., 2023). Accessibility encompasses physical, financial, and cultural dimensions of access (Douthit et al., 2015; Thiede, Akweongo, & McIntyre, 2007).
3. The third attribute is being empathetic. An empathetic health care system prioritizes compassionate care, understanding and addressing the emotional and psychological needs of patients and families (Hardy, 2022; Kerasidou et al., 2020; Moudatsou et al., 2020). This involves training providers in empathic communication and creating environments that support emotional wellbeing.
4. The fourth attribute is being empowering to families. This means families are actively involved in decision-making processes and are provided with the necessary tools and information to manage their health effectively (Coyne, Holmström, & Söderbäck, 2018; Kubb & Foran, 2020; Kuo et al., 2012; Lorig & Holman, 2003). An empowering system recognizes families as partners in care and supports their capacity for self-management (Kuo et al., 2012).
5. The fifth attribute is being integrated. An integrated system promotes seamless coordination and collaboration among various health care providers, services, and sectors to ensure comprehensive and continuous care (American Hospital Association, 2021; American Psychological Association, n.d.; World Health Organization [WHO], 2018). This reduces fragmentation and improves the patient experience across the care continuum.
6. The sixth attribute is being proactive. A proactive system focuses on prevention and early intervention, addressing potential health issues before they escalate (Lobach et al., 2007). This involves population health management strategies and leveraging data to identify and address health risks (Lobach et al., 2007).
7. The seventh attribute is being safe. In a safe health care system, patient safety is paramount, with systems in place to minimize errors, adverse events, and harm to patients. This involves a culture of safety, robust reporting systems, and continuous quality improvement efforts (Agency for Healthcare Research and Quality, 2020; Institute of Medicine [IOM], 2000; WHO, n.d.c.).
8. The eighth and final attribute is being trustworthy. A trustworthy system fosters trust through transparency, accountability, and consistent delivery of high-quality care. This involves clear communication, ethical practices, and responsiveness to patient and community needs (IOM, 2000; Weaver et al., 2013).

These eight attributes collectively aim to create a health care system that is equitable, patient centered, and effective in improving overall population health. By striving to embody these attributes, health care systems can work toward transforming care delivery and addressing long-standing disparities in health outcomes (Riley, 2023).

COMMON CHALLENGES TO COMMUNITY-CENTERED CARE

Existing endeavors to advance health care transformation often fail to address health care system challenges and to include people with lived experience in their development and evaluation, resulting in a misalignment. Using the broad attributes of a thriving system above as a guide, this section explores the existing literature on challenges related to trustworthiness in the health care system; access to health care; and individual-level disempowerment.

Trustworthiness of Health Care Institutions

Trustworthiness has been identified as a key tenet of a health care system that promotes thriving (Riley, 2023). Unfortunately, many children, youth, families, and communities have reason to be wary of health care professionals and the broader health care system. A review of historical polling data by Blendon, Benson, and Hero (2014) on public trust in U.S. physicians and medical leaders from 1966 through 2014 found that public trust and confidence in U.S. medical leaders has declined sharply since the mid-20th century. The authors suggest that the overall decline in trust in U.S. health care is likely attributable to broad cultural changes in the United States, along with concerns around medical system leaders' responses to major national problems impacting the U.S. health care system (Blendon, Benson, & Hero, 2014; Buhr & Blendon, 2011; Hetherington, 2005). These findings are echoed in survey results on trusted sources of health information on COVID-19 (Steel-Fisher et al., 2023).

Mistrust of the health care system, especially in communities of color in the United States, is grounded in current experience with structural inequities that permeate health care and other systems, as well as with the legacy of health care discrimination; medical research exploitation; and unconsented experimentation, particularly for Black, American Indian/Alaska Native, Hispanic, and other communities that have experienced racism in the United States (Frakt, 2020; Gamble, 1997; Hoffman, 2020; National Academies, 2020c). This section discusses encounters with unethical research and medical practices, practitioner bias, and misinformation and disinformation, which have all served to foster mistrust between the health care system and those it serves. Box 3-2 provides an illustrative personal narrative, informed by research and clinical practice, regarding distrust in the health care system and opportunities for building community trust.

BOX 3-2
Illustrative Example: Building Community Trust—Renée Boynton-Jarrett

For Renée Boynton-Jarrett, health care systems, like other institutions, are not automatically entitled to trust. Boynton-Jarrett's view is informed by her deep background in the sociology of health: an associate professor at Boston University School of Medicine, she is trained as both an anthropologist and a pediatrician. From that perspective, the literature is clear: "Trustworthiness is a requisite condition to foster trust," she said—in other words, institutions must earn trust.

In her clinical life, Boynton-Jarrett sees the other side of the coin: populations historically marginalized—and sometimes harmed—by medical institutions may hesitate to pursue recommended care. In some ways, that can be frustrating, she said. At the same time, Boynton-Jarrett gets it. "In the absence of trustworthiness, distrust is only rational," she said. "It's actually really rational to not trust an institution that has time and time again demonstrated a lack of trustworthiness." That distrust too often comes with a double hit. Not only do these communities forgo care that could help them, she continued, but too often these "minoritized and marginalized populations" are stigmatized further when "the blame falls squarely on the[ir] shoulders."

However, the thorny challenge of distrust is solvable, Boynton-Jarrett said. To her, there are three key ingredients:

First, invest in "community power and capacity building," she said. That means setting up structures—closely tied to traditional health care systems—that build up the civic society of communities in ways that support health. Community health worker programs are a common example, she pointed out. Infrastructure networks and safety nets, such as the Boston Breastfeeding Coalition—a member-led initiative that promotes breastfeeding education and access—is another. "When I'm thinking about healing and thriving, I'm thinking about a whole child, person-centered, family-centered [approach]," Boynton-Jarrett said. "I think about it in the context of relationships."

Second, she continued, "Recogniz[e] the abundance of leadership at the ready to actually support thriving and flourishing for children." Investing in organizations alone is insufficient for creating meaningful or long-term impact, she asserted; health care systems must also lift up the people who operate and drive them forward—granting them both "authority" and "agency" in the same ways it uplifts its own employees. "When I think about culturally affirming models of care, I think about wisdom and knowledge that are held in the community with high levels of expertise—without a medical degree or a high set of academic credentials," Boynton-Jarrett said, "and [I think] about us valuing them equally."

Third, she urged, "Recenter voice, story, and experience." These practices are critical for ensuring that health care systems address the right problems—for example, a breastfeeding coalition is useful only on paper if voices from the community say the more pressing needs are elsewhere. Recentering voice, story, and experience is also essential for fostering true inclusion and collaboration between institutions and communities. In this manner, health care systems must "cente[r] dignity to promote equity," Boynton-Jarrett said. "One of our strongest mental models is that health care functions as an independent system," she added; "we c[an] challenge that idea."

(continued)

BOX 3-2 Continued

Boynton-Jarrett is practicing these lessons through the Vital Village Network, an organization built with the three key ingredients in mind—designed, ultimately, to advance trust, rather than any specific intervention. "When we use the words 'child wellbeing and wellness,' it is very problematic to narrow that to a model that is devoted to reducing risk, reducing harm, and treating harm," Boynton-Jarrett said. "I'm very much an advocate for us broadening the scope of how health care contributes to wellbeing." Her goal in fostering trust is not only to understand what lies below the surface of the iceberg of illness when it comes to these communities, but also to understand "what keeps the water cold," Boynton-Jarrett said—the forces that drive negative outcomes. Only then, she said, will health care systems support flourishing childhood—beyond risk reduction and harm alleviation.

Health care "is not just about how someone recovers," Boynton-Jarrett said, "It's about how someone can thrive."

SOURCE: Correspondence with Renée Boynton-Jarrett, prepared by Eli Cahan, health communication advisor to the committee.

Historical and Contemporary Instances of Unethical Research and Medical Practices

Black people have been historically and continually subjected to intentionally inferior health care access and delivery and poor health outcomes; and ongoing health care system disparities and discriminatory events reinforce historical mistrust (Scharff et al., 2010). For instance, eugenic sterilization laws, which promoted forced reproductive sterilization, were prevalent throughout the United States until the mid- to late 1940s and were routinely used to rationalize the mistreatment of non-White individuals, people with attenuated financial means, and those who were neurodivergent (Reilly, 2015). Such practices continued to be used against the same populations beyond the 1940s, and some have suggested that they are still in use.

Between 1920 and 1945, sterilization laws in California were applied to Latinos disproportionately (Novak et al., 2018). From the 1940s to 1970s, the organization Birthright facilitated the sterilization of Black women, women living in rural areas, and women who were economically marginalized (Reilly, 2015). Moreover, the Indian Health Service is accused of using mass sterilization against Native American women throughout the 1960s and 1970s, and studies have shown that between

25% and 50% of childbearing-age Native American women lost their reproductive ability between 1970 and 1976 (Lawrence, 2000). Most recently, immigrant detainees have reported experiencing forced sterilization while in U.S. Immigrant and Customs Enforcement custody (Ghandakly & Fabi, 2021). Forced sterilization negatively impacted individuals, families, and communities, as evidenced by ruptured family and community relationships; increased susceptibility to psychological distress, substance abuse, and mental health impairment; and decreased economic freedom (Lawrence, 2000).

Unethical research practices have significantly contributed to mistrust in health care systems. Notable examples span several decades and highlight the evolution of research ethics, particularly concerning vulnerable populations. The Tuskegee Syphilis Study (1932–1972) stands as one of the most infamous cases of unethical research. Although not directly involving children, it set a precedent for mistrust in medical research. Researchers studied the effects of untreated syphilis in Black men without their informed consent, denying them treatment even after penicillin became available (Centers for Disease Control and Prevention [CDC], 2022a). This study's impact rippled through generations, affecting attitudes toward medical research in minority communities.

A recent study by Alsan and Wanamaker (2018) comparing older Black men with other demographic groups, before and after the information about the Tuskegee study was revealed and in varying proximity to the Tuskegee study's victims, found that the public disclosure of the study in 1972 was associated with increases in both medical mistrust and mortality, and decreases in both outpatient and inpatient physician interactions for older Black men, with the largest effects found for Black men living in closest in geographic proximity to Tuskegee. Alsan and Wanamaker (2018) estimate that life expectancy fell for Black men by up to 1.5 years in response to the public disclosure of the Tuskegee study, accounting for approximately 35% of the reported life expectancy gap between Black and White men in 1980.

Several studies directly targeted children, often without proper consent or consideration for their wellbeing. The 1936 Monster Study, conducted by Wendell Johnson, experimented on orphans by assigning them to "stutter" and "normal speaker" groups regardless of their actual speech patterns (Erard, 2001). Children in the "stutter" group developed speech impediments, withdrawal, and speech refusal as a result. The negative psychological impact on the children labeled as stutterers led to these harmful outcomes, demonstrating the potential for severe adverse effects from unethical research practices on vulnerable populations such as children (Erard, 2001). Similarly, the Robbers Cave Experiment in the 1950s, led by Muzafer Sherif, manipulated 11-year-old boys to study intergroup conflict. The study subjected participants to hostile interactions and psychological distress without parental consent or the option to withdraw (McLeod, 2023).

Other controversial studies involving children include the Little Albert Experiment, where John Watson conditioned an infant to fear harmless objects (Watson & Rayner, 1920), and child aggression studies on Black and Hispanic boys aged 6–10 years, which exposed them to potentially harmful situations (Klitzman & Kelmenson, 2020). The Willowbrook Hepatitis Experiments took ethical concerns to new heights by intentionally infecting institutionalized children with hepatitis to study the disease's progression and potential treatments (Krugman, 1986).

These studies, conducted before the establishment of institutional review boards in 1974, highlight the critical need for strict ethical guidelines in research involving children. They serve as stark reminders of past transgressions and underscore the importance of protecting vulnerable populations in scientific research. The legacy of these unethical practices continues to influence public perception of medical research and emphasizes the ongoing need for transparency, informed consent, and rigorous ethical oversight in all human studies.

Additionally, many children and youth participate in research that is subsequently unpublished and in turn does not help to advance scientific knowledge. Pica and Bourgeois (2016) found that out of 559 randomized clinical trials involving children, 104 were discontinued early and 136 that were completed did not result in publication of findings.

Present-day distrust and mistrust can be attributed to past institutional failures and conceptualized as a rational response aimed at protecting against future harm (Griffith et al., 2021; Nweke, Isom, & Fashaw-Walters, 2022; Platt, Jacobson, & Kardia, 2018). Specifically, Griffith and colleagues (2021) identified an enduring trend of substandard care as one factor contributing to distrust among historically marginalized communities, and they identified unethical research as facilitating mistrust in the current health care system. Moreover, Miller and Miller (2021) argue that this legacy of injustice and violence toward Black bodies feeds into the collective experience of transgenerational trauma within the Black population, which fundamentally undermines trust between Black patients and their physicians.

Finally, Platt, Jacobson, and Kardia (2018) found that a majority of the U.S. population has diminished confidence in the trustworthiness of the overall health care system. Numerous efforts are under way to rectify historical harms while rebuilding trust between the health care system and communities. Yet ongoing patient reluctance and health care disparities suggest these efforts are not achieving their desired outcomes. Future research is needed to elucidate how past mistreatment influences individual-level health care engagement and impacts health equity.

Practitioner Bias

Practitioner bias, frequently intertwined with the racial bias discussed in Chapter 2, can also contribute to mistrust in the health care system among children, youth, families, and communities (see, e.g., Blair, Steinerc, & Havranek, 2011; Canedo et al., 2018; FitzGerald & Hurst, 2017; Hall et al., 2015; Kugelmass, 2016; Vela et al., 2022). In pediatric health care, "practitioner bias" refers to the potential for health care providers to exhibit subjective judgments or preferences that may impact their decision making, diagnosis, and treatment of pediatric patients (Johnson et al., 2017; Schnierle, Christian-Brathwaite, & Louisias, 2019). This bias can stem from various factors, including personal beliefs, cultural background, stereotypes, or lack of awareness about one's own biases (Schnierle, Christian-Brathwaite, & Louisias, 2019). It is essential to recognize bias as a normal but malleable aspect of human cognition, and to address practitioner bias in pediatric health care through targeted solutions that are rigorously tested across all levels of care (Raphael & Oyeku, 2020).

Several studies have explored the concept of bias in pediatric health care, highlighting how implicit and explicit biases contribute to experiences of racism and discrimination. It has been consistently documented that historically marginalized racial and ethnic populations are overrepresented among those who experience substantial pain yet receive inadequate pain management (Goyal et al., 2020; Mossey, 2011; Sabin & Greenwald, 2012). Research conducted in pediatric emergency departments has revealed disparities based on race and ethnicity in the management of analgesics for children who present with acute abdominal pain, sickle cell disease, and appendicitis (Fearon et al., 2019; Goyal et al., 2015; Johnson et al., 2013; Raphael & Oyeku, 2020). Disparities in both process and outcome measures based on race and ethnicity have also been observed in emergency departments' management of pain in children with long-bone fractures (Goyal et al., 2020). Despite a higher likelihood for historically marginalized children to receive analgesics and experience more than a 2-point reduction in pain, they are less likely to receive opioids and achieve optimal pain reduction (Goyal et al., 2020). In addition, research has also shown that some providers perceive Black individuals as less likely than White individuals to adhere to medical advice, a perception that contributes to poor communication and care (Laws et al., 2014; van Ryn & Burke, 2000).

Gender bias is another barrier to achieving health equity, and predominantly impacts two aspects of health care (Carrilero et al., 2023). First, it can influence the diagnosis, affecting medical history, physical examinations, and the implementation of additional tests (Criado, 2019). Second, it plays a role in therapy, as the communication style and dynamics of the professional–patient relationship may vary based on whether professionals and patients share the same gender (Carrilero et al., 2023). Gender-diverse people are also known to be at a greater risk for health disparities and for trauma as a result of mistreatment in a health care setting (Sherman et al., 2021).

Patients and families often cite mistrust of health care practitioners as a barrier to engagement, and evidence shows that practitioners do not always trust their patients (e.g., undertreatment of pain for women and people of color; failure to take health concerns, particularly women's concerns, seriously; failure to listen to patients' initial concerns without interruption; Curtis et al., 2019; Khan, Ramotar, & Landrigan, 2019; National Partnership for Women & Families, 2023). For example, practitioner bias has been shown to be detrimental to Black maternal health because of parents' concerns being minimized or dismissed, resulting in increased infant and maternal mortality within the community (Saluja & Bryant, 2021). Furthermore, some research suggests that Black women are less likely than their White counterparts to receive an epidural during childbirth because of providers' beliefs about the relationship between race and pain tolerance, as well as poor communication in racially discordant provider–patient relationships (National Academies, 2021a,c).

Additional reporting from 2020 by Public Agenda surveyed trust between people with Medicaid and primary care doctors. The report found that many participants from Medicaid focus groups described feeling disrespected or distrusted by their providers because of their race and insurance coverage (Silliman & Schleifer, 2020). However, Silliman and Schleifer (2020) also reported that primary care doctors largely identified patients with Medicaid coverage as equally trustworthy as those with other forms of insurance, and as more trustworthy when they are actively engaged in care. Relatedly, studies have shown that race, ethnicity, and poverty influence child maltreatment reporting in hospital settings (Rebbe, Sattler, & Mienko, 2022). For example, Rebbe, Sattler, and Mienko (2022) conducted a record review of children hospitalized for maltreatment; using diagnostic codes, they found that Native American families and children with public health insurance were more likely than those with private insurance to receive a maltreatment diagnosis code (a strong predictor of being reported to child protective services).

Misinformation and Disinformation

The growing prevalence of misinformation and disinformation[3] has eroded trust between the health care system and children, youth, families, and communities in recent years. As stated by the U.S. Surgeon General,

[3]"Disinformation" refers to false information that is deliberately created and spread with the intention to deceive or mislead (WHO, 2024). Unlike misinformation, which may be shared without malicious intent, disinformation is designed to cause harm, sow discord, or undermine trust in health care institutions, scientific experts, and public health agencies (WHO, 2024).

"Health misinformation is a serious threat to public health. It can cause confusion, sow mistrust, harm people's health, and undermine public health efforts" (Murthy, 2021, p. 3). "Misinformation" is defined as "information that is false, inaccurate, or misleading according to the best available evidence at the time" (Murthy, 2021, p. 3).

For example, the lack of professional consensus regarding treatment and care during the early phase of the COVID-19 pandemic, given the novelty of the virus, exacerbated people's mistrust of the health care system, as new developments necessitated revised guidance (Frenk et al., 2022). During this period, misinformation and disinformation were also amplified across social media platforms leading to additional mistrust of the health care field (Benoit & Mauldin, 2021). National surveys conducted in 2022 and 2023 reflect polarized public opinions about the health care system and its actors (Del Ponte, Gerber, & Patashnik, 2023; Steel-Fisher et al., 2023). In this climate of polarization, misinformation and disinformation can thrive.

For pediatrics, controversy on the care of children with gender dysphoria has also been a flashpoint for polarization and misinformation, with implications for these children and families and far reach to other policies. While gender-affirming care has now been limited by more than 20 state legislatures, its prohibition has been also attached to many other pediatric policies unrelated to gender-affirming care (e.g., funding for graduate medical education in children's hospitals, Medicaid participation).

The National Academies conducted a roundtable in December 2020 on addressing misinformation (National Academies, 2020a), finding that technology use plays a pivotal role, as a high percentage of those who use the Internet search for information around health. Misinformation is disseminated online, which also drives inequity, because the consequences of misinformation "disproportionately affect communities of color, communities with lower socioeconomic status, and queer communities" (National Academies, 2020a, p. 2). The report highlighted several strategies for combatting misinformation, including using fact-checking organizations; promoting health literacy; using digital platforms; and promoting science literacy, specifically "understanding the uncertain and evolving nature of science" (National Academies, 2020a, p. 6).

Access to Health Care and System Fragmentation

Health care experiences vary greatly depending on where families seek care. Presently, health care is a largely fragmented, disjointed system lacking care coordination. Communication across systems is often limited, resulting in minimal reciprocal communication between systems and incomplete information shared with families about next steps. As a result, patients and families are forced to navigate complex, heterogenous health care systems (see Chapter 5). The delivery of health care spread across an excessively large number of poorly coordinated providers is a significant source of inefficiency in the U.S. health care system (Agha, Frandsen, & Rebitzer, 2019). Regional differences in practice styles contribute to varying levels of care fragmentation. Regions with higher levels of fragmentation are associated with increased care utilization and hospitalizations, suggesting that consistent relationships with primary care providers may reduce the demand for hospital care. Recent antifragmentation initiatives aim to reduce costly silos of care by altering provider financial incentives, but the effectiveness of these initiatives remains to be fully understood (Agha, Frandsen, & Rebitzer, 2019; see also Chapter 5).

Other issues regarding access to health care involve the availability, churning, and state variations of health care insurance (see Chapter 6), as well as the proximity and availability of needed health care, particularly for rural communities (see Chapter 5).

Individual-Level Disempowerment: Literacy, Language, and Cultural Congruence

In addition to trustworthiness and fragmentation of the health care system, families have also identified challenges with individual-level disempowerment when engaging with the health care system. Individual characteristics playing into these challenges include limited parenting knowledge and skills (including knowledge about prevention and children's health care needs), limited understanding of diagnosis and treatment options, and level of health literacy.[4] A large body of research focuses

[4]Sykes and colleagues (2013) describe "critical health literacy" as "a set of characteristics of advanced personal skills, health knowledge, information skills, effective interaction between service providers and users, informed decision making and empowerment, including political action" (para. 1). The potential consequences of critical health literacy, under this definition, are "improving health outcomes, creating more effective use of health services, and reducing inequalities in health" (Sykes et al., 2013, para. 1). Using a critical health literacy framework, Gould and colleagues (2020) identified three levels of literacy: functional, interactive, and critical (see also Nutbeam, 2000). The levels can be described using safe sex as an example (National Academies, 2021f):

> Functional literacy would entail providing individuals with facts about having safe sex. Interactive health literacy would be reached when people have learned how to communicate about having safe sex and are able to problem solve and independently make decisions about safe sex. Critical health literacy, which is not taught much in the United States today [...] is about an individual's understanding of the SDOH and their ability to take action at both the individual and the community level (p. 2).

In this example, critical health literacy would come into play when a safe sex problem is identified in the community (e.g., high levels of sexually transmitted infections or unplanned pregnancies) and the question is asked: "How can the community take action on the problem?" (National Academies, 2021f, p. 2).

on health literacy and physician–patient communication and patient outcomes. Belasen, Oppenlander, and Belasen (2020), for example, examined the relationship between provider–patient communication and data in the Hospital Consumer Assessment of Healthcare Providers and Systems, noting that communication between health care providers and patients is a determinant of patient outcomes.

Language barriers have been shown to increase adverse health outcomes, such as having difficulty understanding instructions on how to take a medication (Al Shamsi et al., 2020). Moreover, families have reported language barriers, including lack of professional interpreters or use of informal ad hoc interpreters (Elderkin-Thompson, Silver, & Waitzkin, 2001), nontranslated or incorrectly translated health materials (Flores et al., 2000), and resources that are not tailored to be culturally appropriate or relevant (Falbe et al., 2015; Lopez et al., 2019; McCurley, Gutierrez, & Gallo, 2017). With over a quarter (26.3%) of children under age 18 in the United States living with at least one foreign-born parent, cultural and language challenges are common in the pediatric health care setting (Anderson & Hemez, 2022).

Research has also linked cultural competency or humility, cross-cultural communication (language proficient providers and families), and patient–provider racial/ethnic congruence to increased health care engagement and perception of quality care. For example, racial concordance between patient and physician has been associated with reduced health disparities and increased patient satisfaction (Alberto et al., 2021; Greenwood et al., 2020; National Academies, 2023g; Takeshita et al., 2020). A previous National Academies report, *In the Nation's Compelling Interest: Ensuring Diversity in the Health-Care Workforce,* found that a more diverse health care workforce increases access to care for historically marginalized patients, improves patient choice and satisfaction, results in better patient–provider communication, and ultimately can produce better quality of care for all Americans (Institute of Medicine [IOM], 2004).

In a study of maternal mental health care, Matthews and colleagues (2021) conducted a series of focus groups and structured interviews to identify antiracist solutions to inequities in maternal care. The authors reported (Matthews et al., 2021):

> Several participants expressed the need for services informed by cultural humility and holistic care, which is inclusive of dignified, respectful, humane, and empathetic care. [. . .] Active listening, answering a client's questions, intentionally dismantling power dynamics, creating "brave spaces" (environments that foster critical dialogue and acknowledge varying perceptions and realities of safety) were reported as important strategies to build trust and respond to a client's needs holistically. (p. 1600)

STRATEGIES FOR IMPROVEMENT

Fostering confidence and overcoming mistrust in the health care system requires strong relationships and an infrastructure that supports addressing the structural factors that create disparities in health outcomes. This section summarizes some of the strategies aimed at building trust. These include prioritizing health equity, family and community voice, a cultural humility in the health care workforce, patient- and youth-led services, and leveraging local anchor institutions.

Health care that centers on partnerships, strengths, and equity provides children with the greatest opportunities to receive care and resources to support their lifelong development. The joyful faces of these young Black children in the mural in Figure 3-4 serve as a powerful reminder of the importance of cultivating cultural humility, empathy, and antiracist practices in all areas of health care and social services, to ensure equitable, compassionate, and affirming support for children and families of color.

Advancing Health Equity with Communities

Building trust in health care systems, particularly with communities of color, needs to begin with acknowledgment of existing inequities and pursuits to combat such inequalities in communities (National Academies, 2021b,c). The 2017 National Academies report *Communities in Action: Pathways to Health Equity* shared the significance of the role of communities in promoting health equity. The report concluded that community-driven solutions are necessary, as communities are in a unique position to

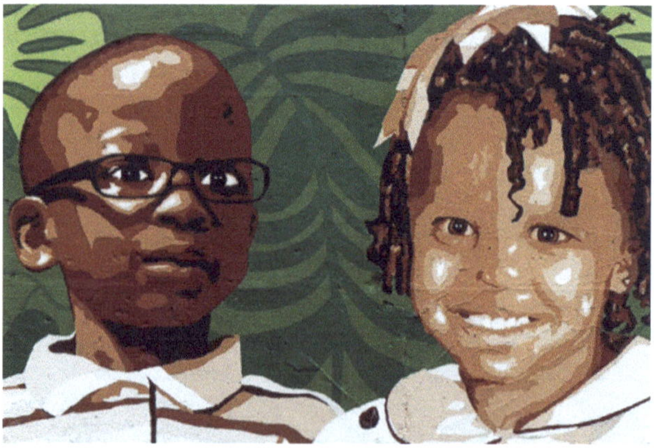

FIGURE 3-4 Childhood hope and sense of pride.
SOURCE: Brent Billingsley, Cincinnati, OH. Photo by Pixxel Designs. Courtesy of the artist.

drive priorities and actions tailored to their needs that address many of the determinants of health (National Academies, 2017a, p. 179). In addition, the report encourages enhanced engagement of patients, families, and communities as a strategy in health policy change, research, and care delivery to improve the quality of care and drive health equity (National Academies, 2017a, p. 237). Reframing the health care system around the experiences, needs, and considerations of patients, families, and communities is a necessary precondition to achieve the values of equity, efficiency, and effectiveness. See Box 3-3 for a personal narrative of Tamela Milan-Alexander as she reflects on linking health care to community experiences.

Children, families, communities, providers, and other engaged stakeholders consistently identify achieving health equity as a fundamental goal. Achieving equity will require multilevel and multipronged strategies and interventions at the policy, system, and program levels to align with science and evidence around equity outcomes and to distribute resources to where they are needed most (National Academies, 2019a,c,d). The Center for Health Care Strategies (CHCS) brief *Engaging Communities of Color to Promote Health Equity* (2022) suggests partnering with patients and community members of color to understand their needs and preferences as an initial step toward improving health outcomes and advancing health equity (Spencer & Ohene-Ntow, 2022). This initial step can facilitate longer-term relationships that may develop into trusting and collaborative relationships between engaged parties. In its assessment of the experiences of learning collaborative participants across New York–based health care organizations, CHCS distilled five broadly applicable lessons for better understanding patient experiences and addressing long-standing health disparities (Spencer & Ohene-Ntow, 2022):

1. Build trust with patient partners over time;
2. Tailor outreach strategies to resonate with patient populations;
3. Use trauma-informed approaches to strengthen relationships with patient partners;
4. Collect and use data in partnership with patients; and
5. Approach patient engagement with humility and patience (p. 2).

Building Trust through Engagement of Children, Families, and Communities

Engaging children, families, and communities is critical to overcoming the challenges identified in the previous section—specifically, engagement is critical to overcoming mistrust and building confidence in the health care system. Building trust requires a strong infrastructure and relationships that support organizing for policy change, providing accessible care, listening to the needs of communities, addressing the structural factors that create disparities in health outcomes, and ensuring measurement and transparent

BOX 3-3
Illustrative Example: Community Engagement—Tamela Milan-Alexander

Tamela Milan-Alexander grew up on Chicago's West Side. "I definitely sought, outside the home, for different forms of recognition and acceptance," Milan-Alexander said, "I felt smothered [. . .] and it was exciting to be out—to be in the hood, so to speak."

"But of course," she added, "that excitement led to some pivotal changes in my life."

By age 17, Milan-Alexander was pregnant. By age 18, she had her first child. By age 20, she was in a relationship riddled with domestic violence. And soon thereafter, she started using drugs, including crack cocaine. Things quickly spiraled as she found herself within the grips of dependency. "At some point it became physically necessary to my existence—the sickness of it became debilitating," Milan-Alexander said, "Every day was a day to use."

It was a challenging time to have a substance use disorder. People using crack cocaine faced harsh judgment. Despite her awareness and insight into her condition, Milan-Alexander did not feel that she could turn to the health care system. She could not share what was going on, and she could not ask for help. If anything, health care itself represented a threat rather than a safety net. "There was this fear of—or distress related to—the system," Milan-Alexander said, "There was this environment of, you know, health care could take your kid."

Eventually, Milan-Alexander did get help for her addiction—and eventually, she was able to overcome it. But she remembers how it felt to be marginalized from—and threatened by—the health care system. Some days, actually, Milan-Alexander still feels it, such as in interactions as simple as a vaccination visit: "That fear factor [is] ever present," she said.

reporting of inequities (National Academies, 2021d). Patients and families generally desire to be involved and engaged in health care decisions; however, this desire varies depending on the individual, the number of treatment options available, and the certainty of those treatment options (Blumenthal Kostick, et al., 2015). Robust trust levels contribute to confidence, peace of mind, and a sense of security. Conversely, shattered trust can result in anxiety, second-guessing, and frustration (Sisk & Baker, 2019).

Most principles of engagement directly promote fostering trust. Frameworks of patient and family engagement can be understood as falling into one of three levels along a continuum: listening and advising, co-creation and co-design (Durrah, 2023a,b,c).

Listening

Listening involves point-of-care interactions where patients, families, and care team members engage in mutual respect, trust, and communication (Durrah, 2023b). This level of engagement is crucial for building trust

So, these days, Milan-Alexander is fighting to connect communities like hers with the health care system in ways she never benefited from. That means ensuring there are "access points" to health care for parents struggling with addiction, such as during a child's routine physical, she said. It could also mean working with the state's department of education to provide foundational care for families in school-based health centers—which are often more physically and emotionally accessible than are hospitals. This is the focus of the initiative her organization, EverThrive Illinois, is undertaking.

Health care systems need to form meaningful partnerships with the specific communities they serve, Milan-Alexander said. That could mean broadening colon cancer screening in one community, medication-assisted treatment in another, or physical therapy in a third. That also means health care systems ought to move from the gospel of the "melting pot" to that of the "salad bowl," she said.

"I can't ask a mushroom what a tomato is doing—I can't be a carrot and a cucumber at the same time," Milan-Alexander said, "the ingredients are very different, very unique to themselves—they [must be] separated out, and acknowledged for the differences they show."

And, practically, it means health care systems need to look outwards for both inspiration and impact. "Look outside the four walls," Milan-Alexander said, "if you don't know what's outside the walls, you don't know what's going on."

Only then, she said—when health care systems truly meet families where they live, when they include the community institutions that families attend as equal partners—will parents, and their children, truly be able to thrive.

SOURCE: Correspondence with Tamela Milan-Alexander, prepared by Eli Cahan, health communication advisor to the committee.

because it ensures that patients and families feel heard and valued. For example, family-centered rounds, where providers include patients and families during bedside rounds, demonstrate respect and openness, which are essential for building trust (Carman et al., 2013; Durrah, 2023b). Effective communication by providers can significantly impact patient satisfaction, willingness to follow medical advice, and adherence to treatment plans (Boudreaux & O'Hea, 2004; Dorsey et al., 2022; Hall, Roter, & Rand, 1981; Herndon & Pollick, 2002; Kaplan, Greenfield, & Ware, 1989; Roter, 1983).

Advising

Advising involves patient and family advisory councils, where patients and families provide input on health care practices and policies. While this level of engagement still places decision-making power primarily with providers, it is a step toward more inclusive practices (Durrah, 2023b). Building diverse advisory councils and compensating advisors can enhance trust by showing a commitment to inclusivity and valuing the contributions of all community members (Durrah, 2023a,b; Van Veen, 2014). Engaging advisors from historically marginalized communities and providing educational opportunities can build trust by ensuring that all voices are heard and respected (Durrah, 2023b).

Eliminating barriers to financially compensate patients and families for their participation in health care improvement efforts is crucial for ensuring diverse representation and meaningful engagement (Spencer & Ohene-Ntow, 2022). Financial compensation acknowledges the value of patients' time and expertise while addressing socioeconomic barriers to participation (Domecq et al., 2014). The Agency for Healthcare Research and Quality (2018) and the Patient-Centered Outcomes Research Institute (2015) both emphasize the importance of this practice for better outcomes. However, health care organizations often face regulatory and administrative barriers in providing such compensation, including concerns about violating antikickback statutes and complexities in accounting (Deverka et al., 2012). Addressing these barriers requires policy changes, clear organizational guidelines, and education of health care administrators. Some health care systems, such as the University of Vermont Medical Center (2020), have successfully implemented compensation programs, leading to increased diversity in advisory councils and more impactful care improvements. By overcoming these barriers and establishing equitable compensation practices, health care organizations can foster more inclusive and effective improvement efforts, aligning with principles of health equity and patient-centered care (National Academies, 2019d).

Co-Creation and Co-Design

Co-creation and co-design represent the highest level of engagement, where patients, families, and communities are equitable partners in health care system transformation (Durrah, 2023a,b,c). This approach is built on shared power and responsibility, fostering active partnerships and shared decision making. By involving stakeholders in the design and implementation of health services, trust is built through transparency, collaboration, and mutual respect (Silvola et al., 2023). Co-creation and co-design ensure that health services are tailored to the real needs and desires of patients, which is essential for building trust (Silvola et al., 2023). These approaches have been used to improve health equity and promote accountability, further enhancing trust within communities (Andrews, Sahama, & Gajanayake, 2014; Reopell et al., 2023; Roche et al., 2020). Co-creation and co-design can be applied at the practice, system, research, and policy levels, but they require leadership support, flexibility and nimbleness, sharing of power and resources, and funding. Box 3-4 describes Southcentral Foundation's Nuka System of Care, an example of a transformative model for a health care system that is coproduced with customer-owners.

BOX 3-4
Southcentral Foundation's Nuka System of Care

Southcentral Foundation's (SCF's) Nuka System of Care is a relationship-based, Alaska Native–owned health care system. Relationships are a core concept within the Indigenous worldview, and the Nuka system was designed to center relationships across the spectrum of care (Healey, 2017). Based in Anchorage, Alaska, SCF's Nuka system evolved out of the consumer-driven overhaul of the formerly centralized health care system overseen by the Indian Health Service (Gottlieb, 2013). Today, the nonprofit organization serves roughly 65,000 Alaska Native and American Indian people across Anchorage, the Matanuska-Susitna Borough, and 55 rural villages in the Anchorage Service Area[a] (Healey, 2017). The Nuka system recognizes health as not just the absence of illness but a comprehensive, interconnected state of physical, emotional, mental, and spiritual wellbeing (Eby, 2023; Southcentral Foundation Nuka System of Care, n.d., 2019).

Upon assuming responsibility for primary care, SFC underwent a transformative process, gathering feedback from the Native community over the course of a year. The Nuka System of Care underwent a complete overhaul, focusing on two key elements: customer ownership and relationships (Transnational Forum on Integrated Community Care [TFICC], 2019). SCF avoids referring to the Alaska Native and American Indian individuals it serves as "patients" because the term is deemed passive and does not align with the high level of engagement SCF seeks. Instead, recognizing that those served are both customers and owners of the health care system, as well as their personal health journeys, they are termed "customer-owners" (Salinsky, 2017). SCF functions within the tribal authority of Cook Inlet Region, Inc., which appoints SCF's seven-member board of directors. This board formulates policies and holds overarching control and management responsibilities for the organization. Notably, all members of SCF's board of directors, the president/CEO, and over 60% of the management and leadership are customer-owners (TFICC, 2019).

SCF aims to involve the entire Native community in the health care system. On an individual level, SCF acknowledges that individuals have more control over their health outcomes than providers do. Building strong, long-term relationships with customer-owners is emphasized, fostering understanding of their health issues and establishing trust (TFICC, 2019). This approach enables providers to more effectively support customer-owners in achieving wellness.

Redesigning behavioral health services was instrumental to the success of the Nuka system; it provided customer-owners with improved access to services, including (Salinsky, 2017):

> group learning circles, individual appointments with a psychiatrist or behavioral health clinician, collocated psychiatrists in primacy care, same day appointments with a master's level clinician in outpatient behavioral health, the integration of behavioral health consultants into primary care, and improved workflows to ensure timely handoffs between primary care and specialty behavioral health service (p. 2).

(continued)

BOX 3-4 Continued

This has been a successful redesign, with participants reporting a nearly 50% reduction in substance abuse, depression, and trauma symptoms and a 25% reduction in anxiety. Nearly two-thirds reported an increase in self-esteem, cultural connectedness, and spiritual wellbeing (Huhndorf, 2017).

SCF actively engages with the community through various initiatives. They organize the Annual Gathering, a free event offering insights into SCF services, live entertainment, and activities for children, along with the opportunity to purchase Alaska Native art. SCF maintains strong connections with community organizations, such as the Alaska Federation of Natives and the Alaska Native Health Board. In addition, the Health Education department collaborates to provide a range of services, including group classes, workshops, health fairs, counseling, cooking classes, and educational demonstrations, fostering community wellbeing and education (TFICC, 2019).

Access to and quality of care for customer-owners has resulted in dramatic improvements since services were transformed under the Nuka system, with SCF reporting the following changes from 2000 to 2017: a 26%, 47%, and 59% drop in deaths due to cancer, heart disease, and cerebrovascular disease, respectively; a 58% drop in infant mortality; a 40% drop in emergency room visits; a 36% drop in hospital admissions; 97% customer-owner satisfaction; and 95% employee satisfaction (Huhndorf, 2017; Routledge, 2020; Salinsky, 2017).

By embracing cultural traditions, emphasizing community engagement, and prioritizing patient-centered care, the Nuka system has transformed health care delivery for Alaska Native communities. SCF has diverse funding streams, with support from, but not limited to, the U.S. Indian Health Service, private insurance, Medicare, Medicaid, private and public grants, and other third-party payers (TFICC, 2019). Its innovative principles and components hold promise for promoting health equity and improving outcomes for populations across the country. Groups such as CareOregon, the Cherokee Nation, the U.S. Department of Veterans Affairs, and Harvard Medical School's Center for Primary Care are a handful of the organizations adopting Nuka's integrated-care approach (Huhndorf, 2017). Funding of SFC and related initiatives is a key concern for scaling up and sustaining the model.

SCF's Nuka System of Care is a primary example of the possibility and power of incorporating patients and communities into extended community-based care teams and co-creating and co-designing health care. Nevertheless, achieving this integration requires time, the establishment of mutual trust, structured recruitment processes, clarification of roles, and sensitivity to professional and institutional barriers. The model emphasizes prioritizing community input and co-design and shaping the health care system based on community preferences. Allowing customer-owners to take ownership of their health care, coupled with a willingness to implement bold and comprehensive changes, facilitates the creation of a high-quality, sustainable system tailored to community needs (Eby, 2023).

[a]The Anchorage Service Area measures approximately 107,413 square miles and extends east to the Canadian border, north to Cantwell, west to the upper Kuskokwim Valley, and southwest to the Aleutian Pribilof Islands. The Anchorage Service Area has the largest urban population in the state, and the most diverse rural population (Indian Health Service, n.d.b).

Children can be encouraged to actively participate in their own health care by voicing their needs and preferences, which can help tailor care to be more child centered (Carter et al., 2024). With proper preparation, older children and adolescents can advocate for their health needs and those of their peers, and promote awareness and education about health issues within their communities, as represented in Figure 3-5 (Lee et al., 2016). Families can act as coordinators of care, ensuring that all aspects of a child's health, including medical, social, and educational needs, are addressed comprehensively (Cady & Belew, 2017; Family Voices, n.d.). They can also be involved in shared decision-making processes with health care providers, ensuring that care plans align with their values and preferences. Additionally, families can provide emotional and practical support to other families navigating the health care system, fostering a community of shared experiences and resources (Gage-Bouchard, 2017). Engagement of children, youth, families, and communities can better address their needs and lead to development of more effective programs.

Communities also play a vital role in health care transformation. Community members can be trained as health workers to provide culturally sensitive care, bridge gaps between health care providers and families, and address social determinants of health (Lloyd, Moses, & Davis, 2020; Schaaf et al., 2020). Communities can also mobilize to advocate for policy changes that support health equity, such as improved access to health care services and antiracist practices. Furthermore, communities can establish

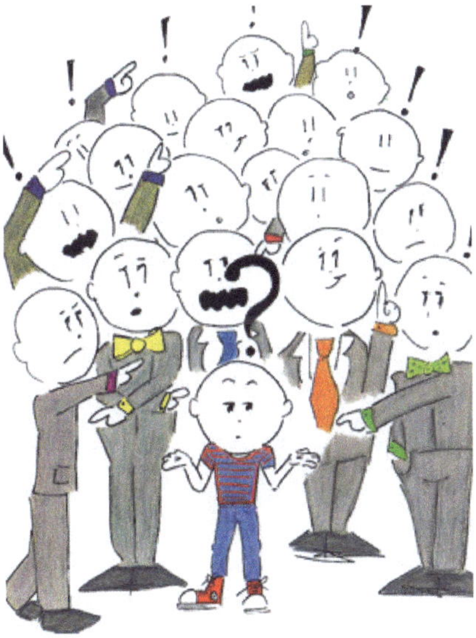

FIGURE 3-5 Making it happen.
SOURCES: Dann Warrick, age 22, United States; © Peace Child International, used with permission.

resource hubs that provide access to health-related information, services, and support, promoting a holistic approach to child health and wellbeing (Gilbert et al., 2023; Manis et al., 2022). Each of these models of engagement can be used to redistribute power, and they value multiple forms of knowledge and can facilitate increased trust and improved outcomes for children, youth, families, and communities.

NAM developed a conceptual model to assess community engagement in the context of health equity and systems transformation, presented in Figure 3-6. This model identifies and defines core principles necessary to produce meaningful engagement, along with four outcome areas to evaluate community engagement efforts toward health equity (Aguilar-Gaxiola et al., 2022).

COMPREHENSIVE WORKFORCE TRAINING

Implementing comprehensive training programs is essential to ensure that the health care workforce is competent, diverse, team oriented, antiracist, and able to promote relational health. This includes efforts to increase diversity in the health care workforce, cultural humility training, and attention to compassionate care (Lloyd, Moses, & Davis, 2020). A well-trained and diverse workforce is better equipped to address the unique needs of children and families from various backgrounds. Research has shown that a diverse health care workforce can improve patient satisfaction, promote better communication between providers and patients, and reduce health disparities (Jongen, McCalman, & Bainbridge, 2018).

The concepts of cultural humility and health equity can be interwoven to all aspects of graduate medical, nursing, and allied health education. For example, case studies in which students learn about the experience of a particular disease or strategies for disease prevention can be designed to model culturally humble approaches in the provision of care and the avoidance of stereotypical thinking (Foronda et al., 2016; Mosher et al., 2017). Research suggests one effective approach to cultivating cultural humility is to accompany experiential learning opportunities or case studies with reflection that expands learning beyond skills and knowledge. This includes questioning current practices and proposing changes to improve the efficiency and quality of care, equality, and social justice (Barton, Brandt, et al., 2020; Barton, Murray, & Spurlock Jr., 2020; Foronda, Liu, & Bauman, 2013). In the case of nursing education, programs designed to develop nurses' cultural sensitivity and humility, as well as cultural immersion programs, have been developed, and research suggests that such programs can effectively develop skills that strengthen nurses' confidence in treating diverse populations, improve patient and provider relationships, and increase nurses' compassion (Allen, 2010; Gallagher & Polanin, 2015; National Academies, 2021e, p. 207; Sanner et al., 2010).

A burgeoning body of research points to the importance of empathy, compassionate care, and empathic engagement in patient care leading to better patient outcomes and improving the patient experience. Empathy involves

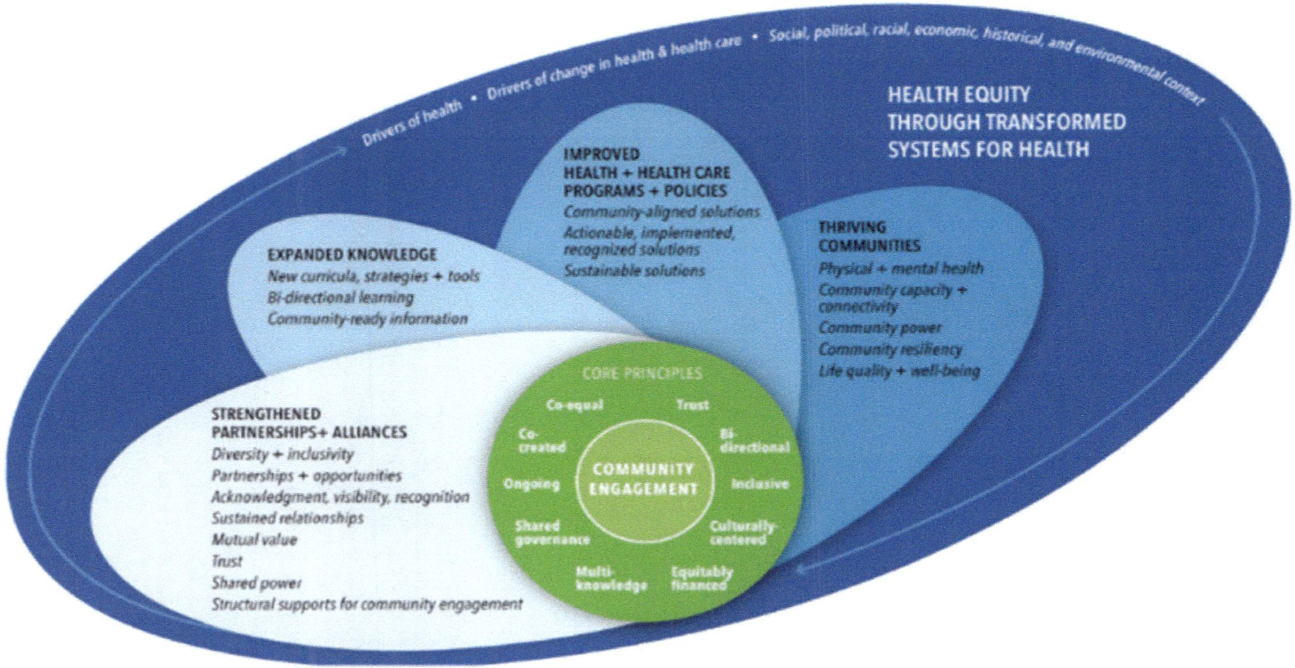

FIGURE 3-6 Meaningful community engagement in health and health care programs and policies.
SOURCE: Aguilar-Gaxiola et al., 2022.

"understanding (rather than feeling) of a patient's concerns, experiences, pain, and suffering combined with a capacity to communicate this understanding and an intention to help" (Hojat, 2007, para. 3). Compassionate care serves as the vehicle for care providers to express empathy toward patients and families, and supports a person-centered and relationship-based care model (Arnold P. Gold Foundation, 2014). Empathic engagement brings together empathy and compassionate care to fully recognize, acknowledge, and validate a larger understanding and appreciation of the experience patients and families (Guidi & Traversa, 2021). Emerging research also demonstrates how compassionate patient care can improve health outcomes and reduce workplace stress and burnout for health care professionals (Cochrane et al., 2019).

Recognize Activities Related to Patient and Family Experience

Accrediting bodies have begun recognizing activities related to assessing and improving patient and family experience. This recognition can drive improvements in care quality and patient satisfaction, ultimately leading to better health outcomes for children (Halfon, DuPlessis, & Inkelas, 2007). Patient and family education has been identified as a critical element in delivering quality health care services, emphasizing its importance in improving overall outcomes for consumers (Bhattad & Pacifico, 2022; Bombard et al., 2018; Patel, 2020). By incorporating patient and family experience metrics into accreditation standards, these bodies encourage health care organizations to focus on patient-centered care and family engagement.

Providing Support and Care through Youth-Led Services

Youth-led services encompass a variety of initiatives where young people take the lead in addressing issues pertinent to their communities, and typically include mental health initiatives, health promotion and education, community service and development, and participatory research (Ozer et al., 2020; Talbert, 2017; YouthPower Learning & YouthPower Action, n.d.). Youth-led mental health initiatives may involve creating safe spaces, reducing stigma through campaigns, and providing peer-support programs (Hogan et al., 2003; Registered Nurses' Association of Ontario, n.d.; World Health Organization, 2023). Health promotion efforts may include, for example, sexual and reproductive health education campaigns or health fairs organized by youth (AmeriCorps, 2024; Yun & Yun, 2023; YouthPower Learning & YouthPower Action, n.d.). Community service initiatives often involve volunteer programs and youth advisory councils that influence local policies (YouthPower Learning & YouthPower Action, n.d.). Participatory research, such as Youth Participatory Action Research, trains youth to conduct research on issues affecting their lives, leading to actionable insights and policy changes (Annie E. Casey Foundation, n.d.;

Ballonoff Suleiman et al., 2019; CDC, n.d.b; Morrel-Samuels et al., 2017; Ozer et al., 2020; Soleimanpour et al., 2008; Youth.gov, n.d.).

Youth-led services are intended to address significant gaps in traditional service delivery models by leveraging the unique perspectives and energy of young people (Talbert, 2017; YouthPower Learning & YouthPower Action, n.d.). Many current efforts are designed to address the growing mental health crisis among youth, which is exacerbated by factors such as the COVID-19 pandemic, racial injustices, and climate change (Bell et al., 2023; National Academies, 2022b; see also Chapter 2). Research shows that peer-to-peer support programs are associated with several positive benefits, including increased self-esteem and confidence, a heightened sense of control in bringing about life changes, and feelings of greater hope and inspiration (California Children's Trust, 2022; Mental Health America, 2018). These positive outcomes are shown to help decrease substance use and depression as well as psychotic symptoms, and reduce hospital admission rates (California Children's Trust, 2022; Mental Health America, 2018).

These services often struggle with sustainability and scalability due to limited funding and resources. Youth-led services require structured support, mentorship, and adequate funding to achieve their full potential and make a lasting impact (AmeriCorps, 2024; Learning to Give, n.d.). Several strategies have been suggested to scale and sustain youth-led services:

1. Integrating youth participatory approaches into health equity initiatives (Ozer et al., 2020);
2. Developing a developmental framework for youth-led programs (Ballonoff Suleiman et al., 2019);
3. Establishing formal certification and training programs for youth peer-support specialists (California Mental Health Services Authority, n.d.);
4. Fostering partnerships with established mental health organizations (American Academy of Child and Adolescent Psychiatry, n.d.); and
5. Implementing rigorous evaluation and research to demonstrate effectiveness (Ballonoff Suleiman et al., 2019; Ozer et al., 2020).

Initiatives such as AmeriCorps's (2024) Healthy Futures provide critical opportunities to expand the workforce of youth leaders and provide consistency in the delivery of youth-led services (see also Talbert, 2017; Wong, Zimmerman, & Parker, 2010). Healthy Futures encompasses multiple projects and initiatives, often partnering with local health organizations, community centers, schools, and other institutions to maximize their impact (AmeriCorps, 2024). Healthy Futures programs have produced favorable outcomes, such as improved food security, increased utilization of health care, improved mental health, and reduced child maltreatment

(AmeriCorps, 2019, 2024). Moreover, these initiatives play a role in sustaining the development of the future health care workforce (Schultz Family Foundation, 2024; Soleimanpour et al., 2008).

Leveraging Anchor Institutions

Since the 1960s, discussions have been ongoing about the role of local community organizations and their abilities to address social determinants of health in cities and localities across the United States (Koh et al., 2020). Community organizations that impact education, health care, and infrastructure, along with public institutions such as local government entities, faith-based groups, and cultural establishments, were first identified as "anchor institutions" in 2001 (Fulbright-Anderson, Auspos, & Anderson, 2001; Harkavy et al., 2014) and described thereafter as "[a] new paradigm for understanding the role that place-based institutions could play in building successful communities and local economies" (Taylor & Luter, 2013, p. 4).

While there is no singular definition of anchor institutions, Taylor and Luter (2013) have identified the following common features: "anchors are large, spatially immobile, mostly nonprofit organizations that play an integral role in the local economy" (p. 8). For-profit hospitals, which are more likely to operate in vulnerable communities, also have the potential to serve as anchor institutions (Cronin et al., 2021; Franz et al., 2021). Because these groups are deeply embedded in their communities (Norris & Howard, 2015, p. 8), they have been described as "sticky capital," a designation implying a vested economic self-interest in actively contributing to the wellbeing and prosperity of the communities where they operate, ensuring safety, vibrancy, and health (Serang, Thompson, & Howard, 2013, p. 4). The mission of anchor institutions has been identified as "a commitment to consciously apply their long-term, place-based economic power of the institution, in combination with its human and intellectual resources, to better the long-term welfare of the communities in which the institution is anchored" (Serang, Thompson, & Howard, 2013, p. 5). Hospitals dedicate significant financial, human, and intellectual assets to tackle societal issues, recognizing the interconnectedness of their future with the community beyond their confines. In 2017, hospitals allocated over $1.1 trillion annually (Koh et al., 2020) and constituted between 7.5% and 10.4% of the U.S. labor force, depending on the region, in 2016 (Koh et al., 2020; Statista, n.d.).

Communities in Action: Pathways to Health Equity discusses at length the significant impact of anchor institutions on their surrounding communities (National Academies, 2017a):

> These institutions, often the largest employers within cities and other localities, play a crucial role in the economic, social, and cultural fabric of their areas (ICIC, 2011; Viveiros & Sturtevant, 2016). With vast economic

> resources and human capital, hospitals and other anchor institutions can influence local well-being (Norris & Howard, 2015). However, challenges arise when the community perceives minimal benefits from these institutions, leading to conflicting relationships and mistrust (Martin, Smith, & Phillips, 2005; Miller & Rivera, n.d.; O'Mara, 2012). Rubin and Rose (2015) have identified that "[m]any anchors have a history of being distant from grassroots communities or of wielding their power and influence in ways that advance their immediate agenda but not that of nearby residents or the broader public" (Rubin & Rose, 2015, p. 2), for example, in terms of their human resources and procurement practices and real estate investments. (p. 393)

Efforts to bolster the role of anchor institutions and improve community trust and engagement have gained traction, emphasizing their responsibility to contribute to community wellbeing (National Academies, 2017a). Projects such as the National Task Force on Anchor Institutions (2010), Healthcare Anchor Network, and the Democracy Collaborative (n.d.) propose altering traditional business practices to leverage the economic power of these institutions for local improvement. This approach highlights the importance of leadership and community involvement, strategic planning, and metrics for tracking community benefits. Unlike past unsuccessful efforts dependent on short-term projects and external funding, the current approach integrates community improvement into the institutional mission, culture, and structure of anchor institutions (National Academies, 2017a), in order to address broad social and environmental factors impacting health (Artiga & Hinton, 2018). To become an "engaged anchor" (Rubin & Rose, 2015, p. 2) and embrace an anchor mission for making a positive impact on local communities, a deliberate and intentional collaborative approach is essential (Harkavy et al., 2014). This involves active participation from leadership at hospitals and other anchor institutions and members of the communities they serve (National Academies, 2017a). Developing operational strategies and creating new organizational structures are crucial steps toward achieving substantial and meaningful change (Harkavy et al., 2014; Rubin & Rose, 2015).

Anchor institutions play a crucial role in enhancing community conditions by leveraging economic power to address social determinants of health, promoting multisector collaboration, and involving community residents. However, it is important to recognize that an anchor institution alone is not a cure-all, particularly if it lacks an equitable approach to economic development that genuinely improves the living conditions of long-standing, economically disadvantaged residents (Artiga & Hinton, 2018; McGinnis & Foege, 2004). Opportunities for non–health care system actors to improve community conditions are explored in Chapters 7 and 8 of this report.

Without intentional efforts to ensure equitable benefits from economic development, there is a risk of contributing to gentrification and the displacement of existing impoverished residents (National Academies, 2017a). Therefore, the central challenge in anchor institution initiatives lies in finding ways to enhance community conditions without causing displacement (National Academies, 2017a; Viveiros & Sturtevant, 2016). The key is to focus on tangible and measurable indicators that demonstrate improvements in living conditions for individuals and families residing in these neighborhoods prior to reinvestment, which is exemplified in Box 3-5.

BOX 3-5
Healthy Neighborhoods Healthy Families (HNHF)

The HNHF initiative by Nationwide Children's Hospital (n.d.a) in Columbus, Ohio, is a community investment program designed to actively engage with and address the needs of the neighborhoods surrounding the hospital. The initiative seeks to improve positive health outcomes in Columbus by increasing the supply of local affordable housing, engaging community residents through workforce development programs, and addressing other community needs (Jones, 2022; National Initiative on Mixed-Income Communities, 2020). HNHF launched in 2008, following the hospital's expansion on the South Side of Columbus. Recognizing the importance of being a good neighbor, the hospital adopted a "Good Neighbor Agreement" and pledged to share plans, listen to feedback, and align its goals with the Columbus community (Jones, 2022).

HNHF is a holistic endeavor dedicated to enhancing community wellbeing by addressing multifaceted concerns beyond the realm of health care, including affordable housing, workforce development, financial counseling, and educational support (Children's National Hospital, 2023b). The initiative actively collaborates with an array of community partners, such as faith-based organizations and civic associations, thereby ensuring a cooperative and community-centric approach. HNHF's commitment to fostering enduring relationships and contributing comprehensively to the overall wellbeing of the communities it serves includes actively listening to community members, addressing their lived challenges, and deploying resources not only in terms of financial capital but also through dedicated staff, time, and expertise (Jones, 2022). A central tenet of the program is the empowerment of community members to guide initiatives, reflecting a commitment to a fully collaborative and co-designed process aimed at enhancing the likelihood of success in community development and health improvement endeavors (Jones, 2022).

In the process of extending this initiative to adjacent locales, such as the Linden area, the hospital places paramount importance on cultivating trust through direct engagement with residents (Nationwide Children's Hospital, n.d.a). Over the initiative's trajectory, HNHF has significantly expanded its scope, garnering investments exceeding $50 million to either develop or enhance more than 500 residences, characterized by their high quality and affordability (Jones, 2022). HNHF emphasizes the evolving role of anchor institutions as active contributors to community wellbeing, with a focus on addressing social determinants of health and fostering genuine partnerships with community residents and organizations.

CONCLUSION

This chapter has summarized common priorities for health care among families and communities. It addressed issues of trustworthiness and offered examples of building trust and ways to engage children, youth, families, and communities in decision making within the health care system. While a lot can be said at a high level about community health needs, it is critical to recognize the diverse and intersecting identities that shape individual, familial, and communal experiences and health outcomes. Effective and transformative changes will need to be tailored to address the unique needs and contexts of different groups.

Child- and family-centered care recognizes unique needs and the importance of developing partnerships between families and providers. It lets families drive their level of involvement. Community-centered care is a way to work collaboratively with or through groups to identify and address issues affecting wellbeing. The goal of this approach is comprehensive, equitable care that addresses holistic family needs and leverages successful community practices.

Shifting to health care that centers child health and lifelong health requires understanding the perspectives of children, youth, families, and communities on their health and health care needs. Issues of trust present barriers to this understanding. Long-standing mistrust is the result of past history of unethical research and medical practices and is compounded by practitioner bias and misinformation. Mistrust of the health care system, especially in communities of color in the United States, is grounded in current experience with structural inequities that permeate health care and other systems, as well as with the legacy of health care discrimination. Challenges with communication and language barriers and lack of cultural humility can also contribute to care that fails to center families and communities.

Strategies aimed at building trust include prioritizing health equity, family and community voice, cultural humility in the health care workforce, patient- and youth-led services, and leveraging local anchor institutions. Each of these strategies requires commitment to long-term, place-based partnerships with the long-term wellbeing of the community in mind.

Conclusion: Reframing the health care system around the experiences, needs, and considerations of children, youth, families, and communities is a necessary precondition to achieve excellent and equitable health outcomes.

4

Children in the United States: Demographics, Health, and Wellbeing

We need a focus on prevention with so many children already experiencing needs for tier 2 and 3 [mental health] intervention.

—Comment to Committee from Educator, Palmyra, Pennsylvania

This chapter builds on the science frameworks explored in Chapter 2 and the evidence that social, environmental, and relational factors influence trajectories in health, wellbeing, and development. Here the committee provides an overview of the health of children and youth in the United States and their demographics, along with the declining birth rate. As shown in recent reports by the National Academies of Sciences, Engineering, and Medicine (National Academies), the chapter describes higher rates of poverty among U.S. children than those of most other industrialized nations. The current state of child and adolescent health and wellbeing is discussed at length, as are significant family and community factors that influence child health. The committee reports that U.S. children are not doing well—they face major health problems with lasting impact on their overall growth and development and preparation for adult life.

CHILDREN AND YOUTH IN THE UNITED STATES

In 2022, there were 72.5 million children under age 18 years in the United States, accounting for nearly 22% of the total U.S. population (Federal Interagency Forum on Child and Family Statistics [FCFS], 2022b;

Kids Count Data Center, 2023b). While the number of children in the United States increased by nearly 2% from 2000 to 2015, the rest of the population grew 9 times faster during that same time (Myers, 2017). The child population has since decreased, from 74.2 million in 2010, to 73.1 million in 2020, to 72.5 million in 2022. This decrease in the child population reflects the decline in U.S. births, with an estimated 3.6 million births documented in 2020, compared with 4.0 million in 2010, resulting in fewer children under age 5 than in 2010 or 2000 (Census Bureau, 2023a).[1]

The Pew Research Center notes that three key demographic forces have reshaped the overall U.S. population recently: growing racial and ethnic diversity, increasing immigration, and rising percentage of older adults (Parker et al., 2018). However, these changes are uneven across the country, with a faster rate of change in urban counties than in suburban areas and smaller cities. Rates in rural counties have lagged the most, with half of rural counties having fewer residents in 2018 than they did in 2000. The number of children living in the 100 largest cities has decreased from 14.2 million in 2010 to 13.9 million in 2020 (a drop of 2.2%), consistent with the decrease in the number of children nationwide during this period (O'Hare & Mayol-Garcia, 2023). Immigration may also influence this reduction of children in urban areas, with settling of immigrants to rural counties steadily increasing over the past 10 years. Of note, the majority of rural counties had fewer U.S.-born residents in 2018 than they did in 2000 (Parker et al., 2018). Nonetheless, immigrants are still more concentrated in cities and suburbs than in rural areas.

Immigration

The overall U.S. population has grown more diverse in recent decades, with especially high rates of diversity among U.S. children. Analysis of child population Census data by the Annie E. Casey Foundation shows that the percentage of children of color has doubled in recent decades, from 26% in 1980 to 53% in 2020 (O'Hare, 2001; O'Hare & Mayol-Garcia, 2023).[2] In 2023, non-Hispanic White children still accounted for the largest racial

[1]Limitation of Census data in 2020: In the 2020 Census, there was a net undercount of 2.1% of all children (birth to age 17 years). Young children (birth to age 4 years) had a higher net undercount—5.4%—than any other age group. Preliminary analysis suggests young Black and Hispanic children were missed at a higher rate than non-Hispanic White children (Census Bureau, 2023a).

[2]To assess demographic change, O'Hare and Mayol-Garcia compare data from the 2020 and 2010 censuses with previous Annie E. Casey Foundation analysis of data on the child population from the 2000 Census (O'Hare, 2001; O'Hare & Mayol-Garcia, 2023, Table 3).

and ethnic group, at 49% (FCFS, 2023a).[3] Hispanic or Latino children represented 26% of children, Black children made up 14%, Asian children 6%, American Indian and Alaska Native 1%, and Native Hawaiian and other Pacific Islander less than 0.5% (FCFS, 2023a).

Regarding their households, in 2019, over a quarter (26.3%) of American children lived with a foreign-born parent (Anderson, Hemez, & Kreider, 2022),[4] and 21% spoke a language other than English at home (FCFS, 2023a). In 2022, an estimated 25% of children lived in immigrant families, either born outside of the United States themselves or living with at least one parent born outside of the United States (KFF, 2023b; Kids Count Data Center, 2023c).[5] In the past 30 years, the growth in the number of immigrant children offsets the decline in the number of nonimmigrant children (see Figure 4-1).

As of 2018, approximately 4 million children who are U.S. citizens lived with at least one undocumented parent; about 6 million in total lived with at least one undocumented family member (American Immigration Council, 2021). Between 2010 and 2021, the number of children with immigrant parents grew by 6%, a significantly slower rate of growth than from 2000 to 2010, when the number grew by 30% (Ward & Batalova, 2023).[6] Almost all children in immigrant families were born in the United States (88% in 2021), yet they are less likely to access health care (Brooks et al., 2020; Keisler-Starkey & Bunch, 2022; Keisler-Starkey, Bunch, & U.S. Census Bureau, 2020) and other health-related services (Haley et al., 2020) than are children with native-born parents.[7]

[3]FCFS (2023a) evaluates many sources of data when developing its yearly report on key national indicators of wellbeing. Sources used in this report, such as data from the U.S. Census Bureau, have implemented the standards for reporting race and ethnicity statistics issued in 1997 by the U.S. Office of Management and Budget.

[4]To explore the living arrangements of children by selected characteristics, Anderson, Hemez, and Kreider (2022) used data from the 2008 and 2018 American Community Survey (ACS), 2007 and 2019 Current Population Survey Annual Social and Economic Supplement, and 2014 Survey of Income and Program Participation.

[5]The Kids Count Data Center at the Annie E. Casey Foundation relied on analysis by the Population Reference Bureau of data from the U.S. Census Bureau, Census Supplementary Survey, and ACS. KFF analysis was performed on a 2022 ACS 1-year Public Use Microdata Sample.

[6]Ward and Batalova (2023) drew on statistics from the Migration Policy Institute, U.S. Census Bureau (using data from the 2021 ACS, 2022 Current Population Survey, and 2000 decennial Census), and the U.S. departments of Homeland Security and State.

[7]More than one in four immigrant children did not have health coverage in 2019 (25.5%, compared with 5.1% of native-born citizen children; Keisler-Starkey, Bunch, & U.S. Census Bureau, 2020). As of January 2020, 35 states and the District of Columbia provided health coverage to lawfully residing immigrant children without a 5-year wait (Brooks et al., 2020), and as of July 2019, six states and the District of Columbia use state-only funds to provide Medicaid coverage to income-eligible children regardless of immigration status (Artiga & Diaz, 2019).

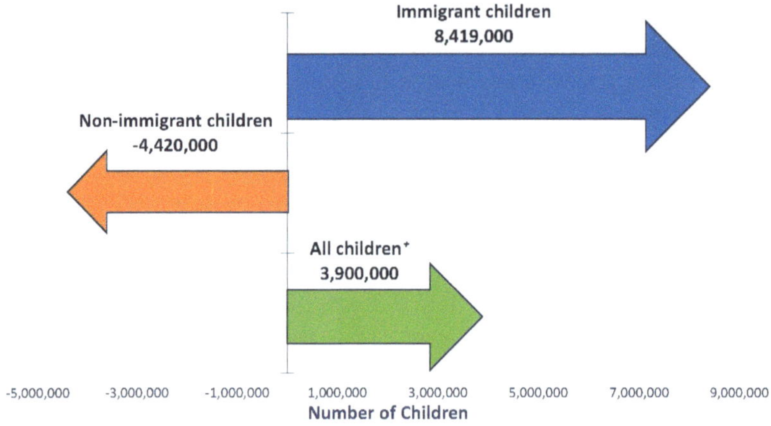

FIGURE 4-1 Growth in the number of U.S. children (under age 18) by immigrant status, 1994–2022.
NOTE: Children who are foreign born or reside with at least one foreign-born parent are considered immigrant children. Foreign-born children with native-born parents are considered nonimmigrant children. "All children" includes ~100,000 children without an immigrant status (i.e., children living in households with no parents present).
SOURCE: American Academy of Pediatrics, 2024, with data from U.S. Census Bureau, Current Population Survey Annual Social and Economic Supplement, and Current Population Reports.

Children migrating with their parents are at higher risk for adverse childhood experiences, chronic health conditions, trauma and exposure to violence, and development of mental health disorders (Alegría et al., 2023; Chang & Slopen, 2023; Claypool & Moore de Peralta, 2021; Linton et al., 2020). Refugee or unaccompanied children have increased levels of anxiety, depression, and post-traumatic stress disorder (PTSD; Frounfelker et al., 2020; Linton et al., 2020). Immigrant families may not have access to services; or, given their cultural views or worries about the cultural congruency of available services, they may not seek treatment because of shame and stigma related to mental health problems (Fendian, 2021; Mohammadifirouzeh et al., 2023). Integrating culturally sensitive mental health services into health care and schools allows for reduction in stigma and ease of access (Phelan et al., 2023).

According to estimates by the Migration Policy Institute and Urban Institute, at least 40% of children of immigrants had parents with limited English proficiency, which can pose challenges for parents in obtaining good jobs, finding and enrolling in public programs, navigating their children's education systems, and communicating with schools (Batalova, 2024; Lou & Lei, 2019). Children of parents who have low English proficiency are at increased risk of receiving suboptimal quality of care and worse health care access, including care for children with special health care needs (Blumberg et al., 2010; Dougherty et al., 2020; DuBard & Gizlice, 2008; Linton et al., 2020). Utilizing trained medical interpreter services appropriately alongside health care providers can improve care for this population (Linton et al., 2020). Additionally, depending on the legal status of the family, families may fear deportation or legal action when trying to seek services (Raphael et al., 2020; Rodriguez & McGrath, 2021). During the COVID-19 pandemic, immigrant families described hesitation in applying for benefits programs out of fear of deportation (Rodriguez & McGrath, 2021).

Poverty

Income level can have a significant impact on the health and wellbeing of children, as it impacts the capacity of their families to meet basic needs and can introduce high levels of family stress that impact important relationships and social interactions in a child's life. Family income influences where a child lives, what they eat, and what child care settings and schools they are able to attend. Living in poverty leaves children vulnerable to environmental, health, educational, and safety risks.

As noted, children in the United States experience high rates of poverty, substantially higher than in almost all other industrialized countries (National Academies, 2019a, 2023g). According to the United Nations Children's Fund (UNICEF), the United States is ranked 6th worst out of 41 countries for childhood poverty outcomes (Ingraham, 2014). Among children living in poverty in the United States, approximately three-quarters are children of color; two-thirds live in working families; and many live in single-parent households, primarily with their mothers (Haider, 2021; Office of Juvenile Justice and Delinquency Prevention, 2022a,b). More than 2 million children live in "deep poverty" (having family income below one-half of the poverty line; National Academies, 2019a). The highest rate of poverty of any age group is children under age 5 (Children's Defense Fund, 2023). Children in the South experience higher poverty rates than in other regions of the country. In 2022, Hispanic children were the largest group of children living in poverty, followed by Black, Asian, and White children (see Figure 4-2; Shrider & Creamer, 2023). Poverty rates among immigrant children, especially Hispanic children, are the highest, with child poverty rates twice as high as among immigrant families as among nonimmigrant families (Acevedo-Garcia et al., 2021). The U.S. Department of Education

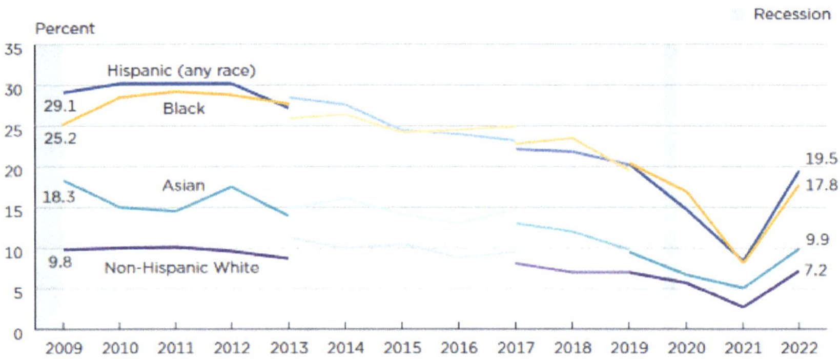

FIGURE 4-2 Child supplemental poverty rates by race and Hispanic origin, 2009–2022.
NOTE: Population as of March of the following year. The supplemental poverty measure estimates for 2019 and beyond reflect the implementation of revised methodology. The data for 2017 and beyond reflect the implementation of an updated processing system. The data for 2013 and beyond reflect the implementation of the redesigned income questions. The data points are placed at the midpoints of the respective years.
SOURCE: Shrider & Creamer, 2023; based on data from the U.S. Census Bureau, Current Population Survey, 2010–2023 Annual Social and Economic Supplements.

indicated a median estimated poverty rate of nearly 14% for children ages 5–17 in U.S. school districts in 2022 (Lui, 2023). This average hides the massive variation across districts, with the poverty rate ranging from just 3.1% in some districts to as high as 42.4% in others.

In 2021, child poverty levels fell dramatically—by nearly half—with the help of pandemic-era government programs and cash assistance not typically seen in other years. However, the end of these pandemic-era social safety net programs led to a doubling of the supplemental poverty measure rate for children from 2021 (5.2%) to 2022 (12.4%), returning to prepandemic levels and affecting about 9 million children (Shrider & Creamer, 2023).

Food security intersects with economic status—children living in households with annual incomes below the official poverty line have higher rates of food insecurity, with rates varying between rural and urban areas (Carson & Boege, 2020; Economic Research Service, 2023a; Marshall et al., 2022). In 2022, approximately 7.3 million children lived in food-insecure households, and the number of food-insecure households with children (insecure at least some point during the year) increased from approximately 6% in 2021 to almost 9% in 2022 (Rabbitt et al., 2023a,b). A growing body of evidence associates the negative consequences of food insecurity with children's health and developmental outcomes (Wight et al., 2014). For example, children in households experiencing food insecurity have rates of lifetime asthma diagnosis and depressive symptoms that were 19.1% and 27.9% higher, respectively, compared with their food-secure counterparts (Thomas, Miller, & Morrissey, 2019).

Housing also affects children's health outcomes. Housing that is inadequate, crowded, or too costly can pose serious problems for children's physical, psychological, and social wellbeing (Breysse et al., 2004; Frederick et al., 2014; Krieger & Higgins, 2002; Kushel et al., 2006). In 2021, 39% of U.S. households with children had one or more of three housing problems: physically inadequate housing, crowded housing, or housing cost burden greater than 30% of household income (FCFS, 2023b). During 2022, an estimated 97,800 children were homeless at a single point in time, and 10% of these children were unsheltered (FCFS, 2023b).

Historically marginalized people and their families are disproportionately impacted by homelessness. Black and Hispanic youth face greater risks, spending more time homeless than their White counterparts (Gonzalez et al., 2021). Among youth aged 13–25, American Indian and Alaska Native, Black, and Hispanic youth experience higher rates of homelessness (11%, 7%, and 7%, respectively) than White, non-Hispanic youth (4%; Gonzalez et al., 2021). The intersection of marginalized identities exacerbates these inequities, with LGBTQ+-identifying Black youth facing especially high rates of homelessness.

An Aging Population and Life Expectancy

Two major demographic changes document the importance of strengthening the health and wellbeing of America's children and youth: (1) major shifts in the population pyramid, with increasing longevity among older Americans and a declining birth rate and (2) major increases in chronic disease, disability, and early mortality among working-age U.S. adults. Numerous reports document the aging of the global population in recent years and in the United States, but few reference how rising lifespans of older populations relate to the decrease in birth rates and what changes in the population pyramid will mean for the country in the coming decades (National Academies, 2022a). In 1970, the population aged 65 and over was 9.8%, growing to 13% in 2010 and to 16.8%, or 55.8 million people, in 2020 (Caplan, 2023; Ortman, Velkoff, & Hogan, 2014). Conversely, the population of children has experienced a notable decline during the same time frame. In 1970, children under age 18 represented 36% of the total population, falling to 25% in 2010 and 22.1% in 2020 (Census Bureau,

1996, 2023a). This trend is expected to continue, presenting both social and economic challenges for policy makers and service providers (Caplan, 2023; Mather & Scommegna, 2024; Ortman, Velkoff, & Hogan, 2014; Urban Institute, 2024; Vespa, Medina, & Armstrong, 2020).

Beyond the dramatic increase in the ratio of older adults to children in the United States, the country has also experienced a marked decline in the fertility rate (Buckles, Guldi, & Schmidt, 2019). Since 2007, the number of U.S. births has declined and the fertility rate has dipped well below the "replacement rate" at which the number of births equals the number of deaths (Kearney & Levine, 2023). The end result of such a long-term trend will be an increasingly aging population and a declining economy as fewer workers care for more and more disabled citizens, a situation already evident in countries such as Japan and now China (Cheng et al., 2022).

Policies for supporting families with children, such as enhanced child leave, tax incentives, and increased educational support, have not coincided with a higher fertility rate in other countries even though they may be associated with improved outcomes for the children that are born (Malak, Rahman, & Yip, 2019). This points to other factors contributing to decreased birth rates, including shifts in social norms and attitudes. In the United States, immigration has maintained population numbers in spite of the declining fertility rates, although current political threats to immigration may limit its influence on numbers of workers and productivity (Pew Research Center, 2015).

The relative shortage of children and greater proportion of older adults in the United States will lead to an unbalanced level of workers and taxpayers supporting retired older adults (see *The New Importance of Children in America*; Myers, 2017). This imbalance will be felt unevenly, as urban areas have seen a sharp growth in the prime-age working population in recent years, while 88% of rural counties have lost prime-age workers since 2000 (Parker et al., 2018).

Trends in U.S. life expectancy also raise concerns and opportunities for the nation. Since 2010, U.S. life expectancy has been decreasing, in stark contrast with other industrialized countries (see Figure 4-3).

Despite increased longevity among older adult populations, U.S. life expectancy experienced notable declines, even prior to the COVID-19 pandemic (Arias et al., 2023; Bastian et al., 2020; Woolf & Schoomaker, 2019). This decline has been driven by increasing mortality rates among younger populations (Woolf & Schoomaker, 2019; Woolf, Wolf, & Rivara, 2023). This change reflects increases in successful suicide, drug overdoses, and gun violence. These in turn reflect growing rates of anxiety and depression in children and youth, which continue into young adulthood, leading to "deaths of despair" among young and middle-aged adults (Case & Deaton,

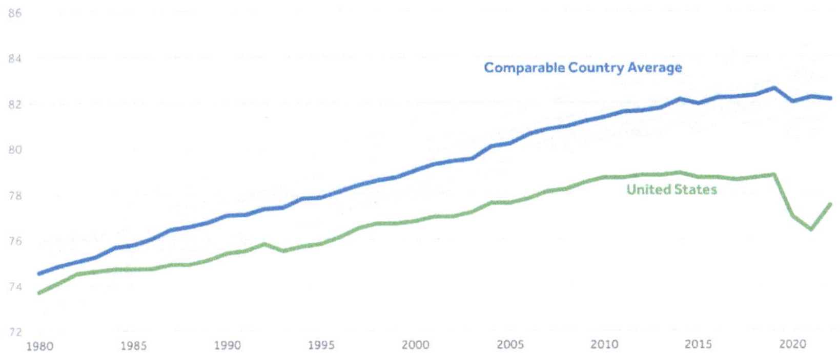

FIGURE 4-3 Life expectancy at birth in years, 1980–2022.
NOTE: Comparable countries include Australia, Austria, Belgium, Canada, France, Germany, Japan, the Netherlands, Sweden, Switzerland, and the United Kingdom. See Methods section of "How Does U.S. Life Expectancy Compare to Other Countries?" (Rakshit, McGough, & Amin, 2024).
SOURCE: Peterson-KFF Health System Tracker, 2022.

2022; see also Brignone et al., 2020). In addition, large increases in chronic conditions, especially obesity (Olshansky et al., 2005), pulmonary disease, and cardiovascular disease, have also made major contributions to increasing mortality. Most of these conditions have onset in childhood and adolescence, when opportunities to prevent them could result in major gains in U.S. life expectancy.

The COVID-19 pandemic accelerated the decline in life expectancy, with the Centers for Disease Control and Prevention (CDC) estimating a drop of 0.1 to 6.6 years due to COVID-19 (Andrasfay & Goldman, 2021; Arias & Tejada-Vera, 2023; Shmerling, 2022). Life expectancy from COVID-19 dropped more among American Indian/Alaska Native, Hispanic, and African American groups, which experienced higher rates of COVID-19 infection, hospitalization, and death than other groups (Andrasfay & Goldman, 2021; Arias & Tejada-Vera, 2023). Of note, however, life expectancy has recently begun to rise again (see Figure 4-3).

CURRENT STATE OF CHILD AND ADOLESCENT HEALTH

Chapter 1 noted that a growing proportion of children have chronic physical, mental, and social conditions and that this growth, particularly around mental and behavioral health, reflects early life experiences and community and environmental exposures. This section takes a closer look at the current state of the health and wellbeing of America's nearly

73 million children and youth, examining adverse experiences, health risks, and protective factors, chronic health conditions, and key causes of mortality.

The United States lags well behind other wealthy Organisation for Economic Co-operation and Development (OECD) countries on numerous indicators of child wellbeing (OECD, 2020, 2022). This analysis ranks the United States near the bottom of dozens of wealthy nations for infant mortality, low-weight births, childhood poverty, and several education and school success indicators. The United States ranked 36th out of 38 countries evaluated in the 2020 UNICEF report *Worlds of Influence: Understanding What Shapes Child Well-Being in Rich Countries*, which focused on children's mental wellbeing, physical health, and academic and social skills (Gromada et al., 2020). The United States ranks lowest among OECD countries for child physical health, including rates of childhood obesity (Fryar, Carroll, & Afful, 2020; Gromada et al., 2020). Additionally, the OECD 2022 Child Well-Being Dashboard ranks the United States well below average on life satisfaction among children, with only 31% of 15-year-old youth reporting high satisfaction with their life as a whole (OECD, 2022).

Consideration of the health status of children and youth must review not only the presence or absence of physical, developmental, and mental health conditions, but also their progress toward flourishing and wellbeing. Compared with ratings of children's overall health status, parents/caregivers tend to rank their children lower on important indicators of flourishing that impact quality of life (Child and Adolescent Health Measurement Initiative [CAHMI], 2024). Flourishing for children ages 6 months to 17 years has been assessed in the National Survey of Children's Health (NSCH) by asking parents whether children show interest and curiosity in learning new things, are able to regulate emotions and behaviors when faced with a challenge, and can focus and persist to complete tasks (Bethell et al., 2019a). Studies using these measures of child flourishing find positive associations with school engagement, health behaviors, wellbeing, and life expectancy. They also note variations in flourishing among children with similar risks (e.g., poverty, disability, adverse childhood experiences) that link to measures of positive family relationship factors. (Bethell, Gombojav, & Whitaker, 2019; Kandasamy et al., 2018). Based on recent findings from the NSCH, only 21.5% of caregivers both report that their child's overall health status is excellent or very good and that their child is also consistently flourishing (CAHMI, 2024).

As delineated in Chapter 2, whole child and family health and wellbeing emerges through a complex and dynamic development process that integrates a range of biological, interpersonal, social, environmental, and behavioral influences. These factors can shape and modify brain development, gene expression, and physiologic, mental, emotional, social, and behavioral functioning. Several social and environmental influences can optimize health and wellbeing, including: (1) positive childhood experiences, whereby children and youth have a sense of being physically and emotionally safe, nurtured, and loved and that they belong at home, school, and in the community; (2) environments that support children's emotional and cognitive engagement, curiosity and interest in learning, and activities for positive social interaction; (3) experiences that develop children's skills for building and maintaining positive relationships and the capacity to sustain a sense of meaning and hope for the future; and (4) environments free from discrimination (La Charite et al., 2023; Sege & Harper Browne, 2017; Wallerich et al., 2023). Such enduring influences and childhood experiences promote wellbeing and can buffer the impact of adverse childhood experiences and other health risks.

Adverse Childhood Experiences

Adverse childhood experiences refer to potentially traumatic events that occur before age 18 years, including, among other forms, physical, emotional, or sexual abuse; neglect; and household dysfunction (CDC, 2019d). These experiences have been shown to have profound and long-lasting impacts on an individual's physical and mental health, as well as their overall wellbeing. Adverse childhood experiences are common across all communities and socioeconomic groups in the United States but are more prevalent among historically marginalized populations (Camacho & Clark Henderson, 2022; Mersky et al., 2021; Sacks & Murphey, 2018).

CDC (2019d) estimates one in six adults have experienced four or more types of adverse childhood experiences, and research has now established numerous linkages between these experiences in childhood and lifelong health risks. Preventing adverse childhood experiences can help children and adults to thrive, reducing health conditions, risky behaviors, and socioeconomic challenges.

The consequences of adverse childhood experiences are far-reaching and can manifest in various ways throughout an individual's life. Children who experience adversity are more likely to struggle with academic performance, behavioral issues, and mental health problems such as depression and anxiety (CDC, 2019d). As adults, those with a history of adverse childhood experiences are at increased risk for chronic health conditions such as heart disease, cancer, and substance abuse disorders, as well as shorter life expectancy and decreased life opportunities (e.g., educational achievement and job potential; Brown et al., 2009; Dube et al., 2003; Elmore & Crouch, 2020; Grummitt et al., 2021; Iverson, Cook, & Iverson, 2024; Walker et al., 2022). Recognizing the impact of adverse childhood experiences, and implementing strategies for preventing and mitigating their effects, has become a public health priority, with efforts focused on promoting resilience and trauma-informed care and addressing the social determinants of health (Jones, Merrick, & Houry, 2020a).

Chronic Conditions and Disabilities

A large and increasing number of U.S. children have some chronic health condition, and many require substantial care by families and the health care system. Rates of chronic conditions have risen dramatically over the past half century, partly because of improved survival rates for more complex conditions that previously would have led to early death (e.g., spina bifida, cystic fibrosis, leukemia, sickle cell disease; Payot & Barrington, 2011). However, a larger contributor has been more common conditions that are not associated with early death—especially asthma, obesity, mental health conditions (especially anxiety, depression, attention deficit hyperactivity disorder [ADHD], and substance use), and neurodevelopmental conditions (especially autism spectrum disorders, cerebral palsy; Jo et al., 2019; Perrin, Anderson, & van Cleave, 2014). Most of these conditions continue into adulthood and help account for growing chronic conditions among working-age adults (Institute of Medicine [IOM], 2007b).

Children who experience diverse conditions can be understood in overlapping categories: The first includes children with complex conditions involving multiple organ systems (e.g., mobility, lungs, feeding) and requiring multiple supports, including technological and equipment support. About 1% of U.S. children are in this category, although their care accounts for much higher expenditures than most other children (estimates range $50–$110 billion annually; Bergman et al., 2020; Berry et al., 2014; Cohen et al., 2011, 2018; Kuo et al., 2011; Murphy et al., 2020). The second category includes children with relatively low-prevalence but usually high-severity conditions (e.g., spina bifida, leukemia, arthritis, sickle cell anemia, cystic fibrosis; Perrin, Anderson, & van Cleave, 2014). These children, who represent at least 2% of the U.S. population, require ongoing support and access to specialized therapies and devices that may not be widely accessible in a child's community or even state. The third category, about 10 times larger than the first two, includes high-prevalence conditions such as asthma, obesity, mental health conditions, and neurodevelopmental conditions (Maenner et al., 2023; Perrin, Anderson, & van Cleave, 2014). These are discussed in more detail below. The last category includes children in apparent good health, without any chronic conditions, although they may face adversity in childhood as discussed above, putting them at risk for later chronic conditions.

Table 4-1 provides a comparative snapshot of national and state data on prevalence of chronic health conditions, special health care needs, and functional difficulties, using data from the 2021 and 2022 NSCH. The U.S. Census Bureau (2024) conducts the NSCH annually for the U.S. Department of Health and Human Services's (HHS's) Health Resources and Services Administration (HRSA) Maternal and Child Health Bureau. All NSCH data collected are self-reported by parents or caregivers.

These data indicate that about 20% of children under age 18 years have a special health care need (HRSA, n.d.e). Over one in four households with children, 28.6%, has at least one child or youth with special health care needs (HRSA, n.d.e). These children are more likely to live in low-income neighborhoods and rely more on public health insurance; over half also have a co-occurring behavioral or mental health diagnosis such as ADHD or anxiety (Kids Count Data Center, 2023a). Among low-income children with special health care needs, about 85% of children do not receive needed health care, mainly because of cost and lack of access (Houtrow et al., 2020; Kids Count Data Center, 2023a).

Special Needs, Medical Complexity, and Functional Disability

Various agencies and clinical groups use different terms to describe chronic conditions among children, such as "disability," "special health care need," "functional limitation," "complex medical condition," and others. These terms describe overlapping groups, and in turn various strategies exist for identifying children and youth with these conditions. Some strategies use lists of specific conditions (Agency for Healthcare Research and Quality [AHRQ], 2022b; Berry et al., 2015; Goodman et al., 2013; Simon et al., 2018). Others use a series of screening questions based on characteristics of chronic conditions, arising from the body of evidence regarding common needs or impacts across various conditions (McPherson et al., 1998; Stein et al., 1987; World Health Organization [WHO], 2013). In most cases, these approaches have been validated through studies of chronic physical conditions, with varied evidence of their ability to identify young people with chronic mental and behavioral conditions.

The definition of "children with special health care needs" emerged in 1998 to assist leaders in health policy, payment, and state programs in planning service delivery for this patient population (Kuhlthau et al., 2022). Children with special health care needs were defined as those "who have or are at increased risk for a chronic physical, developmental, behavioral, or emotional condition and who also require health and related services of a type or amount beyond that required by children generally" (McPherson

TABLE 4-1 National and State-Level Child Prevalence of Chronic Health Conditions, Special Health Care Needs, and Functional Difficulties

Chronic Health Condition, Special Health Care Need, and Functional Difficulty Indicators	National Prevalence, % (Across State Prevalence Range)	Children with Any Public Health Insurance, %	Children with Private Health Insurance, %
Children with one or more of 24 chronic or lifelong health conditions[a]	38.8 (30.6–45.9)	42.9	37.7
Children diagnosed with one or more physical or genetic health conditions[b]	28.9 (23.1–34.6)	31.7	28.1
Children diagnosed with one or more mental, emotional, and/or behavioral health conditions	18.4 (12.4–27.6)	22.9	16.6
Children diagnosed with one or more developmental health conditions	12.5 (9.4–15.8)	17.4	10.2
Children with any chronic condition who also require an above-routine type/amount of health care services	20.0 (13.9–25.3)	25.9	17.5
Children born premature and/or with a low birth weight (less than 2,500 grams at birth)	15.3 (11.1–21.1)	17.6	13.7
Children with obesity (body mass index–for–age equal to or greater than the 95th percentile), ages 6–17 years	18.1 (11.6–26.1)	26.2	13.2
Children experiencing one or more of 12 functional difficulties[c]	23.9 (16.7–30.7)	32.0	19.3

[a]The 24 conditions asked about in the National Survey of Children's Health (NSCH) include (1) physical or genetic health conditions: allergies (food, drug, insect, or other), arthritis/autoimmune disease, asthma, blood disorders (e.g., sickle cell disease, thalassemia, hemophilia), cerebral palsy, cystic fibrosis, diabetes, Down syndrome, epilepsy or seizure disorder, genetic or inherited condition, heart condition, frequent or severe headaches including migraine (3–17 years), hearing problems, and vision problems; (2) mental, emotional, and/or behavioral conditions: anxiety problems (3–17 years), depression (3–17 years), autism or autism spectrum disorder (3–17 years), attention deficit disorder or attention deficit hyperactivity disorder (3–17 years); (3) developmental health conditions: Tourette syndrome (3–17 years), behavioral or conduct problem (3–17 years), developmental delay (3–17 years), intellectual disability (3–17 years), speech or other language disorder (3–17 years), or learning disability (also known as mental retardation; 3–17 years).
[b]Children with any chronic condition and need and/or use of an above-routine type or amount of health care services (national definition of "children and youth with special health care needs") is assessed using the validated Children with Special Health Care Needs screener.
[c]The 12 functional difficulties asked about in the NSCH include (1) physical limitations: frequent or chronic difficulty with breathing or other respiratory problems; eating or swallowing; digesting food (including stomach/intestinal problems, constipation, or diarrhea); repeated or chronic physical pain (including headaches or other back or body pain); deafness or problems with hearing; blindness or problems with seeing, even when wearing glasses; (2) activity limitations: using their hands (0–5 years); coordination and moving around (0–5 years); serious difficulty walking or climbing stairs (6–17 years); difficulty dressing or bathing (6–17 years); difficulty doing errands alone, such as visiting a doctor's office or shopping (12–17 years); (3) socioemotional difficulties: serious difficulty concentrating, remembering, or making decisions (6–17 years).
NOTES: "Public insurance" is defined as Medicaid, Medical Assistance, or any kind of government assistance plan for those with low incomes or a disability. "Private insurance" is defined as insurance through a current or former employer or union, insurance purchased directly from an insurance company, TRICARE or other military health care, or coverage through the Affordable Care Act or other private insurance.
SOURCE: 2021 and 2022 NSCH (CAHMI, 2024).

et al., 1998, para. 11; see also HRSA, n.d.a). The Children with Special Health Care Needs screener is used most commonly (Bethell et al., 2015, see Table 4-1).

The National Academies Committee on Improving Health Outcomes for Children with Disabilities (National Academies, 2018) defined "disability" as "an environmentally contextualized health-related limitation in a child's existing or emergent capacity to perform developmentally appropriate activities and participate, as desired, in society" (National Academies, 2018, p. 23; see also Halfon et al., 2012). Its report notes also that the varied definitions and lack of a consistent framework led to different estimates of the size of the population of children with disabilities (Currie & Kahn, 2012; National Academies, 2018). In one estimate, the U.S. Census Bureau reports that the percentage of children in the United States with one of six types of functional limitations as a disability increased between 2008 and 2019, from 3.9% to 4.3%, to around 3 million children under age 18 (Young, 2021; Young & Crankshaw, 2021). In other surveys, an estimated 13–15% of children experience a larger range of functional difficulties that impact daily living (2020–2021 National Health Interview Survey; NSCH; see also Table 4-1).[8]

Government agencies that provide services for individuals with disabilities define "disability" in a way that is specific to their legislative mandate. For example, the Individuals with Disabilities Education Act (2004) defines disability more broadly than does the Social Security Administration (SSA), given the agencies' disparate purposes. The Supplemental Security Income program, administered by SSA, provides cash support for children and other people with severe disabilities. To determine eligibility, SSA uses a combination of diagnoses with specific indicators of severity, along with some functional measures for people who may have severe disability but who do not meet the specific diagnostic criteria (National Academies, 2015). Given the complexity of multiple systems with different eligibility requirements, families face barriers and challenges in navigating the various programs that provide health, education, social, emotional, employment, and financial supports (National Academies, 2018).

[8]The FCFS 2023 *America's Children* report considers a child to be disabled if their daily activities are consistently impacted by any one of the 13 functional difficulties assessed through the 2020–2021 National Health Interview Survey (NHIS), whether or not the child also experiences a diagnosed health condition. This method identifies 13% of children ages 5–17 as having a disability. The functional difficulties evaluated through the NSCH comprise a similar list as those used in the NHIS disability indicator. Yet, rather than label children as having a disability due to the presence of any functional difficulty, the NSCH identifies children with chronic conditions and special health care needs due to their condition and enables assessing whether or not these children also experience functional difficulties. Such a calculation results in identifying 15.2% of children ages 6–17 as having any chronic or lifelong health condition that requires above-routine health care services and who also experience one or more functional difficulty.

Chronic Conditions

Rates and types of chronic conditions vary across populations. For example, immigrant children have a notably lower likelihood of having one or more chronic conditions compared with native-born children (Singh, Yu, & Kogan, 2013), with a prevalence of 6.8% in Asian immigrant children, compared with 30.6% in native-born non-Hispanic Black children. Children living in English-speaking households are more than twice as likely to have a mental, emotional, or behavioral health diagnosis than those living in non-English-speaking households. Hispanic children have higher rates of obesity; dental caries; and some congenital conditions, such as spina bifida (Berry, Rock et al., 2013; Ogden et al., 2020; Palfrey et al., 2004). For some chronic conditions, such as autism spectrum disorder, rates of diagnosis continue to increase, in part because of better awareness of these conditions and improvement in screening practices.

Substantial variations are also observed consistently in the prevalence of chronic health conditions across communities, and these variations remain after adjusting for differences in the sociodemographic characteristics of children across states and align with variations in access to and quality of health care services and systems (Bethell et al., 2014; Blumberg et al., 2010). The severity of chronic health conditions varies across conditions, impacted by underlying medical factors, natural variation, the quality of health services children receive, and a range of social and environmental factors (Bethell et al., 2014).

Five conditions of high prevalence provide examples of how chronic conditions affect children and families and often persist into adulthood: asthma; overweight and obesity; neurodevelopmental conditions; mental, emotional, and behavioral health disorders; and substance use disorders. There are notable disparities in prevalence, outcomes, and care management for each condition. Certain populations, such as children in foster care and those in contact with the juvenile justice system, have elevated rates of chronic conditions, particularly mental, emotional, and behavioral health disorders. A high proportion of children and youth in foster care and those incarcerated have lapses in preventive care and unmet physical, developmental, and mental health needs. This is often the result of frequent changes in living situations and disruptions in continuity of care and access to health care coverage (Barnert et al., 2020; Committee on Adolescence, Braverman, & Murray, 2011; Deutsch & Fortin, 2015; Owen et al., 2020).

These conditions are preventable or manageable and offer opportunity for policy interventions and cross-sector collaboration. It is also important to recognize that among children with any one chronic condition most experience another condition as well. For example, 77% of children with asthma and most children with depression (93.5%) also experience at least one other condition (CAHMI, 2024). Common comorbidities have led to health care system efforts to integrate pediatric health care and related services.

Asthma

Asthma, a chronic lung disease, can affect people of any age, but it is one of the most common chronic conditions for children (WHO, 2023). In 2021, 6.5% of children under age 18 years were estimated to have an asthma diagnosis (CDC, 2023a; Federal Interagency Forum on Child and Family Statistics, n.d.), with wide variation across population groups, from 3.3% of Asian-American children to 5.9% of Hispanic children, to 11.6% of Black children (CDC, 2021d). With good care, most children manage their asthma well. However, if not properly managed, children may require emergency department visits and hospitalizations. In 2021, approximately 38.7% of children in the United States under age 18 years with asthma had one or more asthma attacks in the past 12 months (Elflein, 2023). This statistic underscores the persistent challenges in achieving optimal control over this chronic respiratory condition among the pediatric population. Data on asthma are collected through a variety of methods, leading to robust asthma surveillance across the country, including prevalence, medications used, emergency room visits, and days of work or school lost.

Many studies document disparities in asthma medication use (Amin et al., 2020; McQuaid, 2018), health care utilization (Fitzpatrick et al., 2019), and outcomes in low-income and racial/ethnic minority patients (Federico et al., 2020; Perez & Coutinho, 2021; Redmond et al., 2022). These disparities led to the creation of a federal task force to examine root causes and recommend remediations. The task force recommended controlling environmental exposures to air pollutants and environmental hazards, and improving access to care for communities with high asthma prevalence (Environmental Protection Agency [EPA], 2012). Current efforts to address environmental asthma triggers involve controlling environmental factors in schools, homes, and communities (EPA, 2012; Matsui, Abramson, & Sandel, 2016).

Asthma is a leading cause of school absenteeism (Qin et al., 2022). Students with asthma miss an average of 2.3 more days of school each year than those without asthma. Asthma is the most common cause of pediatric emergency department use (Butz et al., 2013; CDC, 2023c; Yoong et al., 2021). Morbidity remains high, especially among inner-city children (Butz et al., 2013; Poowuttikul, Saini, & Seth, 2019). Poor urban communities face higher rates of pollution and infestations that can exacerbate asthma, as well as other characteristics associated with higher rates of asthma (Aryee et al., 2022).

Overweight and Obesity

CDC (2024f,g) defines "obesity" as having a body mass index (BMI) greater than or equal to the 95th percentile for children overall. Data from the National Health and Nutrition Examination Survey (Fryar, Carroll, & Afful, 2020) indicate that nearly two in five children ages 2–19 (almost 40%) have obesity, a rate that has increased greatly from 13.9% in 2000. An additional 16% are "overweight," defined as having a BMI between the 85th and

95th percentiles (Fryar, Carroll, & Afful, 2020). Rates of being overweight are highest among Hispanic and non-Hispanic Black children (26.2% and 24.8%, respectively; CDC, 2024e,f). The COVID-19 pandemic worsened the obesity epidemic, especially among children (World Obesity Federation, 2023). Childhood obesity has been linked to higher increased total medical costs, outpatient visit costs, and hospitalization costs than childhood overweight. By 2050 the annual direct costs related to childhood obesity will be $13.62 billion and the indirect health care costs will be $49.02 billion (Ling et al., 2023).

A complex interplay of genetic, environmental, and socioecological factors affects the development of obesity (Aris et al., 2022; Hampl et al., 2023), and higher rates are associated with low socioeconomic status, exposure to adverse childhood experiences, and high needs related to other social determinants of health (Bethell et al., 2014; Hampl et al., 2023). Contributing factors include food insecurity, restricted availability of healthy food choices, limited time and access to opportunities for physical activity and recreation, and discrimination and stigma (Williams, Burns, & Rudowitz, 2023). Notably, the rate of obesity continues to increase for children in low-income households (Hampl et al., 2023; Iacopetta et al., 2024; Lange et al., 2021). Obesity is associated with increased prevalence of later serious conditions, including hypertension, diabetes, metabolic dysfunction–associated fatty liver disease (previously termed "nonalcoholic fatty liver disease"), and obstructive sleep apnea (Dietz et al., 2015; Hampl et al., 2023).

U.S. children have low rates of physical activity, exacerbating the obesity epidemic. In 2021, over 54% of high schoolers said they were physically active for less than 60 minutes for 5 days of the week. Nearly 16% were physically active for less than 60 minutes on just 1 day (CDC, 2021c). According to 2021 NSCH data, only 20.3% of children ages 1–5 years experience at least five of the six evidence-based health behaviors associated with childhood obesity prevention, including daily consumption of fruits and vegetables, sufficient sleep and outdoor play, limited consumption of sugary drinks, and less screen time (HRSA, 2023k). This number increased to 30.7% for children living in households with incomes 400% or more above the federal poverty level (HRSA, 2023k). Children covered by Medicaid are more than twice as likely to experience obesity compared with those with private insurance: 26.0% of Medicaid-enrolled children have obesity, in contrast to 11.4% among children with private insurance alone (Estabrooks & Shetterly, 2007).

Obesity is a serious public health issue, associated with both immediate and long-term health problems (BeLue, Francis, & Colaco, 2009; Dietz, 1998; Ebbeling et al., 2002; Freeman, Walker, & Vrana, 1999; Gilliland et al., 2003; Luppino et al., 2010; Reilly et al., 2003). Children with obesity are five times more likely to be obese in adulthood and experience elevated risk for other illnesses and early death (Ferraro, Thorpe, & Wilkinson, 2003; Simmonds et al., 2016; Tsoi et al., 2022). Severe obesity was more common among individuals aged 40–59 than other age groups (Hales et al., 2020).

Neurodevelopmental Conditions

Neurodevelopmental conditions affect cognition, communication, behavior, and/or motor skills, stemming from irregularities in brain development (Mullin et al., 2013); they include intellectual disabilities, communication disorders, autism spectrum disorder, specific learning disorders, and movement disorders (Cainelli & Bisiacchi, 2023).

Autism spectrum disorder, a lifelong developmental disability, is associated with difficulties with social communication and interaction, and repetitive or restricted behaviors or interests, affecting one's learning, cognitive organization, attention, and adaptive skills (Drmic, Szatmari, & Volkmar, 2017). Diagnoses of autism spectrum disorder have increased in recent decades, and prevalence of diagnoses among children has risen markedly in the United States between 2000 and 2020—in 2020 an estimated 2.8–3.5% of children were identified as having autism spectrum disorder (Li et al., 2022b; Maenner et al., 2023; Rice et al., 2012).

Autism spectrum disorder is almost four times more common among boys than among girls (Maenner et al., 2023). Before 2016, more White children than Black or Hispanic children were diagnosed with autism by age 8 years (CDC, 2019c, 2023g). However, these disparities have decreased, with no overall difference observed in the percentage of Asia Pacific or Pacific Islander, Black, Hispanic, or White children identified with autism by age 8 in 2018. In 2018, however, a new trend emerged, with higher rates of 4-year-old Black and Hispanic children diagnosed with autism compared with their White counterparts (CDC, 2019c, 2023g). This pattern persisted in 2020 among 4-year-olds and was noted for the first time among 8-year-olds. These findings suggest potential advances in autism awareness, identification, and access to services for Black, Hispanic, and Asia Pacific children, indicating a need to investigate factors such as social determinants of health that may contribute to higher disability rates in historically underserved populations (CDC, 2019c, 2023g). Autism spectrum disorder presents with a diverse range of characteristics, including onset, symptoms, and severities, with needed variation in appropriate health care (Malik-Soni et al., 2022). Many children with autism also have ADHD, adding complexity to health and educational interventions (Zablotsky et al., 2023).

Intellectual and developmental disabilities constitute a broad group of differences that are usually present at birth and affect the trajectory of the individual's physical, intellectual, and/or emotional development (National Institute of Child Health and Human Development [NICHD], n.d.). Intellectual disability starts any time before age 18 years and involves limitations to both intellectual functioning or intelligence (e.g., ability to learn, problem solve) and adaptive behavior (e.g., everyday social and life skills). Developmental disabilities include a broader category of often lifelong challenges that can be intellectual, physical, or both. The term "intellectual and developmental disabilities" is often used to describe situations in which both intellectual disability and other disabilities are present (NICHD, n.d.). Children with these disabilities from historically marginalized and ethnic backgrounds often encounter barriers to care related to negative social determinants of health, leading to unfavorable health outcomes (Magaña, Heydarian, & Vanegas, 2022; Parish et al., 2013).

Mental, Emotional, and Behavioral Health

Concerns with children's mental, emotional, and behavioral health have been growing in recent years, with greater recognition of its contribution to child wellbeing (see Chapter 2; see also Shim & Compton, 2020; Whitney & Peterson, 2019). Children's mental health conditions are typically characterized by disruptions or alterations in thinking, behaviors, social skills, or emotional regulation (American Academy of Pediatrics [AAP], 2021a; CDC, 2024q). These challenges interfere with the ability to function effectively at home, in school, or in other social settings. Common childhood mental health disorders include ADHD, anxiety (manifesting as fears or worries), depression, substance use, and behavior disorders (Bethell, Garner, et al., 2022; CDC, 2024q). In 2018–2019, 13.2% of U.S. children ages 3–17—just over 8 million—had a diagnosis of at least one of the following: depression, anxiety, ADHD, or a behavioral or conduct disorder (Census Bureau, 2024), with somewhat higher rates for non-Hispanic White and non-Hispanic Black children. The conditions diagnosed most often were ADHD and anxiety, each affecting approximately 1 in 11 children (CDC, 2024r).

More than 19% of adolescents (ages 12–17) reported a major depressive episode in the past year (Substance Abuse and Mental Health Services Administration [SAMHSA], 2022a,b); 13.5% had serious thoughts of suicide, with 6.5% making a suicide plan, and nearly 4% attempting suicide. From 2019 to 2021, female adolescents had increased prevalence of seriously considered suicide (from 24.1% in 2019 to 30% in 2021), an increase in making a suicide plan (from 19.9% to 23.6%), and an increase in suicide attempts (from 11.0% to 13.3%; CDC, 2024k).

Typically, ADHD is first diagnosed in childhood and often persists into adulthood (Nigg et al., 2020; Salari et al., 2023; Wilens & Spencer, 2010). In 2018, nearly 10% of children ages 3–17 years had a diagnosis of ADHD (CDC, 2018). For Black children, this number was nearly 13%, but for Hispanic children, it was less than 7%, and for Asian children it was only 3.2%. Many evidence-based pharmacological and psychosocial treatments for ADHD exist, with increased utilization linked to enhanced acute and long-term outcomes (Baweja, Soutullo, & Waxmonsky, 2021); nonetheless, long-term results are often less optimal, as many individuals do not access multimodal treatments and many stop care prematurely (Froehlich & Brinkman, 2018; National Institute for Health and Care Excellence, 2018; Wolraich et al., 2019). Over the life course, ADHD increases the risk for serious secondary mental health issues, such as substance use disorder, depression, psychosis, and anxiety. The condition also affects life outcomes such as school and occupational underachievement, unemployment, poor overall health, housing instability, injuries, and suicide (Agnew-Blais & Seidman, 2013; Forte et al., 2020; Groenman, Janssen, & Oosterlaan, 2017; Kessler et al., 2006; Lee et al., 2011; Nigg et al., 2020).

The many children with mental health challenges face difficulty obtaining necessary diagnostic and treatment services (CDC, 2023e). Adolescents are more likely to receive any form of mental health treatment than younger children, although less than 20% in either group received services (Zablotsky & Ng, 2023). Across the lifespan, mental health and mental disorders are often comorbid with physical conditions and chronic diseases (Bitsko et al., 2022; Merikangas et al., 2015), indicating the need for integrated services that address both physical and mental health needs of children and youth (Arrojo et al., 2023; Catalano & Kellogg, 2020).

Mental and behavioral health conditions are often chronic. Half of all lifetime cases start by age 14 years and three-fourths start by age 24 years (National Research Council & IOM, 2009). Childhood mental health problems, if not addressed, may persist into adolescence and adulthood. Adverse childhood experiences, such as trauma or neglect, can further exacerbate mental health challenges (Ceccarelli et al., 2022). An accumulation of adverse childhood experiences raises the likelihood of developing psychopathology in adulthood, along with impairments in social functioning (Gu et al., 2022).

Substance Use Disorders

The initiation of substance use is common during adolescence and emerging adulthood. After seeing a decrease in youth substance use between 2020 and 2021, in 2022 substance use rates either remained stable (cannabis use and nicotine vaping) or returned to prepandemic levels (alcohol use). Rates of use vary by age with 15% of 8th graders and 52% of 12th graders using alcohol within the last 12 months (Miech et al., 2023). For some youth, early substance use can become problematic and result in substance use disorders as early as during adolescence and early adulthood.

Substance use disorders include the misuse or excessive use of drugs or alcohol (Nationwide Children's Hospital, n.d.b; Thomasius, Paschke, & Arnaud, 2022) and are prevalent among adolescents, spiking during early adulthood. According to the 2022 National Survey on Drug Use and Health, more than 17.3% of people (48 million) aged 12 and older had a substance use disorder in the previous year (SAMHSA, 2022a,b). Young adults ages 18–25 had the highest rates (25.6% or 8.6 million) of past-year substance use disorders, including binge drinking in the past month and heavy alcohol, marijuana, or prescription pain medication abuse. And 8.5% of adolescents ages 12–17 reported having a substance use disorder (2.2 million people; SAMHSA, 2021). Among youth, alcohol use disorder is the most common type, followed by marijuana use disorder. Prevalence of misuse of prescription pain relievers among adolescents ages 12–17 was 1.9% and 3% among young adults ages 18–25 (SAMHSA, 2021). Beyond those diagnosed with substance use disorders, many more young people use substances regularly, an opportunity for prevention before use becomes a disorder. Among people aged 12 or older in 2022, nearly 60% (168.7 million) used tobacco products, vaped nicotine, used alcohol, or used an illicit drug in the past month ("current use"; SAMHSA, 2022a,b,d).

Rates vary among population groups, with illicit drug use disorder higher among those reporting two or more races (5.0%) and among American Indian/Alaska Native individuals (4.8%; Center for Behavioral Health Statistics and Quality, 2021). American Indian/Alaska Native individuals had higher rates of alcohol use disorder (8.3%) than other racial/ethnic groups; White individuals had higher rates (5.8%) than Black, Hispanic, and Asian individuals (4.8%, 5.2%, and 3.3%, respectively).

Substance use disorders often coexist with mental health conditions such as depression or anxiety (Alsheikh et al., 2020; Perrin et al., 2019). In 2021, nearly 4% of adolescents (ages 12–17) had both a substance use disorder and a major depressive episode in the previous year, with most reporting severe impairment to ability to function. Higher rates were found among multiracial, Hispanic, and White adolescents than among Black adolescents (SAMHSA, 2021). Adolescents with a past-year major depressive episode were more likely (27.7%) than their peers without such an episode (10.7%) to use illicit drugs, including marijuana use (20.3% vs. 8.0%; SAMHSA, 2021) and to binge alcohol and use tobacco products in the past month.

Addressing substance use in childhood, adolescence, and young adulthood through prevention, early identification, and treatment is crucial for their health and wellbeing (Camenga et al., 2022; Fadus et al., 2019; HHS, 2016; Hsiung et al., 2022). Failure to intervene early or provide age-appropriate substance use services can lead to significant and long-term adverse consequences for individuals and families, and across generations (Straussner & Fewell, 2018).

Typically, initial substance use begins during childhood or adolescence (Bahl et al., 2023; Forouzanfar et al., 2015). Individuals who initiate substance use at an early age face elevated risks of psychosocial problems across multiple life domains—including behavior patterns, psychiatric disorders, family dynamics, peer relationships, leisure and recreation, and work adjustment—compared with those who start substance use later in life (Poudel & Gautam, 2017). Promisingly, programs aimed at preventing adolescent substance use have the potential to cultivate lasting individual and interpersonal resilience factors (Camenga et al., 2022; Feinberg et al., 2022). These factors not only enable participants to navigate unforeseen periods of acute stress and adversity but also contribute to the wellbeing of both participants and their future children, with reduced deterioration in health and overall wellbeing.

Leading Causes of Mortality and Injury

Childhood mortality rates had decreased for decades until 2020, when the all-cause mortality rate for those between ages 1 and 19 increased by nearly 11% from the previous year (Woolf, Wolf, & Rivara, 2023). It then rose another 8.3% between 2020 and 2021. Although COVID-19 played an important role, the increase can be attributed mainly to injuries, including suicide, homicide, drug overdoses, transportation-related deaths, and fires or burns (CDC, 2021c; Woolf, Wolf, & Rivara, 2023). In 2020, the absolute increase in injury deaths alone for ages 1–19 was nearly 12 times higher (2.80 deaths per 100,000) than the mortality rate due to COVID-19 (0.24 deaths per 100,000; Murphy et al., 2021). Among children ages 1–9, injuries explained two-thirds (64%) of the increase in all-cause mortality in 2020. Suicide is the second-leading cause of death among children ages 10–14 and the third leading cause of death, behind homicide, for youth ages 14–18 years (Woolf, Wolf, & Rivara, 2023).

These risks and rates differ across population groups, with greater increases in injuries among males. Non-Hispanic Black youths accounted for nearly 63% of homicide victims ages 10–19 in 2020 (Woolf, Wolf, & Rivara, 2023). Notably, as well, the child mortality rate in the United States has been higher than other wealthy nations since the 1980s (Thakrar et al., 2018). This section continues with a focus on the top contributors to child mortality and injury: infant mortality, gun violence, self-harm and suicide, and child abuse and domestic violence.

Infant Mortality and Low Birth Weight

According to CDC, in 2022, the United States had 20,538 infant deaths, a 3% increase from 2021 (Ely & Driscoll, 2022), representing 5.6 infant deaths per 1,000 live births, with variation across the states. In 2019, Massachusetts had the lowest rate at 3.8 deaths per 1,000 live births and Mississippi had the highest at 8.6 deaths per 1,000 live births. Similar to maternal mortality, infant death rates also differ by race (see Figure 4-4). Leading causes of death were typically related to maternal complications and bacterial sepsis of newborns (Ely & Driscoll, 2022). Other causes include low birth weight, circulatory system diseases, unintentional injury, and respiratory distress of the newborn. The United States has around 3.6 million live births annually, with approximately 10% categorized as preterm births (delivery before 37 weeks gestational age; WHO, n.d.b) and 8–9% as low birth weight (less than 2,500 grams or 5.5 pounds; Hamilton, Martin, & Osterman, 2023; National Academies, 2023f; Osterman et al., 2023). Most infants born preterm or with low birth weight have no severe developmental impairments; however, some may experience increased rates of mild to moderate chronic health issues, such as cognitive and behavioral

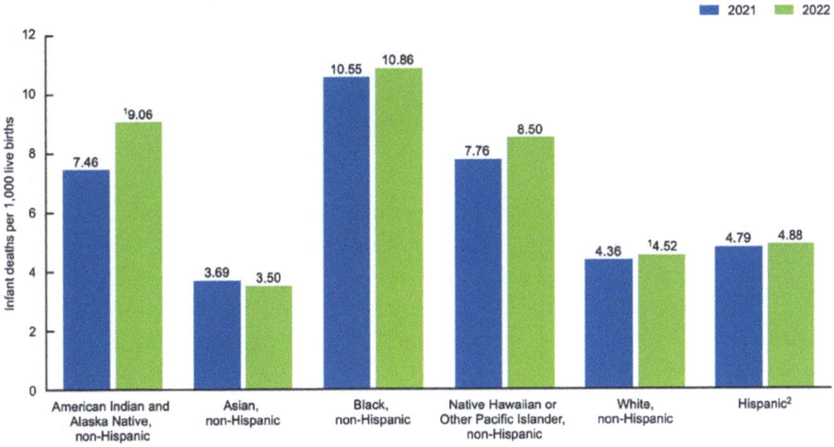

FIGURE 4-4 Infant mortality rate, by race and Hispanic origin: United States, 2021 final and 2022 provisional.
NOTES: (1) The increased rate for American Indian and Alaska Native, non-Hispanic, is significantly different from 2021. (2) Infants of Hispanic origin may be of any race.
SOURCE: National Center for Health Statistics, National Vital Statistics System, linked birth/infant death file (Ely & Driscoll, 2022).

impairments, ADHD, autism spectrum disorder, cerebral palsy, hearing loss, vision loss, and chronic lung disease. These conditions can have significant functional impacts throughout the life course (Busque et al., 2022; National Academies 2023e; Orchinik et al., 2011).

Injury and Gun Violence

Nearly half of the increase in all-cause mortality in children has resulted from firearm-related injuries, the leading cause of death among young people ages 1–19 (CDC, n.d.d; Goldstick, Cunningham, & Carter, 2022; Woolf, Wolf, & Rivara, 2023) and more than 8% of U.S. deaths for those under the age of 20 (Leach-Kemon, Sirull, & Glenn, 2023). When infants less than 1 year of age are excluded, this number jumps to 15% of all deaths under age 20.

The United States also has experienced record levels of school shootings and mass shootings, which have become more deadly since the turn of the century (Mariño-Ramírez et al., 2022). In 2018–2019 alone, more than 100,000 children attended a school where a shooting took place (Mariño-Ramírez et al., 2022). School shootings occur in the United States 27 times more than all other major industrialized nations combined. These events have lasting impacts on children and adolescents, who are more likely to abuse drugs and alcohol, suffer from mental illness, and engage in criminal activity (Finkelhor et al., 2009). Students who experience these events are also less likely to graduate high school, attend college, and graduate college; are less likely to be employed; and are more likely to have lower earnings into adulthood (Rossin-Slater, 2022). The toll of gun violence is both human and financial, with about $1 billion spent each year treating gunshot wounds, more than 50% of which was paid by Medicaid (Government Accountability Office, 2021). Compared with similar countries, the United States is an extreme outlier in childhood deaths (see Figure 4-5; Leach-Kemon, Sirull, & Glenn, 2023). Age-adjusted firearm homicide rates in the United States are 33 times greater than in Australia and 77 times greater than in Germany.

However, the risk of death from firearms is not evenly distributed around the country, and deaths due to firearm injuries occur disproportionately for children living in poverty and children from historically marginalized groups. Black children and adolescents accounted for approximately 46% of youth

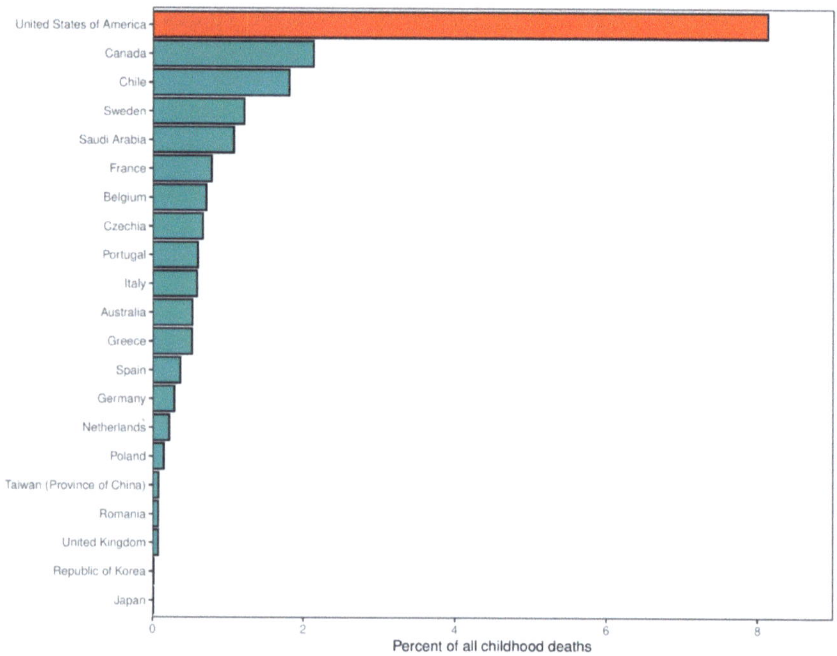

FIGURE 4-5 Percentage of childhood deaths caused by firearms among high-income countries with populations over 10 million, 2021.
SOURCE: Scott Glenn, Institute for Health Metrics and Evaluation (Leach-Kemon, Sirull, & Glenn, 2023).

firearm deaths in 2021 (Mariño-Ramírez et al., 2022; Panchal, 2022). Specifically, gun-related deaths are highest among non-Hispanic Black youth ages 10–19, with rates doubling from 2018 to 2021, following a modest decrease in 2018 (Mariño-Ramírez et al., 2022; Panchal, 2022). The firearm suicide rate among young people has increased to its highest rate in more than 20 years, with White youth ages 10–19 and American Indian/Alaska Native youth having the highest rates of suicide (Everytown Research & Policy, 2022). Although not as high as rates among White youth, rates of suicide among Hispanic and non-Hispanic Black youth have also increased since 2018 to their highest level (AHRQ, 2022a; CDC, 2023b, 2024k).

Compounding the dire problem of child deaths by firearms, almost 6,000 additional children and adolescents each year suffer injuries and disabilities from guns (Sun et al., 2022). Health care settings have been on the front line in coping with the immediate aftermath of firearm injuries (Sakran & Bulger, 2023). Emergency room visits, trauma surgeries, and rehabilitative services related to firearm injury have all increased. In addition, there is a growing recognition of frontline health care workers dealing with firearm victims as secondhand victims themselves, with associated stress, emotional reactivity, and burnout (Elwell, Krichten, & Mattocks, 2015; Ozeke et al., 2019; Salston & Figley, 2003).

Self-Harm and Suicide

Self-harm includes both suicide and other situations in which individuals intentionally hurt themselves without the intention of ending their lives (Klonsky, 2007; Klonsky, Victor, & Saffer, 2014; Nock & Favazza, 2009). The latter conditions have been labeled "nonsuicidal self-injury," describing cutting and other forms of self-harm (AAP, 2023). Nonsuicidal self-injury occurs most commonly among adolescents and young adults (UNICEF, n.d.), potentially as a means for children to assert control over their bodies in situations where they perceive a lack of control or feel overwhelmed (Hampl et al., 2023). While nonsuicidal self-injury can lead to suicidal behaviors, it is often a coping tool used to feel better rather than an attempt to end one's life (Whitlock & Lloyd-Richardson, 2019).

Suicide is a serious public health problem, responsible for more deaths among youth ages 10–24 years than any single major medical illness (AAP, n.d.; Asarnow, 2020). Suicide risk arises from a complex interplay involving underlying psychiatric conditions, family history of mental disorders, and family conflicts; it can be mitigated with support from friend networks and access to outpatient psychiatric resources. Specific life events such as interpersonal losses, academic stress, bullying, and physical/sexual abuse can set off a suicide attempt (CDC, 2021c, 2024k; Sekmen et al., 2023). Nonfatal attempts are more common, with roughly 100–200 suicide attempts for every suicide death. The suicide rate for people ages 10–19 increased by 56% between 2007 and 2016 (Curtin et al., 2018; Lindsey et al., 2019). Adolescent boys complete suicide three times more often than girls, although girls make twice as many attempts (Miranda-Mendizabal et al., 2019). American Indian and Alaska Native males have the highest suicide rate, and Black females have the lowest (Shain et al., 2016).

FAMILY, CAREGIVER, AND COMMUNITY HEALTH

Parental, household, and community factors all influence children's health and wellbeing.

Maternal Health

The first 1,000 days of development, from conception to age 2 years, is a particularly critical period. It is a time of incredible growth and development, crucial for the development of all body systems, such as the brain, metabolism, and immune system (Likhar & Patil, 2022). Nutrition, relationships, and physical environment during this time have long-term effects on the child's health, development, and wellbeing. The health of mothers is a critical determinant to children's health trajectory (De Genna et al., 2007; National Academies, 2019d). However, after many years of decline, rates of maternal morbidity and mortality in the United States have increased in recent years (Fleszar et al., 2023). The risk of death related to pregnancy and childbirth in the United States more than doubled between 1999 and 2019 (Fleszar et al., 2023). The United States is one of the only countries with an increase in this indicator in the past few decades, with mortality rates more than double that of similar countries, such as Canada, France, and Sweden, in 2018 (Kennedy-Moulton et al., 2022). Dramatic disparities in mortality exist between Black mothers (69.9 deaths per 100,000 live births) and those who identify as non-Hispanic White (26.6 per 100,000) and Hispanic (28 per 100,000; Joseph et al., 2021). In addition, approximately 60,000 women experience severe morbidity from labor and delivery each year, affecting their physical and mental health and making it difficult to provide the nurturing and healthy environment their child needs (Declercq & Zephyrin, 2021; Flagg et al., 2023). The 2020–2021 NSCH indicates that only 60% of children ages 0–17 have mothers who rate their overall physical and mental health status as being excellent or very good, with variation across racial/ethnic subgroups of children. For example, Hispanic (54.5%) and Black (55.2%) children are the least likely to have mothers reporting excellent or very good physical and mental health. Racial and ethnic variations are largely driven by physical health status differences, with more consistent reporting across subgroups on mental health status (Williams, 2018).

Community Health Crises

The recent opioid crisis is another example of a health phenomenon that has significantly affected U.S. children and families over the past decade. In 2019, 1.4 million children and adolescents lived with a parent with an opioid use disorder (Brundage & Levine, 2019). These children are at increased risk for being removed from the home and having a parent incarcerated because of opioids. Additionally, children of parents with a substance use disorder are more likely to experience maltreatment (Kepple, 2018). Parents also may overdose, with growing rates in recent years. Children of parents who overdose experience further consequences from bereavement, including an increased incidence of depression, primarily during the first 2 years, along with PTSD and functional impairment (Hulsey et al., 2020; Pham et al., 2018). It is estimated that by 2030, the cumulative lifetime cost of the "ripple effect" of the opioid crisis on children will be $400 billion (Brundage & Levine, 2019), based on additional spending in health care, special education, child welfare, and criminal justice.

Similarly, the COVID-19 pandemic affected parent and caregiver mental health, which increased difficulties coping with parenting demands (Hartley et al., 2021). In addition, during the pandemic, more than 229,000 children lost one or both parents due to COVID-19; 252,000 lost a primary caregiver; and 291,000 lost a primary or secondary caregiver (Hillis et al., 2021). Families and communities of color, including tribal communities, experienced the negative impact of these losses disproportionately. Compared with White children, American Indian and Alaska Native children were 4.5 times more likely to lose a parent or primary caregiver; Black children were 2.4 times more likely; and Hispanic children were nearly twice as likely (Coker et al., 2023; Hillis et al., 2021; National Academies, 2023c).

Relational and Social Health Risks

For some children, the home context and living conditions present social and relational health risks. Social health risks for children include economic hardship, food insecurity, living in unsafe neighborhoods with exposure to violence, and experiencing discrimination due to race or ethnicity. Over one-quarter of U.S. children and youth experience one or more of these risks, and more than 40% of those with chronic conditions face these risks (Bethell, Blackwell et al., 2022; Bethell, Garner et al., 2022).[9] Relational

[9]The Social Health Risk Index identifies children who sometimes or often could not afford enough food to eat; somewhat often or very often found it hard to cover the costs of basics needs, including housing; lived in an unsafe neighborhood or where the child was a victim of or witnessed violence; and witnessed their child being treated or judged unfairly due to his or her race or ethnic group (CAHMI, 2024).

health risks for children include having two or more adverse childhood experiences in the home environment, low parental coping, insufficient caregiver emotional support, and high levels of parental aggravation with their child (Merrick et al., 2019). Nearly 40% of U.S. children and more than 50% of children with chronic conditions experienced one or more of these risks (Bethell, Blackwell et al., 2022; Merrick et al., 2019).[10] These findings and other studies link both social and relational health risks to higher prevalence of poor physical and mental health (Bitsko et al., 2022; Ghandour et al., 2018; O'Loughlin et al., 2022; Umberson & Montez, 2010) and point to the value of mitigating negative impacts of home contexts and living conditions. Studies on national trends in child wellbeing find that poor caregiver mental health and lower parental coping (both relational health risks) have increased in recent years (2016–2020) and household-based adverse childhood experiences (e.g., alcohol/substance abuse, domestic violence) have remained consistently high for all children (31.3% in 2021; Ceccarelli et al., 2022; Cree et al., 2018; Hutchins et al, 2022; Lebrun-Harris et al., 2022; O'Loughlin et al., 2022; Swedo et al., 2023).

Family and domestic violence affect approximately 10 million individuals each year, including child abuse, intimate partner violence, and elder abuse (Huecker et al., 2024). In 2020, 1,750 children in the United States died as a result of abuse and neglect (CDC, 2022b). Domestic violence can include economic, physical, sexual, emotional, and psychological abuse directed toward children, adults, or elders, and can lead to deteriorating psychological and physical health, reduced quality of life, diminished productivity, and mortality. Parents or caregivers involved in a turbulent relationship may think that the relationship does not affect their children; however, even children shielded from witnessing domestic violence can experience distress because of familial conflict (American Academy of Child & Adolescent Psychiatry, 2023; Office on Violence Against Women, 2023). Child abuse and exposure to domestic violence increase the risk of emotional and behavioral issues in children. Children living in poverty are more susceptible to abuse and neglect because of the stress associated with poverty (CDC, 2022b). Low-income families have child maltreatment rates five times higher than those of other families. The economic impact of child abuse and neglect in the United States was approximately $592 billion in 2018, rivaling the costs of prominent public health problems such as heart disease and diabetes (CDC, 2022b).

---

[10]The Relational Health Risk Index identifies children who experienced two or more of six household-level adverse childhood experiences (serious parental mental illness, household substance, drug or alcohol abuse; witnessed domestic violence, parental death, divorce/separation, or incarceration), had one or two caregivers with fair/poor mental health, had a caregiver report frequent aggravation with their child, and had a caregiver who lacked emotional support or was not coping well (CAHMI, 2024).

CONCLUSION

This chapter has aimed to show that children in the United States face major health problems. The full extent of today's child health challenges will become apparent later in life. The rates of adult physical, mental, and behavioral health problems and decreases in adult life expectancy have roots in childhood health and experiences (Case & Deaton, 2017, 2022; Knifton & Inglis, 2020; Muennig et al., 2018), a concept explored in-depth in Chapter 2 of this report. As discussed, having certain health conditions as a child or exposure to certain factors or adverse experiences can affect an individual throughout the life course.

Key findings regarding the current state of health and wellbeing of children and youth include the following:

- The United States continues to rank near the bottom in child well-being globally.
- Health disparities in the wellbeing of America's children and youth are apparent when comparing population subgroups and geographic areas.
- Child populations at higher risk of poor health and mental health conditions include those living in poverty, from historically marginalized groups (e.g., Black, Hispanic, and American Indian/Alaska Native children), living in foster care, and/or in contact with the juvenile justice system.
- A small portion of children (1–2%) have complex medical needs. A larger portion of children (~20%) have functional difficulties either from complex conditions, more prevalent chronic conditions, or socioemotional challenges.
- Many chronic conditions in children (such as asthma and mental, emotional, and behavioral health conditions discussed in this chapter) are preventable and manageable. The presence and management of these chronic conditions are heavily influenced by family and community factors.
- Increasing mortality rates in children and adolescents have been linked primarily to injuries related to gun violence, suicide, and substance abuse. There is also a child mental health crisis.
- Attention to relational health risks (low parental coping, high levels of caregiver aggravation) has been shown to be just as important as attention to social health risks (poverty, violent neighborhoods, discrimination).
- Population trends underscore the importance of improving child health: the increasing longevity of older Americans; a declining birth rate; and increases in chronic disease, disability, and early mortality among working-age adults.

The committee concludes that persistent and worsening health of U.S. children and a shrinking child population calls for substantial change in health care services, notably increasing focus toward prevention to address the wide-ranging issues affecting the health and wellbeing of children and youth. As discussed throughout this report, the committee emphasizes the need to address whole child and family health and build supports for protective factors that can be employed to mitigate negative effects. Given the range of social and relational issues affecting health and wellbeing, a more integrated approach among the health care system, public health, and community services is needed.

Without a focused strategy for optimizing the health trajectory of children and adolescents, young people will continue to enter adulthood with poor physical and mental health, a greater burden of chronic disease, and diminished capacity to contribute economically. The poor state of children's health threatens society's future workforce and economic prosperity.

While the lifelong effects of early childhood adversity have become well established in recent years, growing evidence documents the potential for interventions to minimize early adversity. Many of these interventions center the importance of social and environmental factors that impact the life course, with a focus on fostering family and community protective factors and ensuring early identification, treatment, and support for children, youth, and families. The committee explores these concepts and interventions further in subsequent chapters. The health care system is well positioned to leverage its strengths in optimizing the quality of preventive health care and integrated services for children and youth, and it can utilize knowledge of the health status of children and adolescents to best address the many social, environmental, and relational conditions that impact the health and wellbeing of the nation's children and youth. The next chapter examines the contexts in which children and youth receive health care and the various providers of such care.

5

Health Care for Children and Youth

Elevate the role of the [health care] system beyond disease prevention and caring for sick children [. . .], design a better system with the patient and their caregiver in mind [. . . and support] the family system as the key pathway to promoting child health.

—Comment to committee from health
foundation employee, Houston, Texas

Generally, the U.S. health care system is fragmented and uncoordinated, and it typically responds to diseases and health problems after they arise. Despite shifts to managed care and forms of capitation at the payer level, the fee-for-service payment model still dominates in payments to clinicians and provider organizations, incentivizing inefficient, inequitable, and unnecessarily costly care (see Chapter 6). Overall, the system is optimized to maximize visits, procedures, profits, and treating medical problems after they occur, rather than preventing them from occurring in the first place. This payment model provides little support for health promotion, team care, and coordination (National Academies of Sciences, Engineering, and Medicine [National Academies], 2023a).

As for adults, health care for children and youth in the United States is delivered in a patchwork of settings with little coordination among multiple insurers and siloed delivery systems. Children, youth, and their families find and receive care from a complex array of providers that differs based on geography, community, clinical and social need, and financing. The child health care system has largely been modeled after the adult system; however, as discussed in Chapter 1, five important factors (the "5 Ds"—developmental change, disease/differential epidemiology, dependence, demographics, and dollars—indicate unique aspects of care delivery for children that require attention.

Despite the needed improvements, health care for children has seen innovations and improvements in many communities over the past few decades, providing a clear and evidence-based strategy for transformation. Advances have included greater attention to various social, family, and community factors influencing health outcomes; changing the content of pediatric care; building connections with other programs to enhance child and family development; coordinating care broadly; and linking families with other critical community resources. Yet bringing these strategies to scale and implementing them consistently have been hampered by payment and other factors. Even with this progress and well-evidenced strategies for change, the health status of children and young families in America is considerably inferior to that in comparable developed countries (see Chapter 4). Several prior reports have noted progress in implementing a life course approach, integrating mental and behavioral health into pediatric care—both primary and subspecialty—and integrating within community systems, although without broad and adequate uptake (National Academies, 2019d, 2022b, 2023c,f,j, 2024b).

Given this complexity, defining the scope of and discussing all the health care system's elements and issues are difficult. This chapter focuses on a high-level review of health services for children and families and the clinical settings in which they are provided, with a specific examination of the opportunities and challenges for providing mental and behavioral health care. It spans primary care for preventive, acute, and chronic care services, emergency care, chronic care, subspecialty care, inpatient and intensive care, and rehabilitation. The chapter describes innovative expanded advanced primary care and specialty team care models that integrate physical and mental health care and provide a wider set of services to aid families and strengthen child development and wellbeing.

Most of this chapter focuses on transforming primary care to strengthen health promotion and disease prevention, but it also reviews innovations in inpatient and specialty care for children with acute and complex chronic conditions. The chapter concludes with a review of the pediatric health care workforce. Subsequent chapters discuss financing for health care (Chapter 6), care in conjunction with investments in population health (Chapter 7), care in school-based settings (Chapter 8), and measurement and accountability approaches to support an improved focus on health promotion and prevention and integrated, team-based care (Chapter 9).

The child and adolescent health workforce is diverse, including physicians (those with an MD or DO in pediatrics, family medicine, or general medicine), nurse practitioners and physician assistants, nurses, mental health care providers, community health workers, and others. General pediatricians provide most primary care visits for U.S. children across all pediatric age groups, including adolescents (76% in 2019, 72% in 2020, and 72% in 2021; Hong, Huo, & Desai, 2023). Almost all U.S. children and youth have identified sources of primary care and insurance coverage, although the nature, quality, and accessibility of the services vary, and low-income children often report the local emergency room as their usual source of care. Residents of rural areas often lack access to many services, especially specialized services for children.

Some primary care providers offer mainly the essentials of traditional practice—immunizations, some screenings, identification and treatment of common acute conditions—and refer patients to other providers for needs beyond these basic efforts. In other cases, following the model of the family-centered medical home, primary care has evolved into a multidisciplinary team-based program, with integrated mental and behavioral health and links to other community programs and supports through extended team members, such as community health workers and social services providers. This shift toward team-based care presents a critical opportunity for medical providers and community partners (e.g., caregivers, schools, dietitians and/or nutritionists, specialists, pharmacies, nursing agencies, vendors of durable medical equipment, other home care agencies and counselors) to respond to the unique and evolving needs of children and youth by drawing on a variety of support systems (Katkin et al., 2017). Given the increasingly fragmented and complex landscape of health care, team-based care can serve as a catalyst for fostering more effective patient care and improving the experience of those in the workforce (Smith et al., 2018). In settings that support integrated care, screening and intervention with families has evolved from traditional screenings, such as for lead and anemia, to greater attention to relationships, child development and behavior, and social determinants of health.[1] Increasingly, pediatric primary care providers have worked to identify and provide resources for addressing broader influences on child health, although financing rarely incentivizes such changes (see Chapter 6). Although these developments are not the norm, efforts to shift emphasis from diagnosis and treatment to prevention and health promotion require centering individual needs while simultaneously promoting population and community health (see Chapter 7).

Hospitals that provide care to children and adolescents offer a wide array of often very specialized services, building from extensive research advances and new diagnostic and treatment methods. As noted in Chapter 1, most pediatric subspecialists work in academic medical centers. Such placement

[1]Such screenings are recommended through the national Bright Futures Guidelines (American Academy of Pediatrics [AAP], 2017).

has facilitated advances in medical care with astonishing impacts on disease management and children's survival. The growth of excellent subspecialty care (e.g., for childhood cancers) has also moved a significant amount of specialized care from inpatient to outpatient settings. Today, pediatric inpatient care typically serves children who have relatively rare conditions or marked instability requiring more intensive care (Agency for Healthcare Research and Quality, 2021b, 2022b; Weiss, Liang, & Martin, 2022).

Children and families receive mental health screenings and services in several settings, including traditional practice; community-based mental health centers; schools and preschools; and, increasingly, primary care settings that integrate mental and behavioral health professionals and include community health workers as part of the mental health team. Children and youth also receive some mental and behavioral health services in juvenile justice settings and inpatient hospital settings—some of which are part of a children's or general hospital, while others are focused solely on psychiatric and mental health. Finally, as an intermediate level between hospital and community settings, residential care provides supervised care at lower acuity levels than hospitals. Despite this array of settings, many children and youth do not receive needed mental and behavioral health care, and there is limited coordination among these settings or with the rest of the health care system, including primary care.

HEALTH CARE AND CRITICAL PERIODS OF DEVELOPMENT

Chapter 2 described sensitive and critical developmental periods, including preconception and prenatal periods; infancy, childhood, and adolescence; and the transition into adulthood. Understanding and optimizing these developmental periods—and ensuring that the health care system provides developmentally appropriate care as children and youth transition across these stages—are essential for children to thrive.

Preconception and Prenatal Health

Health during the preconception and prenatal periods is crucial to minimize the risk of adverse birth outcomes, such as preterm or low birth weight, and to optimize the healthy development of children (including organ formation, fetal growth, epigenetic changes, and long-term health outcomes) and their families (Keikha, Jahanfar, & Hemati, 2022; Khekade et al., 2023). These periods are critical because they lay the foundation for the health and development of the child, influencing outcomes from birth through adulthood (see Chapter 2). Preconception care involves health care interventions and services provided to individuals or couples before pregnancy to optimize their health and promote favorable outcomes for both the pregnant person and the baby (Keikha, Jahanfar, & Hemati, 2022; Khekade et al., 2023). The Centers for Disease Control and Promotion (CDC), American Association of Family Physicians, and the American College of Obstetricians and Gynecologists provide guidance on prepregnancy or interconception care and counseling (Jack et al., 2008; Wise, 2008). This care includes health promotion and lifestyle adjustments, risk assessment, and management of preexisting conditions. Key components include health education on maintaining a balanced diet and folate supplementation, exercising, and avoiding harmful substances, as well as regular checkups and screening for health risks, medical conditions, genetic counseling, and ensuring immunizations are up to date (Herval et al., 2019; Peahl & Howell, 2021; Soucy et al., 2023). Health and lifestyle choices made before conception can have a profound impact on the health outcomes of future offspring (Atrash et al., 2006; Khekade et al., 2023). Preconception care helps to mitigate risks and support healthy development from the earliest stages, influencing long-term health outcomes for the child and family.

Optimizing preconception health requires broad strategies to reach the population at risk for pregnancy; multiple health care interventions have shown promise (Hemsing, Greaves, & Poole, 2017). Pediatric primary care can support preconception care among parents in their practice who are interconceptional for their next child. A multisite cluster randomized trial of a maternal health screener and brief intervention in primary care was found to be feasible and effective in increasing folate use and decreasing smoking (Chilukuri et al., 2018; Upadhya et al., 2020).

Early Childhood and Family Health

Families have more encounters with pediatric primary care in the first 3 years of life than with the education sector; thus, pediatric primary care represents a critical leverage point in promoting early relational health, in addition to focusing on health creation, prevention, and wellbeing for those with access. Most families bring their children to a health care provider for preventive care, with visits starting just after birth. Preventive care visits can be frequent in the first years of life—12 well child care visits are recommended to be provided to children in their first 3 years of life based on the national Bright Futures Guidelines—offering multiple touchpoints with families; preventive care is nonstigmatizing because it is a universal intervention in the United States (Roby et al., 2021). However, current trends in visits fall short of these national guidelines (see below).

Early intervention services for supporting the health and wellbeing of young children and families have been a focus for improving outcomes.

Home visiting programs starting prenatally or after birth demonstrate improved child, maternal, and family outcomes (see Chapter 7). Integration of home visiting programs with the health care system has been variable, and data sharing and more collaboration are needed (Tschudy, Toomey, & Cheng, 2013). The importance of early childhood preventive care and its impact on long-term health outcomes is well established. Several models have been proposed and studied to transform the delivery of preventive care during this critical period.

The Parent-focused Redesign for Encounters, Newborns to Toddlers (PARENT) model incorporates a culturally responsive parent coach as part of the care team for children aged 0–3 years. PARENT has been shown to improve the receipt of well-child care, enhance parent experiences, and reduce emergency department utilization (Coker et al., 2016; Mimila et al., 2017). The 3-2-1 Integrated Model for Parents and Children Together (IMPACT) program, launched by New York City Health and Hospitals in 2020, provides a comprehensive two-generation program integrating mental health, pediatrics, and women's health to improve the long-term trajectory for each family unit (NYC Health + Hospitals, 2020). The program offers a personalized approach to care with routine screenings for mothers during pregnancy and postpartum follow-up and pediatrics visits, employing Healthy Steps workers to engage families during visits (HealthySteps, n.d.a,c). Screening identifies when a family has additional medical or nonmedical social needs, such as mental health care or food or income support, with interventions provided in addition to universal parenting supports within health care (Filene et al., 2013; NYC Health + Hospitals, 2020). Preliminary evidence indicates that the 3-2-1 IMPACT model can improve health outcomes among low-income populations (McCord et al., 2024).

School-Age Children

As children start school, health care visits decrease in frequency, occurring annually unless health issues require more frequent follow-up (AAP, 2023; Freedman, 2020; Riley, Morrison, & McEvoy, 2019). During this period, children can learn basic positive health behaviors. It is also a time when several behavioral and mental health disorders can manifest, and screening and early intervention for those conditions is critical for long-term mental and behavioral health (Abramson, 2022). Given the fewer primary care visits during this period (as well as limited access to care for some children), school-based health monitoring, including for mental and behavioral health problems, in collaboration with health care systems provides key preventive services and intervention (see Chapter 8).

Adolescents and Young Adults

Health care services during adolescence and emerging adulthood are critical for ensuring both their present and long-term health and wellbeing. Adolescence is an opportune time to address health-related habits—including diet, exercise, sexual and reproductive health, and substance use—that can impact longer-term health. However, many adolescents, particularly those from historically marginalized groups, face a variety of barriers to accessing health care services, including financial barriers, privacy concerns, lack of culturally responsive care, and timely availability of services. Adolescents also have needs that are distinct from those of children. Health services for adolescents and young adults need to prepare youth and their families for the developmental changes (physical, cognitive, and social) that take place during adolescence and address these changes with culturally informed services that are attentive to the needs of all adolescents (National Academies, 2019c).

Adolescents need access to models of care that consider the entirety of their needs—from medical to social—and other factors in their lives (e.g., social determinants of health, the cultural and social content in which they live; National Academies, 2019d, 2020b). Models of care need to promote communication, collaboration, and coordination among physical health and mental health care providers, youth, and their families.

With increasing independence and autonomy, adolescents need confidential care and preparation for navigating the health care system independently, particularly the transition into adult health care systems, although many do not receive preventive health counseling and key preparatory advice (Akers et al., 2014). Confidentiality concerns remain a critical barrier for adolescents seeking appropriate medical services (Pathak & Chou, 2019). Adolescents who have time alone with clinicians have higher rates of screening and discussion of sensitive topics, more opportunity to navigate the clinic setting and engage with their own health care, and receive confidential care (Al-Shimari et al., 2022; Brown & Wissow, 2009, 2010; Chung et al., 2024; Committee on Adolescent Health Care, 2020; Ford, English, & Sigman, 2004; Klein & Wilson, 2002; McKee, Rubin, & Campos, 2011). Many youth underuse behavioral health services, despite expressed interest and need for such services (Boyd, Butler, & Benton, 2018; MacDonald, McGill, & Murphy, 2018). Like younger children, many adolescents may first seek help for mental health concerns from primary care providers. Others may rely on schools, mental health providers, or crisis centers, or they may seek care at emergency departments or other treatment facilities (National Academies, 2019c).

While adolescent health care addresses health risks such as substance use, risky sex, and poor mental health, care encounters are also opportune for exploring and supporting an adolescent's goals and strengths (Calabrese et al., 2022; Lindstrom Johnson, Blum, & Cheng, 2014; Lindstrom Johnson, Jones, & Cheng, 2015). Further, as adolescents and young adults enter childbearing years, sexual and preconception health is of critical importance, as is gender-affirming care.

The transition from pediatric to adult health care is particularly important for adolescents with special health care needs and/or chronic health conditions (Bloom, Cohen, & Freeman, 2012; National Academies, 2018; Stein, Perrin, & Iezzoni, 2010), who, while transitioning within the health care system, also face typical adolescent life transitions and challenges (e.g., postsecondary education or employment, leaving home, parenthood). Factors during the transition into the adult health care system affect not only the uptake of services, but also the adolescents' ongoing physical and mental health, overall wellbeing, quality of life, and educational and employment outcomes. Many youth and young adults with special health care needs and/or chronic or complex health conditions and their families do not receive the support they need in the transition from pediatric to adult health care (White et al., 2018). Medical care models that are purposeful and planned are critical at this stage in life; such care models prepare the adolescent and their family for the transition from child-centered to adult-oriented health care in a way that considers typical developmental processes as well as access, appropriateness, and continuity of services (Calabrese et al., 2022). Strong evidence supports a continuum approach to health care transitions that incorporates multiple elements of preparation, planning, tracking, and follow-through for all youth and young adults beginning in early adolescence and continuing into young adulthood (Calabrese et al., 2022; Cooley & Sagerman, 2011; Jones, Merrick, & Houry, 2020a; Lemke et al., 2018; Schmidt et al., 2020; White et al., 2018).

PEDIATRIC PRIMARY CARE

Primary care forms the base for every health care system. A report by the National Academies titled *Implementing High-Quality Primary Care: Rebuilding the Foundation of Health Care* defines "high-quality primary care" as "the provision of whole-person, integrated, accessible, and equitable health care by multidisciplinary teams who are accountable for addressing the majority of an individual's health and wellness needs across settings and through sustained relationships with patients, families, and communities" (National Academies, 2021b, p. 4). The report notes that its definition does not describe what most people in the United States experience today, an observation supported by data from the National Survey of Children's Health on indicators of quality of care (see Table 5-1). Table 5-2 summarizes data compiled by the committee on children's health care utilization.

TABLE 5-1 Quality-of-Care Indicators for Children's Health Care in the United States

Performance Indicator	National Prevalence, % (Across State Prevalence Range)	U.S. Children with Any Public Health Insurance,[a] %	U.S. Children with Private Health Insurance,[b] %
Percent of children ages 0–17 years who have adequate and continuous health insurance	68.0 (59.2–81.0)	84.5	66.3
Percent of children ages 0–17 years who received care in a setting that met core criteria for being a medical home[c]	46.1 (33.8–57.1)	36.3	55.6
Percent of young children ages 9–35 months who received screening for their development	33.7 (24.5–49.1)	28.7	39.0
Percent of children ages 3–17 years with a mental health condition who received treatment or counseling	52.8 (31.9–67.6)	52.0	54.9
Percent of children ages 0–17 years whose health insurance and health care met criteria for being a well-functioning system of care[d]	17.3 (11.6–23.8)	14.8	21.2
Percent of children enrolled in Medicaid/CHIP who had at least 6 of 9 recommended well-child care visits before age 15 months	Not available (N/A)	55.7 (30.1–77.4)	N/A
Percent of children enrolled in Medicaid/CHIP who had at least 2 of 4 recommended well-child care visits between ages 15 and 30 months	N/A	64.9 (36.5–82.3)	N/A

[a]Public insurance is defined as Medicaid, Medical Assistance, or any kind of government assistance plan for those with low incomes or a disability.
[b]Private insurance is defined as insurance through a current or former employer or union, insurance purchased directly from an insurance company, TRICARE or other military health care, or coverage through the Affordable Care Act or other private insurance.
[c]The presence of a medical home was measured based on five components: personal doctor or nurse, usual source for sick care, family-centered care, problems getting needed referrals, and effective care coordination when needed.
[d]A well-functioning system of care was assessed based on children's experience across several measures: (1) the family feels like a partner in their child's care, (2) the child has a medical home, (3) the child receives medical and dental preventive care, (4) the child has adequate insurance, and (5) the child has no unmet need. A sixth measure is included for adolescents (ages 12–17 years): preparation for transition to adult health care.
SOURCE: 2021 and 2022 National Survey of Children's Health (CAHMI, 2024); 2022 Child Core Set Report (Centers for Medicare & Medicaid Services, n.d.a).

TABLE 5-2 Children's Health Care Utilization

Health Care Effectiveness Data and Information Set				
Utilization Measure[a]	Year	Commercial HMO, %	Commercial PPO, %	Medicaid HMO, %
At least 6 well-child visits in first 15 months	2022	81	80.8	56.8
At least 2 well-child visits between 15 and 30 months	2022	87.3	88.2	66.7
At least 1 well-child visit in past year (ages 3–6 years)	2019	79.1	77.7	74.1
At least 1 well-care visit in past year (children and adolescents)	2022	57.6	56.2	48.6

National Center for Health Statistics, National Health Interview Survey				
Utilization Measure	Age Group	Year	Characteristic	Value
Visits to physician offices and hospital emergency departments[b]	Under age 18 years	2018	Number of visits (thousands)	128,781
People with hospital stays in the past year[c]	1–17 years	2019	% with 1 or more hospital stay	2.6
	1–5 years	2019	% with 1 or more hospital stay	3.2
	6–17 years	2019	% with 1 or more hospital stay	2.4
Emergency department visits in the past 12 months among children under age 18 years[d]	All children[e]	2018	% with 1 or more emergency department visit	17.6

[a]The percentages indicate the proportion of eligible children who met the criteria for each measure and are based on national averages.
[b]Data are based on reporting by a sample of office-based physicians and hospital emergency departments
[c]Data are based on household interviews of a sample of the civilian noninstitutionalized population.
[d]Data are based on household interviews of a sample of the civilian noninstitutionalized population.
[e]Includes all other races not shown separately and those with unknown health insurance status.
NOTE: HMO = health maintenance organization; PPO = preferred provider organization.
SOURCE: Generated by the committee, based on data from National Committee for Quality Assurance, n.d., and National Center for Health Statistics (n.d.) CDC Data Finder.

Pediatric primary care includes a broad range of services (National Academies, 2019d), with a priority on provision of comprehensive age-specific physical and mental health promotion and preventive services, particularly as outlined in *Bright Futures: Guidelines for Health Supervision of Infants, Children, and Adolescents* (AAP, 2017).[2] The guidelines cover monitoring physical, cognitive, and socioemotional growth and development. They include screening for metabolic and genetic conditions in the newborn period; developmental screenings at specific ages; screenings for health conditions, such as autism, anemia, and vision or hearing impairment, and exposures, such as lead; screening for socioemotional issues and maternal and adolescent depression; and screening for social and/or other nonmedical drivers of health. There are also resources for age-specific guidelines to educate and counsel parents/caregivers on promoting the healthy development of their children. Pediatric primary care supports health promotion and disease prevention by providing immunization, dental fluoride varnish, and anticipatory guidance on topics related to physical and mental health, as well as physical and emotional development. In addition, a growing number of practices screen for social determinants of health and provide referrals and links to community services to address family needs.

Primary care also includes diagnosing and treating acute health conditions, such as infectious illnesses and injuries, as well as identifying and caring for children with special health care needs and chronic illnesses, such as asthma and attention deficit hyperactivity disorder (ADHD). Depending on the level of complexity of a child's illness, the primary care clinician may diagnose and treat such conditions or may refer to and coordinate care with pediatric medical and surgical subspecialists. Primary care practices also help coordinate care with households in managing insurance coverage and access to prescriptions; diagnostic testing; subspecialty care; physical, occupational, and speech therapies; and other services. Primary care clinicians often link families to services in other sectors that are important for the overall health and wellbeing of children, such as nutrition programs (e.g., Special Supplemental Nutrition Program for Women, Infants, and Children) and early education programs (e.g., Head Start, school-based preschool programs).

Children and youth obtain primary care in multiple settings: independent pediatric and family medicine practices, larger private group practices (single and multispecialty), health centers (federally qualified health centers [FQHCs] and similar community health centers, Indian Health Service [IHS] facilities, and school-based health centers [SBHCs]), hospital or health care system–based practices, and military treatment facilities (clinics located on

---

[2]The Bright Futures Program is funded through a cooperative agreement from the Health Resources and Services Administration with the American Academy of Pediatrics to create and share clinical national guidelines for pediatric well-child visits from birth to age 21.

military installations). Nonemergency acute care is also provided through urgent care facilities and retail-based clinics. Although in the previous century, U.S. primary care tended to occur in smaller, independent practices, over time delivery has shifted toward community clinics, hospital outpatient clinics, and health care system practices (Simon et al., 2015).

Primary care office visits are declining both across adult populations (Ganguli, Lee, & Mehrotra, 2019) and among commercially insured children and adolescents, where visits fell approximately 13% between 2008 and 2016 (Ray et al., 2020). Problem-based visits dropped 24%, while preventive care visits increased by 10%, visits to nonprimary care settings increased, and out-of-pocket costs for problem-based visits increased (Ray et al., 2020). This is consistent with findings that the number of FQHCs and the number of patients they serve have increased since 2001 (National Association of Community Health Centers [NACHC], 2014).

The next section reviews some specific settings for primary care for children and youth, including community health centers, settings for specific populations, and SBHCs, and concludes with a discussion of the growing area of telehealth.

Community Health Centers

Community health centers provide primary care and other services for 30 million people, including 12% of all U.S. children (NACHC, 2022). Health centers often serve communities with otherwise limited access to health care and high social need. Most community health centers are FQHCs. Through the Health Resources and Services Administration (HRSA, 2022b), the federal government supports about 1,400 health centers and similar organizations with more than 14,000 service delivery sites across the United States. FQHCs have governance boards with more than 50% patients served by the health center and are designed to meet the specific needs of the communities they serve. Many community health centers offer integrated behavioral health services, dental care, pharmacy, cancer screening, vision and eye care, pharmacy, and diagnostic and laboratory services. They also offer case management and referral to specialty care and social services, if necessary. While community health centers are not all the same, many provide more comprehensive, whole health services that focus on prevention, social needs, and upstream factors than are available in other settings (National Academies, 2023a). FQHCs provide services to about 14% of those in marginalized racial/ethnic groups in the United States, as well as 20% of the country's individuals who are uninsured, 33% of those living in poverty, and 20% of those in rural areas. Almost 80% of FQHC patients have either public insurance or lack insurance; approximately 90% of patients had income less than 200% of the federal poverty level (NACHC, 2023a,b).

Special Population Health Care Providers

Families and children may access primary care in other settings, including IHS clinics and on-base military treatment facilities. These facilities offer comprehensive and culturally competent care tailored to the specific needs of these populations, address health disparities, and ensure access to essential health services. IHS clinics offer comprehensive services akin to community health centers and are important access points to care for American Indian/Alaska Native tribal nations (see further discussion of the IHS in Chapter 6, see also IHS, n.d.a).

Pediatric clinics located within military treatment facilities are accessible to active-duty and retiree families who are TRICARE beneficiaries (Hero et al., 2021). TRICARE is the Department of Defense insurance program for eligible service members, retirees, and their dependents. On-base pediatric clinics follow a patient-centered medical home model of care (Defense Health Agency, 2019). TRICARE beneficiaries can also access care through the broader TRICARE network of civilian providers.

School-Based Health Centers

SBHCs, located on or near primary and secondary school campuses, may provide primary and preventive medical care, behavioral health services, diagnostic care such as routine screenings, and/or preventive dental care (Medicaid and CHIP Payment and Access Commission, 2018b). SBHCs vary in services provided, accessibility, degree of integration with the school, and quality of care. Although most SBHCs are operated by an FQHC, others receive support from school districts or a combination of local health care systems, public health departments, and community-based organizations. A 2016–2017 census indicated that the number of SBHCs doubled in the previous 20 years, with more than 2,500 SBHCs operating in the United States in 2016, serving 10,629 schools and more than 6.3 million children (Love et al., 2019). As of 2019, 40% of SBHCs served elementary school–age children, 30% middle or high school–age youth, and 30% children in all other grade combinations (Love at al., 2019). While this number represents only about 13% of schools nationwide and services vary widely, these facilities are typically located in areas of higher need, where communities face greater barriers to health care access (Love et al., 2019; Soleimanpour, 2020). SBHCs are more common in schools with larger proportions of socially and economically disadvantaged youth (Love et al., 2019) who may also experience disproportionate academic challenges (Chetty et al., 2019) because of structural inequalities that extend far beyond what SBHC services can influence directly (Soleimanpour, 2020). This complexity adds to the challenge of demonstrating impacts on not only health outcomes but also educational success.

SBHCs are associated with positive short- and long-term outcomes, including increased access to health services for children, families, and communities; improved health including increased use of cost-effective preventive care, such as immunizations, family planning, well-child visits, and behavioral health care; improved clinical quality scores in areas such as well-child visits, immunizations, chlamydia screening, depression screening and follow-up, and asthma control; increased health equity through access to culturally competent, high-quality, first-contact primary care; and increased number of regular patient groups and community engagement for FQHCs, school districts, and other health care providers (Arenson et al., 2019; California School-Based Health Alliance, 2022; Key, Washington, & Hulsey, 2002; Knopf et al., 2016). SBHCs have been shown to manage and treat chronic health conditions effectively, improve prenatal care and pregnancy outcomes for pregnant teens, and decrease teen pregnancy rates (Arenson et al., 2019).

Nearly 70% of SBHCs offer mental health services. Despite limitations, SBHCs can be an important access point for screening and treatment of mental health conditions, especially for children with no insurance or public insurance, who are more likely to seek mental health services at SBHCs than those with commercial insurance (Arenson et al., 2019; Keeton, Soleimanpour, & Brindis, 2012; Knopf et al., 2016). Mental health services in schools improve mental health access and outcomes (see further discussion in Chapter 8).

Overall, for children with access to them, SBHCs are an important source of primary care, chronic condition management, and mental health services. Expansion of SBHCs, particularly in resource-limited settings, is an important strategy for improving equitable access to high-quality care for children and is an approach recommended by CDC's Community Guide and the Community Preventive Services Task Force (2021) as a means of advancing health equity.

Telehealth

Telehealth is the provision of health services remotely via video, phone, or mobile device. Telehealth can increase patient access; improve care coordination; strengthen the role of the primary care clinician; and allow subspecialists the time to provide inpatient and outpatient care in a manner that is feasible, fulfilling, and financially sustainable and best for children (Curfman, Hackell et al., 2021; Curfman, McSwain et al., 2021a,b; National Academies, 2023c,g,i). The COVID-19 pandemic led to rapid and widespread expansion of telehealth in pediatric primary care, where its use had not been common previously (Curfman, Hackell et al., 2021; Curfman,

McSwain et al., 2021a,b). With the public health emergency, policy changes allowed children with acute and chronic illnesses to connect via telehealth services to their usual source of care for management of their conditions. Many states allowed preventive care using a hybrid model that combined virtual and in-person visits (Hsu et al., 2023). During the pandemic, telehealth improved access to care for many children and youth, although disparities in access to technology and digital infrastructure related to poverty, systemic racism, and other inequities were also highlighted (Zhang et al., 2023). A review of prepandemic studies of the use of telehealth in pediatric care in specific contexts—including asthma, obesity, ADHD, and skin care—found low- to moderate-quality studies with outcomes for telemedicine interventions that were comparable to or sometimes modestly better than routine care, with positive results for parent satisfaction (Shah & Badawy, 2021).

Many mental health care systems have used telehealth to provide virtual consultations with child and adolescent psychiatrists, psychologists, and therapists (University of Texas Rio Grande Valley School of Medicine, n.d.). For example, the Texas Child Health Access Through Telemedicine program links school staff evaluating students to appropriate telehealth services (University of Texas Rio Grande Valley School of Medicine, n.d.) Telehealth allows mental health providers to collaborate with primary care physicians for early detection and treatment of conditions such as anxiety and depression. Virtual visits also make it easier for busy families to access care, reducing transportation barriers and the time between symptom onset and treatment (CDC, n.d.e). Telehealth is proving to be an effective and scalable solution to the pediatric mental health workforce shortage and improving outcomes for children and adolescents (Archer et al., 2021; deMayo et al., 2022; Gajarawala & Pelkowski, 2021; Guthrie & Snyder, 2023; Thomas et al., 2023; Totten, McDonagh, & Wagner, 2020).

Telehealth virtual visits with patients or teleconsultation across specialties are likely to continue to grow as will remote patient monitoring. New technology and the use of artificial intelligence have the potential to increase the efficiency of practice by decreasing documentation time, managing patient communications, synthesizing data, or prereading images. Virtual visits and remote patient monitoring (e.g., for failure to thrive, diabetes management, asthma, hospital follow-up) will keep more patients at home. New models of care building from telehealth are exploring "hospital at home" and "going to where the kids are" with expanded connectivity and services in schools, child care, and in the home (including home visiting). Ethical and equity considerations for patients and the workforce must be central as these innovations evolve. With children being "digital natives," and given the developmental origins of health and disease early in the life course, inclusion of pediatrics in these innovations is essential.

Recently, many state Medicaid programs have introduced new telehealth policies and payment opportunities, telehealth portals, telepsychiatry consultations, and collaborative care as solutions to help overcome challenges of geographical access, with a notable increase in the implementation of such models during the COVID-19 pandemic (Federation of State Medical Boards, 2023; Kwong, 2024). Prior to the pandemic, the use of telehealth in Medicaid was becoming more common; in particular, most states offered some coverage of behavioral health services delivered via telehealth, and the majority of telehealth utilization was for behavioral health services and prescriptions. However, Medicaid policies regarding allowable services, providers, and originating sites vary widely across states, with often unclear payment policies. To increase health care access and limit risk of viral exposure during the pandemic, all 50 states and the District of Columbia expanded coverage and/or access to telehealth services in Medicaid (Federation of State Medical Boards, 2023; Kwong, 2024). Many have permanently adopted telehealth policy expansions, although some states have limited coverage of audio-only telehealth. Regionalization of pediatric specialists makes coverage of telemedicine services across state lines of particular importance.

At the federal level, the Bipartisan Safer Communities Act (2022) directed the Centers for Medicare & Medicaid Services (CMS) to issue guidance to states on expanding access to telehealth in Medicaid. In 2023, CMS (2023j) published *Telehealth for Providers: What You Need to Know*, which outlines various provisions and flexibilities that CMS has issued, including those impacting Medicaid services delivered via telehealth. It provides detailed information on state policies, Medicaid coverage, and best practices for telehealth services, which align with the directive from the Bipartisan Safer Communities Act (CMS, 2023j).

Retail Clinics

Retail clinics, which have spread in many regions, provide easy access for minor illnesses and often advertise convenience and lower costs in providing such services as immunizations or sports physicals (Garbutt et al., 2013; Wong et al., 2017). Among the fastest-growing components of ambulatory care for children and adults, up to 90% of retail clinic pediatric visits focused on ten common conditions, including immunizations (Mehrotra et al., 2008). While increasing access to care, they are ill equipped to provide continuity of care and comprehensive services such as those mandated under Medicaid's Early and Periodic Screening, Diagnostic, and Treatment services (see discussion in Chapter 6).

INNOVATION AND CHANGE IN PEDIATRIC PRIMARY CARE

Primary care in pediatrics has evolved substantially over the past several decades, from early work by the U.S. Children's Bureau to the development and growth of the medical home model (National Academies, 2019d), aiming to transform pediatric primary care from individual-centered, treatment-focused care to whole child, family, and community health care as reviewed in Chapter 1. Active implementation of the medical home model began in 1967, with greater recognition of the importance of early life and child and community factors in the development and wellbeing of children (Sia et al., 2004). The medical home transformation called for pediatricians and pediatric clinicians to provide guidance to young families, coordinate their care and access to needed additional services, and serve as a main point of care that families can easily access for help with the broad range of services that they and their children need. The medical home model calls for comprehensive, high-quality primary care for children and youth, emphasizing characteristics of accessibility, family-centeredness, continuity, coordination, compassion, and cultural proficiency (AAP, 2022; Boudreau et al., 2022). The federal Maternal and Child Health Bureau has long championed the medical home concept, collaborating actively with the AAP in its support and development. And the medical home concept underlays key aspects of primary care reform in the Patient Protection and Affordable Care Act (2010).

Medical home models differ in their focus and content for different age groups, but they generally follow a broad set of definitions and standards recognized by several professional organizations such as the AAP and the National Committee for Quality Assurance (Domino, 2021). The AAP, American Academy of Family Physicians, American College of Physicians, and American Osteopathic Association have jointly outlined seven core principles of a patient-centered medical home[3] (American Academy of Pediatrics, American Academy of Family Physicians, & American College

[3]The AAP earlier outlined four principles for pediatric medical homes, described as "a family-centered partnership within a community-based system that provides uninterrupted care with appropriate payment to support and sustain optimal health outcomes" (Ad Hoc Task Force on Definition of the Medical Home, 1992, p. 774; see also AAP, 2007; Buka et al., 2022). These principles include: (1) Family-centered partnership: Providing family-centered care through a trusting, collaborative partnership with families, respecting diversity and recognizing families as constant in a child's life. (2) Community-based system: The medical home is part of a coordinated network of community services designed to promote healthy child development and family wellbeing. (3) Transitions: Facilitating smooth transitions along the continuum of care as the child moves through different systems and into adulthood. (4) Value: Appropriate financing to support and sustain medical homes that promote quality care, optimal health outcomes, family satisfaction, and cost efficiency (AAP, 2007, p. 1).

of Physicians-American Society of Internal Medicine, 2002; see also AAP, 2007; Kellerman & Kirk, 2007):

1. Personal physician: Each patient has an ongoing relationship with a personal physician trained to provide first contact, continuous, and comprehensive care.
2. Physician-directed medical practice: The personal physician leads a team of individuals that collectively takes responsibility for the ongoing care of patients.
3. Whole person orientation: The personal physician is responsible for providing all the patient's health care needs or taking responsibility for appropriately arranging care with other qualified professionals.
4. Coordinated and integrated care: Care is coordinated and integrated across all elements of the complex health care system.
5. Quality and safety: Quality and safety are hallmarks of the medical home, with a focus on evidence-based medicine and clinical decision-support tools.
6. Enhanced access: Enhanced access to care is available through systems such as open scheduling, expanded hours, and new options for communication.
7. Appropriate payment: The payment structure appropriately recognizes the added value provided to patients who have a patient-centered medical home.

These principles developed nearly 20 years ago by physician organizations center the role of physicians. More recently, as discussed in this chapter, a wider range of clinicians provide primary care; however, the principles of a medical home still emphasize continuity of care, in alignment with the concept of whole person health (National Academies, 2023a; see also Chapter 2). Although the medical home model has helped improve care generally, its impact on families living in poverty has been limited because they often do not receive care that aligns with the principles of the medical home (Liljenquist & Coker, 2021; MacArthur & Blewett, 2023).

Nonetheless, development of the medical home concept over the years has led to innovation and testing of new and expanded models of high-performing pediatric primary care. These changes reflect a growing understanding of important characteristics and content of pediatric primary care (see Figure 5-1). Main advances have taken place in the content of primary care, improved coordination of care, and providing access to other services that support whole child and relational health (CMS, n.d.e; InCK Marks, 2020). Advances in the content of care have included increasingly sophisticated screening for social determinants of health and broader assessment of behavior and development. Addition of programs such as Reach Out and Read (Jimenez et al., 2023) and

WELL-CHILD VISITS - Redesigned visits and content, office organization and practice	• **Developmental surveillance:** Many validated tools (e.g., ASQ, PEDS, SWYK, SEEK, WVP) • **Social determinants of health screening:** Many validated tools (e.g. We Care) and referral linkages and clinic food pantries • **Universal promotion activities** (Reach Out and Read, Prescription for Play) • **Redesign well-child visits** (e.g., group well child visits, CenteringParenting, PARENT, DULCE) • **Technology-assisted approaches supporting and engaging families** (Cycle of Engagement, Small Moments Big Impact, Vroom) • **Training/coaching enrichments** (ECHO, mental health consultation)
ENHANCED CARE COORDINATION - Additional team members and sectors	• **Explicit structures to support referral and follow-up, effective referrals and linkages to programs and services, community-based organizations and associations, and voluntary networks and groups** (e.g., Help Me Grow, medical-legal Partnerships, food banks) • **Relational care coordination and accompaniment to provide coaching and connections to support and strengthen families in their roles and part of medical home team** (e.g., community health workers, doulas, promotores, family coaches)
INTEGRATION OF HEALTH- RELATED SERVICES - Whole child and family, developmental, place-based, and relational health	• **Primary care integration of services and co-located programs** to promote development and relationships (e.g., HealthySteps, VIP, 3-2-1 IMPACT) • **Parenting programs** and Infant, Early Childhood Mental Health programs from universal to targeted (e.g., Circles of Security, Triple P, Parent-Child Interactive Therapy, Preconception Women's Health) • **Home visiting programs** from universal to targeted (e.g., Family Connects, Family Check-Up, Child First) • **School-based health centers and services** • **Behavioral health integration into care across care settings** • **Social care in health settings and public health partnerships**
DATA COLLECTION & QUALITY IMPROVEMENT - Information technology advancement and measurement of quality and safety outcomes	• **Learning health networks** with the goal of improving health outcomes, transparency of outcome measures, and a flexible and adapted collaborative learning system (e.g., Children's Hospitals' Solutions for Patient Safety, ImproveCareNow Network, National Pediatric Cardiology Quality Improvement Collaborative NPC-QIC, Autism Treatment Network) • **Technology innovations with electronic health records, apps, artificial intelligence**

FIGURE 5-1 Examples of evidenced-based programs and practices grouped by child health transformation elements.

NOTES: This figure is not exhaustive of all evidence-based innovations in child health care transformation but reviews some areas of innovation to the traditional health care model, including redesigned well-child care, integration of systems and added services, personnel, and technology. The maturity of these innovations is variable, with some in their infancy and others progressing rapidly. ASQ = Ages & Stages Questionnaire; DULCE = Developmental Understanding and Legal Collaboration for Everyone; ECHO = Extension for Community Healthcare Outcomes; NPC-QIC = National Pediatric Cardiology Quality Improvement Collaborative; PARENT = Parent-focused Redesign for Encounters, Newborns to Toddlers; PEDS = Parents' Evaluation of Developmental Status; SEEK = Safe Environment for Every Kid; SWYK = Survey of Well-being of Young Children; VIP = Video Interaction Project; WVP = Well-Visit Planner.

SOURCE: Generated by the committee based on InCK Marks, 2024.

Prescription for Play have enhanced support for parents (Weitzman Institute, 2023). Coordination of care efforts include strategies to help households link to community resources and support, through programs such as medical–legal partnerships or StreetCred (both providing legal counseling and help with accessing various benefit programs in primary care settings), and Help Me Grow, which helps link families with a broad array of community resources (American Hospital Association [AHA], 2020; Boston Medical Center, 2023). Programs such as Healthy Steps (2024) enhance pediatric care by connecting early childhood workers with young families. Others have developed parent behavior training programs through pediatric practices. Box 5-1 describes the initiative Pediatrics Supporting Parents, aimed at using early well-child visits as an opportunity to support relational health. Box 5-2 describes several promising programs with innovative approaches to pediatric team care.

Healthy Steps is among the better-studied programs, with good evidence that the program improves up-to-date well-child visits and immunizations and more family-centered care. Parents also report improved strategies for

BOX 5-1
Opportunities for Centering Relational Health in Pediatric Care

Recognizing the great importance of early childhood and wellbeing—and the importance of supporting relationships within young families—several programs have developed to strengthen and support efforts in pediatric primary care. Well-child visits (usually there are 12 between birth and age 3 years) present a unique context for interacting with and supporting families to promote relational health. In 2017, the Silicon Valley Community Foundation launched Pediatrics Supporting Parents (PSP), with support from five early childhood funders (Cohen Ross et al., 2019; Cornell, 2019). Given the importance and critical nature of early childhood experiences, PSP emphasizes enhancing pediatric care in the early years to help improve socioemotional development through support of the primary caregiver–child relationship (Cohen Ross et al., 2019; Cornell, 2019; Cornell, Therriault, & Dworkin, 2021; PSP, n.d).

The PSP initiative centers on collaboration among health care professionals, educators, and community organizations (Cohen Ross et al., 2019; Cornell, 2019). Pediatricians, child psychologists, and experienced parenting coaches work in tandem to provide evidence-based strategies and practical advice on various aspects of child-rearing. From addressing common concerns such as sleep routines, discipline techniques, and developmental milestones, to tackling more complex issues such as behavioral challenges and special needs, the program offers a comprehensive suite of services tailored to each family's unique circumstances.

Early work focused on implementing an integrated platform, incorporating tools such as the Survey of Well-Being of Young Children, Well-Visit Planner, Promoting Healthy Development Survey, Welch Emotional Connection Screen, and FINDconnect (Cornell, 2019), and identifying 14 common practices for promoting managing their young children's behaviors (HealthySteps, 2024; Minkovitz et al., 2007; Piotrowski, Talavera, & Mayer, 2009). The Video Interaction Project, begun at New York University, uses video tapes of parent–child interactions also to help parents learn strategies to address their children's behaviors and learn how to support the child's development (Canfield et al., 2015; Mendelsohn et al., 2005, 2011; Video Interaction Project, n.d.). Reach Out and Read has a substantial evidence base, showing significant improvement in children's literacy (High et al., 2000; Sinclair et al., 2019). More recent work has documented improvements in parenting stress and parent–child relational interactions (Canfield et al., 2020). All of these (and several other) innovations have developed good evidence for their effects on care and outcomes, and many have seen substantial growth in their uptake in pediatric primary care over the past decades. Nonetheless, as indicated in Chapter 6, financing has not transformed to support these key advances and bring them to scale.

Increasingly, the medical home model has moved to team-based care, supporting the changing and expanding content of pediatric primary care

socioemotional development (Center for the Study of Social Policy & Pediatrics Supporting Parents, 2018; Cornell, 2019). Later work has aided practices with strategies for implementing and financing these changes (CSSP, 2018).

Two California programs exemplify the lessons from the earlier PSP work. Built in part on specific California benefits that support whole family health and dyadic care for young families, these two programs have enhanced connections of primary care with other early childhood activities. The LIFT/ACEs LA Medical-Financial Partnership (MFP) and Network of Care addresses the complex social and financial situations of low-income and working-class families by providing clinic-based financial coaching (Bell et al., 2020; Holguin et al., 2023). Existing studies, while limited, have shown that MFPs improve both health outcomes and family finances (Bell et al., 2020; Holguin et al., 2023). The MFP approach provides structured financial counseling and helps families identify their strengths, priorities, goals, and actionable steps aimed at improving economic stability. The University of California, Los Angeles's MFP assists with connecting families to resources that can assist them in navigating social systems and structures that can otherwise prove prohibitively difficult to engage with. The MFP helps affiliated clinics develop and maintain networks of financial and social resources, which are available to all families served at the clinics (Holguin et al., 2023; Spiker, 2023).

The University of California, San Francisco Center for Child and Community Health and the Ready! Resilient! Rising! (R3) Network serve to transform early childhood health care for low-income children. R3 includes educators, health plans, health providers, and social service agencies collaborating to improve whole child health through trauma-informed screening for basic needs and expanded behavioral health care in pediatric primary care. These trauma-informed programs create pathways for families to combat and overcome toxic stress in early childhood.

BOX 5-2
Models Supporting Early Child Wellbeing in Pediatric Primary Care

Several programs have innovated models for strengthening pediatric teams and staffing in early childhood care. Each helps pediatric primary care transform to team-based care.

DULCE

Developmental Understanding and Legal Collaboration for Everyone (DULCE) is a team-based approach to pediatric care that transforms how families experience health care (Center for the Study of Social Policy [CSSP], n.d.). Based in the pediatric care setting, it proactively addresses social determinants of health, promotes the healthy development of infants, and provides support to their parents during the critical first 6 months of their child's life (Center for the Advancement of Youth [CAY], n.d.). DULCE introduces into the care team a family specialist trained in child development, relational practice, and problem solving. Family specialists attend well-child visits with families and providers, get to know the families, provide peer support, and collaborate with the team to connect families with resources and support. The DULCE program includes family specialists, medical providers, legal partners, early childhood systems representatives, and mental health representatives, along with a project lead and a clinic administrator. By addressing the accumulated burden of social and economic hardship, the DULCE team reduces family stress, giving families more time and energy to bond with and care for their new child (Monahan, McCrae, & Arbour, 2024). The DULCE approach to social determinants of health recognizes the inequities in the distribution of power and resources, rooted in a history of racism (McCrae et al., 2021), and uses community health models to create a more equitable distribution of power and resources (CAY, n.d.; CSSP, n.d.a,b).

HealthySteps

HealthySteps is a three-tiered model that integrates developmental and behavioral services into pediatric primary care for children from birth to age 3 years (HealthySteps, n.d.b, 2022; Piotrowski, Talavera, & Mayer, 2009; Valado et al., 2019). It employs HealthySteps specialists, who are experts in child development and behavioral health, to work alongside pediatric providers. These specialists offer services such as developmental screening, positive parenting guidance, care coordination, and referrals to community resources. Evaluations have provided evidence for the model's effectiveness in promoting healthy child development and family wellbeing (HealthySteps, 2022; Piotrowski, Talavera, & Mayer, 2009; Valado et al., 2019). HealthySteps improves the quality of care and the capacity of pediatric practices to operate as institutional resources within their communities (Barth, 2010; Valado et al., 2019). The model also improves child health outcomes, including breastfeeding rates, age-appropriate nutrition, timely developmental screening and intervention, and socioemotional development (HealthySteps, 2022; Piotrowski, Talavera, & Mayer, 2009; Valado et al., 2019). Other findings include enhanced parenting practices and maternal mental health (Forum on Promoting Children's Cognitive, Affective, and Behavioral Health, 2014; Minkovitz et al., 2003, 2007; Valado et al., 2019).

Help Me Grow

Help Me Grow (HMG) leverages and expands upon existing resources to create a comprehensive approach to early childhood system-building within any community (HMG National Center, n.d.). The model provides a centralized access point to enhance utilization of existing community resources rather than creating new programs. Research shows HMG positively impacts child and parent factors by improving understanding of child development and increasing access to supportive services (Bogin, 2006; Dworkin & Kelly, 2022; Hill & Hill, 2018; HMG National Center, 2023; Hughes et al., 2016; Therriault et al., 2021). The model integrates with broader child and family-serving systems, addressing complex social needs that impact development. HMG employs targeted universalism to ensure equitable access to quality services. The Centers for Disease Control and Prevention endorsed HMG as a strategy for achieving equity, which bolsters the model's foundation in targeted universalism and supports its validity and importance (Robinson et al., 2017).

Reach Out and Read

The Reach Out and Read program is a nationally recognized early literacy intervention implemented in pediatric primary care settings across the United States (Garbe et al., 2023; Klass, Dreyer, & Mendelsohn, 2009). Founded on the principle that promoting early literacy is essential for children's cognitive and socioemotional development, the program integrates literacy promotion into routine pediatric visits by providing developmentally appropriate books to children during well-child checkups and offering guidance to parents on the importance of reading aloud (Garbe et al., 2023; Miller et al., 2023). Participation in Reach Out and Read is associated with numerous positive health outcomes, including improved language and literacy skills, enhanced parent–child bonding, increased school readiness, and reduced developmental disparities among children from low-income families (Garbe et al., 2023; Jimenez et al., 2023; Klass, Dreyer, & Mendelsohn, 2009; Needlman et al., 1991).

PlayReadVIP

PlayReadVIP, originally known as the Video Interaction Project, is an evidence-based parenting program developed by a team at the New York University Grossman School of Medicine (NYU Langone Health, n.d.; PlayReadVIP, 2024). The program aims to enhance early child development and literacy by utilizing videotaping and developmentally appropriate toys, books, and resources to help parents engage in pretend play, shared reading, and daily routines with their children (Center for Parents & Children, n.d.; Institute of Human Development and Social Change, n.d.). PlayReadVIP sessions involve one-on-one coaching during routine well-child visits where parents receive feedback on their interactions with their children. Participation in PlayReadVIP improves children's socioemotional, cognitive, and language development (Cates et al., 2018; Mendelsohn et al., 2011; Miller et al., 2023; Piccolo et al., 2023; Roby et al., 2021), increases parental engagement, and reduces parenting stress and depression (Berkule et al., 2014; Canfield et al., 2023; Cates et al., 2016; Miller, 2023). The program's integration into pediatric primary care provides a strategic platform for reaching high-risk families and promoting school readiness skills among low-income children.

by basing care in a multidisciplinary team. Teams support more care for behavioral and developmental needs, coordination of care with greater numbers of children and youth with chronic health conditions, and connection to community resources for nonmedical drivers of health. Well-designed team-based models optimize existing resources and personnel to deliver care and leverage the expertise of all team members; address the total whole person needs of the community; and focus on the upstream drivers of health, disease prevention, and health promotion (National Academies, 2023a). Team-based health care has been linked to improved health care quality, patient outcomes, and cost savings, with increasing evidence that it also improves clinician wellbeing (Jacob et al., 2015; Pape et al., 2011; Roberts et al., 2001; Tiel Groenestege-Kreb, van Maarseveen, & Leenen, 2014).

Traditional pediatric office practices typically include one or more clinicians, with support from nurses or medical assistants, and office staff. Extended teams include a variety of additional staff (often depending on community needs) that may include advanced practice nurses (to help coordinate chronic care), mental and behavioral health professionals, and community health workers, as well as care managers, interpreters, nutritionists, lactation specialists, school liaison staff, health educators, health coaches, and attorneys and other medical–legal partnership staff. Figure 5-2 provides examples of an extended health care team and extended community care team, with the patient and the family at the center of the core team.

Team approaches to care, when adequately staffed and resourced, have many benefits in clinical settings. For example, team-based care is associated with reduced workload, increased efficiency, improved quality, improved patient outcomes, reduced fragmentation, and decreased clinician burnout and turnover (National Academies, 2019e, 2021b). Expanding teams addresses some of the major time constraints faced by usual physician-run primary care—where time available to address social, community, and developmental issues can limit services. Well-designed teams can also support nurturing, longitudinal, person-centered care (Mitchell et al., 2012; Sullivan & Ellner, 2015), a key feature of high-quality primary care (National Academies, 2021b). Effective teams are designed to meet the specific needs of the communities they serve. Ideally, teams reflect the diversity of the communities they serve (Katkin et al., 2017) and evolve with the changing needs of the community over time (National Academies, 2021b, p. 182; see also Bodenheimer, 2019; Bodenheimer & Smith, 2013; Brownstein et al., 2011; Coker, Thomas, & Chung, 2013; Coker et al., 2009, 2014; Fierman et al., 2016; Grumbach, Bainbridge, & Bodenheimer, 2012; Katkin et al., 2017; Margolius et al., 2012).

Recent studies have shown the particular value of community health workers (and related workers such as peer counselors and family coaches) in improving health and outcomes (Bruner & Kotelchuck, 2023). Reviews of studies (though mainly among adult populations) found improved treatment adherence and decreased hospitalization and more attention to social

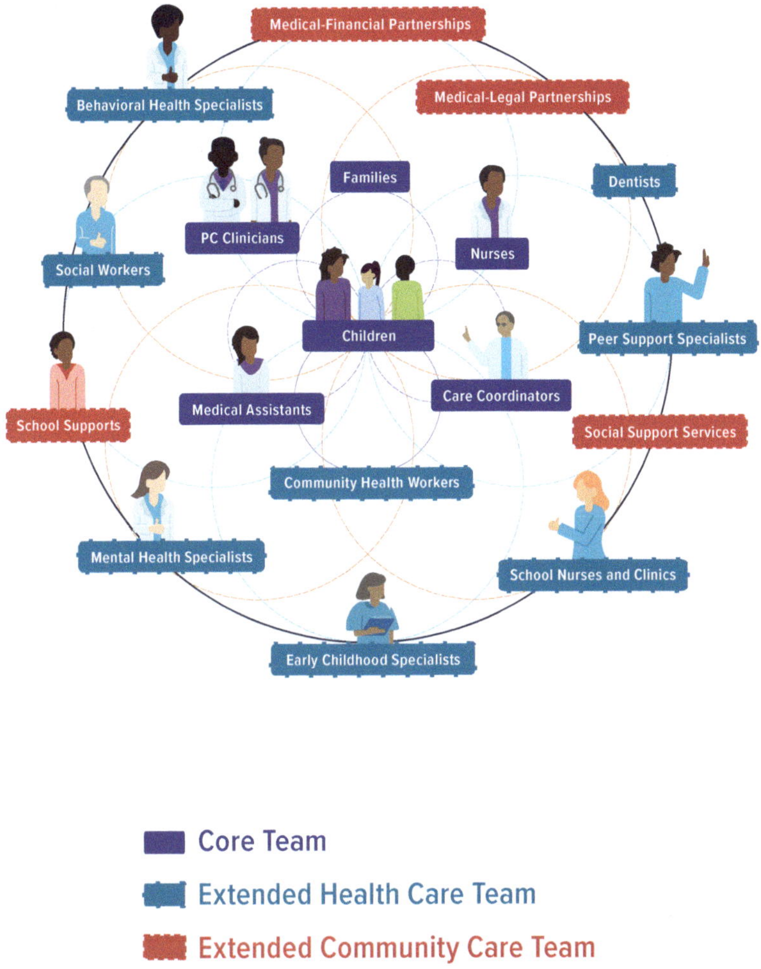

FIGURE 5-2 The composition of a multidisciplinary primary care team.
NOTE: PC = primary care.
SOURCE: Adapted from National Academies, 2021b.

determinants of health (Kangovi et al., 2020; National Academies, 2021b; Vasan et al., 2020). The PARENT intervention has documented how family coaches reduced emergency department use and increased preventive care services (Coker et al., 2016; Mimila et al., 2017).

The extended community care team in Figure 5-2 involves clinical–community partnerships and cross-sector, multidisciplinary programs such as medical–legal and medical–financial partnerships, clinic-based food pantries, and embedded and school behavioral health services. Screening for child and family needs and social determinants of health have accompanied

BOX 5-3
Medical–Legal Partnerships (MLPs)

MLPs integrate legal advocates into health care settings to address health-related social needs of the child and family. There are more than 400 MLPs across the United States where legal advocates work with clinicians to co-design social risk screening, educate health care professionals about legal remedies, and intervene to address health-harming legal issues (e.g., housing, public benefits, utilities, educational needs; Beck et al., 2021). Legal advocates are powerful allies in driving upstream changes to promote health, and MLPs enable broader, system-level pattern recognition and advocacy in pursuit of health equity and justice. A retrospective cohort study examining the effect of referral to an MLP on hospitalization rates among urban, low-income children in Greater Cincinnati, Ohio, found that the median predicted hospitalization rate for children in the year after referral was almost 40% lower if children received the legal intervention than if they did not (Beck et al., 2022). Clinicians report that MLPs also increase their self-efficacy for addressing child and family needs by improving their awareness of the social determinants of health and health-harming legal issues, empowering them to engage in systemic advocacy and improving their relationships with patients' families (Murillo et al., 2022).

team-based care. However, the effect of such screening is often limited without further assistance with referrals, navigation supports for families, and monitoring of follow-up. When linked to facilitated referrals, a comprehensive program can help families increase access to community services. Systematic screening and closed-loop referrals for social determinants during well-child care lead to larger initial enrollment in community resources for families (Garg et al., 2015). Box 5-3 describes the growth of medical–legal partnerships to support pediatric transformation addressing social determinants of health.

While there is compelling evidence that team-based approaches to primary care can foster high-quality, efficient, continuous, and relationship-based care (National Academies, 2021b), making the transition to a team-based approach to care delivery often requires additional support. Many practices—especially independent small to medium-sized practices and those located in resource-limited communities—find the transition challenging, both logistically and financially. Dominant fee-for-service payment offers few incentives for this transformation, not only in terms of paying for additional multidisciplinary team members, but also in terms of financing the development of the clinic-level infrastructure needed to make the shift to team-based delivery. Most team-based care expansions have come from a combination of some billed services (especially for mental and behavioral treatments), grants, and philanthropy (Assistant Secretary for Planning and Evaluation, 2023a). A few state Medicaid programs have allowed billing for various nonphysician personnel or have restructured payment with incentives to develop team-based care (MassHealth, 2022). Additionally, in 2023, the Centers for Medicare & Medicaid Services (2023c) implemented rule changes designed to improve equity, including a change that makes it easier to cover community health workers on care delivery teams. Most, but not all, states currently allow Medicaid payment for community health workers (see Box 5-4; Haldar & Hinton, 2023).

BOX 5-4
Community Health Workers (CHWs)

CHWs have critical roles in improving access to health care and addressing social determinants of health for children and families, particularly in underserved communities. CHWs serve as trusted liaisons between health care systems and the communities they serve, bridging cultural and linguistic gaps, and providing culturally appropriate support and education (Coker et al., 2016; Rogers et al., 2023). In pediatric care settings, CHWs support caregivers of children with special health care needs, helping them understand and manage their child's condition, navigate the health care system, and address clinical and social needs (Moheize et al., 2024). CHWs and family coaches have helped reduce hospitalizations and emergency department visits for children with asthma, promoting medication adherence, and empowering families to better manage chronic conditions (Costich et al., 2019). By connecting families with community-based organizations and resources, CHWs address social determinants of health, including transportation, food insecurity, housing instability, and financial strain (Costich et al., 2019; Moheize et al., 2024; Rogers et al., 2023).

Peer- and family-support specialists are nontraditional workforce additions who can also help teams provide comprehensive support and improve health outcomes (Hayhoe et al., 2018; Malcarney et al., 2017; Department of Health and Human Services [HHS], 2007). Peer-support specialists are individuals with lived experience of mental health conditions or substance use disorders who use their personal recovery stories to inspire hope, provide emotional support, and assist others in navigating the recovery process. They facilitate support groups and skill-building activities, and advocate for individuals' needs and rights, promoting self-determination and empowerment. Research has shown that peer-support services can improve engagement in treatment, reduce hospitalizations, and enhance overall recovery outcomes (Hayhoe et al., 2018; HHS, 2007; Malcarney et al., 2017).

Family-support specialists, also known as family peer advocates or family partners, are caregivers or family members of individuals with disabilities, mental health conditions, or other special health care needs (National Indian Child Welfare Association [NICWA], 2014; Robertson et al., 2023; Substance Abuse and Mental Health Services Administration [SAMHSA], 2017). They leverage their personal experiences to support other families by providing emotional understanding, helping them navigate complex service systems, advocating for family-centered care and rights, facilitating peer-support groups and skill-building workshops, and promoting family empowerment and self-advocacy. The involvement of family-support specialists has been associated with improved family functioning, increased access to services, and better outcomes for children with special health care needs (NICWA, 2014; Robertson et al., 2023; SAMHSA, 2017).

Still, many practices, particularly small and medium-sized independent practices, face both space limitations and difficulty finding needed multidisciplinary personnel, especially in rural areas. Workforce demands and burnout have especially affected the supply of mental and behavioral health personnel. One tactic that small and medium-sized practices can take is banding together to pool resources and sharing certain personnel or community resources (e.g., social services) across multiple practices (Mostashari, 2016).

MENTAL AND BEHAVIORAL HEALTH CARE PROVIDERS AND SETTINGS

The mental health care system is also diverse, including multiple settings, with limited coordination among the several sectors involved. Behavioral health services are provided across six general sectors: behavioral health care systems, schools, child welfare, substance abuse services, medical and primary care clinics, and juvenile justice. Services focus on treatment rather than prevention and often do not meet the basic population-level behavioral health needs of children and youth in the communities they serve (American Psychological Association Task Force on Evidence-Based Practice for Children and Adolescents, 2008).

Traditional models of outpatient mental health services may focus primarily on mental health diagnosis and its intra- and interpersonal complications rather than on the interaction of a diagnosis with physical health and health-maintenance behaviors. Services may take place in the offices of a physician, psychologist, social worker, or mental health counselor and increasingly virtually. Often, such mental health services are out of network or paid for out of pocket, as finding in-network behavioral specialists, particularly psychiatrists, can be more difficult than finding other types of specialists (National Alliance on Mental Illness, 2016, 2017; Overhage et al., 2024).

Other settings may involve a multidisciplinary team of professionals—including psychologists, psychiatrists, developmental and behavioral pediatricians, social workers, and therapists—who collaborate to provide assessment, diagnosis, and treatment (Haines et al., 2018). Clinics may be publicly funded as community mental health centers or may take only commercial insurance (or private pay). Clinics often tailor therapeutic interventions to each child's specific concerns, utilizing evidence-based approaches such as cognitive-behavioral therapy, dialectical behavior therapy, and play therapy (Bhide & Chakraborty, 2020; Hoagwood et al., 2001; Kaminski & Claussen, 2017). Additionally, these settings may offer medication management as needed. With an emphasis on creating a supportive and nurturing environment, clinicians strive to empower children to explore their emotions, develop coping skills, and foster resilience (Masten & Barnes, 2018; Ronen, 2021). Family involvement is often encouraged to promote holistic healing and facilitate long-term stability and wellbeing for the child (Berger

& Font, 2015; Hogue et al., 2021). Regular monitoring and follow-up ensure that interventions remain effective and adaptable to the child's evolving needs (Almirall & Chronis-Tuscano, 2016; Colizzi, Lasalvia, & Ruggeri, 2020). Disparities in access for children seeking mental, emotional, and behavioral health care in the United States stem from differences in insurance coverage, geographic availability of services, cultural barriers, and stigma, leading to unequal access to care based on financial resources, location, ethnicity, and perceptions of mental illness (Hoffmann et al., 2022; Mongelli, Georgakopoulos, & Pato, Toure et al., 2022).

School-based mental health programs have emerged as integral components of the children's mental health care system, providing on-site counseling services, behavioral interventions, and crisis support to students within the familiar environment of their educational settings (see Chapter 8). These programs facilitate early identification and intervention for mental health issues and promote collaboration among educators, mental health professionals, and families to create supportive learning environments conducive to emotional wellbeing.

Inpatient psychiatric treatment provides acute care for those experiencing serious mental health and/or behavioral concerns that require a higher level of care for safety, treatment management, and supervision. Inpatient care provides intensive treatment services ranging from milieu therapy to medication management and a high level of supervision in a restricted, controlled environment. Children and youth may be hospitalized at the recommendation of a physician, mental health provider, or family following assessment. Follow-up outpatient therapy and services are essential for continued stabilization and alleviation of symptoms following inpatient psychiatric treatment, including residential treatment and other options.

The current U.S. child mental health crisis has contributed to a notable shortage of pediatric inpatient psychiatric treatment facilities, especially in rural states (Feuer et al., 2023; Gulliver, Griffiths, & Christensen, 2010; Ibeziako et al., 2022, 2024). This has resulted in pediatric mental health boarding of youth in emergency departments or admitted to inpatient medical/surgical units, awaiting placement in psychiatric treatment programs (Dalton et al., 2023; Feuer et al., 2023; Ibeziako et al., 2022, 2024; Zipursky et al., 2023). Interventions to address this have included enhanced crisis stabilization services, bridge programs to safely discharge patients with a bridge to expedited follow-up, and treatment initiation in the emergency department and on inpatient medical/surgical units for boarding patients awaiting placement.

Residential treatment centers offer longer-term therapeutic interventions for children with persistent mental health challenges, providing structured programming, individualized treatment plans, and opportunities for skill-building and rehabilitation (CMS, 2023h). Partial hospitalization programs provide structured and intensive psychiatric treatment for children and adolescents experiencing acute mental health crises or significant functional impairment (CMS, n.d.f). These programs typically offer a comprehensive range of therapeutic interventions, including group therapy, individual counseling, medication management, and educational support, while allowing participants to return home each day. Residential treatment and partial hospitalizations programs designed for children are in short supply.

To meet growing needs for mental health services, the health care system has evolved to expand access to services through a range of providers and settings that best serve families and children, including a wide variety of mental health professionals. Many of these professionals specialize in child and family health, and some provide team-based care for children and families. Furthermore, efforts are increasing to train other health care professionals, including physicians and primary care providers, to recognize and identify mental health issues and treat mild to moderate issues when possible and/or refer to specialized care. Some health care systems have even engaged, trained, and funded those with lived experience with mental health issues to help others (Levine, 2023).

Extension for Community Healthcare Outcomes (ECHO) programs have emerged as a promising strategy for improving mental health services for children especially in under-resourced areas (Hager et al., 2018; Zhou et al., 2016). These programs leverage technology to connect specialists with primary care providers, behavioral health experts, and other health care professionals allowing them to collaborate, share expertise, and build capacity to effectively address children's mental health needs. Project ECHO employs a model that connects a specialist team, the "hub," with providers, or "spokes," across a wide area using videoconferencing technology (Lalloo et al., 2020). ECHO programs improve providers' knowledge, confidence, and competence in diagnosing and treating various mental health conditions in children, including depression, anxiety, and behavioral disorders (Sockalingam et al., 2018). Additionally, ECHO programs promote a collaborative and multidisciplinary approach to care, which can lead to more comprehensive and holistic treatment plans that address the unique needs of each child. ECHO programs contribute to reducing disparities in mental health care access and outcomes among underserved populations, ensuring that children receive the support and treatment they require for optimal mental health and wellbeing.

Barriers to Pediatric Behavioral and Mental Health Services

Untreated mental health disorders in childhood have a high likelihood of persisting into adulthood (Mulraney et al., 2021). Yet families face many barriers when trying to engage services, with long delays in accessing care or receiving no care at all. More than half of children with mental health problems do not receive care from a mental health clinician for more than 3 years after a problem arises (Whitney & Peterson, 2019). In all, only about 20% of children with mental and behavioral health disorders receive care from a mental health clinician (Martini et al., 2012). Accessibility (e.g., distance to agency, coordination of services, knowledge of available services), availability (e.g., mental health workforce shortage, limited scope of services), affordability (e.g., care cost, insurance coverage, copay), and acceptability (e.g., stigma, dual relationships) create barriers, especially for rural communities (National Rural Health Association [NRHA], 2015).

Medicaid and the Children's Health Insurance Program (CHIP) are the dominant payors for behavioral health services for children and adolescents in the United States (Counts, 2022; Dieleman at al., 2020). However, many behavioral health providers do not accept Medicaid payments, and penetration rates of Medicaid-funded services remain low, with over half of children who need services not accessing care (Pires, McLean, & Allen, 2018). While Medicaid and CHIP provide comprehensive behavioral health services, children with commercial insurance tend to access these services more frequently, likely due to fewer access barriers and higher utilization rates of specific services, such as psychotherapy (Ali et al., 2019; Doupnik et al., 2020; Haley et al., 2023; Kalmin et al., 2023). Many behavioral health providers, including psychiatrists and psychologists, work in private settings and accept no insurance (Bishop et al., 2014; Hamp et al., 2016). Services provided through private practices vary in terms of quality and availability, with little systematic information available on the structure of these services.

The current availability and financing of substance use prevention, assessment, and treatment services fall short of meeting the needs of young people. In 2019, only 8% of adolescents and young adults who required substance use treatment received it, according to data from the Substance Abuse and Mental Health Services Administration (2020). This disparity in treatment access is linked to social, economic, and criminal justice inequities, as well as stigma within the health care system toward substance use (Jordan, Mathis, & Isom, 2020; Marrast, Himmelstein, & Woolhandler, 2016; National Academies, 2016b). Black and Hispanic adolescents and young adults with substance use disorders are particularly affected by these inequities, being less likely than non-Hispanic White youth to receive specialty substance use treatment as of 2021 (Cummings, Wen, & Druss, 2011; Pinedo & Villatoro, 2020). Furthermore, the majority of adolescents and young adults with opioid use disorder do not receive medications for it, and non-Hispanic Black and Hispanic youth are less likely to receive medications than non-Hispanic White youth (Alinsky et al., 2020; Bagley et al., 2020; Mauro et al., 2022; Society for Adolescent Health and Medicine, 2021).

Several reasons explain the lack of availability of treatment. One barrier is the stigma that surrounds mental health. Even in places where resources and mental health supports are available, there can be reluctance to promote them and to make use of them. Another primary barrier is that most communities lack sufficient providers. There are shortages of qualified mental health providers across the spectrum of all licensed practitioners (especially psychologists, psychiatrists, developmental and behavioral pediatricians, addiction counselors, mental health counselors, and psychiatric–mental health nurse practitioners). A 2018 analysis estimated that 9,956 child and adolescent psychiatrists were practicing actively (approximately 15 practitioners per 100,000 children under age 18 years; Beck et al., 2018). Distribution of clinical child and adolescent psychiatrists and psychologists is uneven across the country, with the majority located in the Northeast and on the West Coast (Andrilla et al., 2018; Lin & Stamm, 2020). Particularly troubling for children and youth is the projected shortage of 21,030 school counselors over the next 15 years; these estimates are based on current use of behavioral health services in the United States and do not consider that significant needs for the same services are currently going unmet (National Center for Health Workforce Analysis [NCHWA], 2023). Children and youth from rural areas have less access to mental health care than their urban peers (NRHA, 2015). Many rural counties have no practicing psychiatrists or social workers at all (Counts, 2023). With such shortages, families often have to travel long distances, endure long wait times to receive services, or go without services.

Disparities in Pediatric Mental and Behavioral Health

Compared with White children and adolescents, children from historically marginalized racial/ethnic groups have a higher prevalence of many mental and behavioral health conditions and are less likely to receive services for them (Hoffmann et al., 2022). Compared with White children, Black and Hispanic children have fewer mental and behavioral health visits, are less likely to be seen by specialists, have lower expenditures, are less likely to be prescribed psychotropic medication, and are less likely to receive evidence-based care for common mental and behavioral health conditions (e.g., anxiety, depression, ADHD, substance use). This unequal access to services and treatment is thought to have led to the poorer outcomes discussed in Chapter 4.

Stark racial/ethnic disparities are evident in diagnosis and care for autism spectrum disorder. Reports from the Autism and Developmental Disabilities Monitoring (ADDM) Network (CDC, 2020c) have consistently found disparities in diagnosing autism in children in Black and Hispanic populations. Potential barriers leading to these disparities include stigma, lack of access to health care services due to noncitizenship or low income, and non-English primary language (ADDM, 2018; CDC, 2019c). What is more, Black children with autism often experience a delay in diagnosis, are underidentified, or are misdiagnosed with a disruptive behavior disorder (Hoffmann et al., 2022).

Literature on disparities in mental health care receipt among U.S. children and adolescents is nuanced and complex. Several studies have highlighted variations in the nature and direction of disparities across different mental health conditions and over time. While racial/ethnic disparities in

ADHD diagnosis and treatment have narrowed in recent years (Coker et al., 2016; McKay & Perente, 2019), disparities persist for conditions such as depression and anxiety, with minority youth being less likely to receive outpatient mental health services (Cummings & Druss, 2011; Hodgkinson et al., 2017; Hoffmann et al., 2023; Lê Cook et al., 2019; Marrast, Himmelstein, & Woolhandler, 2016). Children from low-income families and those without adequate insurance are also less likely to receive needed services (Hodgkinson et al., 2017; Kirkbride et al., 2024). The specific mental health condition, age group, and geographic region studied can influence the nature and direction of disparities, highlighting the complexity of the issue (Hoffmann et al., 2023).

While the many societal, political, and economic factors that created and continue to perpetuate a system of unequal treatment go beyond what the health care system can do alone, the mental health care system can take steps at both the delivery and larger systems levels, to help minimize disparities. At the clinician level, understanding implicit biases and taking steps to minimize them, such as by using standard screening and diagnostic instruments and standardizing their implementation, is one way of reducing disparities (Viswanathan et al., 2022). Similarly, ensuring that the care delivered is culturally competent and trauma informed can help as well (Trent, Dooley, & Dougé, 2019). At an organizational level, eliminating any race or ethnicity considerations that are used in detrimental ways in treatment algorithms or practice guidelines is another way to reduce treatment disparities based on race or ethnicity (Wright et al., 2022). Progress toward reducing disparities must be tracked over time (Harrington et al., 2021).

Integrating Mental and Behavioral Health Care with Primary Care

Integration of behavioral health services into primary care has grown over the last few decades, partly in conjunction with the exponential rise of the mental health challenges children and families face, but also from recognition that prevention and early detection can help avoid more serious conditions later. Early experimentation took place about 50 years ago, with slow but definite growth since that time. In *Child Health and the Community,* Haggerty (1975) documented the growing mental and behavioral health issues in pediatrics (the "new morbidity"). Integration has the added benefit of improving access to care, improving equity, and reducing silos between service lines and thus managing a workforce more efficiently. Having mental and behavioral health clinicians as part of team-based care also expands the range of care available and can link mental and behavioral health providers with community health workers and others to improve community prevention and treatment strategies. Numerous organizations advocating for children's health support greater integration of mental and behavioral health into pediatric primary care (Ader et al.,

2015; American Academy of Child and Adolescent Psychiatry, 2023b; National Academies, 2019b).

Pediatric settings are well suited for early identification and intervention of childhood mental and behavioral health concerns (Talmi et al., 2016), as families seeking mental health services often seek care initially from their pediatric clinician. Consequently, mental health symptoms and disorders are among the most common concerns addressed in pediatric care (Yonek et al., 2020). Integrating mental and physical health can help with care coordination, access, efficiency, and outcomes for children and their families (Reiss-Brennan, 2014; Reiss-Brennan et al., 2016; Walter et al., 2019). Team-based integrated behavioral health supports primary care clinicians and families by improving providers' skills in engaging families to discuss mental and behavioral health concerns, comanaging identification and treatment, sharing information that facilitates coordination and communication across providers, and using evidence-based screening tools for developmental and behavioral disorders (Hine et al., 2017; Talmi et al., 2016; Tyler, Hulkower, & Kaminski, 2017). Operationally, integration can range from simple coordination and colocation of clinical services to a more robust collaborative care model (Asarnow et al., 2015). With collaborative care, primary care and behavioral health professionals, often supported by a care coordinator and other team members, work on a single treatment plan with both behavioral and medical elements in a single system of care that addresses whole child and family health (Gerrity, 2016; National Academies, 2021b,c).

One of the benefits of integrated behavioral health is streamlining the provision of needed services. A common challenge faced by families with mental health needs is navigating the behavioral health care system, referral to appropriate and/or culturally appropriate services, and limited follow-through on community-based mental health referrals (Hine et al., 2017; Talmi et al., 2016). With integrated mental and behavioral health services, most mental and behavioral health needs can be addressed within a single system. In instances when additional services are needed, providers identify and connect patients and families to community resources and programs to address their needs and provide individualized, person-centered care that incorporates family members and caregivers into the treatment plan.

Integrated behavioral health care is a worthwhile investment because it addresses gaps in care seen with traditional models, increases access to specialty care, and improves behavioral health outcomes (Tyler, Hulkower, & Kaminski, 2017). Kolko and Perrin (2014) found positive effects on children's mental health problems (greater reductions in externalizing and internalizing problems), parent–child interactions, parental distress, and lowered treatment costs per patient, when comparing integrated with usual care. In a follow-up paper, the authors emphasize more distal indicators of effectiveness in measures of "feasibility, clinical effectiveness, heightened consumer satisfaction, coordination and continuity of care over time, and potential cost savings related to less use of restrictive and costly placements or other services" (Yu, Kolko, & Torres, 2017, p. 57).

Despite the many benefits of integration, the transition to integration can be challenging, requiring supports different from those needed for adult care (National Academies, 2021b). Because child mental health concerns are most often linked to parental mental health and family psychosocial needs, successful pediatric behavioral health integration requires mechanisms for identifying and addressing the mental, social, and parental–child interaction needs of the entire family (Wissow, Platt, & Sarvet, 2021). Relatedly, child mental health is often more behavioral focused and time intensive (and thus resource intensive) than adult care, which is more commonly addressed with medication.

HOSPITAL-BASED AND SPECIALIZED CARE

Hospitals provide a wide range of health services for children and youth, including hospital-based primary care activities and specialty outpatient, urgent, and emergency care. They also provide inpatient care when needed for critical acute conditions, when chronic conditions become unstable, or for severe trauma and injuries. Various surgical procedures require treatment and follow-up in hospitals or surgical centers. Most U.S. births occur in hospitals, including specialized neonatal intensive care for sick newborns.

Consolidation has characterized the hospital sector over the past several decades, including consolidated locations for hospital beds for children and youth, which has contributed to rising costs and reduced access (Goodwin, Levinson, & Hulver, 2023; Levins, 2023). With the decreasing rates of childhood conditions requiring hospitalization (e.g., decreased rates of infectious disease, increasing outpatient care) along with cost concerns in maintaining a pediatric unit where low Medicaid payment compromises revenues, the hospital industry for children and adolescents has seen a continuing decline in numbers of pediatric beds and consolidation of hospital inpatient services in a smaller number of often larger hospitals (Cushing et al., 2021; Leyenaar et al., 2016, 2023; Perrin, Valvona, & Sloan, 1986). Over the past decade more than 200 hospitals in rural areas of the United States have closed labor and delivery units, reducing access to maternity and neonatal care. These closures have been due to financial and workforce issues and result in long drive times to receive care.

One study categorized hospitals as Tier A hospitals that provided care only to children; Tier B hospitals that had key pediatric services, including pediatric emergency departments and pediatric and neonatal intensive care units; Tier C hospitals that provided limited pediatric services; and Tier D hospitals with no key pediatric services. Classifications were then validated by using publicly available data on hospital membership in various pediatric programs as well as Health Care Cost Institute claims data. Fifty-one hospitals were classified as Tier A; 228 as Tier B; 1,721 as Tier C; and 1,728 as Tier D (Piper et al., 2020). In 2019, a majority of U.S. pediatric hospitalizations occurred at general hospitals, as opposed to freestanding children's hospitals or high-volume hospitals (Steiner et al., 2023; Weiss, Liang, & Martin, 2022). The number of U.S. hospitals with pediatric units declined from 1,753 in 2008 to 1,418 in 2018, a drop of around 19% (Leyenaar et al., 2023). There has also been an increasing trend of interfacility transfers from general hospital emergency departments to other hospitals for admission for certain pediatric conditions, such as asthma and croup (Cushing, Bucholz, & Michelson, 2020; Leyenaar et al., 2016, 2023).

This redistribution and regionalization of pediatric care influences access to care for pediatric patients because of geographic distance to service (Karamlou et al., 2020; Lorch, Myers, & Carr, 2010; Mahant & Guttmann, 2023; Ramos et al., 2020; Turner, Ricketts, & Leslie, 2020). However, some evidence suggests that regionalization can improve quality of care for certain populations, such as reducing mortality for infants with very low birth weights (Phibbs et al., 2007). Regionalization may also reduce costs in some circumstances (Lorch, Myers, & Carr, 2010). A recent National Academies report on low birth weight babies and disability noted the clear risks associated with premature birth and low birth weight and emphasized that specialized programs can improve outcomes for these babies (National Academies, 2023f; see also Aubin et al., 2023; Nguyen et al., 2013; Rouse et al., 2008; Wilson et al., 2022). Numerous studies demonstrate an association between volume and outcomes in pediatric cardiology with lower volumes associated with higher operative mortality, particularly for highly complex cases (Backer et al., 2023). Multiple professional societies have recommended categorizing centers as either essential care centers (essential services for any program, minimum of 75 index cases per year) or comprehensive care centers (services to optimize comprehensive and high-complexity care), based on structure, process, and outcome metrics (Backer et al., 2023).

Hospitals also provide critical services such as emergency and trauma care, with capacity well beyond that of retail clinics or community urgent care centers. They also provide specialized medical and surgical services and intensive care for children with more severe and complex conditions. As noted in Chapters 1 and 4, pediatric chronic conditions are relatively rare, other than a small number of high-prevalence conditions. Although primary care has a substantive role in the care of these children, they often need regular access to pediatric subspecialists, usually housed in hospital settings and larger cities.

Many low-income patients with chronic conditions have barriers to health care access, at times using multiple health care settings or systems for care, leading to fragmented care and worse outcomes. Managed care networks increasingly deny claims for needed services (see Chapter 6), disallowing patients from receiving needed care in nearby sites or from out-of-network providers. Hospital closures and higher costs in consolidated markets have exacerbated access problems for many children, especially those from low-income families (Cushing et al., 2021; Levins, 2023; Leyenaar et al., 2023). Research examining the impact of integration of hospitals and clinic systems on costs show increases in health care prices and spending. These increases have been associated with minimal to no improvements in quality of care and potentially worse outcomes for vulnerable adult patient populations (Levin, Komanduri, & Whaley, 2023). A recent study of reports from the AHA annual survey, which included 1,088 hospitals (235 of which joined a larger health care system), found a significant association of joining a health care system with a loss of inpatient services within 5 years (Joseph, Davis, & Kahn, 2023). Less is known about the impact of hospital closures on access to pediatric acute care for children with chronic conditions and medical complexity, or the effects of consolidation on family experiences, child health outcomes, and costs.

Inpatient Care

Hospitals provide inpatient care for acutely ill children who require interventions and monitoring not available in outpatient settings. Most hospitalized children and those with highly complex needs receive care in children's hospitals or general hospitals with pediatric programs, and the following text uses "children's hospitals" to refer to both. Most of these two groups are teaching hospitals. Pediatric hospitals serve as regional centers, provide resource-intensive care to the sickest children, and are staffed by health care personnel with specialized training in children's health (Piper et al., 2020). There are approximately 250 Tier A and B children's hospitals in the United States (Children's Hospital Association, n.d.). While children's hospitals comprise less than 5% of all hospitals in the United States, they account for 40% of pediatric inpatient days and 50% of national pediatric costs (Cohen & Patel, 2014; Piper et al., 2020; Raval, Reiter, & McCarthy, 2022). They provide more than 95% of specialized care to treat acute and chronic conditions, including 97% of all organ transplants and 90% of all pediatric cancer care (Children's Hospital Association, 2023; Raval, Reiter, & McCarthy, 2022) and are uniquely equipped with specialized staff, technology, and multidisciplinary teams designed to meet the specific needs of children.

Without hospitals designed to serve children, highly complex pediatric care would be more random and uncertain. Complex chronic care hospitalizations make up a growing share of inpatient care and resource utilization (Simon et al., 2010). While the total number of pediatric admissions has declined in recent years, the percentage of admissions for children with complex chronic conditions increased by 5.7% from 2010 to 2016, and unadjusted readmission rates for patients with complex chronic conditions increased from 6.26% to 7.02% (Bucholz, Toomey, & Schuster, 2019). In 2018, pediatric patients with complex chronic care conditions accounted for 9% of all hospitalized patients, and 23% of all hospitalizations (Oztek Celebi & Senel, 2021).

Although they are far more accessible than children's hospitals to most families, most community hospitals do not have the necessary resources, such as medical equipment and health care providers trained in pediatric care, for treating pediatric populations, especially when treating mental health conditions or addressing needs of children with disabilities (CDC, 2023d; HRSA, 2023b; National Academies, 2018). In contrast, children's hospitals provide subspecialty hospital services to children with disabilities who may be hospitalized for an acute illness, chronic illness exacerbation, procedure, or surgery related to their underlying condition. Since only 1 in 20 U.S. hospitals is a children's hospital, children with disabilities and complex medical conditions often must travel far distances to access services (National Academies, 2018).

Specialized children's hospitals are also essential for children from disadvantaged backgrounds. Approximately 50% of all care provided in children's hospitals goes to low-income children, 6% of whom have medically complex conditions (Casimir, 2019). Neighborhood-level characteristics, including household income, overcrowding, exposure to environmental toxins, poverty, and violence, are potential risk factors for hospitalization and illness severity. Using the Child Opportunity Index (COI), a validated tool that incorporates neighborhood-level factors that impact child health (Acevedo-Garcia et al., 2014; Aris et al., 2021), a 2023 study showed that 28 diagnoses (including diabetes mellitus, sickle cell disease, asthma, sleep apnea, COVID-19, and respiratory failure) were significantly more common in hospitalized children from low low-COI neighborhoods (Heneghan, Goodman, & Ramgopal, 2023). Hospitalized children from low-COI neighborhoods also had more severe illness compared with those from more advantaged neighborhoods (Heneghan, Goodman, & Ramgopal, 2023). These findings suggest the need to address disparities in neighborhood characteristics and access to care, especially for children with chronic medical conditions, when allocating resources or developing targeted programming.

Inpatient settings, including critical care units, present an opportunity to screen for and address social determinants of health that impact patient outcomes. Implementing screening for food, housing, and transportation needs in an urban safety-net hospital documented significant correlations between positive screens and race and ethnicity, insurance type, and clinical characteristics like substance use disorder (Byhoff et al., 2017; Chukmaitov et al., 2022). Fritz et al. (2020) surveyed caregivers of hospitalized pediatric patients and found many were comfortable with and accepting of social determinants of health (SDOH) screening during the inpatient stay (Gayle et al., 2023).

Screening for SDOH in the inpatient setting can inform discharge planning, facilitate referrals to community resources, and potentially improve post-discharge outcomes (Chukmaitov et al., 2022; Gayle et al., 2023).

For more than 20 years, a focus on quality improvement and learning health networks in pediatric inpatient care has improved health outcomes. For example, the Children's Hospitals' Solutions for Patient Safety Network is an unparalleled, collaborative effort among children's hospitals working to transform pediatric patient and employee safety in pursuit of eliminating serious harm and improving outcomes across all children's hospitals. Begun in the 1980s from the Ohio Children's Hospital Association, it grew to a network of 140+ pediatric hospitals today working together to help each individual hospital make progress on implementation of the network's best practices reporting. From 2012 to 2024, this national effort estimates 27,509 children saved from serious harm and cost savings of $585.9 million, with a consistent upward trend in harm prevented every month.[4] The quality improvement learning network approach includes focused goals, a theory of change, data sharing and communication, strategic partnerships with families, and a relentless focus on results (Terao et al., 2019). Multiple positive patient outcomes have been documented from reductions in hospital-acquired infections and serious safety events to unplanned extubations (AHRQ, n.d.; Klugman et al., 2020; Lyren et al., 2017; Tripathi et al., 2023). This learning network is also focusing on racial/ethnic disparities in quality and safety (Lyren et al., 2024). Learning networks have proliferated as a successful model for innovation and quality improvement for inpatient care and specific disease conditions (Terao et al., 2019).

Subspecialty and Surgical Care

Pediatrics currently has 22 associated pediatric subspecialties accredited by the Accreditation Council for Graduate Medical Education[5] (2023a,b); these, along with pediatric subspecialties in other areas,[6] provide acute and chronic care expertise and skills for the highest-quality care for children.

[4] See https://www.solutionsforpatientsafety.org/publications

[5] The subspecialties are addiction medicine, adolescent medicine, child abuse pediatrics, clinical informatics, developmental-behavioral pediatrics, hospice and palliative medicine, internal medicine-pediatrics, neonatal-perinatal medicine, pediatric cardiology, pediatric critical care medicine, pediatric emergency medicine, pediatric endocrinology, pediatric gastroenterology, pediatric hematology oncology, pediatric hospital medicine, pediatric infectious diseases, pediatric nephrology, pediatric pulmonology, pediatric rheumatology, pediatric transplant hepatology, sleep medicine, and sports medicine.

[6] Additional specialties with subspecialties for pediatrics include anesthesiology, dermatology, neurology, obstetrics and gynecology, orthopedics, otolaryngology, pathology, physical medicine and rehabilitation, psychiatry, radiology, surgery, thoracic surgery, and urology.

Health care of children with chronic illnesses, when they are not acutely ill or requiring inpatient care, generally takes place in primary care clinics and subspecialty clinics specific to their health condition. As noted in Chapter 4, children's chronic conditions have different characteristics from chronic conditions among adult populations. Most children with chronic conditions have high-prevalence conditions, such as asthma, obesity, and mental and developmental conditions, and most receive health care in primary care or other community settings. A smaller number of children have low-prevalence conditions, such as cystic fibrosis, arthritis, cancer, sickle cell disease, or congenital heart disease, and most of these children see pediatric subspecialists regularly while receiving their primary care in community settings (Perrin, Anderson, & van Cleave, 2014).

About 10–20% of U.S. children visit a pediatric subspecialist each year (National Academies, 2023e). Pediatric subspecialty care has expanded over the past few decades because of changing epidemiology of children with medical complexity (including better survival), development of many new treatments, increased demand from parents and primary care providers, and development of new subspecialties within pediatrics. With advances in medicine, some children with conditions that were previously fatal in childhood are now living into adulthood. For instance, 45 years ago children with cystic fibrosis and sickle cell disease had a life expectancy in the teen years and most did not see adulthood; now life expectancy for children with these conditions is over 40 years of age (Cheng, Monteiro, et al., 2016). This success has required focus on transition of care to adult subspecialists and the advent of new adult subspecialties (e.g., adult congenital heart disease). The relative rarity of most pediatric chronic conditions creates different care patterns from those of most adults with chronic conditions (see the 5 Ds in Chapter 1); this differential epidemiology results in care centered at regional specialized children's hospitals where there are pediatric subspecialists. The smaller number of children with each condition has led to regionalization of that care (unlike for older populations), and few pediatric subspecialists work outside of hospital settings (National Academies, 2023e).

Children with more complex conditions almost always require subspecialists to manage their care or collaborate with primary care providers, depending on the condition (Mosquera, Gonzalez, & Leeds, 2014; Perrin, Anderson, & van Cleave, 2014). Many children's hospitals have established complex care clinics and programs to provide both outpatient and inpatient coordination and management for youth and young adults with medical complexity (White et al., 2018), with growing use of telemedicine. Some of these programs are disease specific (e.g., sickle cell disease clinic) and multidisciplinary (e.g., cerebral palsy clinic staffed with orthopedic surgeons, neurologists, and developmental pediatricians), while others are not;

this structure is driven by local resources and needs (National Academies, 2018). Clinical trials have shown cost reductions in establishing care coordination programs within hospitals or outpatient clinics (Cohen & Patel, 2014; Cohn et al., 2020; Mosquera, Gonzalez, & Leeds, 2014; Simon et al., 2017), albeit with mixed findings. Care coordination improves quality of care (Simon et al., 2017) and family perceptions of the family-centeredness of care (Hill, Knafl, & Santacroce, 2017; White et al., 2018).

Managing care for youth with intellectual development disorders or autism spectrum disorder provides an important example of needed coordination across subspecialties and services (Brookman-Frazee et al., 2009; McClain et al., 2020; Parker, Diamond, & Guercio, 2019) and with the primary care setting. Specialized care for children with intellectual development disorders is often based at academic children's hospitals, requiring families to travel long distances to access specialty care (National Academies, 2022c). Programs such as ECHO, described earlier in this chapter, train clinicians in best practices for treating children with autism, making care more accessible in rural areas (Mazurek et al., 2017). More recent models for supporting individuals with intellectual development disorders throughout their lifespan emphasize a medical home that can span an individual's lifetime from childhood.

Pediatric subspecialists work in partnership with primary care providers in caring for children who have rare health conditions or require technical procedures. Primary care clinicians may also refer to a subspecialist if the patient has not responded to conventional therapy in primary care settings or if they lack time or expertise to initiate care for patients with complex care needs (National Academies, 2023e). Primary care and subspecialty pediatric clinicians often work closely together to deliver comprehensive care for children who require subspecialty care. Team-based care among pediatric subspecialties has been associated with decreased acute health care utilization, greater patient satisfaction, and higher quality of care (National Academies, 2023e).

Many families experience long wait times or limited access to subspecialty care, especially in rural settings. An estimated 1 million to 39 million children (2–53%), depending on subspecialty, reside 80 miles or more from a subspecialist. Across hospital referral regions, there are 1 or fewer subspecialists per 100,000 children for 11 subspecialties (Turner, Ricketts, & Leslie, 2020). The shortage of subspecialty pediatricians limits the ability of health care systems to provide comprehensive, high-quality, and integrated care for children with chronic and complex medical conditions (Orr et al., 2024; Patel & Raphael, 2023; Vinci, 2021). Almost 50% of children's hospitals reported vacancies in adolescent and child psychiatry and developmental and behavioral pediatrics, and more than 30% reported vacancies in child neurology and genetics (Orr et al., 2024;

Pediatric Nursing Certification Board, 2021; Strianese et al., 2020; Vinci, 2021). This subspecialty supply and demand mismatch also creates barriers to integrating genomics, precision medicine, and biomedical research into clinical care pathways and addressing the high rates of mental, emotional, and behavioral concerns among children and youth (see Chapter 2 and National Academies, 2023e). Genetics, developmental and behavioral pediatrics, pain management, palliative care, and child and adolescent psychiatry are the subspecialties with the longest appointment wait times. Use of telemedicine and electronic consults may mitigate some of the barriers to accessing subspecialty care (National Academies, 2023e).

Type of insurance, out-of-pocket payments, and insurance status can also affect access to subspecialty care, with children insured by Medicaid often finding longer wait times or other barriers compared with children with commercial insurance (Bisgaier & Rhodes, 2011). Other factors contribute to disparities in timely access to subspecialty care, such as language barriers and parental ability to take time off work to bring their child to appointments (National Academies, 2023e). Finally, insurance coverage across state lines can also limit access to specialized care and telemedicine. With a growing proportion of children with chronic and complex illness increasingly cared for at regional specialized children's hospitals that may be geographically distant, maintaining care in their community can be challenging.

Coordinated care for young people with chronic conditions is also necessary for the complex transition from pediatric care to adult care (Lollar, 2010). The goals of health care transition are to (1) improve the ability of youth and young adults with and without special health care needs to manage their own health care and effectively use health services, and (2) ensure an organized process in pediatric and adult health care practices to facilitate transition preparation, transfer of care, and integration into adult-centered health care (White et al., 2018). Without an effective transition, youth with chronic conditions may face discontinuity of care, poor health outcomes, and increased rates of emergency room visits and hospitalizations (White et al., 2018). Health transitions often coincide with other events in youths' lives, such as going away to college, starting a new job, changing living arrangements, shifting roles of parents/caregivers, and forming new relationships (Vaks et al., 2016). Common barriers to transition include lack of pediatric and adult provider skills and knowledge, lack of communication and coordination between pediatric and adult providers, lack of infrastructure and limited system supports, the patient's difficulty in separating from their primary care provider, and lack of skilled adult specialty providers (Hergenroeder, Wiemann, & Cohen, 2015; White et al., 2018).

A structured multidisciplinary transition program may be effective in improving health outcomes for adolescent and young adult patients post-transition (Zhou et al., 2016), especially with consistent tracking to accurately monitor patient outcomes post-transition (Prior et al., 2014;

White et al., 2018; Zhou et al., 2016). These models focus on building specific self-management skills in patients, engaging the receiving team, and guiding patients through the transition, which can be particularly helpful for adolescents and young adults with complex chronic conditions (Vaks et al., 2016).

Two programs, Project SEARCH and Rising Ground, have been successful in supporting the transition from pediatric to adult care for youth and young adults with intellectual development disorders. Project SEARCH (2018), an international network developed at Cincinnati Children's Hospital Medical Center in 1996, primarily seeks to secure competitive employment for people with disabilities. It includes a 1-year employment preparation program, featuring workplace immersion with hands-on training, classroom instruction, and career exploration. The efficacy of the Project SEARCH model in acquiring competitive employment after graduation has been evaluated in youth with autism (Wehman et al., 2017, 2020). Rising Ground is a human services organization based in New York City that offers support to individuals with intellectual developmental disorders. It features day and community programs, community residencies, and employment training to help acquire skills needed for independence (Rising Ground, n.d.).

Urgent and Emergent Care

In addition to hospital inpatient services, children also receive acute urgent and emergent care in urgent care centers and retail clinics, as well as emergency care centers. Children have specific health care needs that require specialized training, equipment, and facilities to ensure proper care (see Chapter 1; Institute of Medicine [IOM], 1998; Newgard et al., 2023). However, many general hospitals lack the necessary resources to adequately address these needs, a situation that can lead to tragic consequences (Owusu-Ansah et al., 2015). IOM conducted two major studies, including *Emergency Care for Children: Growing Pains* (IOM, 2007a), highlighting the deficiencies in emergency care for children and calling for systemic improvements (IOM, 1993; see also Foster et al., 2022; Newgard et al., 2023; Whyte & Evans, 2023; Woolf, Wolf, & Rivara, 2023).

Urgent care centers typically provide acute care, but at a lower level of severity than in hospital emergency centers. Retail clinics, usually staffed by nurse practitioners or physician assistants, are often co-located at pharmacies or large retail outlets and offer lower-acuity care than urgent care clinics. They can treat minor illness, administer vaccines, and treat other minor conditions. As with urgent care centers, most retail clinics are not designed to offer the whole child and family health care described in Chapter 1, which is longitudinal, relationship-based, continuous, and coordinated. While urgent care centers and retail clinics may provide convenient access at particular times of need (such as after regular office hours), they do not replace primary care and generally do not offer routine screening, developmental surveillance, or other services characteristic of ongoing primary care in a medical home (Conners et al., 2017). In 2019, at least 25% of children (26.4%) had visited an urgent care center or retail health clinic in the previous 12 months. Non-Hispanic white children (29.2%) had higher utilization of urgent care centers and retail health clinics than non-Hispanic Black children (24.9%) and Hispanic children (22.6%; Black & Zablotsky, 2020). Commercially or publicly insured children had higher utilization than uninsured children (27.6% and 25.3% vs. 19.3%, respectively). Older children used retail clinics more than younger children, especially those under age 2 years (Mehrotra et al., 2008).

Emergency care centers that care for children may be housed within community, regional, or urban hospitals or as freestanding emergency departments, providing broader services than urgent care centers. These centers vary dramatically in the staff available to care for children, including family-trained providers working in smaller, community emergency care centers, and other staff who may be trained in other disciplines (e.g., general surgery). The level of care provided to children depends on the skill and training of providers who may care for children.

Community emergency departments frequently refer to regional specialized children's hospitals and designated pediatric trauma centers when the care extends beyond the general care boundary outlined above in urgent or retail care settings. Regional hospital–based pediatric emergency care centers can provide specialized acute, emergent, and critical care to children of all ages. These centers are frequently staffed by board-certified emergency medicine or pediatric emergency medicine physicians, along with advanced practice registered nurses and physician assistants. Pediatric emergency care centers can provide a number of services to children, ranging from meeting the gaps in care in community settings to critical care, including intubation and ventilation; resuscitation; subspeciality consults; and transfer to inpatient care, operating room, or intensive care unit, as dictated by the patient's condition.

This spectrum of service sites can be difficult to navigate, and parents may bring a sick child to a site that does not have the capacity to provide needed services. Earlier National Academies reports call for improving and clarifying access to emergency services, to avoid potentially tragic results (IOM, 2007; Jenkins et al., 2023; Newgard et al., 2023; Whyte & Evans, 2023).

Emergency department utilization patterns can identify high-risk patient groups, as well as areas of disparities or information gaps of patients and/or parents/caregivers. Of parents surveyed in two studies, children with asthma, disabilities, and behavioral health complaints had higher rates of urgent care and emergency department utilization than children without acute care needs (Montalbano et al., 2017). However, pediatric patients continue to utilize emergency departments for reasons that caregivers note include perceived lack of access to their regular clinic and the perception that emergency room staff can help their child's medical problem (Perrin et al., 1996; Pethe et al., 2019). Additional evidence has shown no association between the strength of the patient–provider relationship and nonurgent emergency department visits (Kirby, Connell, & Linneman, 2021). Likewise, children with public insurance, Black caregivers, or caregivers with lower educational attainment were significantly less likely to seek out care from their primary care provider before accessing emergency care (Ravi et al., 2021). Greater access to primary care is associated with decreased emergency department visits among the insured (Cowling et al., 2013; Johnson et al., 2021; van den Berg, van Loenen, & Westert, 2016; Vogel at al., 2019). Strategies addressing these specific high-utilizing groups need to be considered in the transformed health care system and when designing strategies to address whole population health.

PEDIATRIC HEALTH CARE WORKFORCE

A range of practitioners is responsible for the health care of children. For example, general pediatricians and pediatric subspecialty physicians focus exclusively on the health and development of infants, children, adolescents, and young adults. Historically, general pediatricians have served as the usual source of care for most U.S. children, although in rural areas family medicine physicians provide a key source of primary care for children, related in part to the fact that 95% of pediatricians practice in urban areas (Willis et al., 2020). Apart from pediatricians, primary care clinicians such as nurses (including registered and advanced practice registered nurses, nurse practitioners, and physician assistants) increasingly provide care for children, particularly in multidisciplinary team-based models of care. While many of these clinicians are involved in addressing psychosocial needs of their patients, professionals such as psychiatrists, psychologists, mental health counselors, and social workers focus their attention primarily on mental health, behavioral health, and psychosocial care needs. Many other professionals specialize in the care of children, such as dentists, pharmacists, podiatrists, and a broad array of therapists. While these members of the overall pediatric workforce are not the main focus of this report, many are active at the front lines of care and play a critical role in integrated multidisciplinary team-based care described above, as well as referral and access to health care more generally. Communication and integration of team-based care is critical for the whole child and family health care approach described in Chapter 1. Table 5-3 highlights some of these professionals and their roles.

The COVID-19 pandemic underscored the critical role of a robust and sustainable health care workforce in supporting essential health care infrastructure. The pandemic highlighted severe existing workforce shortages and

TABLE 5-3 Types of Providers for Pediatric Health Care

Pediatric Clinicians	
Pediatricians (MD, DO)	General pediatricians focus exclusively on the health and development of infants, children, adolescents, and young adults. They often form ongoing relationships with children and their families to support their development into adulthood with unique understanding of all the factors that affect their wellbeing.
Pediatric subspecialists, pediatric surgeons	Pediatric subspecialists (physicians who typically complete a pediatric residency and then receive additional fellowship training in discrete areas) and pediatric surgeons are critical to ensuring state-of-the-science care and pursuing research to improve prevention, diagnosis, and treatment for children. Pediatric subspecialists augment the care provided by primary care clinicians, such as general pediatricians, advanced practice providers (e.g., advanced practice registered nurses, physician assistants), and family medicine physicians by caring for children who require technical procedures or have health conditions that occur too infrequently for primary care clinicians to gain and maintain up-to-date clinical knowledge. Approximately 10–20% of U.S. children visit a pediatric subspecialist each year (National Academies, 2023e).
Registered nurses	Registered nurses (RNs) are critical members of the pediatric health care team who assume numerous roles to meet a variety of care needs across diverse care settings (International Council of Nurses, 2022; National Academies, 2021e). RNs can assume essential responsibilities related to (1) caring for children with special health care needs; (2) leading teams to improve the care and reduce the costs of high-need, high-cost patients; (3) coordinating the care of children with special health care needs between primary and subspecialty clinicians; (4) assessing problems to educate and plan with patients and families; and (5) evaluating outcomes (National Academies, 2021a,b). RNs can also lead transition initiatives between pediatric and adult care. In general, nurses cover a broad continuum of care—from health promotion and disease prevention, to curative care and care coordination, to palliative care (IOM, 2011). With appropriate education and training, RNs may provide the same care traditionally delivered by other clinicians, such as "diagnostics, treatment, referral to other services, health promotion, management of chronic diseases, or management of acute problems needing same-day consultations" (Laurant et al., 2018, p. 2). In acute care settings, RNs assume care management responsibilities, supporting management of changing patient conditions, preparing patients and families for discharge by providing education and self-management support, facilitating transitions from acute to outpatient settings, and coordinating follow-up care and resources (Gonçalves et al., 2022; Semanco, Wright, & Rich, 2022).

Nurse practitioners	Nurse practitioners (NPs) are advance practice nurses with additional education and clinical training in the care of a specific patient population that enables them to provide care to patients autonomously (National Organization of Nurse Practitioner Faculties, 2022). While most NPs are trained in and practice in primary care settings, many pediatric NPs work in hospital and inpatient settings and one-third work in ambulatory and clinical settings, providing pediatric subspecialty care (American Association of Nurse Practitioners [AANP], 2022; Gigli et al., 2021). NPs increase children's access to care by practicing in settings that include federally qualified health centers, retail clinics, home health and telehealth settings, schools and school-based health centers, nurse-managed health centers, ambulatory care clinics, and community and tertiary care hospitals (Pediatric Nursing Certification Board [PNCB], 2022). Most NPs who care for children are not certified specifically in pediatrics (e.g., family or psychiatric mental health NPs), and the extent of their contribution to the delivery of pediatric subspecialty care is not well known (Gigli et al., 2021). Less than 4% of NPs specialize in pediatrics (2.4% primary care pediatric NPs, 0.6% acute care pediatric NPs; AANP, 2022); the majority are family NPs (70.3%). Pediatric acute and primary care NPs report working in multiple subspecialties with pediatric patients, including adolescent care, cardiology, critical care, emergency care, gastroenterology, hematology and oncology, neonatology, and pulmonology (PNCB, 2022).
Clinical nurse specialists	Clinical nurse specialists (CNSs) have additional education and clinical training and follow requirements for licensure and certification. According to a 2008 report, "The CNS has a unique APRN role to integrate care across the continuum and through three spheres of influence: patient, nurse, system" (APRN Joint Dialogue Group, 2008, p. 8). CNSs may provide direct patient care, but they also collaborate with other professionals to promote evidence-based care and processes, particularly for patients with complex care needs, and they provide support and education to other health care workers and promote quality improvement initiatives (Lewandowski & Adamle, 2009; Saunders, 2015; Valdivia, 2022). In a study of the 9,470 CNSs who were registered with a national provider identifier, only 6% indicated a specialty as oncology/pediatrics, pediatrics, perinatal, or neonatal, and an additional 3% indicated a specialty in either child and adolescent or child and family psychiatric or mental health. The same study showed that the number of new CNSs specializing in pediatrics with a national provider identifier decreased between 2015 and 2019 (Reed, Arbet, & Staubli, 2021).

(continued)

TABLE 5-3 Continued

School nurses	An estimated 132,300 school nurses care for children in U.S. schools (Willgerodt, Brock, & Maughan, 2018). School nurses are frontline health care providers, serving as a bridge between the health care and education systems. Hired by school districts, health departments, or hospitals, school nurses attend to the physical and mental health of students in school. As public health sentinels, they engage school communities, parents, and health care providers to promote wellness and improve health outcomes for children. School nurses are essential to expanding access to quality health care for students, especially in light of the increasing number of students with complex health and social needs. Access to school nurses helps increase health care equity for students. For many children living in or near poverty, the school nurse may be the only health care professional they access regularly (National Academies, 2021e, p. 108). Schools are increasingly being recognized not just as core educational institutions, but also as community-based assets that can be a central component of building healthy and vibrant communities (National Academies, 2017a). Accordingly, schools and, by extension, school nurses are being incorporated into strategies for improving health care access, serving as hubs of health promotion and providers of population-based care (Maughan, 2018; National Academies, 2021e).
Physician assistants	Physician assistants (PAs) have the potential to play an important role in the care of children in the United States, and the National Commission on the Certification of Physician Assistants (NCCPA, 2023) offers a certification of added qualifications in pediatrics. However, the impact of PAs is limited by their relative scarcity in pediatric practice (Freed et al., 2010). According to a survey of 3,373 PAs who were certified for the first time (in 2019), 23.1% work in primary care (i.e., family medicine, internal medicine, general pediatrics; NCCPA, 2020). However, only 59 (1.8%) reported a principal clinical practice area in general pediatrics and an additional 53 (1.6%) worked in the pediatric subspecialties; none reported a principal clinical practice area in adolescent medicine. Few studies exist on the actual or conceptual use of PAs in pediatrics (Doan et al., 2012, 2013; Freed et al., 2011; Mathur et al., 2005).
Family medicine physicians	As part of their training, family physicians learn how to provide neonatal and routine newborn care, manage children who are acutely ill, and provide preventive health services to children (Accreditation Council for Graduate Medical Education [ACGME], 2022). ACGME has program requirements for family medicine residency programs regarding the preparation of family medicine physicians in the care of children, but most program directors report challenges in meeting the required number of encounters (Krugman et al., 2023).

Mental Health, Behavioral Health, and Social Care Professionals	
Child and adolescent psychiatrists	A child and adolescent psychiatrist (CAP) "specializes in the diagnosis and treatment of disorders of thinking, feeling, and/or behavior affecting children, adolescents, and their families" (American Academy of Child & Adolescent Psychiatry, 2023a, para. 1). CAPs work with patients and families to develop care plans that may include individual, group, or family psychotherapy; medication; and/or consultation with other physicians or professionals from schools, juvenile courts, social agencies, or other community organizations. CAPs also act as advocates for the best interests of children and adolescents and perform consultations in a variety of settings (e.g., schools, juvenile courts, social agencies).
Developmental-behavioral pediatricians	Developmental-behavioral pediatricians (DBPs) have had pediatric specialty training in child development and behavior. Often working in multidisciplinary settings in close collaboration with other professionals, DBPs evaluate, treat, and manage infants, children, and adolescents with a wide range of developmental and behavioral concerns and conditions, as well as physical complaints that are best addressed via a biobehavioral approach. DBPs also evaluate and monitor progress in children at risk for developmental and behavioral disorders on the basis of biological and social factors, adding understanding of the social, educational, and cultural influences on children. DBPs help train general pediatricians and other pediatric subspecialists to understand child development and behavior and improve early screening and identification. A developmental and behavioral pediatrician assesses children's development, learning skills, and behavior and suggests remedies. They try to find underlying causes for deviations in development and behavior and coordinate treatment to move children toward the expected development pathway.
Psychologists	Roberts and Steele (2017) define "pediatric psychology" as a multidisciplinary field that includes "both research and clinical practice that address a range of issues related to physical and psychosocial development, health, and illness among children, adolescents, and their families" (p. 3). Psychologists possess the expertise and clinical proficiency to assist individuals in acquiring better coping strategies to manage mental health issues and various challenges in life through therapy (American Psychological Association, 2023). Psychologists can be integrated in pediatric health care settings and systems (e.g., hospitals, pediatric subspecialty clinics, primary care) to help meet the needs of children and families facing chronic illnesses or disabilities (White & Belachew, 2022). Areas of expertise for pediatric psychologists include "psychosocial, developmental and contextual factors contributing to the etiology, course and outcome of pediatric medical conditions; assessment and treatment of behavioral and emotional concomitants of illness, injury, and developmental disorders; prevention of illness and injury; promotion of health and health-related behaviors; education, training, and mentoring of psychologists and providers of medical care; improvement of health care delivery systems and advocacy for public policy that serves the needs of children, adolescents, and their families" (Society of Pediatric Psychology [SPP], 2023, para. 4). Psychologists can also receive specialty training in clinical child and adolescent psychology (Lin & Stamm, 2020).

(continued)

TABLE 5-3 Continued

Social workers	For children, social workers can play a critical role on health care teams, and can contribute to coordinating care, integrating behavioral health and primary care, and providing psychosocial support for inpatient and outpatient pediatric patients and their families (Children's National Hospital, 2023b; Hospital for Special Surgery, 2023; Johns Hopkins Medicine, 2023; Jones et al., 2018; Ross et al., 2018). The National Association of Social Workers (NASW; 2023a) offers a Specialty Practice Section for supporting the development of children, adolescents, and young adults. The section has a particular focus on physical, emotional, and behavior disorders and supporting transitions through young adulthood. Furthermore, social workers play a key role in children's wellbeing through their involvement in child welfare (e.g., child protective services, case management; NASW, 2023b). In general, including social workers in primary care settings has been associated with improved health outcomes (Cornell et al., 2020; Rehner, Brazeal, & Doty, 2017).
Additional mental and behavioral health clinicians	While they also have specialized training and assist with delivering clinical care, these clinicians often focus on prevention and recovery. They sometimes work in partnership with licensed providers, who may refer patients to them. Clinical supporters include social workers, mental health counselors, occupational therapists, certified addiction counselors, nurses, certified peer specialists, and recovery coaches. They generally focus on educating clients about their conditions; building educational, occupational, housing, and social skills; coordinating care; advocating for patients; and providing social supports to achieve behavioral health recovery goals (Counts, 2022, 2023).
Other Related Health Professionals	
Care coordinators	A variety of individuals with various titles and overlapping responsibilities help patients to coordinate their care needs across providers and to navigate the health care system overall. Some of the most common titles include care coordinators, care managers, case managers, and patient navigators. These roles are often filled by nurses or social workers. In these roles, care coordinators help to overcome barriers to care at the level of the patient, their socioeconomic environment, and the larger health care system. Activities may include patient education; assistance with insurance, transportation, or legal issues; referral to community resources; and encouragement to adhere to follow-up care (Joo & Huber, 2017; Kelly et al., 2015; Paskett, Harrop, & Wells, 2011; Woodward & Rice, 2015). While there are discrepancies in the definitions, scopes of practice, or qualifications for these individuals, there is evidence that care coordination contributes to improved outcomes in health care broadly (Berry et al., 2013; Gorin et al., 2017; NEJM Catalyst, 2018; Ruggiero, Pratt, & Antonelli, 2019).

Community health workers	Community health workers (CHWs) are also known as outreach workers, community health advocates, community health representatives, and patient navigators (Rosenthal, 1998; Rosenthal et al., 2010). There are more than 60,000 paid CHWs in the United States (Bureau of Labor Statistics [BLS], 2023), as well as many volunteers (HRSA, 2023a; Rosenthal et al., 2010). There is no standardized education, training, or scope of practice, for CHWs (Catalani et al., 2009). CHWs provide a wide range of services, including health education and coaching, medication adherence, care coordination, social support, outreach and engagement, health assessment and screenings, patient navigation, case management, program implementation, and referral management for medical and social services (BLS, 2023; HRSA, 2023a; National Academies, 2020b). CHWs also play an important role in addressing health disparities and improving health outcomes, particularly for underserved and marginalized populations (Cosgrove et al., 2014; HRSA, 2023a; Lewin et al., 2010; Vasan et al., 2020). Research has shown that CHWs increase disease knowledge, self-management, and health outcomes for children and youth with chronic diseases (Coutinho et al., 2020; Fox et al., 2007; Lewin et al., 2010; Randolph, 2021; Viswanathan et al., 2010). CHWs work collaboratively with clinicians, social workers, and other professionals to improve the health and wellbeing of the communities they serve; they work in a variety of settings, such as community clinics, federally qualified health centers, hospitals, schools, and public health agencies. They also often make home visits and serve an important role in engaging communities with health care services and improving access to care.
Child life specialists	Child life specialists (CLSs) play a crucial role in pediatric health care by providing developmentally appropriate support to children and their families. They use therapeutic play, age-appropriate communication, and preparation strategies to help children understand and cope with medical experiences, reducing anxiety and stress. CLSs collaborate with health care teams to offer psychosocial support, prepare children for procedures, and educate families about treatments. Their work contributes to improved patient satisfaction, better clinical outcomes, and enhanced overall health care experiences. By addressing the emotional and developmental needs of pediatric patients, CLSs significantly improve the quality of care and support provided in health care settings (Rosenblatt et al., 2024).

SOURCE: Adapted from National Academies, 2023b.

burnout across health care professions in the United States. It also exacerbated discrepant workforce distribution, leading to severe systemic disparities across geographic, racial, and socioeconomic divides (ASPE, 2022b). It magnified the barriers to timely and appropriate health care access in uninsured, rural, low socioeconomic, under-resourced, and historically marginalized communities. The COVID-19 pandemic did drive the explosion of innovative telehealth services supporting existing health care infrastructure and services, but further development may be limited by existing inequities in funding and shortage of staff to support these services (Association of American Medical Colleges, 2021; Boudreau et al., 2022). The pandemic also emphasized the value of coordinated, multidisciplinary team-based models of care, which, as discussed earlier in this chapter, can link families with needed community resources. In addition to improving patient outcomes, team-based care may help improve clinician wellbeing and mitigate burnout (Mijakoski et al., 2015; Smith et al., 2018; Welp & Manser, 2016).

The pediatric health care workforce faces a number of challenges, including a shortage of well-distributed, trained professionals for primary care and subspecialty care; maldistribution of professionals and lack of representativeness in the workforce (see Chapter 3); and reduced health care worker wellbeing and increased burnout. Optimal pediatric care requires teams of clinicians and professionals, including the breadth of relevant practitioners, that specialize in whole child and family health care, are skilled in management of childhood conditions, and are knowledgeable in child development and child, adolescent, and family needs.

The recent National Academies report on the pediatric subspecialty workforce (National Academies, 2023e) documented shortages of pediatric primary care and subspecialty care physicians. The 2024 National Resident Matching Program accentuated concerns with an increase in unfilled pediatric positions and less than 8% of medical students choosing pediatrics as their specialty (Schering, 2024). Popularity of pediatrics has waned, as pediatricians are among the lowest-paid physicians and educational debt is rising. Of pediatric residents graduating with educational debt, the average debt increased to $264,000 in 2020 (after adjusting for inflation) and half of all residents reported $200,000 or more in debt (AAP, 2024a). Unfortunately, this is consistent with the lower pay of other professions who care for children, the nation's most treasured resource (e.g., schoolteachers, child care workers, child life specialists).

Shortage and Maldistribution of Pediatric Health Care Professionals

Shortages in the pediatric health care workforce reflect the current and projected landscape of severe health care worker shortages across the nation and the need to expand the workforce, especially in primary care, pediatric subspecialty care, and mental health. Through 2036, the NCHWA projects a shortage of 3,100 pediatricians, especially in nonmetro areas, where the projected supply is only 69% for pediatricians (vs. 101% in metro areas; HRSA, 2023a). Family medicine physicians provide 16–21% of children's visits to physicians (Jetty et al., 2021; National Academies, 2023d; Phillips et al., 2005); they also have significant projected shortages (HRSA, 2022a) and often spend less time caring for children than pediatricians (Bazemore et al., 2012; Eden et al., 2020; Freed, Segalowitz, & Dewey, 2004; Freed et al., 2010; Wasserman et al., 2019).

Similar to concerns about primary care shortages, growing demands of the pediatric population may outpace the growth of the pediatric subspecialty workforce (see National Academies, 2023e). The nationwide epidemics of mental illness and substance use disorders have highlighted the dramatic shortage (discussed earlier in this chapter) of qualified professionals across the spectrum of all licensed practitioners (especially psychologists, psychiatrists, addiction counselors, mental health counselors, and psychiatric and mental health nurse practitioners), for both adults and children and youth.

The lack of diversity in the pediatric workforce contributes to health care disparities and the maldistribution of providers in underserved areas (Montez, 2021; Vinci, 2021). Physicians from under-represented racial/ethnic groups are more likely to practice in areas with higher proportions of underserved populations. For example, Xierali and colleagues (2021) found that Black, Hispanic, and American Indian/Alaska Native physicians were more likely to care for larger shares of underserved populations compared to their White counterparts. Increasing workforce diversity can therefore help address provider shortages in underserved communities (Guevara et al., 2023). Furthermore, patient–provider racial/ethnic concordance can improve communication, increase patient satisfaction, and enhance adherence to treatment recommendations (Montez, 2021; Orr et al., 2024). As the pediatric population in the United States becomes increasingly diverse, it is crucial for the workforce to reflect this diversity to provide culturally competent care and build trust with patients and families from diverse backgrounds. Efforts to enhance diversity in the pediatric pipeline, such as pipeline programs, holistic admissions processes, and inclusive institutional climates, are essential to cultivating a workforce equipped to meet the needs of all children (Guevara et al., 2023; Orr et al., 2024).

Workforce Wellbeing and Burnout

The pediatric workforce, like other parts of the health care workforce, has faced substantial burnout, exacerbated by the pandemic. While burnout has been a growing problem for years (National Academies, 2019e), the COVID-19 pandemic was a serious stressor on an already fragile workforce. A 2022 AAP report noted that burnout among pediatricians increased from 35.3% in 2011 to 46.3% in 2014 (McClafferty et al., 2022), with reports of more than 50–60% in 2022 (Lucy et al., 2023).

Burnout affects productivity in the workforce, with reduced efforts among health workers (Dyrbye, Satele, & West, 2021). Conversely, clinician wellbeing supports improved patient–clinician relationships, a high-functioning care team, and an engaged and effective workforce (National Academies, 2019e). Some groups experience additional stressors that can increase burnout. Doctors of color and those working in underserved communities face disproportionate amounts of stress because of the socio-political-economic challenges of the particularly vulnerable children in the disenfranchised communities they serve (McClafferty et al., 2022). Women, who make up two-thirds of pediatric doctors, report higher levels of burnout than male physicians (Lyubarova, Salman, & Rittenberg, 2023; McClafferty et al., 2022), especially in emotional distress measurements, with higher risk of suicidality. Long hours of practice are compounded by carrying the bulk of family responsibilities; women who are employed full time spend an additional 8.5 hours per week on domestic care (Jolly et al., 2014). One-third of physician mothers reported discrimination related to their role as a mother, primarily regarding pregnancy or maternity leave (Adesoye et al., 2017; Halley et al., 2018). Women in pediatrics, notably women of color, also report gender-based harassment in the workplace (McClafferty et al., 2022). Expressing fatigue and the desire for self-care remains stigmatized in a workforce culture that discourages asking for help with mental health.

Several strategies exist for diminishing burnout, including team-based care, environments that support providers in their mental health, and improved work hours. A 2019 systematic review of about 50 studies concluded that strategies that promoted team-based care and incorporated medical assistants or scribes to complete electronic health record documentation and other administrative tasks were strongly linked to reducing clinician burnout and stress (DeChant et al., 2019). Other aspects of teamwork that reduced burnout included improved communication among physicians and expanded team member responsibilities that allowed team members to work at the top of their skills and better allocate clinical workload. The following section continues the discussion of strategies to address workforce challenges.

Strategies for Addressing Workforce Challenges

Multiple strategies are needed to address pediatric workforce shortages, maldistribution, and burnout. As described earlier, team-based care in both primary and subspecialty pediatrics can both transform care and address some workforce challenges. Building teams with the capacity to address the array of social, educational, developmental, health, and community needs of children and families, including those with chronic conditions, can improve care and decrease demands on pediatric clinicians to meet these varied needs alone. The growth of teams—with adequate and appropriate financing—provides one of the most promising approaches to meeting child health workforce needs.

Among several strategies, a focus on fixing salary disparities between pediatrics and other specialties and improving workforce diversity is needed. Additional strategies must include training of the broad array of participants in the child health workforce, increased focus on evidence-based practices, innovating new models of care including upstream prevention, and using new technology to increase care efficiency and reach.

Pediatric primary care clinicians have increased their capacity to address some subspecialty and mental health issues, a strategy promoted for additional expansion in the National Academies subspecialty workforce report. Pediatric nurse practitioners have increased in primary and subspecialty care in outpatient and inpatient settings with further growth expected (Gigli et al., 2019; Toia et al., 2024). The workforce of community health workers as part of the team has grown with increasing evidence of improved outcomes and reduced disparities (Coker et al., 2014). New models of team care such as the use of genetic counselors with nurse practitioners will be necessary to address shortages (Stewart & Svihovec, 2022). A focus on upstream primary prevention emphasized in this report can reduce the need for more intensive and costly health services.

CONCLUSION

This chapter described the nature of health care in clinical settings, changes occurring with the settings and workforce, resulting opportunities and challenges, and the progress made in strengthening the content of pediatric primary and subspecialty care for children and youth. Progress has included growth in early intervention and mental and behavioral health services, improved coordination of care among multiple providers, and greater inclusion of community health workers and similar staff to help families develop skills, find resources, enhance their children's lives, and build lasting relationships. These recent trends all include strategies for better addressing the needs of children across the life course.

The pediatric health care system is broad and diverse. Main components of the system include primary care, hospital care, subspecialty care, and their interaction. Primary care comes from a diverse array of programs, from traditional office practice to community health centers, large medical groups, hospitals, and various public clinics. The mental and behavioral health care system, comprising office practices, hospital care, community programs, and more, has long had only limited integration and interaction with the rest of the pediatric care system, although increasing efforts to integrate mental health into primary and subspecialty care have shown promise. Schools too (see Chapter 8) provide substantial amounts of prevention and treatment, especially for mental and behavioral health issues. Progress in improving health and wellbeing outcomes has occurred in all these sectors; however, health care financing has not kept pace with these advances and has prevented their widespread and coordinated uptake (see Chapter 6).

In addition, the health care system in general suffers from a workforce shortage, exacerbated by increased demand for services, workforce stress and burnout, geographical disparities, and training gaps. Most components of the pediatric health care system have faced similar challenges with burnout and workforce shortages. Projections indicate that these shortages will worsen, necessitating innovative approaches to payment, recruitment, training, and retention of pediatric health care providers and teams, as well as new health care delivery models for addressing the evolving needs of children and families.

The transformation of child health care practices has involved adopting more holistic, preventive, and developmental approaches that integrate health care practice with community services. Innovations in primary care, especially broadening the scope of services to include new ways of supporting families and identifying issues of concern, often built from interdisciplinary teams, have shown success in improving child health and wellbeing and decreasing unnecessary care. Supporting upstream prevention in pediatric care has helped to address root causes of health issues before they manifest as clinical symptoms or conditions. This approach recognizes the influence of social, economic, environmental, and relational factors that affect child health and wellbeing, and includes interventions at the earliest stages to promote optimal health and wellbeing in children and their life trajectories. The several stages in child development, including pregnancy and childbirth, infancy, early childhood, school age, adolescence, and young adulthood, each require different strategies and activities for health care. There is evidence to support the ability of these holistic approaches to address health disparities and community health concerns—the need now is to bring these many advances to scale.

Hospital and subspecialty care have also changed in recent years, with fewer hospitalizations; more concentration in urban centers; and greater capacity for subspecialty care, coordinated with the primary care community. The tremendous growth in new science and the understanding of many chronic conditions have made hospital-based subspecialty care ever more complex and sophisticated in pediatric evaluations and treatments. Telehealth has proven to be a valuable tool in pediatric care, offering flexibility, increased access, and improved outcomes with recent growth in other forms of remote monitoring and communication. There is a need for consistent coverage policies across states and payers to ensure equitable access to these services. Effective coordination between primary and specialty care, essential for managing complex cases, requires robust care coordination mechanisms, integrated health information systems, and collaborative care models to ensure seamless transitions and comprehensive care. Learning health systems offer key strategies for improving quality and lowering costs.

6

Insurance and Other Financing for Clinical Services

Long-term fiscal effects of Medicaid spending on children could offset half or more of the program's initial outlays.

—Congressional Budget Office[1]

As discussed in prior chapters, children's health care includes proactive care designed to prevent disease and promote health, as well as medical care designed to screen, diagnose, and treat health conditions. The former is often referred to as "primary prevention" and the latter as "secondary prevention" (identifying conditions as soon as possible); "tertiary prevention" is managing and minimizing consequences of worsening conditions. The nation's investment in children's health care, from primary to tertiary prevention, is financed through multiple and interweaving funding streams; a central example is commercial and public health insurance. Another stream occurs outside of the insurance mechanism through the federal grant-in-aid system for community and state initiatives related to child health.[2] See Table 6-1 for an overview of federal investment in children's health through insurance, health clinics, population health initiatives, and school-based services.

Federal funding for all health care programs in the United States leans heavily on insurance mechanisms. Funding for Medicare, Medicaid, and other health insurance assistance was $1.7 trillion in 2022, whereas other health-related expenditures totaled $242 billion, excluding U.S. Department

[1]Ash et al., 2023.

[2]The grant-in-aid system of federal support to states and communities includes several types of mechanisms, such as categorical grants, block grants, and general revenue sharing (Congressional Research Service, 2019).

TABLE 6-1 Major Federal Investments Addressing Children and Youth Health and Wellbeing

Program	Federal Agency	Appropriation, in billions	Fiscal Year	% to Children and Mothers
Insurance Mechanisms and Clinical Care Services (discussed in this chapter)				
Medicaid	CMS/HHS	$699	2021	15.2%
Children's Health Insurance Program	CMS/HHS	$15.8	2021	100%
Tax subsidies for employer-sponsored health insurance		~$299	2022	
Community health centers (federally qualified health center/rural health clinic/look-alike)	HRSA/HHS	$5.6	2022	12%
Certified community behavioral health clinics	SAMHSA/HHS	$0.3	2022	27% (upper limit)
School-based health centers	HRSA/HHS	$0.03	2023	100%
	CMS/HHS	$0.05	2024	
Indian Health Service	IHS/HHS	$6.96	2023	NA
Public Health Initiatives (Child Care, Maternal and Early Child Health Care, Vaccines, Nutrition, Mental Health (treatment for stress, trauma, substance use disorder) (discussed in Chapter 7)				
Child care and development block grant	ACF/HHS	$5.9	2022	100%
Head Start (HS), Early HS, American Indian/Alaska Native HS, Migrant Worker HS	ACF/HHS	$11	2022	100%
Vaccines for children	CDC/HHS	$5.5	2022	100%
National Center on Birth Defects and Developmental Disabilities	CDC/HHS	$0.2	2022	100%
Preventive Health and Health Services Block Grant	CDC/HHS	$0.1	2020	~29%
Racial and Ethnic Approaches to Community Health	CDC/HHS	$0.04	2022	NA
Good Health and Wellness in Indian Country	CDC/HHS	$0.04	2022	NA
Maternal and Child Health Block Grant (Title V)	HRSA/HHS	$0.7	2022	NA
Maternal, Infant, and Early Childhood Home Visiting	HRSA/HHS	$0.2	2022	NA
National Child Traumatic Stress Initiative	SAMHSA/HHS	$0.08	2022	100%

TABLE 6-1 Continued

Program	Federal Agency	Appropriation, in billions	Fiscal Year	% to Children and Mothers
Residential Treatment for Pregnant and Postpartum Women	SAMHSA/HHS	$0.03	2022	100%
Project LAUNCH (Linking Actions for Unmet Needs in Children's Health)	SAMHSA/HHS	$0.02	2022	100%
Tribal Behavioral Health Grants	SAMHSA/HHS	$0.02	2022	NA
Infant and Early Childhood Mental Health Grants	SAMHSA/HHS	$0.01	2022	100%
Supplemental Nutrition Assistance Program	FNS/USDA	$120	2022	44%
Special Supplemental Nutrition Program for Women, Infants, and Children	FNS/USDA	$6.9	2022	100%
School-Based Services (health promotion, nutrition, management of chronic conditions) (discussed in Chapter 8)				
Healthy Schools Initiative	CDC/HHS	$0.02	2022	100%
National School Lunch & Breakfast programs	FNS/USDA	$26.9	2022	100%
Child and Adult Care Food Program	FNS/USDA	$3.9	2022	High

NOTES: This table lists major federal investments; many other, smaller programs also invest in child and youth health and wellbeing. ACF = Administration for Children and Families; CDC = Centers for Disease Control and Prevention; CMS = Centers for Medicare & Medicaid Services; FNS = Food and Nutrition Service; HHS = U.S. Department of Health and Human Services; HRSA = Health Resources and Services Administration; IHS = Indian Health Service; NA = not available or not applicable; SAMHSA = Substance Abuse and Mental Health Services Administration; USDA = U.S. Department of Agriculture.
SOURCE: Generated by the committee.

of Defense (DoD) and U.S. Department of Veterans Affairs (VA) Medical Care.[3] Another $287 billion in federal support goes to employer-sponsored health insurance through tax subsidies (Congressional Budget Office [CBO], 2019). This heavy reliance on insurance as a funding stream impacts how care is organized by valuing disease-focused medical services (delivered one-to-one) over universal or wellness-focused prevention services (delivered

[3]Per the Office of Management and Budget (n.d.), Table 15.1, "Outlays for Health Programs: 1962–2028 (in billions)": Medicare ($905.6), Medicaid ($591.9), Federal Employees Health Benefits Program ($61.0), health insurance assistance ($79.5), other health ($24.02); excludes DoD ($55.4) and VA ($110.7).

one-to-many), which traditionally do not fit well into insurance models. Over the past four decades, the United States significantly expanded its investments in child health care through the health insurance financing mechanism to provide insurance coverage to all children. By 2015, health insurance coverage for children had stabilized at 95% in 2021 (Keisler-Starkey & Bunch, 2022; Census Bureau, 2021), although the pandemic increased coverage slightly, followed by the recent "unwinding" of Medicaid eligibility with the end of the pandemic public health emergency that reduced rates of children's coverage.[4] This coverage is a major policy success for children, yet the overall picture in the nation masks areas and populations with larger uninsured rates, such as children in the South (6.8%) and in states that have not expanded Medicaid (8.1%), as well as Hispanic children (9.5%) and children who are foreign born (22.6%) (see Figure 4 in Census Bureau, 2023b).

Changes to insurance coverage and financing are more likely to impact disease-focused than wellness-focused services. The share of spending through insurance as opposed to other funding streams varies depending on the type of care—primary, secondary, or tertiary prevention. The majority of secondary and tertiary prevention is delivered through the health care system and financed through insurance. By contrast, primary preventive health care can be delivered through the health care system and financed through insurance, but it is also delivered outside of the health care system and paid for with federal grants-in-aid.

The terms "clinical primary prevention" and "community-" or "population-based primary prevention" highlight the distinction in the delivery and financing of primary preventive care (Institute of Medicine [IOM], 2010). Clinical primary prevention usually involves services that are delivered one-to-one in a medical office setting by health care professionals and are covered by insurance and/or out-of-pocket payments by those receiving the services. Community-based primary preventive health care services can be provided one-to-one or one-to-many—such as a teacher providing socioemotional learning to a class of students, a community health worker providing multigenerational care to a family unit, or a community program or intervention sponsored by a local health department—and often involve health care delivered by nonmedical professionals, such as community health workers, peers, teachers, and other community members (Cuellar & Calonge, 2022). As discussed in Chapter 7, financial support for community-level services comes from federal grants, in addition to local and state

[4]Insurance coverage for children was 0.6% higher in 2021 than in 2020 because of congressional efforts to retain access to insurance during the COVID-19 pandemic (Mykyta, Keisler-Starkey, & Bunch, 2022). With the unwinding, coverage has returned to prepandemic levels.

funding mechanisms. These definitional boundaries are soft, the actors can overlap, and the multiplicity of actors and types of activities speaks to the importance of coordination and communication across clinical and community services.

The long horizon of some investments in children's health has implications for framing strategies for federal budgeting and fund allocation across competing priorities. In scoring the fiscal impact of federal legislation, CBO has generally considered savings within only a 10-year projection period based on its statutory requirements. This long-standing approach leads to undervaluing longer-term investments and disproportionately impacts fiscal calculations around prevention in general and child health investments in particular (Ash et al., 2023; CBO, 2020). CBO can score legislation across multiple budgets, not limited to health care, and doing so could improve results for Medicaid and other investments. Lack of CBO outlays by age group also hampers assessment of investments and returns for children.

At the national level, spending on primary prevention is aimed at protecting against poor future health states among the nation's population and their attendant costs. While not all health conditions are preventable, many have modifiable risk factors. Health care costs associated with such conditions are substantial. For example, a recent *Lancet* analysis estimated that in 2016, U.S. health care spending attributable to modifiable risk factors—including high body mass index, high blood pressure, high glucose, dietary risks, and tobacco use—was $730.4 billion, or 27% of total health care spending. Some of these costs are paid publicly through programs such as Medicare and Medicaid (Bolnick et al., 2020). Another example is mental health disorders, which are among the costliest of health conditions in terms of health care spending (Roehrig, 2016). Moreover, poor mental health in childhood has a range of lasting impacts on later-life outcomes, ranging from educational completion to employment and early death (Currie & Stabile, 2006; Fletcher & Wolfe, 2008, 2009; Goodman, Joyce, & Smith, 2011; Salm & Schunk, 2012; Wang, Frank, & Glied, 2023). Thus, federal spending on primary prevention can be seen as insurance against future costs for both health and nonhealth care (e.g., productivity) that can be attributed to preventable conditions.

This chapter's discussion of spending on children's health care focuses on clinical care funded mainly by insurance. Chapter 7 examines the role of investment in child health through population- and community-level primary prevention.[5]

[5] As a practical matter, drawing a line between what spending falls into public health (related to social determinants of children's health) and what spending can be construed more narrowly as health care spending can be fraught.

HEALTH INSURANCE FOR CHILDREN

Health and medical care provided to children on an individual basis is paid for primarily through health insurance. Today, although some communities continue to have low rates of coverage, in many communities, nearly all children have health insurance coverage, the result of a series of child-related health policies spanning six decades (Cohen, Martinez, & Zammitti, 2015). This policy achievement has removed a major barrier to health care for most children and has positive short- and long-term health and education impacts. Remaining issues with primary insurance for children pertain to those who lack coverage, including undocumented children; intermittent loss of coverage; coverage for parents; access to providers willing to accept insurance, especially for children with Medicaid and for behavioral health and dental care; underinsurance, especially for middle-income children; and limitations of certain provider payment mechanisms.

Importance of Health Insurance for Children

Research has examined whether health insurance coverage improves short- and long-term child outcomes, largely based on expansions in Medicaid (Brown, Kowalski, & Lurie, 2015; Currie & Chorniy, 2021; Hakim, Boben, & Bonney, 2000; IOM, 1998; KFF, 2023b; Meyer & Wherry, 2012; Wherry et al., 2015). For example, a 1998 IOM report, *America's Children: Health Insurance and Access to Care*, provided substantial evidence of the value of health insurance for children's health. Buchmueller, Levy, and Valletta (2019) summarized the literature related to Medicaid expansions for children, concluding that the Medicaid expansions for children increased coverage, net of any reductions in commercial insurance due to crowd-out, and also increased access and utilization of care for children. Other studies found improvements in school achievement (Wehby, 2022). Early studies on Medicaid coverage expansions for pregnant women in the 1980s concluded that the expansions increased enrollment and modestly improved birth outcomes, but showed mixed evidence on prenatal outcomes (Howell, 2001). Improvements were greatest for families with very low incomes (Bellerose, Collin, & Daw, 2022; Currie & Gruber, 1996; Howell, 2001).

More recent studies have assessed the long-term impacts of the Medicaid expansions on children, suggesting that Medicaid plays an important role not only in increasing utilization of health care at young ages, but in improving health outcomes over the long term (Currie, Decker, & Lin, 2008; Miller & Wherry, 2019; Thompson, 2017). Studies have also found that Medicaid eligibility in childhood improves labor market and educational outcomes, including high school and college completion (Brown et al., 2020; Cohodes et al., 2016; Currie & Chorniy, 2021; Groves, 2020; Miller & Wherry, 2019; Wherry et al., 2015). The mechanism by which Medicaid eligibility at young ages drives these long-term effects is not entirely clear, but candidate explanations include direct impacts of health insurance on health care and improved maternal physical and mental health (Guldi & Hamersma, 2023) and birth outcomes. Indirect explanations could include increased access to treatment for substance use disorder and decreased crime (Wen, Hockenberry, & Cummings, 2017); lower financial strain and stress on mothers or families, including reductions in mother's employment changes during early childhood; increased connection to other social supports; and decreased rates of poverty (Aizer, Stroud, & Buka, 2016; Currie & Duque, 2019; Currie & Rossin-Slater, 2015; Sommers & Oellerich, 2013; Wherry, Kenney, & Sommers, 2016). As noted above, many of these longer-term impacts are not captured within the time frame in which legislation is proposed and scored in Congress. A recent CBO report modeled how a different approach could take these economic and budgetary gains into account explicitly and thus enable more comprehensive fiscal assessment of proposals to change health insurance for children (Ash et al., 2023).

Overview of Children's Health Insurance

To clarify the role of health insurance for children, it is important to understand that children's medical expenditures are, on average, very low (Figure 6-1), even among those with any expense (Figure 6-2), and much lower than for adults. Children under age 5 years who have a medical expense have higher spending than children ages 5–17, in part because of the high cost of some births. At the same time, as Figure 6-3 shows, conditional on having a medical event, the mean cost of a medical event can be very high, even for children.

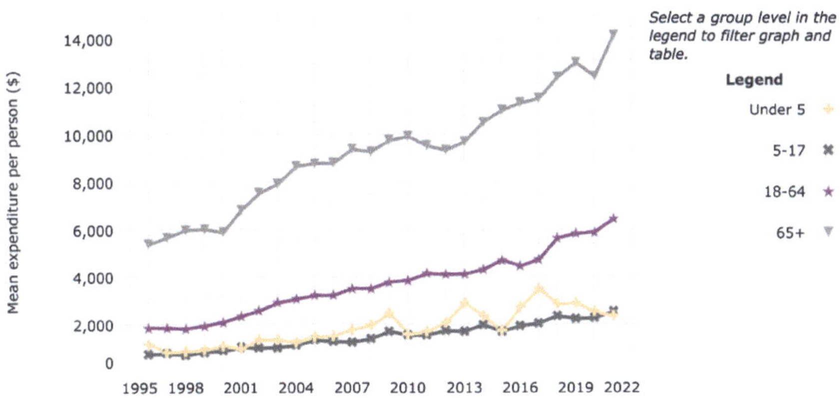

FIGURE 6-1 Mean expenditure per person by age group, United States, 1996–2021.
NOTE: Confidence interval is 95%.
SOURCE: AHRQ Medical Expenditure Panel Survey (https://datatools.ahrq.gov/meps-hc).

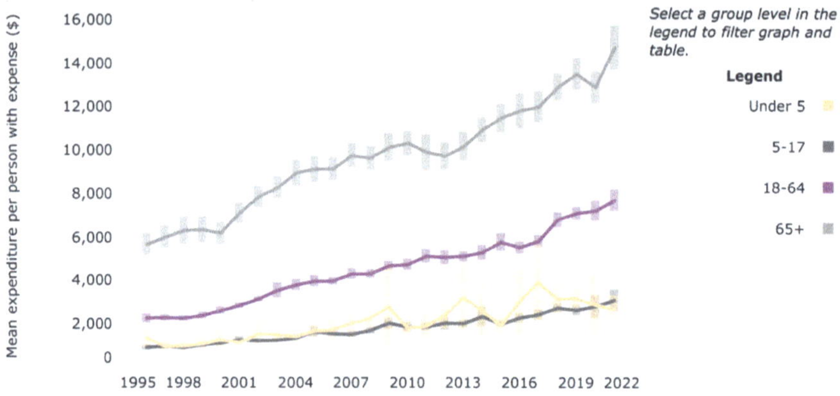

FIGURE 6-2 Mean expenditure per person with expense by age group, United States, 1996–2021.
NOTE: Confidence interval is 95%.
SOURCE: AHRQ Medical Expenditure Panel Survey (https://datatools.ahrq.gov/meps-hc).

More than half of children (54.7%) have commercial health insurance through a parent's employer-sponsored plan. In some cases, employees pay the full premium costs and in other cases employees share the premium costs with their employers; however, employer premium contributions can also be viewed as being paid for by the employee in the form of reduced wages. In general, employers subsidize employee coverage at a higher rate than they subsidize dependent coverage. Employer-provided health insurance is also

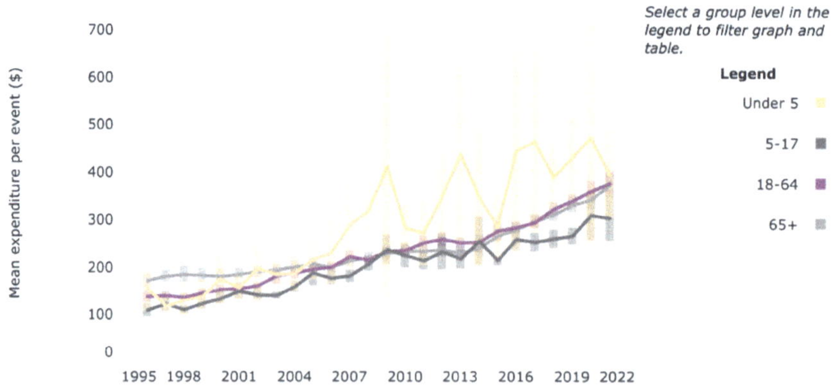

FIGURE 6-3 Mean expenditure per event by age group, United States, 1996–2021.
NOTE: Confidence interval is 95%.
SOURCE: AHRQ Medical Expenditure Panel Survey (https://datatools.ahrq.gov/meps-hc).

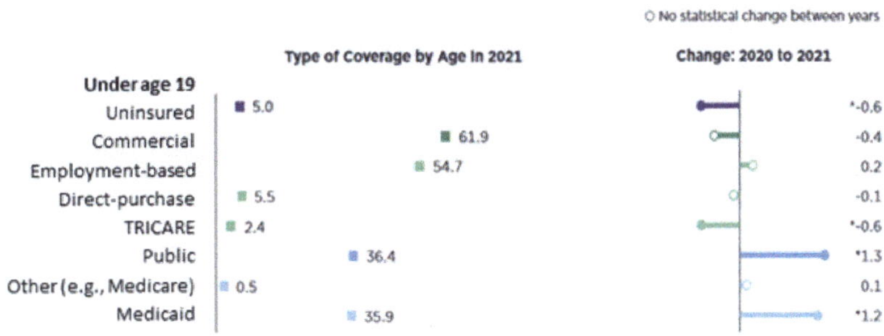

FIGURE 6-4 Percentage of children under age 19 with selected coverage types, 2021.
SOURCE: Based on data from the Current Population Survey; Keisler-Starkey & Bunch, 2022.

publicly subsidized through foregone tax revenue because these benefits are not considered taxable income. CBO (2019) and the Joint Committee on Taxation estimate that federal subsidies via tax benefits for employer-covered insurance for all ages totaled $287 billion in 2019, almost as high as the $314 billion in federal subsidies for Medicaid and the Children's Health Insurance Program (CHIP).[6] Another 5.5% of children are covered through direct-purchase commercial insurance (Keisler-Starkey & Bunch, 2022; see Figure 6-4). Since implementation of the Patient Protection and Affordable Care Act (2010), children are eligible for health insurance coverage as a dependent on a family's plan that is purchased directly from the insurer or through a federal or state health insurance marketplace (e.g., healthcare.gov). Premiums for these plans can be paid for privately by a family or may be subsidized publicly, depending on the family's income level, and thus combine private and public funding. Since 2019, the share of children with employer-sponsored or direct-purchased coverage has been stable, while Medicaid coverage increased especially during the pandemic (Federal Interagency Forum on Child and Family Statistics, 2023a).

Prior to the COVID-19 pandemic, just over one-third of U.S. children (36.9%) had health insurance coverage through one of two publicly funded health insurance programs: Medicaid, which is targeted to low-income and/or disabled children, and CHIP, created in 1997, which is targeted to children in families with somewhat higher income levels (CMS, n.d.b, 2024f). With the COVID-19 public health emergency and changed Medicaid rules, that percentage rose to over 50% (35.1 million on Medicaid; 4.3 million on CHIP). With the end of the public health emergency and the related "unwinding" of Medicaid coverage, that number decreased by about 3.8 million as of February 2024.[7]

---

[6]These estimates include children and adults under age 65.
[7]See https://ccf.georgetown.edu/subtopic/unwinding-phe

The mix of public and commercial insurance for children is anything but uniform. In 2021, 58.7% of non-Hispanic Black or American Indian/Alaska Native children had public coverage, as did 38.1% of non-Hispanic multiracial children, 53.7% of Hispanic, 28.0% of non-Hispanic Asian children, and 28.1% of non-Hispanic White children (Branch & Conway, 2022). The differences in public and commercial coverage across race and ethnicity likely arise from a combination of factors associated with systemic disadvantage, including income; type of parental employment; immigration policy; and geographic factors, such as living in the South, where few states have expanded Medicaid, or living in states where the marketplace exchange is enrolling potential beneficiaries less actively than other states (Snowden & Graaf, 2023).

Regardless of the funding of an insurance plan (commercial, public, or a combination), the costs of health care services provided are typically shared between the insurance plan and the enrollee through outlays for copayments, deductibles, and noncovered services. However, unlike other insurance products, Medicaid allows almost no copays or deductibles for covered services.

PUBLIC HEALTH INSURANCE FOR CHILDREN

Publicly funded insurance coverage for children has expanded in three major waves, based on families' income levels and children's ages. Initially, in 1965, Medicaid coverage was limited to children enrolled in welfare, as well as children who were blind or disabled. The link to public welfare meant that income eligibility was very low—well below the federal poverty level (FPL). From 1980 to 1990, Medicaid expanded incrementally to cover all children under the FPL (National Research Council & IOM, 1998). Under the Balanced Budget Act (1997), the newly established CHIP allowed states to cover children up to age 19 whose parents were working and had incomes above the state Medicaid levels; it also permitted states to collect premiums and copays from enrolled families for coverage. In 2014, the Patient Protection and Affordable Care Act (ACA) created health insurance exchanges through which all individuals under age 65 with family incomes between 100% and 400% FPL became eligible for premium subsidies, and those with incomes below 250% FPL became eligible for reduced cost-sharing. Even though few children have direct-purchased commercial insurance through marketplaces, the broad-based enrollment activities supported by the ACA help both families and their children, with many families learning of their children's eligibility for Medicaid through the ACA enrollment process. Furthermore, the ACA established a mandatory minimum Medicaid eligibility threshold for children at 133% FPL, regardless of the child's age group. This shifted older children in some states from CHIP to Medicaid.[8]

[8]Prior to the ACA, the mandatory eligibility levels for children in Medicaid differed by age: States were required to cover children ages 0–5 years in Medicaid with family incomes up to 133% FPL and children ages 6–18 years with family incomes up to 100% FPL (MACPAC, n.d.).

Arguably, the COVID-19 public health emergency created a fourth wave of children's health insurance coverage by expanding premium subsidies for families with incomes up to 600% FPL and incentivizing state's continuous coverage for Medicaid and some CHIP programs. The extended Medicaid/CHIP coverage—under which enrolled persons stayed covered unless they voluntarily disenrolled, moved, or died—persisted for 3 years until passage of the Consolidated Appropriations Act (2022). Continuous coverage ended with states resuming eligibility assessments and coverage terminations as early as April 2023 (Wikle & Wagner, 2023). Under the law, states had up to 12 months to return to preemergency eligibility and enrollment operations, resulting in significant administrative chaos and lost coverage for eligible children (Bohra, 2023; Heberlein, 2023). The Consolidated Appropriations Act also requires Medicaid and CHIP to cover children up to age 19 who are enrolled in Medicaid or CHIP for 12 months continuously beginning January 2024 (Daugherty et al., 2024).

Medicaid and CHIP represent federal–state partnerships with joint funding but have different financing formulas. In both cases, the federal government, through the Centers for Medicare & Medicaid Services (CMS), provides the majority share of funds, a share that varies based mainly on the level of poverty in the state; this is called the Federal Medical Assistance Percentage (FMAP), which ranges from 50% to 83% (Medicaid and CHIP Payment and Access Commission [MACPAC], 2023a).[9] States pay the remainder and, within federal parameters, they can manage their spending through decisions on eligibility, benefit scope, optional coverage, quality standards, and provider payment. In contrast, state CHIP programs are funded through a capped federal block grant to states, with an FMAP that is always higher than that of Medicaid. The corresponding fiscal commitment by states is also fixed.

Medicaid is an entitlement (i.e., states are required to enroll any eligible applicant). With the CHIP block grant, however, states can refuse enrollment once they reach the end of their grant funding. In contrast to CHIP, Medicaid is countercyclical, requiring more spending during recessions, but also offering greater protection when more individuals lose their jobs and poverty rates are higher. States are required to have balanced budgets, and the countercyclical nature of Medicaid is challenging for state governments, with increased demand and lower revenues in recessions. In the 2001 recession, the Great Recession, and the recent COVID-19 pandemic, Congress appropriated additional federal fiscal relief to state Medicaid programs to ameliorate the budgetary impact of these major economic disruptions (see, respectively, Jobs and Growth Tax Relief Reconciliation Act, 2003; American Recovery and Reinvestment Act, 2009; Families First Coronavirus Response Act, 2020).

[9]The FMAP was increased by 6.5 percentage points for 4 years from 2020 through 2023 as part of the federal COVID-19 pandemic response (Families First Coronavirus Response Act, 2020).

Medicaid

From the lens of Medicaid policy making, children are the largest group of Medicaid enrollees (39%), but they account for a smaller proportion of total spending than other groups (16%; Figure 6-5). All states currently offer Medicaid to low-income children. Child coverage is offered in 2 states for family incomes of 138–200% of FPL; in 30 states for 200–300% of FPL; and in 18 states and the District of Columbia for 300–405% of FPL. Some states offer coverage under federal options and others use "waiver authority" to expand coverage or add benefits to selected groups. For example, Michigan covers pregnant women and children up to 400% of FPL under waiver authority; five states have used the federal option to cover children with disabilities up to 300% of FPL (KFF, 2016; Musumeci et al., 2022).

As the major insurers of U.S. children and youth, Medicaid and CHIP provide a broad base of health insurance coverage for large numbers of children who would otherwise lack any health insurance. Children and youth of color are overrepresented among those with Medicaid coverage; thus, problems and progress in Medicaid and CHIP can either exacerbate or address major inequities in care and access (Michener, 2021). Medicaid improves equity by ensuring a strong health insurance base for large numbers of low-income children of color. As noted above, Medicaid coverage has been associated with a wide variety of short- and long-term improved

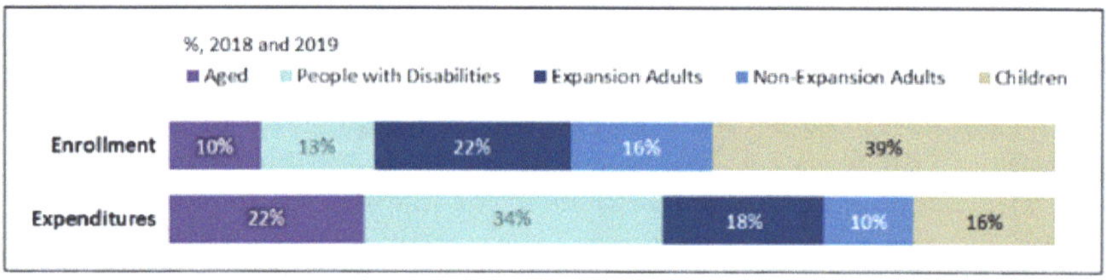

FIGURE 6-5 Estimated Medicaid enrollment and expenditures for benefits, by enrollment group as a share of total (2018 and 2019).
NOTES: The Centers for Medicare & Medicaid Services (CMS) calculated these figures for calendar years 2018 and 2019 using Transformed Medicaid Statistical Information System data to determine the percentage of total Medicaid expenditures accounted for by each beneficiary category; it then applied that percentage to the net total Medicaid expenditures (federal and state) states reported to the Medicaid Budget and Expenditure System using form CMS-64. These national estimates include state-reported data from the 50 states; Washington, DC; Puerto Rico; and the U.S. Virgin Islands. Total net expenditures exclude spending for administrative expenses and Medicaid disproportionate share hospital payments. May not sum to totals due to rounding.
SOURCE: CMS, 2022b; Congressional Research Service, 2023b.

health outcomes, as well as lower health care costs and needs in later life—in these ways, it has improved equity. But Medicaid and CHIP have limitations that make access and care more difficult for many children; thus, they may exacerbate inequities too.

States have several choices or options in designing and implementing their programs. Although they must meet base CMS standards for income eligibility, provider payment, quality measures, and enrollment procedures, they have flexibility beyond these basic standards. State choices lead to major variations in all these items across state lines. Children's access to services therefore depends on where they live and not so much on what they need. A child in Kansas City, Kansas, may need specialized services for a relatively rare chronic condition available in Kansas City, Missouri—but the Kansas Medicaid program network may not include the Missouri provider in its network, may not include the service among its benefits, and may restrict that child's access to appropriate services. State variations, coupled with the geographic concentration of certain racialized communities, Black and Hispanic in particular, have led to significant racial inequities in both health insurance coverage and the services received by a Medicaid- or CHIP-enrolled child. States also have different standards of quality measurement, although, as of fall 2024, CMS (2024a) began requiring a minimum common set of child health measures for the states.

About 85% of children covered by Medicaid receive their basic coverage through a comprehensive managed care organization (MCO), rather than the traditional fee-for-service system (MACPAC, 2023a). Through these MCOs, states contract out many Medicaid functions, including elements of enrollment; provider credentialing, networks, reimbursement, and rate setting; quality reporting and monitoring; service authorization and grievance processes; and utilization review, among others. For comparison, 52% of Medicare beneficiaries are enrolled in managed care plans (MedPAC, 2023a,b,c). Unlike most children with Medicaid coverage, all Medicare beneficiaries can choose to stay in the traditional fee-for-service system or enroll in an MCO, where they can select among an average of 41 plan choices (MedPAC, 2023c). Medicaid beneficiaries are less likely to have a choice of plans. In both Medicare and Medicaid, MCOs are paid a fixed monthly amount per enrolled person, although the payment details differ. Medicaid MCOs must provide services in the same "amount, duration and scope" as would be available under Medicaid fee-for-service (Coverage and Authorization of Service, 2024) and may not deny care because of a patient's diagnosis, type of illness, or condition. Whereas Medicare plans operate largely under uniform national rules set and overseen by CMS, Medicaid rules at the federal level are broader, giving states the flexibility to make key design decisions.

In choosing to privatize major program functions through MCOs, governments must balance giving MCOs the flexibility to innovate and at the same time ensure efficiency, quality, and access. In the Medicaid managed care program, states fall along a continuum of specificity and flexibility. By law, however, a state's managed care program must follow federal Medicaid rules and carry out all elements of the state's approved Medicaid plan.

In some states, the MCO contract becomes a significant vehicle that details expectations and performance provisions and promotes accountability (Rosenbaum & Johnson, 2023). Once a contract is awarded, MCOs have substantial leeway in their interpretation of the federal and state rules. States vary substantially in public inclusion and transparency in developing and reviewing contracts, as well as their strategies and mechanisms for ensuring that MCOs meet their contractual obligations (MACPAC, 2022). Federal regulations require that states have a managed care monitoring system (42 CFR § 438.66), which addresses 14 areas ranging from enrollment to encounter data, provider networks and grievances, among others (State Monitoring Requirements, 2024). Several oversight entities have proposed greater uniformity and transparency in states reporting on key managed care provisions, such as payments and grievances (MACPAC, 2015a, 2022). In general, states and MCOs have provided little evidence regarding how MCOs have met their obligations, and few data exist to determine how well MCOs meet their requirements regarding benefits and coverage for children and youth. New and proposed CMS rules seek to address some of these issues (CMS, 2023d, 2024a; Lopez et al., 2020).

Medicaid Physician Payment Levels and Structures

By law, Medicaid programs should pay providers (physicians, hospitals, and others) sufficiently to produce participation—and ensure that access to care is comparable to that of the general population.[10] Other than state affirmation, however, CMS has little documentation of how well states meet this requirement.

Medicaid fee-for-service rates tend to be lower than Medicare rates for similar procedures (Zuckerman, Skopec, & Aarons, 2021; Zuckerman, Williams, & Stockley, 2009). In part, these lower fees have a long history in Medicaid policy (Fein, 2015; Ford & Michener, 2022). In 2019, Medicaid physician fees for 27 common procedures were estimated to be 72% of Medicare physician fees, with the Medicaid-to-Medicare fee index lower for primary care (0.67) than for obstetric care (0.80; Zuckerman, Skopec, & Aarons, 2021). These comparisons have been published sporadically in the research literature (Rosenbaum,

[10]See Social Security Act, State Plans for Medical Assistance (2024, § 1396a[a][30][A]): "payments are consistent with efficiency, economy, and quality of care and are sufficient to enlist enough providers so that care and services are available under the plan at least to the extent that such care and services are available to the general population in the geographic area."

2014; Zuckerman, Skopec, & Aarons, 2021; Zuckerman, Williams, & Stockley, 2009), but the data are not routinely collected and made public by states or CMS. Recent Medicaid access rules require states to compare their Medicaid and Medicare payment rates for specific services, including primary care, obstetrical and gynecological services, and outpatient behavioral health (42 CFR Parts 430, 438, and 457). Notably, however, children's specialty services are not covered under the proposed rule, nor is there a requirement that the rule be adjusted for volume of care, which would provide a more comprehensive picture of differences in payment rates and service mix, as well as the relative attractiveness of different payers to providers.

Several proposals have been made in the past to benchmark Medicaid-to-Medicare rates (Allen, Golberstein, & Bailey, 2022), in part because of the administrative simplicity of such a proposal. Given that half of children are covered by commercial insurers, a comparison between Medicaid and commercial rates for child-relevant services, such as primary care, obstetric, and specialty care services, would be more relevant to children. Gaps in payment rates for Medicaid versus commercial insurance particularly affect children from racially marginalized and rural communities, as both have high rates of Medicaid insurance coverage. Existing studies have not explored differences between Medicaid fee-for-service and commercial clinician rates, a notable gap in the literature on the child health care system.

A recent review found commercial rates for physician services 118–179% higher than Medicare rates (Lopez et al., 2020; MACPAC, 2015a). The range of estimates likely reflects the differences in the services examined (e.g., procedures vs. evaluation and management), the market power of the insurance plan, the market power of the physician group, the timing of the data (2010–2017 across the studies reviewed), and other geographic differences. Few studies examined rural areas. In a related study pediatric subspecialists seeing many patients with Medicaid insurance reported highly discounted fees (Forrest et al., 2024). These studies, combined with the Medicaid-to-Medicare studies, imply strongly that Medicaid fee-for-service rates for children's services are also lower than commercial rates.

Most relevant to children's coverage are rates paid to clinicians by MCOs. Medicaid MCOs, some nonprofit and many for-profit,[11] are contracted to state Medicaid agencies to receive capitated payments. They have considerable autonomy in setting provider rates, although many continue enhanced fee-for-service payments for providers, sometimes with end-of-year adjustments for certain performance indicators. Little work documents the adequacy of MCO payments. While states use population-level capitation payments for MCOs, the many providers receiving fee-for-service

[11]Five for-profit entities (Centene, Elevance, CVS, United, Molina) control 50% of the MCO Medicaid market, and their profits are quite sizable.

payments from MCOs have limited incentives to improve care or appropriateness. States can impose provider payment schemes on MCOs (Hinton & Raphael, 2023; MACPAC, 2019, 2021a,c) and have demonstrated increasing interest in payment schemes that offer alternatives to fee-for-service payments to address misaligned incentives. Unfortunately, no data explore whether the alternative payment arrangements that MCOs have tested have increased Medicaid payments beyond average fee-for-service levels or improved quality.

The recent CMS access rules require states to submit an annual payment analysis that compares MCO payment rates for routine primary care, obstetrical and gynecological care, and outpatient mental health and substance use disorder services as a proportion of Medicare payment rates. While not required, similar analysis of Medicaid and commercial rates could also be performed. In 2021, Congress passed the Health Care PRICE Transparency Act (2021), making enormous amounts of hospital and insurer price data available to the public. The sheer quantity of data has been part of the challenge, since it is difficult to summarize and process, and, unfortunately, Medicaid MCOs are not included under the transparency mandate, limiting the value of this act for children's care. The rule offers an alternative for obtaining MCO rates, assuming state reporting is reasonably complete and consistent.

Further complicating payment-rate comparisons is the fact that more than half of states make add-on Medicaid payments to providers outside of the regular payment formula (MACPAC, 2022). These "supplemental" and "directed" payments (discussed below) are captured as lump sums in public reporting and cannot be tied back to individual services in ways that facilitate a rate comparison with another payer (MACPAC, 2022). These additional payments are significant, with supplemental add-on payments accounting for $4 billion (or 33% of total fee-for-service payments to physicians) in fiscal year (FY) 2022 (MACPAC, 2023b), although the state variation here is wide, with Texas providing over half of the national total and California and Florida providing other large amounts. Most states provide relatively little physician and other provider supplemental funding. The total size of supplemental payments, relative to physician payments made by MCOs, is not reported. Also not available is the share of directed payments (totaling $38.5 billion) that are paid by MCOs and go to physicians (Government Accountability Office [GAO], 2023d).

Physician Participation

The central reason for policy concern around provider payment is to ensure that Medicaid programs can enlist enough providers such that their enrollees have access to covered services. By law, beneficiaries' access should be the same as for the general population in the same geographic area (Congressional Research Service, 2023a,b), regardless of whether coverage is by fee-for-service, through MCO fee-for-service to clinicians, or through an MCO alternative payment model. However, lower provider participation in Medicaid arises in large part from lower provider payment rates (Hing, Decker, & Jamoom, 2015; Zuckerman, Skopec, & Aarons, 2021), on top of disproportionate administrative burdens imposed by Medicaid programs.

Evidence that Medicaid rates are too low relative to commercial rates is bolstered by findings that providers are less willing to participate in Medicaid or accept new patients than in Medicare or commercial plans (Holgash & Heberlein, 2019; Tang et al., 2018). Clinicians may even misstate their willingness to see Medicaid patients in surveys because they may feel scrutinized (Rankin et al., 2022). "Secret shopper" studies, wherein researchers contact providers posing as patients, corroborate prevalent access problems for Medicaid patients. Across several children's specialty services, Medicaid patients were less likely to receive appointments than patients with other forms of insurance; furthermore, even when the provider accepted Medicaid patients, their appointment delays were longer (Bisgaier & Rhodes, 2011; Chaudhry et al., 2013; Galbraith et al., 2005). Low payment leads to low revenue which also impacts providers' ability to sustain innovation in pediatric health care delivery, particularly models focused on health equity. Challenges with MCO provider networks, and how they are monitored to ensure robust provider participation, are discussed at greater length below.

MCOs must meet federal and state provider networks' adequacy provisions, but these networks also have potentially important gaps. A recent four-state study of Medicaid MCOs found skewed patient loads, with 50% of participating pediatric primary care providers seeing 150 or more Medicaid-enrolled clients per year (Ludomirsky et al., 2022). At the same time, 29% of listed pediatric Medicaid MCO providers saw just 10 or fewer clients, and roughly half of these saw zero clients. Listed providers who see zero patients are sometimes called Medicaid "ghost" providers, and while they are problematic in pediatric primary care, they are also common in adult primary care (15%), particularly in psychiatric care (35%). Low actual participation of providers in an MCO network may indicate that a network meets a state's requirements on paper but does not provide adequate access in practice.

Low payment rates and low provider participation have generally led to recommendations to increase rates. Payment rate increases could enhance access in several ways: more providers could participate, providers could serve more Medicaid enrollees, or providers could extend visit length. However, the evidence is somewhat mixed on whether historical payment rate increases have been successful. A recent systematic review identifies seven studies of Medicaid fee changes and likelihood of provider participation

(Saulsberry, Seo, & Fung, 2019). Of these seven, five were conducted before 2001 and two examined the effects of the ACA fee increase for primary care physicians, which was relatively modest and temporary. One study found positive effects of fee increases on the probability of participation; one found a slightly negative effect; and three studies found no significant association, including two studies that examined the ACA fee bump. Among the seven studies, six examined Medicaid fee changes and the impact on patients seen per physician. Two studies found positive associations between fees and volumes, including one study of obstetrical care and one of physicians seeing children, and four studies found no significant effects. Unfortunately, the older studies predate large expansions in insurance coverage, and major increases in the consolidation and integration of physicians with hospitals, meaning the results may not apply today. Moreover, these studies examined Medicaid fee increases but did not account for payment increases of the magnitude associated with recent state supplemental payments, which could affect provider participation differently (as was the goal). Few studies address payment rate changes for subspecialty care (see National Academies, 2023e), although several hospital-based subspecialties, especially those with high hospital usage, receive supplemental payments, as discussed below.

Access to Clinicians

Another indicator that provider rates may be too low is consumer-reported access to care. A recent study by Haley and colleagues (2023) used 2016–2019 data from the National Survey of Children's Health (NSCH) and the 2016–2018 National Health Interview Survey (NHIS) to examine access barriers for children enrolled in Medicaid/CHIP (before the COVID-19 pandemic). These researchers reported that 4.0% of Medicaid/CHIP-enrolled children ages 17 and under had at least one unmet need for medical, dental, vision, hearing, mental health, and/or other services (with dental care the highest at 2.0%); in the NHIS, 8.2% of Medicaid/CHIP-enrolled children ages 2–17 had some sort of need for care being unmet because of cost (most commonly dental care). In the NSCH the most common reasons for not receiving needed care were problems getting appointments (2.0%) and cost (1.9%), comparable to similar barriers reported in the NHIS. In the NHIS 6.6% of parents with children covered by Medicaid/CHIP reported delays in care from appointment waits, compared with 3.6% for commercially insured and 4.4% for uninsured children (Haley et al., 2023, Table 2), with 8.2% of Medicaid-covered children reported to have an unmet need due to cost, compared with 4.8% and 26.6% for commercially insured and uninsured children, respectively.

Haley and colleagues (2023) found that 23% of parents with children covered by Medicaid/CHIP experienced at least some frustration when trying to get care for the children in the past 12 months, compared with 13% for commercially insured children, and 28% for uninsured children. At the same time, 22% of all children were reported to have no preventive medical visit in the previous 12 months (Haley et al., 2023), with stark variations by race and ethnicity (38.2% for American Indian/Alaska Native children; 32.0% for non-Hispanic Asian children; 21.9% for non-Hispanic Black children, 25.4% for Hispanic children, and 18.4% for non-Hispanic White children). These rates fall well below the American Academy of Pediatrics (AAP)/Bright Futures goal of all children receiving an annual preventive visit and the CMS goal of at least 80% of children receiving such visits (AAP, 2017). Arranging appointments can be frustrating and add to parental stress, and the presence of frustrations and stress may indicate that they lack alternatives. Haley and colleagues (2023) also found that children insured by Medicaid/CHIP had higher rates of access to preventive care than uninsured children but lower rates than commercially insured children.

Early and Periodic Screening, Diagnosis, and Treatment

Medicaid pioneered coverage of preventive services, particularly for comprehensive prenatal care and early and periodic screening, diagnosis, and treatment (Wiley, 2016).[12] The statute titled Early and Periodic Screening, Diagnosis, and Treatment (EPSDT, 1968) provides a consistent, national standard for covered benefits, and states are required to use it as the base for children's benefits. EPSDT's statutory language refers to coverage of services necessary to "correct or ameliorate" physical or mental health conditions (42 USC § 1396d, 2024)—that is, if screening and diagnosis identify a problem needing services not included in the state's benefit package, the state must still provide that service for children and youth up to age 21 years (42 USC § 1396d, 2024). Nonetheless, CMS and the states have administered and enforced the EPSDT benefit inconsistently and inequitably. Concerns about the regulatory base of EPSDT and its implementation in the states led to language in the Bipartisan Safer Communities Act (2022) to require CMS to review state implementation of EPSDT. That review is under way, along with calls to modernize EPSDT regulations (Rosenbaum & Johnson, 2023).

The lack of a national definition for "medical necessity" allows states and MCOs flexibility, which has led to many denials of services, especially for children and youth with long-term health care needs and autism spectrum disorder (Baseman & Zettle, 2024; Grimm, 2023). EPSDT provides an important base for the services that children and youth need and has helped

---

[12]For additional information, see https://www.medicaid.gov/medicaid/benefits/early-and-periodic-screening-diagnostic-and-treatment/index.html

many receive services; nonetheless, issues in its implementation have limited access for many. A recent GAO report reviewed MCO prior authorization decisions restricting care and called for additional systematic oversight from the states. Specifically, the GAO asked CMS to provide guidance for whether MCOs can set their own EPSDT medical necessity standards when the state lacks an EPSDT standard (GAO, 2024).

Children and Youth with Chronic Conditions and Special Health Care Needs

Medicaid plays an important role for children with disabilities and special health needs in several respects (Berry et al., 2021). It is the sole form of health insurance for approximately 36% of the total 13.9 million children estimated to have special health care needs, according to 2019 NSCH data (Williams & Musumeci, 2021). Low-income households have disproportionately higher rates of children with special health care needs, in part because parents are less likely to work or more likely to work less, in order to meet their child's care needs, but also because of the long-term effects of poverty on health and birth weight leading to higher rates of chronic conditions and disability among low-income populations (Kuhlthau & Perrin, 2001; Thyen, Kuhlthau, & Perrin, 1999). Furthermore, the EPSDT benefit requires states to support a broad array of services that commercial insurance often does not cover, especially long-term care services, including institutional and noninstitutional services provided in the home or community, such as attendant care, assistive technology, and case management services (National Academies, 2018), encouraging some families to seek Medicaid coverage for their child with chronic conditions. Thus, while EPSDT applies to all children in Medicaid, it can be particularly important for children with special needs and children in foster care, many of whom also have special health care needs.

While the core Medicaid program supports some long-term services, others are covered through waivers available to states,[13] again leading to wide variation among states (Manatt & Phillips, 2022; Williams & Musumeci, 2021). Main waivers that apply to home and community services include 1915c waivers and a specific "Katie Beckett" waiver that is meant to reduce hospitalizations for people under age 19 with disabilities.

Medicaid also supports populations of young children with disabilities through a wraparound program, in which children with commercial

---

[13]An important waiver supports states' coverage of noninstitutional services for children with disabilities who are under age 19 who without these services would be placed in an institution. This so-called "Katie Beckett" option (Tax Equity and Fiscal Responsibility Act waiver) is available in 49 states and Washington, DC. States can also apply for 1915c waivers, which support home- and community-based services for people with disabilities (not limited to younger populations), and some states include children and youth in their waiver population.

insurance that does not pay for home- and community-based services may receive Medicaid support for those services. As a result, 8% of children with special health care needs nationally have both commercial and wraparound Medicaid coverage, with Medicaid covering long-term services and supports. This proportion varies by state depending on state coverage rules, and children typically must meet a fairly high level of severity to receive such support (Alker et al., 2015; Gusmano & Thompson, 2018; MACPAC, 2018a). Because coverage of long-term services and supports for children is more extensive under Medicaid than with commercial insurance, families with children and youth with special health care needs are more likely to report reasonable out-of-pocket costs, greater benefit adequacy, and greater provider access if they have supplemental Medicaid coverage than if they have commercial coverage only. Nevertheless, families of children with special health care needs with Medicaid coverage more commonly report trouble covering basic needs, including not being able to afford enough to eat, compared with those who have commercial coverage (Williams & Musumeci, 2021).

Children's Health Insurance Program

As noted earlier, CHIP was created in 1997 to expand coverage of children in low-income families by including eligibility to those below 200% of FPL but above the state Medicaid coverage level. This program permits states to collect premiums and copays from enrolled families for coverage. While Medicaid is an entitlement program with specified income eligibility and spending that reflects changes in enrollment, payment rates, and benefits, CHIP is not. CHIP funding is distributed as block grants to states, each receiving a fixed funding allotment that must be matched with state funds (Schneider, Klukoff, & Lehan, 2023). The matching requirement is lower than that for Medicaid (MACPAC, 2023a,b).[14]

CHIP is a significantly smaller program than Medicaid. In FY2020, children enrolled in CHIP totaled 9 million, while 35.2 million were enrolled in Medicaid (CMS, n.d.g). Nationally, 89% of CHIP-enrolled children are in families with incomes under 250% of the FPL (MACPAC, n.d.). Because CHIP programs do not have a federally imposed mandatory minimum or maximum income eligibility (other than the state's Medicaid income base), states vary widely in their CHIP eligibility rules, ranging from 170% FPL in North Dakota to 400% FPL in New York. Under CHIP, states also have the option to cover pregnant women and unborn children (CMS, n.d.a; Social Security Administration [SSA], n.d.).

States choose how to implement CHIP funding. Some states use CHIP to expand Medicaid eligibility levels, while others cover children through

---

[14]https://www.medicaid.gov/chip/financing/index.html

a separate state CHIP program; still others use a combination of the two approaches. Forty percent (40%) of CHIP-enrolled children are in a state program that is separate from Medicaid (MACPAC, 2020).

When CHIP is structured as a separate program, it can differ greatly from Medicaid, in that (1) states can require copays, (2) EPSDT is not mandated, and (3) states need not enroll eligible applicants if they have already used up the current year funding allotment. Stand-alone CHIP programs must offer "benchmark coverage" that is substantially equal, in actuarial terms, to the health benefits coverage in selected federal or state plans, and they must offer well-child care, dental coverage, behavioral health care, and vaccines (CMS, n.d.h). Many states use Bright Futures recommendations, developed jointly by the Health Resources and Services Administration (HRSA) and AAP (AAP, 2017), as their guide to well-child coverage.

Of the 34 states that operate stand-alone CHIP programs, 27 also contract with MCOs (Schneider, Klukoff, & Lehan, 2023). CHIP MCO contracts are not subject to the Medicaid protections, such as minimum loss ratios, provider network adequacy provisions, transparency requirements, or quality monitoring, unless managed care plans enroll both CHIP and Medicaid enrollees under the same contract (Schneider, Klukoff, & Lehan, 2023).

Commercial Insurance

Most commercial insurance for children is employer based and is funded by premium contributions from employers and individuals. When firms offer health insurance coverage, 77% of workers accept that coverage (KFF, 2021; note that because these data are based on surveys of large and small employers, covered children cannot be examined separately from adults). The employee take-up rates vary by firm size and by workers' income and age. Most employers (75%) who offer coverage offer just one plan choice. Twenty six percent (26%) of workers were in firms where the single plan was a high-deductible health plan. Larger firms are more likely than small firms to offer two or more health plan options. Overall, 46% of covered workers were enrolled in preferred provider organizations; followed by 28% in high-deductible health plans, which have lower premiums but higher cost-sharing than other plans; and 25% in health maintenance organizations or point-of-service plans, which limit provider choice through narrow provider networks. For young families with limited incomes, high-deductible health plans are attractive—premium costs are low and, in general, preventive services are excluded from cost determinations. Children with chronic conditions, however, are subject to higher out-of-pocket costs in a high-deductible health plan for the same set of services, and families may forgo needed treatment because of costs. For these families, high-deductible health plans may not be a good financial choice (Galbraith et al.,

2009, 2010, 2011; Kullgren et al., 2010; Kusma & Davis, 2021; Larson et al., 2021).

Based on employer surveys, the average annual premium in 2022 was $22,221 for family coverage, compared with $7,739 for single coverage (KFF, 2021). Employees contributed on average 28% of the premium for family coverage and 17% of the premium for single coverage. The premium amount depends on the type of coverage and is lower for plans with tighter provider networks, such as health maintenance organizations, and for plans with high deductibles (Figure 6-6). Premiums are also lower for private than for public firms, firms with more low-wage workers, and firms with many young workers. On average, differences in family premiums across firm size, worker age, low and high incomes, and firm ownership are under 15% (KFF, 2021a). However, the full range of family premiums is wide, with 15% of employers offering family coverage at $16,500 per year and 10% of employers offering family coverage at premiums of $29,000 per year or more (KFF, 2021).

The ACA eliminated out-of-pocket costs for selected preventive clinical services for employer- and exchange-based commercial insurance (Seiler et al., 2014). The specific services identified in the ACA must be offered without any form of cost-sharing (e.g., deductibles, coinsurance,

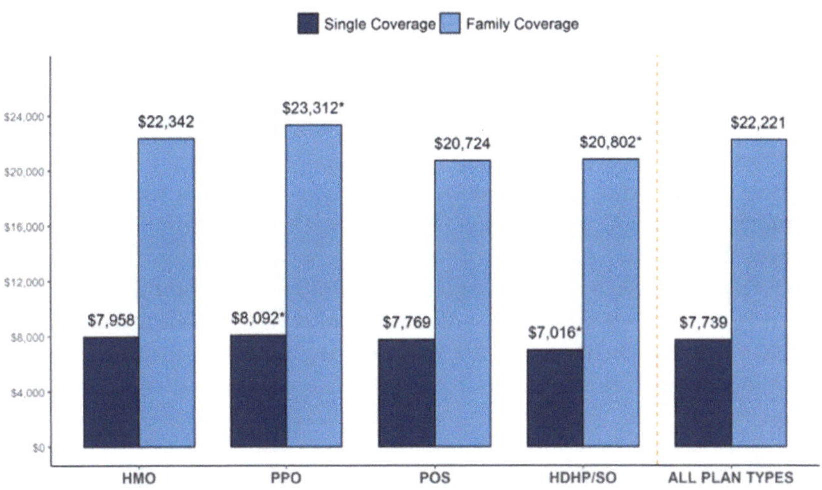

FIGURE 6-6 Average annual premiums for covered workers, single and family coverage, by plan type, 2021.
NOTES: *Estimate is statistically different from "all plan types" ($p < .05$); HDHP/SO = high-deductible health plan/savings option; HMO = health maintenance organization; POS = point of service; PPO = preferred provider organization.
SOURCE: Employer Health Benefits Survey (KFF, 2021).

copayments) and are sometimes referred to as "Section 2713 services" after the relevant paragraph in the Public Health Service Act (Coverage of Preventive Health Services, 2023). They include services with a grade of A or B from the U.S. Preventive Services Task Force; immunizations recommended by the Advisory Committee on Immunization Practices; services recommended for infants, children, and adolescents by Bright Futures; and services for women recommended in the Women's Preventive Services Guidelines (CMS, 2024a; HRSA, 2024b).

Insurance Coverage for Parents

Adults caring for young children play a critical role in ensuring their children's access to clinical care. They are responsible, for example, for ensuring their children have health insurance, identifying providers, navigating the health care system, making appointments, transporting children to care, paying for care, and obtaining needed prescription drugs or otherwise following up on a treatment plan. Whether a parent has health insurance is a key factor in children's access to health care—including whether or not the child is insured (Hamersma, Kim, & Timpe, 2019; Hudson & Moriya, 2017), receives recommended preventive care (Venkataramani, Pollack, & Roberts, 2017), or goes without needed health care (DeVoe, Tillotson, & Wallace, 2009). Furthermore, the health and wellbeing of parents are key elements of support needed by children (see National Academies, 2019e, and earlier chapters in this report). Children raised by healthy parents have better health and outcomes.

Despite the importance of parental insurance coverage for children, an estimated 27.5 million individuals were uninsured in 2021, including 12.2% of adults under age 65 (Tolbert, Drake, & Damico, 2023). For low-income families who live in non-Medicaid expansion states, the median income for Medicaid eligibility is lower than the FPL (Tolbert, Drake, & Damico, 2023). And parents with incomes above the Medicaid eligibility threshold may lack access to premium tax credits for coverage through the Health Insurance Marketplace, which are designed to make that insurance more affordable (Drake et al., 2024). Ensuring access to affordable—and continuous—health insurance coverage for parents is a critical component of transforming the health care system for children. Increased health care coverage of adults increases health care coverage of children.

The 10 states that have yet to adopt the ACA Medicaid expansion (KFF, 2024) as of the writing of this report are predominately in the Southeast region of the country (see Figure 6-7). And in 2021, 44% of low-income Black adults and 37% of low-income Hispanic adults lived in the 12 states that had yet to expand Medicaid at that time (Baumgartner, Collins, & Radley, 2023). These inconsistent Medicaid policies for adults prior to, during, and after pregnancy impact children and child health even before conception and well after delivery.

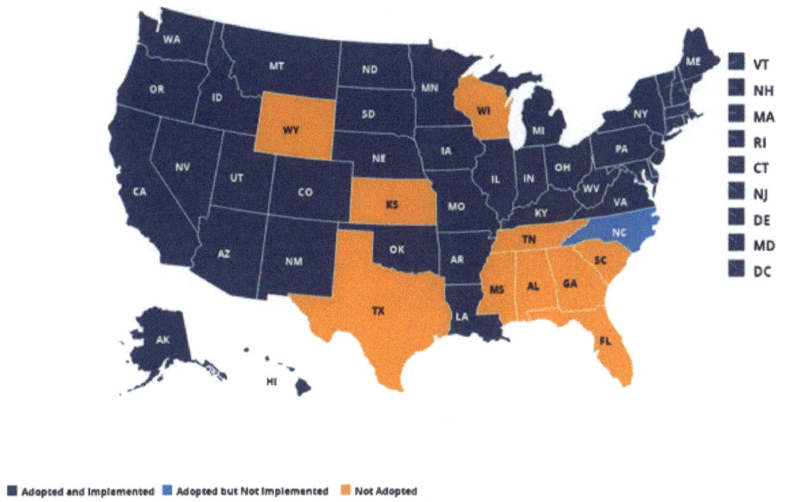

FIGURE 6-7 Status of state action on Medicaid expansion decision.
SOURCE: KFF, 2024.

Direct Clinical Services Support

Community Health Centers

First launched in 1965 as "neighborhood health centers," the goal of community health centers is to improve the health and lives of Americans regardless of their ability to pay for medical services. Funding for these centers is determined annually by Congress and is discretionary. Community health centers receive funding through insurance-enhanced payment and funds administered through HRSA to provide additional resources for capital expenditures, training, and other support. In addition, they receive funding from Title X for family planning services and revenue from public and commercial payers, as well as through a sliding scale for out-of-pocket payments established by a board of directors (National Academies, 2021b). Community health centers (which include federally qualified health centers [FQHCs], rural health clinics, school-based health clinics, migrant health centers, health centers for residents of public housing, and look-alikes[15]) have consistently received bipartisan support and expanded significantly since 2010, more than doubling their number of locations and removing

[15] "Look-alikes" is a term used by HRSA. Health center program look-alikes are HRSA-designated health centers that provide comprehensive, culturally competent, high-quality primary health care services while meeting all health center program requirements, but they do not receive federal award funding (HRSA, 2023e).

barriers to care in many communities (Behr et al., 2022; HRSA, 2023e). However, not all communities have experienced increased access to community health centers equally; studies show that recent expansions were less likely to occur in rural areas or areas of high poverty (Chang, Bynum, & Lurie, 2019; Varshney, 2022).

As noted in Chapter 5, community health centers provide a comprehensive array of services to predominantly low-income populations who are uninsured or have Medicaid insurance. In 2021, community health centers served about 33% of individuals living in poverty and 20% of individuals living in rural areas (National Association of Community Health Centers [NACHC], 2022); FQHCs served more than 30 million patients, including about 12% of all children in the United States (NACHC, 2022).

Medicaid uses a prospective payment system for FQHCs rather than a fixed per-visit rate, as is common in fee-for-service systems. Rates are based on various indicators of center costs and prevailing health center rates in the area. Centers can achieve higher payment rates when they increase staff—for example, adding mental and behavioral health practitioners. The additional costs are then included in the negotiated rates for the prospective payment. States may use alternative payment models other than the prospective payment system for their contracts with FQHCs, but only if the resulting payment will be at least as high as it would be in the prospective payment system. Although usually not labeled as an alternative payment model, the prospective payment system has the advantage of supporting practice transformation with movement to teams for clinical care. The growth of managed care has also affected the payment arrangements for FQHCs, with many MCOs not following the prospective payment system rules of Medicaid.

Notably, FQHC governing boards are required to be composed of at least 51% of people who live in the communities served by the center and reflect the demographic characteristics of its population, making them uniquely community oriented. Community health centers must also complete a community needs assessment every 3 years, make and maintain relationships with other clinicians in their catchment to help coordinate care outside their center, and annually assess the geographic boundaries of their patient population. These centers must provide service to everyone regardless of their ability to pay.

Community health centers offer several important advantages and improved outcomes over traditional delivery systems for some populations with previously limited access (Heisler, 2017; Rieselbach et al., 2019). FQHCs offer transportation, translation, and case management services in addition to on-site care and referral to specialty care. These services help decrease disparities in access and outcome by race and ethnicity, and income and insurance status (Topmiller et al., 2023). HRSA-funded health center members who utilize enabling services such as transportation or translation are more likely to get routine checkups, receive primary care, and report higher patient satisfaction than those who do not utilize such services. Overall, FQHC members have fewer hospitalizations than comparable populations, and FQHCs spend less on inpatient and specialty care while outperforming other delivery systems across measures of quality and outcomes, cost-effectiveness, and patient satisfaction (National Academies, 2021b). In caring for children, community health centers save 35% in emergency services, prescription drugs, and ambulatory care, compared with other types of providers (Bruen & Ku, 2017). Mothers receiving care at FQHCs, despite tending to be more at-risk individuals, are less likely to have an infant with a low birth weight compared with national averages across racial/ethnic groups (NACHC, 2020). For children, integrated behavioral and primary care at FQHCs improves detection and treatment of behavioral health conditions, such as attention deficit hyperactivity disorder (ADHD; Sheldrick et al., 2022). Communities with a new FQHC have had an associated 5% drop in teen birth rates, with declines largest among Black teens and in counties with more than one FQHC (Farid, 2020).

The community health center model has been successful in meeting primary preventive care needs, but its growth (serving 24% more individuals from 2015 to 2021) has not kept pace with community needs (the number of individuals without a usual source of primary care has doubled since 2014; NACHC, 2023b). Some challenges in expanding the model relate to workforce shortages and financing. Although community health centers provide services nationally for roughly 16% of Medicaid recipients, they receive less than 2% of Medicaid payments (National Academies, 2021b). Moreover, their funding has not kept pace with medical care inflation (Brill, 2023).

Certified Community Behavioral Health Clinics

The Community Mental Health Act (1963) established community mental health centers across the United States. However, initial efforts resulted in a fragmented system that did not meet community needs (National Academies, 2024a). The certified community behavioral health clinic (CCBHC) model—administered by the Substance Abuse and Mental Health Services Administration (SAMHSA) in partnership with the Office of the Assistant Secretary for Planning and Evaluation (ASPE) and CMS—has evolved to provide coordinated, comprehensive behavioral health care based on community needs assessments. CCBHCs have been designed for mental health and substance use disorders to reach individuals across the lifespan with developmentally appropriate care. They are required to serve anyone who requests care, regardless of their ability to pay, place of residence, or age. CCBHCs must meet standards for the range of services they provide, including those for screening, family-centered treatment, and peer- and family-support services, and they are required to get people into care quickly. Such features include 24/7 access to crisis services, mobile crisis response within 3 hours, urgent noncrisis need seen within a day, and routine care within 10 days (National Academies, 2024a). CCBHCs must provide clinicians with training on cultural competency; person-centered, family-centered, and recovery-oriented services; and trauma-informed care. Trainings must also be aligned with the National Standards for Culturally and Linguistically Appropriate Services (U.S. Department of Health and Human Services, n.d.). Furthermore, governing boards of CCHBCs are to have members representing individuals and families with lived experiences of mental health conditions and/or substance use disorders. A 2020 report to Congress noted that CCHBCs in participating states outperformed state Medicaid benchmarks in quality metrics for children and adolescents receiving an initial evaluation within 10 days, and for follow-up care after mental health hospitalization and after ADHD medication initiation and continuation (ASPE, 2020a).

An evaluation of the initial 2 years of the CCBHC demonstration found that, depending on the state, 8–27% of CCBHC clients were children or adolescents, 3–22% were African American, <1–8% were American Indian and Alaska Native, and 5–41% were Hispanic. Services provided to children and families were reported to include community wraparound services; dialectical behavioral therapy; peer support for families; and supported employment, housing, and education. Subgroup findings in this evaluation did not suggest that the CCBHC model systematically impacted service use differently for children and adolescents across the participating states (Brown et al., 2022).

CCBHCs can be supported through the Section 223 CCBHC Medicaid Demonstration of the Protecting Access to Medicare Act through SAMHSA-administered CCBHC expansion grants, or through independent state programs separate from the Section 223 CCBHC Medicaid Demonstration. In FY 2022, CCHBCs were appropriated $315 million through SAMHSA (2022c).

Currently, more than 500 CCBHCs are operating across the country, as either CCBHC expansion grantees, as clinics participating in their states' Medicaid demonstration, or as a part of independent state CCBHC programs (see Figure 6-8). The CCBHC model has been designed to integrate a number of promising approaches discussed in this report. The effects of the model and expansion on child and family mental health have yet to be determined. Appropriate oversight will be necessary to ensure these centers make progress toward health equity and mental health goals and reach communities most in need.

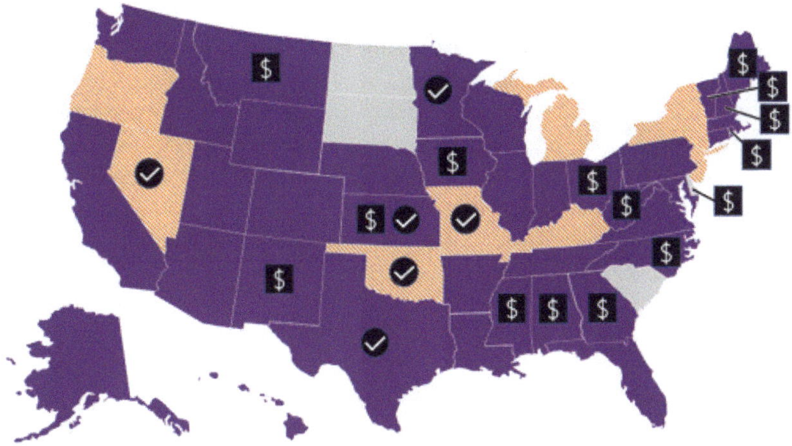

FIGURE 6-8 Certified community behavioral health clinics (CCHBCs) across the United States (as of March 6, 2023).
NOTES:
Federal CCBHC Medicaid Demonstration (and Substance Abuse and Mental Health Services Administration [SAMHSA] Expansion grants)
State contains at least one local SAMHSA expansion grantee in the state
Centers for Medicare & Medicaid Services–approved payment method for CCBHCs via state plan amendment or 1115 waiver separate from Demonstration
$ Chosen to receive 1-year planning grant needed to join Medicaid Demonstration starting in March 2023
SOURCE: SAMHSA, 2023a.

School-Based Health Centers

School-based health centers are important settings where children can receive clinical care; moreover, centers located in low-income areas improve children's health and education outcomes (Community Preventive Services Task Force [CPSTF], 2016a). For schools specifically, Medicaid allows simplified processes for calculating payment rates, for documenting services delivered, for determining Medicaid coverage (using estimated ratios of eligible children applied to services delivered, rather than person-specific eligibility determination), and for qualifying participating providers. In addition, through administrative matching funds, schools can support Medicaid outreach, enrollment, and care coordination (CMS, 2023c). In 2023, CMS released guidance on how Medicaid can fund services in schools (e.g., preventive, behavioral health, physical therapy). While Medicaid and commercial insurance can be billed, barriers exist including lack of effective billing infrastructure and at times primary care approval or preauthorization for certain school-based services.

Despite this flexibility, the fundamental structure of Medicaid as an insurance program does not support other effective school-based interventions, aside from school-based clinical services (Moore et al., 2024), such as schoolwide positive behavior supports, universal school-based programs to reduce violence or increase mental health (CPSTF, 2019b), enhanced school-based physical activity, school-based nutritional interventions, or multitiered services (Moore et al., 2024), or approaches that support school staff and teachers. See Chapter 8 for further discussion of school-based care services.

Indian Health Service

The Indian Health Service (IHS) provides direct health care services to eligible Native American individuals and Alaska Natives. About half of Native American individuals are eligible for this program, and in 2020, the IHS served 64% of the eligible population (National Academies, 2023d). IHS clinics include federal, tribal, and urban Indian health organizations that provide comprehensive care across the lifespan in rural areas; on reservations; and, increasingly, in urban population centers (IHS, 2020a). Some have been designated as FQHCs (IHS, 2005, 2020b).

IHS receives funding through congressional appropriations (mainly discretionary), which are supplemented by a small share of reimbursement collections from Medicaid, CHIP, and commercial insurance. Financing of IHS through annual discretionary allocation with specific spending limits is very different from Medicaid as an entitlement program with no annual spending caps. This impacts not only the year-to-year delivery of health care services but its long-term sustainability and the ability to update infrastructure and respond to public health crises (e.g., COVID-19 pandemic) or other unexpected events. IHS's global budget structure also means that as the number of community members served increases, the per capita spending declines. It is also notable that Medicaid, with its relatively low reimbursement rates, comprised nearly 70% of third-party collections at IHS facilities during the federal FY2019 (MACPAC, 2021b). This creates a compounded and insidious inequity in how health care services for Native Americans are financed.

Currently, funding for IHS has been estimated to address only 48.6% of the health care needs of Native Americans (ASPE, 2022b). IHS funding for urban health has been only around 1% of the current allocation, even though 70% of Native Americans live in urban areas (ASPE, 2022a; National Council of Urban Indian Health [NCUIH], 2023). In 2018, the funding gap for direct care services for children and mothers eligible for IHS was estimated to be $7.8 billion (National Academies, 2023f). See the recent report by the National Academies titled *Federal Policy to Advance*

Racial, Ethnic, and Tribal Health Equity for a broader discussion of IHS structure and inadequate funding levels, its history and federal responsibility, and policy solutions for addressing health inequities for all ages of American Indian and Alaska Native people (National Academies, 2023e).

More than 60% of IHS appropriations are administered by tribes through self-determination contracts (25 USC § 5301; IHS, 2020b). The self-determination option allows tribes to leverage tribal leaders' knowledge to assess needs and tailor services to their communities. The self-determination approach could be useful for providing child, family, and community-oriented care; however, as discussed above, the IHS to date is chronically underfunded (GAO, 2018; Heisler & McClanahan, 2020; Lofthouse, 2022; National Academies, 2021e; Tribal Budget Formulation Workgroup, 2022; United States Congress, 2024).[16]

Hospital Supplemental Payments

Policy discussions about Medicaid hospital payment include both Medicaid base payment rates but also several special payment programs (MACPAC, 2017), with a significant share of Medicaid hospital payments routed outside the usual fee-for-service or MCO payment system. These supplemental payments tie to various policy goals (MACPAC, 2021a, 2023b). Some payments are used to "top up" Medicaid base rates, while others support the care of uninsured groups, and still others are tied to quality or access goals.

One type of hospital supplement is the Disproportionate Share Hospital (DSH) program, which was originally designed to strengthen financing for hospitals with large proportions of low-income, especially uninsured, patients. However, a recent MACPAC (2024a) report found low correlation between DSH payment amounts and uncompensated care at the hospital level, suggesting that these funds may not be well targeted. Other supplemental payments go to hospitals, physicians, or other large providers (mental health centers, nursing homes; MACPAC, 2021a).

One important distinction across providers is that supplements to physicians are not tied to upper payment limits (MACPAC, 2021a, 2023a), whereas several hospital supplements are capped at Medicare equivalents (i.e., with the goal of raising Medicaid rates to the upper limit of prevailing Medicare rates). Most supplements are tied to provider fee-for-service payments, but a rapidly growing category of special payments, called "directed

[16]"The 2023 omnibus spending package provided IHS with $6.96 billion for FY 2023, and, in a historic change, also included advance appropriations totaling $5.13 billion for FY 2024 (NCUIH, 2023). However, it is not clear if advance appropriations will continue past 2024" (National Academies, 2023c, p. 268).

payments," targets MCOs, with the major growth of MCOs replacing fee-for-service Medicaid arrangements. With these arrangements, states can direct MCOs to pay certain state-selected providers additional sums (GAO, 2023d; MACPAC, 2022). In total, supplemental payments constituted 52% of total fee-for-service Medicaid payments to hospitals (MACPAC, 2023b) and 33% of total payments to physicians and other practitioners (MACPAC, 2023b). GAO (2023d) estimates that providers received a net $32 billion from directed payments in 2022.

As with many dimensions of Medicaid policy, the national averages mask large underlying state variation. Furthermore, the data do not distinguish pediatric from other hospitals. States differ in the total amounts, mix, goals, and distribution of funding to providers (MACPAC, 2021c, 2023b). To illustrate, physician supplements most often benefit public (state or county) academic medical centers or teaching hospitals (MACPAC, 2021c), but 20 states have no supplemental payments to physicians, and shares in other states range from less than 1% to over 92% (MACPAC, 2023a). All but five states with MCOs have directed payments ranging from under $100 million to more than $1 billion.

One appeal of supplemental payments, relative to increasing the base payment levels, is that supplements are capped in aggregated, more predictable ways, and they are less likely to rely on state general funds (GAO, 2023d). Hospitals frequently share in the financing of the supplemental payments (i.e., putting up a portion of the state share through intergovernmental transfers, health care provider taxes, or certified public expenditures), again with large state variation. For government-owned (county or state) health care systems, states can also increase their federal match through intergovernmental transfers, providing substantial financing for public institutions (GAO, 2023d). Once these health care systems contribute a share of the costs, those funds are then reimbursed through the supplement.[17]

Historically, states did not report supplemental payment amounts at the provider level, making it difficult to assess which providers benefit and where payment gaps remain (MACPAC, 2023a). Federal law (Consolidated Appropriations Act, 2022) now requires provider-level reporting for certain supplemental payments, although this provision has not yet been implemented through regulations and it omits several kinds of supplemental payments. The lack of transparency and insufficient evaluation surrounding supplemental (and directed) payments have been raised repeatedly as policy challenges: neither their impact on the child health care system nor on the distribution of health care resources to reduce child health disparities is

[17]GAO (2023d) estimates that 75% of intergovernmental transfers are returned to local government providers and 80% of provider taxes are returned to the same providers.

clear (GAO, 2021, 2023d). However, many of these mechanisms likely have major impact on the financing of children's inpatient care. In some cases, a children's hospital may be the only provider of specialized pediatric services in a community, and it may therefore qualify for DSH payments. In other cases, the upper-payment-limit strategy can improve hospital financing; and in still others, state pediatric inpatient units can receive additional funds through the Medicaid pass-through program.

MACPAC (2017) published a seminal analysis of hospital payment rates in Medicaid, including comparisons with Medicare rates, finding that hospital fee-for-service rates, overall, were comparable or higher than Medicare for a selected set of common services, once adjustments were made to the Medicaid fees based on supplemental hospital payments. These supplemental payments on average accounted for 49% of total Medicaid payments to hospitals. This general conclusion aligned with estimates from the American Hospital Association (AHA, 2016). As anticipated, large state-specific differences emerged: for 18 selected conditions, the average Medicaid payment was higher than Medicare in 25 states and lower than Medicare in 22 states (AHA, 2016). MACPAC (2017) also documented very large differences in hospital payment rates within and across states, within and across individual hospital services, and in the distribution of supplemental hospital payments.

KEY CHALLENGES OF HEALTH INSURANCE

On the positive side, children have high rates of insurance coverage. However, high out-of-pocket costs; gaps in covered benefits; limited provider participation, particularly for mental health and dental care; and periodic gaps in coverage and other administrative burdens create uncertainty and financial stress in families, with detrimental effects for child health. Several persistent challenges remain in providing equitable health insurance coverage for children.

Racial and Geographic Variation

Employer-Sponsored Insurance

Most children's commercial health insurance financing is tied to their parents' employer; consequently, the choices employers make about the insurance policies they offer to their employees can perpetuate structural racism and health inequities for children. A 2022 analysis of health disparities among employer-sponsored insurance enrollees found that those with low to moderate incomes had high rates of both difficulty paying medical bills and emergency department utilization; overall, among individuals with employer-sponsored insurance, racial disparities persisted in areas such as maternal and behavioral health (Morgan Health & NORC, 2022).

Because employer-sponsored insurance plans are not required to cover mental health, dental care, or other preventive services not required in Section 2713 (29 CFR), coverage of these services becomes an employer-specific decision, leading to wide variability in the experience of children and families. For example, 54% of employer-sponsored plans do not cover pediatric dental services, half do not cover applied behavioral analysis therapy, and 31% of small employer plans and 20% of large employer plans do not cover autism services (MACPAC, 2015b). Currently, few data describe differences among employer-sponsored plans in coverage or access to speech, physical, or occupational therapies for children (MACPAC, 2016). However, an analysis of children continuously enrolled for 1 calendar year in an employer-sponsored insurance plan found that children with noncomplex and complex chronic disease and those who sought behavioral health services experienced significantly higher rates of out-of-network care and associated higher rates of cost-sharing.

Employer-sponsored insurance has clear benefits, including coverage of young adults through their parents' insurance up to age 26 (Conway, 2020). This provision effectively publicly subsidizes (because the value of employer-sponsored benefits such as insurance are not taxed) young adults from wealthier families, who are more likely to have access to employer-sponsored insurance than those in lower-income families, extending the impact of structural racism on economic opportunity (McMorrow et al., 2015). Figure 6-9 (Hill, Artiga, & Damico, 2024) illustrates that Asian and White children and their families are more likely to get insurance coverage through employers. A previous National Academies report states, "This policy creates tax inequity, as it benefits those with employment and provides greater subsidies to those with higher incomes" (National Academies, 2023e, p. 229). Large employers are more likely to offer employer-sponsored health insurance; employers with a large percentage of low-wage workers are less likely to offer health insurance (MACPAC, 2016). Previous data show that 74.9% of White children's parents were offered employer-sponsored insurance, compared with 60.7% of Black and 51.4% of Hispanic children's parents (Pylypchuk & Selden, 2008). This is consistent with more recent data that also found that only a few firms that offer coverage to employees do not offer it to other dependents and that low-wage workers with families are more likely to be employed in small firms and so less likely to be offered employer-sponsored health insurance. Around 19% of employers offered health benefits to part-time workers in 2015, and only 3% offered any coverage to temporary workers (MACPAC, 2016). A Brookings Institution report found that Latino/a, Black, and women workers were overrepresented in the low-wage workforce, with White and

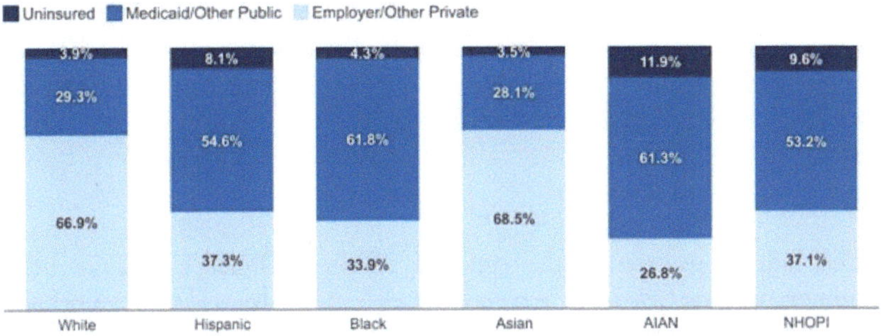

FIGURE 6-9 Health care coverage of children by race and ethnicity, 2022.
NOTES: Includes children ages 0–18 years. Persons of Hispanic origin may be of any race but are categorized as Hispanic for this analysis; other groups are non-Hispanic. AIAN = American Indian and Alaska Native; NHOPI = Native Hawaiian or Other Pacific Islander. Totals may not sum to 100% because of rounding.
SOURCE: KFF (2024) analysis of 2022 American Community Survey, 1-year estimates.

Asian Americans underrepresented (Ross & Bateman, 2019); additionally, 40% of low-wage workers were noted to be raising children.

Uninsured Children

The complexity, inconsistency, variations, and structural racism inherent in the system of health care financing for children means that 5.4% of children remain uninsured (Alker & Osorio, 2023). These numbers are notably higher in American Indian and Alaska Native (13.3%), Hispanic (8.6%), and Native Hawaiian and other Pacific Islander (7.1%) communities, which have the highest rates of uninsured children and youth (Branch & Conway, 2022).

Compare these with uninsurance rates for adults ages 65 and older, which have been below 1% since 2019 (Cohen & Cha, 2023)—although disparities exist even among older populations, with increased rates in older people from Hispanic (3.6%), Native Hawaiian and other Pacific Islander (2.0%), and Asian (2.3%) communities (Branch & Conway, 2022). This high rate of coverage largely comes from the financing and structure of Medicare, which is an entitlement program with eligibility based primarily on age and citizenship status. Medicare has full federal financing, with funding stemming from a combination of general revenues, payroll taxes, income taxes, premiums for those not eligible for premium-free coverage, and interest earned on the two trust fund accounts set up and held by the U.S. Treasury exclusively for Medicare, with little to no variation in coverage among states or territories.

In contrast, Medicaid relies on general revenues. In 2021, federal Medicare spending for the 63,964,675 enrolled members was $900 billion, while spending on the 85,809,179 individuals in Medicaid and CHIP was $734 billion (CMS, 2021a,b, 2023i, n.d.g).

Disparate COVID-19 Relief

The federal government's response to the COVID-19 public health emergency illustrates how current health care financing undervalues pediatric care and exacerbates long-standing racial and health inequities. In addition to the continuous Medicaid and CHIP eligibility policies noted earlier, as part of the Coronavirus Aid, Relief, and Economic Security (CARES) Act (2020), Congress provided direct funding to eligible hospitals and providers (Schwartz & Damico, 2020). Funding included targeted Medicare distributions through a "high-impact distribution," which went out automatically in two rounds. Payments were determined through a formula set by CMS, relying in part on the hospital's share of fee-for-service Medicare payments out of total Medicare payments in 2019 for the initial round (Franco, 2020). A similar formula was used for the Provider Relief Fund administered by HRSA (n.d.d), relying on revenues from 2018. The stated intent was to assist hospitals that had significant decreases in the volume of care. However, given that the formula for distribution of funds relied on a prepandemic health care system with known inequities, the result of these initial allocations was that funding went disproportionately to larger, wealthier health care systems that were less likely to serve Medicaid and uninsured patients or those from rural or racially marginalized communities (Rau, 2020a,b). This initial allocation of funding by revenue instead of by need had a disparate impact on Black populations in particular (Kakani et al., 2020). Subsequent analyses showed that hospitals with a larger proportion of Medicaid patients saw relatively increased pandemic relief funding; however, critical access hospitals and those in rural communities saw lower levels of CARES Act funding (Cantor et al., 2021).

Immigration Status and Health Insurance

A child or their caregiver's immigration status also impacts their likelihood of having health insurance and accessing care (Norris, 2023; Pillai et al., 2023; Rosenberg et al., 2022). In 2021, approximately 44.7 million immigrants lived in the United States, including 20.8 million noncitizens (both documented and undocumented individuals) and 23.9 million naturalized citizens (KFF, 2023a,b). Many families have mixed immigration status—that is, citizens and documented and undocumented individuals living in the same home. Twenty percent (20%) of children have at least one parent who is an immigrant; 12% of children who are U.S. citizens have at least one noncitizen parent (KFF, 2023a,b).

Legislation enacted by Congress in 1996 prohibited federal funding of Medicaid for individuals who have had legal permanent-resident status (often referred to as having a "green card") for 5 years or less (Broder & Lessard, 2023). Certain groups, such as refugees and asylees, veterans, and their families, do not have to wait 5 years. States are allowed to cover these individuals with state-only funds; 29 states—plus Washington, DC, and the Commonwealth of the Northern Mariana Islands—have chosen to cover pregnant women and children in these groups through Medicaid without a 5-year waiting period, while 21 of those states also cover them through CHIP (Health Insurance Marketplace, n.d.). Individuals in these groups can also get coverage for emergency care for certain conditions through Medicaid. Additionally, all documented individuals are eligible for coverage through the federal health insurance marketplace, as well as emergency Medicaid.

Although noncitizen immigrants have high employment rates, they frequently have low-wage jobs in industries that do not offer employer-sponsored insurance. States that have extended coverage to children regardless of immigration status have found a decline in forgoing preventive or needed medical and dental care. Similar expansion of coverage for pregnancies through Medicaid was associated with improved birth weights and average gestation for newborns (KFF, 2023a,b).

However, recent federal policy changes, notably "public charge" rules regarding entry to the United States and/or eligibility for a green card or citizenship (Pillai & Artiga, 2022), have contributed to declines in enrollment in Medicaid among mixed-status and immigrant families. Indeed, many noncitizen immigrants pay taxes that support the very programs they cannot access. In 2018 undocumented immigrants contributed an estimated $20.1 billion in federal taxes and $11.8 billion in state and local taxes (New American Economy, n.d.).

Continuity of Health Insurance Coverage for Children

Even with four waves of health insurance coverage expansion for children over multiple decades, 2.5 million children (Tolbert, Drake, & Damico, 2023) were eligible but never enrolled in Medicaid, even during the public health emergency. These eligible families may not have enrolled out of lack of awareness of eligibility, administrative burdens, or for other reasons (Buchmueller, Ham, & Shore-Sheppard, 2016). State and federal rules often create administrative barriers to continuous enrollment in Medicaid, requiring frequent redetermination of eligibility, which is often a time-consuming task for parents (e.g., time spent gathering relevant information). Thus, many children lose coverage for administrative reasons; in other words, they are disenrolled from Medicaid despite being eligible (this is also called "churn"). Churn is a persistent challenge in insuring children (ASPE, 2022c; Corallo et al., 2021; Frenier & McIntyre, 2023), as was made starkly clear during the recent Medicaid "unwinding." As of May 2024, more than 5 million children and youth had lost Medicaid coverage, often through administrative problems rather than ineligibility (Center for Children and Families, n.d.).

The ACA requires states to coordinate eligibility and enrollment across Medicaid, CHIP, and coverage on health insurance exchanges with an eye toward reducing coverage gaps as families' incomes and other circumstances change. Despite common income, application, and electronic data transfer provisions, several nuanced differences among the health insurance programs' rules and paperwork requirements can lead to gaps in coverage (MACPAC, 2022). A recent MACPAC study (2022) examined gaps in coverage for children with Medicaid or CHIP. After a coverage gap, one-third to half of children did not transition to new coverage within 12 months (this rate was lower than that of adults; 65%).

As the recent Medicaid unwinding has also documented, administrative barriers create major problems for families who must regularly provide information about their continuing eligibility. Additionally, immigrant parents who are concerned about public charge rules (e.g., applications for U.S. citizenship face scrutiny if an adult uses various public programs) may avoid enrolling their (often U.S. citizen) children in Medicaid (Gonzales, Haley, & Kenney, 2023; Raphael et al., 2020). Many states require burdensome eligibility checks, and in recent years, federal assistance with enrollment has been reduced. What is more, reauthorization of CHIP funding was delayed in 2017 (Brooks, Park, & Roygardner, 2019). Entities such as MACPAC (2022) have made numerous recommendations for marginal administrative changes that would reduce churn and loss of coverage in transitions.

Another policy lever for reducing gaps in coverage is for states to expand the length of continuous coverage for Medicaid and CHIP. Federal policy made a significant step toward coverage continuity in 2023. Whereas 17 states previously did not have continuous 12-month eligibility for Medicaid or CHIP, beginning in 2024, all states must do so for children under age 19 years (Consolidated Appropriations Act, 2023). In addition, states may cover pregnant women for 12 months postpartum. States may also opt to further extend continuous coverage. In 2023, Oregon began offering multiyear coverage through age 6 years, plus 2-year continuous eligibility for children over age 6 (Buettgens, Nichols, & Dorn, 2023; KFF, 2023d). Washington and New Mexico now also offer multiyear coverage, and several other states (California, Colorado, Illinois, Minnesota, North Carolina, New York, Ohio, and Pennsylvania) are in the process of developing relevant policies (Burak, 2023). Rationale for these policy innovations includes the low cost to federal and state budgets (0.1%; Buettgens, Nichols, & Dorn, 2023) and relatively low rates of change in eligibility in younger families (Oregon Health Authority, 2021), as well as evidence that gaps in health care insurance coverage for children lead to higher likelihoods of unmet medical, prescription, and dental needs; delays in accessing urgent care; and lower likelihoods of attending well-child visits or having a usual source of care (Cassedy, Fairbrother, & Newacheck, 2008). Additionally, policy makers have pointed to the well-documented critical window of the first 5 years in a child's development, as well as the priority for continuous coverage for communities that historically experience the brunt of structural racism and inequity (Burak, 2018; Chomilo, 2022).

Underinsurance

While the problem of uninsurance among children has declined, the challenge of underinsurance has risen. "Underinsurance," when individuals with health insurance coverage still face financial risk (Lavarreda, Brown, & Bolduc, 2011), can be caused by coverage that stops and starts and from limited covered benefits, limited provider networks, or high out-of-pocket costs—challenges especially common to children with commercial insurance and in stand-alone CHIP programs. From 2016 to 2019, the proportion of U.S. children experiencing underinsurance rose from 30.6% to 34.0%, representing an additional 2.4 million children (Yu et al., 2022). Many families with commercial insurance face high out-of-pocket costs for health care. In fact, underinsurance is particularly notable among commercially insured children (Daw et al., 2023), likely because of the more limited benefits and higher copayments and premium costs than in Medicaid. In 2021, 33.0% of commercially insured children reported inadequate coverage (i.e., experiencing gaps in benefit adequacy, provider access, or out-of-pocket costs), compared with 12.2% of publicly insured children (Daw et al., 2023).

The risk of underinsurance also depends on children's health status (Kogan et al., 2010; Perrin, Kenney, & Rosenbaum, 2020; Yu et al., 2022). Children with disabling conditions or special health care needs face greater underinsurance challenges than other children (40% vs. 30.8%; Validova et al., 2023). Children in these groups represent 13.3%, or 9.7 million children, according to the NSCH (Census Bureau, 2024).[18] Another group at risk of underinsurance is children in families with middle incomes, meaning

[18]The category of "children with chronic conditions" is defined as those experiencing one or more of the following health consequences: (1) elevated need or use of medical services; (2) limitations in day-to-day activities; (3) need or use of specialized therapies (e.g., physical and occupational therapy); and/or (4) need or use of treatment of an emotional, behavioral, or developmental condition (as defined in Bethell et al., 2015).

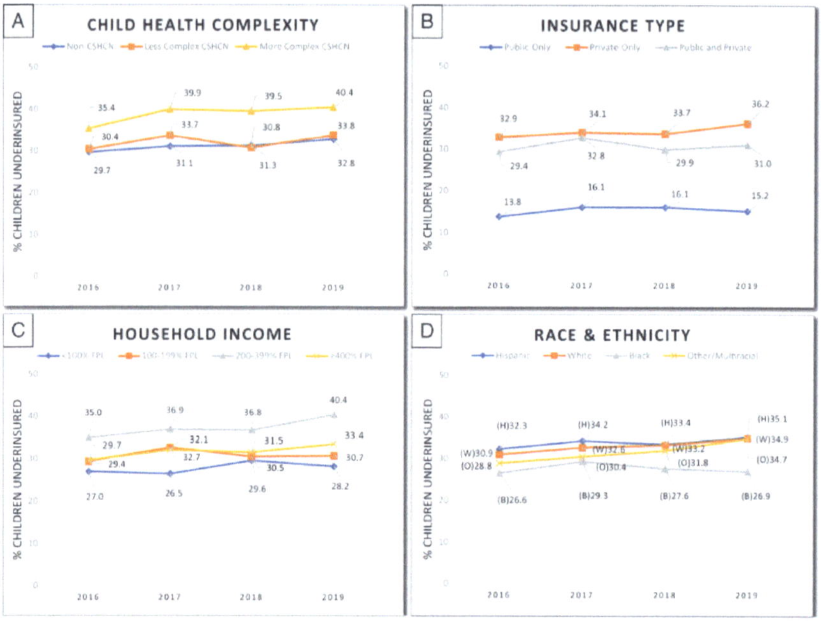

FIGURE 6-10 Percentage of children underinsured by demographic characteristics.
NOTE: CSHCN = children with special health care needs; FPL = federal poverty level.
SOURCE: Yu et al., 2022.

households earning 200%–399% FPL (36.7% are underinsured). The concentration of underinsurance among middle-income families underscores how commercial insurance can leave families vulnerable to financial insecurity (see Figure 6-10).

Variations in Medicaid and CHIP Policies in U.S. Territories

Although not often included in conversations about health care system and policy changes, approximately 3.5 million individuals live in the territories of the United States. All five territories offer both Medicaid and CHIP, and the percentage of their populations covered by Medicaid/CHIP varies widely based on different policies and social conditions within the territories. However, "under the Social Security Act (the Act) the territories are considered states for the purposes of Medicaid and CHIP, unless otherwise indicated (§ 1101(a)(1) of the Act)" (MACPAC, 2021b, p. 1). Two of the five territories, American Samoa and the Commonwealth of the Northern Mariana Islands (CNMI), utilize a Section 1902 waiver uniquely available to them that "allows the Secretary of the U.S. Department of Health and Human Services to waive or modify any Medicaid requirement except for the statutory annual limit on federal Medicaid funding, the federal medical assistance percentage (FMAP), and the requirement that payment can only be for services otherwise coverable by Medicaid" (MACPAC, 2021b, p. 1). As a result, these two territories are not required to provide all of Medicaid's mandatory benefits; the other territories must follow the same Medicaid rules as states.

The percentage enrolled in Medicaid or CHIP in U.S. territories was highest in American Samoa, at 68.4%, and lowest in Guam, at 21.2%, as of June 2019 (MACPAC, 2021b)—in spite of the fact that the rate of poverty has historically been higher among communities in the territories than in the states (Hall, Rudowitz, & Gifford, 2019). Financing plays a significant factor in this variability, as although individuals born in the U.S. territories are citizens or considered U.S. nationals, their public programs are financially differently from the programs in the 50 states and Washington, DC (Hall, Rudowitz, & Gifford, 2019). Annual Medicaid funding for the territories has been fixed in statute with a cap on the FMAP, whereas funding for the 50 states and DC is uncapped and adjusted annually based on state per capita income. The FMAP for territories was increased from 50% to 55% with the passage of the ACA in 2014 (along with a higher FMAP for nondisabled adults without children); the 2023 Consolidated Appropriations Act increased the FMAP to 83% for American Samoa, CNMI, Guam, and the U.S. Virgin Islands (USVI), and extended Puerto Rico's FMAP of 76% for 5 years. However, because of a block grant or capped funding, territories still have less Medicaid funding per capita than states with comparable or lower per capita incomes. Once a territory has spent all of its funds, unless it received temporary relief funding, it no longer receives federal matched funding for the remainder of the fiscal year. This impacts decisions around who is offered coverage; notably, three territories—Guam, Puerto Rico, and USVI—are "statutorily exempt from providing Medicaid coverage to certain mandatory coverage groups including poverty-related children and pregnant women" (MACPAC, 2021b, p. 1). This also impacts the availability of certain services, as not all territories are required to offer mandatory Medicaid benefits, such as nonemergency medical transportation. Additionally, recent natural disasters, due in part to human-driven climate change, have significantly impacted the territories' ability to meet the health care needs of Medicaid and CHIP members because of destruction of facilities and erosion of the health care workforce (Michaud & Kates, 2017; Seervai, 2017; Velázquez, 2022). So while all territories offer the EPSDT benefit; prescription drugs; and clinic, dental, and eye services, they have also seen increased costs, as members must increasingly seek their care off island.

Access to Providers in Networks

Access concerns for children and youth covered by Medicaid include whether a given MCO offers an adequate provider network. The state's MCO contract provides a vehicle for establishing provider adequacy and related provisions (SSA, n.d.), but federal and state monitoring of pediatric network adequacy has been limited. Although CMS access rules require states to document adequate network and service access, reporting is left to the states, which mainly need to affirm satisfactory or adequate access.

Importantly, as discussed in previous chapters, subspecialty network needs are very different for children than for adults. Most childhood chronic conditions are rare, while adults experience relatively high rates of common chronic conditions. Thus, knowledgeable pediatric subspecialists are far less common than for adults. MCOs typically develop "narrow" networks for adult care as one way to curb costs. However, while children needing subspecialty care require a larger network geographically to ensure access (e.g., to a specialized pediatric cardiologist), few MCOs offer different networks for specific populations.

Adequacy requirements are measured in several ways—for example, time–distance requirements relative to beneficiary locations, provider-to-beneficiary ratios, appointment wait times, and geographic comparisons (Lipson et al., 2017). These requirements may vary by service specialty or apply differentially to urban and rural areas, although states typically do not call out specific network adequacy for younger populations (Cuellar, 2022). Recent federal regulations call for improving access in several ways. First, they require assessing and improving wait times for three areas: primary care, maternity care, and outpatient mental/behavioral health care. They require improvements in provider directories and their accessibility to enrollees, including secret shopper strategies to assess access. These approaches also address network adequacy (whether beneficiaries have similar access to services as others in the community), although these requirements do not address different needs for network capacity for children compared with adults.

The new rules also call for transparency in payment rates in the three areas and comparison with prevailing Medicare rates for the same services. New rules also address access to home- and community-based services, as well as states' use of directed payments through their MCOs. Finally, the rules clarify and expand opportunities to use nontraditional services that can improve health ("in lieu of service and setting" rule; e.g., certain allowable housing and nutritional supports that are medically appropriate and cost effective; CMS, 2024a,b; Georgetown University Center for Children and Families, 2024; Whitener, 2024).

Access to Mental Health Providers

Many children and adolescents face challenges locating a provider willing to treat them, even when they have insurance. This is a particularly acute problem in mental health care as illustrated in a recent secret shopper study (King et al., 2024). Secret shopper studies seek to capture the experiences of families seeking treatment, in this case for an adolescent with substance use disorder. The focal child in the study case was uninsured but likely eligible for Medicaid. Notably, using a variety of search engines and listings, the study identified only 160 residential treatment centers across the United States that, when called, would accept a patient under age 18 who had a recent nonfatal fentanyl overdose. In 10 states researchers found no residential treatment center for adolescents. Furthermore, the findings related to access by Medicaid versus self-pay are striking. Fifty-seven percent (57%) of facilities called accepted Medicaid, but in 23 states researchers were not able to identify any adolescent residential treatment centers that accepted Medicaid. What is more, most centers accepting Medicaid had waitlists (57% of all facilities that accepted Medicaid reported a waitlist, compared with 19% of facilities that did not accept Medicaid; King et al., 2024).

Access problems in mental health are not limited to residential care; and they are not limited to Medicaid. Similar secret shopper studies found that pregnant women were more likely to face challenges when seeking care for substance use treatment than nonpregnant women and that many behavioral health providers accepted only cash and no insurance (Patrick et al., 2020). Moreover, over one-third of patients with Medicaid or commercial insurance were unable to make appointments (Patrick et al., 2020). For pregnant women, the provider access challenges were not statistically significant between Medicaid or commercial insurance, pointing to systemic problems in behavioral health care beyond the bounds of insurance. Other studies support the widespread nature of this problem. The percentage of psychiatrists accepting commercial insurance declined over time from 70.7% in 2007–2008 to 59.6% in 2015–2016 (Carlo et al., 2024), while Medicare participation among psychiatrists also declined from 68.0% to 62.7%. In contrast, commercial insurance acceptance by nonphysician mental health specialists remained at 88.0% over time. Medicaid acceptance rates are lower than other types of coverage (46.8% for psychiatrists and 77.5% for nonpsychiatrists in 2015–2016), with no statistically significant change since 2007–2008 (Carlo et al., 2024). Medicaid expansion for adults, despite the large reduction in uninsured rates, has not increased Medicaid acceptance among psychiatrists or nonpsychiatrists (Carlo et al., 2024; Wen et al., 2019).

NEW PROVIDER PAYMENT MODELS TO TRANSFORM INSURANCE PAYMENT FOR CHILDREN'S HEALTH CARE

As discussed, traditional payments to providers use a fee-for-service arrangement, with providers rewarded when they increase the volume of care, all else equal, even when such care is of marginal value. While this model is administratively straightforward and promotes access to care, it also incentivizes more health care utilization, which can lead to unnecessary treatment and higher costs that are not associated with improvement in the health of the population. Fee-for-service payments rarely and inconsistently cover many services that children and families need, such as coordination of care, school liaisons, and community connections, although some payers have included some of these services. Adding services to current fee systems requires substantial effort, usually involving the American Medical Association's (n.d.) Relative Value Scale Update Committee (RUC), followed by CMS approval. The structure and constraints of the RUC value surgical procedures and interventions over many cognitive services, a major barrier to reforming fee-for-service payments. Some have called for a specific pediatric RUC as a strategy for adapting fee-for-service models for pediatric contexts (Committee on Coding and Nomenclature et al., 2014).

The limitations of the fee-for-service model have led to interest in alternative payment models. Most of the efforts to change payment arrangements have come from programs for adults, where overall costs are higher than for populations under age 20. The driving goals of alternative payment for older populations have been to increase quality and patient satisfaction with care and to lower costs. Variations in spending in different areas of the country without obvious health benefits have also motivated the search for more cost-effective ways of paying for care (Bronner & Skinner, 2022).

CMS (2021c, 2022b), through the Center for Medicare and Medicaid Innovation (CMMI), has stimulated a number of alternative payment models, mostly under Medicare, with variable results in cost savings and quality improvement (CMS, 2022a, 2024d,j). The alternative models range from fixed, per-patient payments for primary care physicians, to service- or disease-specific bundles, to payments to larger health care systems via accountable care organization (ACO) payments. Narrower alternative payment models that focused on reducing acute or specialty care or that targeted specific populations were more likely to show favorable savings and utilization results than broader models.

The appeal of the various payment designs is that they seek either to tie payment to outcomes or to control spending relative to fee-for-service payment, or both; but the potential returns for children and youth differ substantially from those for older populations. ACO models for Medicare beneficiaries have generated savings relative to annual benchmarks from reductions in postacute care, inpatient care, tests, and imaging; however, child health care has fewer opportunities for such savings (Medicare Payment Advisory Commission, 2018). The total health care expenditures for children and youth are lower than for adults, and their use of expensive treatments and hospitalizations is lower as well, which limits the potential, short-run financial return on investment to ACOs and to payers.

Medicaid programs in 12 states have implemented ACO payment programs under which coordinated groups of health care providers come together to improve quality of care, patient experience, and efficiency of care delivery over a defined, broad population of beneficiaries (KFF, 2023d). Six states include both children and adults in their ACO programs, and three of these six contract with child-only ACOs, meaning ACOs that have children's hospitals and pediatric providers (Center for Health Care Strategies, 2022). In addition, in Ohio, three exclusively pediatric Medicaid ACOs sponsored by children's hospitals now contract with the state's MCOs for regional Medicaid pediatric care (see Chapter 9 for an illustration of innovations under way in Ohio). In some states, ACOs have formed specifically for subpopulations of children covered by Medicaid, such as children in foster care (e.g., Texas) (Perrin et al., 2017). While early conceptualizations of ACOs occurred in the Medicare program for adult populations, the Medicaid program has more flexible rules regarding their design and implementation. For example, Medicaid states can mandate coverage through an ACO, as is the case in Oregon (Oregon Health Authority, 2023).

A recent review summarized 32 studies of Medicaid ACOs, 10 of which evaluated outcomes for infants, children, or maternal health and the majority of which focused on Oregon, Minnesota, and Ohio (Holm, Pagán, & Silver, 2024). Findings on quality, utilization, and costs were mixed. Results across studies suggest improved primary care and well-child care for children, improved prenatal care, reduced readmissions after childbirth, mixed evidence with respect to infant and maternal morbidity, and evidence of lower costs for some services. However, the substantial variability of the populations analyzed and differences in implementation made identifying elements associated with success difficult (Holm, Pagán, & Silver, 2024).

Beyond Medicaid ACOs for children, CMMI launched demonstrations of the Integrated Care for Kids (InCK) model in seven locations across the country, seeking to promote comprehensive, multidisciplinary, team-based care for children that coordinates with multiple service sectors (Alley, Ashford, & Gavin, 2019; CMS, n.d.e), improves child health, and reduces hospitalizations and out-of-home placements (Jones & Lucienne, 2023). The InCK model also emphasizes health-related social needs and locally designed delivery models that seek to coordinate care across health care and other child services. including early childhood care, education, food, housing, Title V, child welfare, and mobile crisis response (CMS, 2024f).

Furthermore, the demonstrations were charged with implementing at least some form of alternative payment model, either broad or focused. For example, in North Carolina's InCK, MCOs give incentives to integrated networks of providers based on standard measures such as depression screening and emergency department visits, and also on measures such as promotion of kindergarten readiness and screening for housing and food insecurity (but not outcomes from other sectors; CMS, 2024e; James et al., 2023).

A major challenge to applying adult-designed alternative payment models, such as ACOs, to children is that adult models have a relatively narrow focus on changing delivery of physician and hospital services, improving quality and patient experience in these domains, and recovering savings from the health care system. By comparison, better child health can lead to improved education and employment outcomes for children, as well as savings to special education and criminal justice sectors (Flanagan, Tigue, & Perrin, 2019). As this report reiterates, health and wellbeing in early life help establish a positive life course trajectory. Currently, neither fee-for-service arrangements nor alternative payment models provide incentives to achieve improvement in these longer-term outcomes. This represents an opportunity to design and evaluate different payment approaches to shape health care to meet the needs of children and youth.

Several considerations are important when designing alternative payment models for children (Perrin et al., 2017). One is an ex ante, actuarial exercise to understand how much spending falls on primary care, specialty physician care, hospital care, nonhospital facility care, medication, and other services. This includes, for example, assessing the average level of per-person spending, determining the variation in spending that creates financial risk, and further assessing spending by population or patient condition. Alternative payment rates are generally based on historical overall fee-for-service payment levels, meaning that they may not lead to higher revenues for providers where access challenges are greatest. Another design element are the ex post economic incentives, which are created once a payment scheme is in place. For instance, payers generally engage in greater monitoring of overutilization under a fee-for-service payment model, but the focus would shift to greater monitoring of underutilization with payment schemes that have more financial risk and incentivize providing less care. A recent National Academies report calls for partial capitation payments for primary care, providing flexibility to achieve the report's goals including whole person care and team-based care, while maintaining fee-for-service incentives for specific desired services (National Academies, 2021b). The recent Massachusetts 1115 Medicaid waiver implements a similar partial capitation approach, also incentivizing certain specific services (Brykman, Houston, & Bailey, 2021). Capitation covers most services (with an effort to adjust risk for more complex patients), along with additions to the capitation rates for including various practice enhancements, such as integrated mental and behavioral health staff, community health workers, or school liaison personnel. Such models may provide guidance for new payment arrangements for child health care.

Other design elements to weigh for child populations are whether to separate adult and child populations entirely (Brykman, Houston, & Bailey, 2021), how to incorporate existing school-based or other clinical services in the community (CMS, 2024b) to avoid incentives to shift costs, and how to leverage existing population screening that is performed, for example, in schools around food insecurity and school lunch programs. Furthermore, in order to anticipate the likelihood of desired and undesired behaviors, models also need to assess nonhealth outcome measures carefully, both from an ex ante, actuarial perspective, which would tally costs across sectors, and from an ex post economic perspective, including whether the providers in question have meaningful control over the outcome (Counts, Mistry, & Wong, 2021a). Holding health care providers financially accountable for home visiting to promote early attachment or medical screening to promote school readiness have very different implications from holding health care systems financially accountable for grade-appropriate reading levels or high school graduation rates, which are primarily under the control of the education system. Novel models could test combinations of alternative payment to providers and simultaneous investment in community prevention—for example, around school-based mental health or physical activity—to see which approaches generate the greatest improvements in child health.

A further payment model design consideration is which population subgroups are more likely to be treated (or undertreated) under one scheme versus another. For example, schemes that reward better health outcomes may incentivize providers to focus on those subgroups that are most likely to succeed, all else equal—typically those who are healthier or face fewer social disadvantages. Payers resort to adjusting payments for this risk, although most risk adjusters so far do not work well for younger populations, other than the small number of children with quite severe conditions (National Academies, 2016a).

Transformation from fee-for-service to health outcome–based payment is complex (Farmer et al., 2016; Tieder et al., 2018). Population-management payment models may need fairly long time windows to succeed, to allow for investments in care coordination, team staffing, information technology, and data analytics to ultimately achieve improvements in health and other outcomes (CMS, 2021c; Perrin et al., 2017). Such changes place significant demands on providers and require a level of technical sophistication and investment that many providers currently lack.

Adjusting payments for social needs also requires careful consideration, as shown for adults. In a recent Medicare study, researchers found that populations with higher social needs had similar or lower spending after adjusting for health risk, compared with populations with lower social risk. This finding suggests forgone care for higher-risk patients and that adjusting for social risk in this manner would increase, not reduce, disparities (McWilliams et al., 2023). Oregon and Washington have experimented with improving social risk assessment for children. Massachusetts, recognizing the perverse incentives of allocating more resources to higher users, has also worked to pay for care needed rather than basing pay on previous utilization (Alcusky et al., 2023; Ash & Ellis, 2012; Dyer et al., 2023).

While alternative payment models may hold some promise over fee-for-service models for improving the health of children, fundamental challenges associated with their design and implementation must be recognized and potential solutions for addressing them must be developed and tested. These considerations include the longer-term nature of potential cost savings for children in the case of alternative payment models (vs. shorter-term cost savings for adults from reduced health care spending), the optimal design of payment rates, decisions about what children's health outcomes to measure and prioritize, the need for strategies that avoid inadvertently incentivizing a narrow focus on youth populations whose health status may more amenable to improvement, consideration of social risk adjustment, and ensuring providers are able to manage technical aspects of implementation.

CONCLUSION

Children's health insurance coverage comes from a mix of commercial, employer-sponsored, and public health insurance through Medicaid and CHIP, which cover a large majority of children, along with a few other sources. Current health insurance coverage for children is high—around 95% have some insurance, although major periodic fluctuations in Medicaid and CHIP can change coverage levels significantly, as seen in the recent loss of coverage by millions of children with the unwinding at the end of the pandemic public health emergency.

During the pandemic, Medicaid and CHIP alone provided coverage for about half of all U.S. children and youth—a higher percentage for any age group dependent on public health insurance, other than populations over age 65 with Medicare coverage. Medicare and Medicaid/CHIP have very different administrative structures. Medicare is fully funded by the federal government and administered nationally. Medicaid and CHIP, in contrast, have joint federal and state funding (although the federal government provides at least 50% of each state's Medicaid costs), and the states administer the programs under federal guidelines and requirements.

Key Medicaid strengths include that it is an entitlement—i.e., any eligible person applying must be included. Furthermore, Medicaid has no copays or premiums and has a statutory benefit for children and youth up to age 21—the EPSDT program that guarantees access to medically necessary services that children need, even if that service is not usually included in the state's allowed services. CHIP programs, however, need not follow the same requirements as Medicaid.

Public insurance through these programs follows a complex series of rules and options that can help or hinder access to needed pediatric services. Opportunities exist to standardize key characteristics across states, including eligibility, enrollment, scope of services, payment, and quality. The poor state of health of U.S. children and youth and the lasting impact of child health on adult morbidity and mortality (see Chapter 4) threaten the readiness of the nation's military and workforce and, in turn, economic stability. These findings support the need for Medicaid and CHIP reform to eliminate inequities in access to care and improve care and outcomes for all children and the adults they will become. Reform will require decreasing state variation in program policy and administration, strengthening the critical EPSDT program, and ensuring adequate payment for services.

Many states have carried out innovative strategies for improving their programs, providing some guidance for payment reform and the changes recommended by the committee. However, many current payment reform efforts have ignored younger populations and have incentives that are better directed to older patients. There is a critical need for experimentation and analysis of new strategies for improving payment for children's health care.

7

Investing in Child Health through Population- and Community-Level Primary Prevention

Finding resources is an ongoing struggle for our families. It is impossible for parents to focus on the [health] struggles that their children are having if they are first unable to meet their basic needs. Mental health care, access to enough food, and transportation are all huge factors which can affect follow-through and compliance.

—Comment to committee from registered nurse in Iowa

The previous chapter discussed the role of health insurance and financing for clinical services. This chapter examines noninsurance financing toward public health and its influences on children's health and wellbeing. "Public health" has been variously defined but is commonly thought of as the science and pursuit of promoting and protecting the health of all people and their communities. This definition makes clear two important dimensions of public health—its focus on (primary) *prevention* and its focus on the health of a *population* (Wiley, 2016). As described in Chapter 6, primary prevention can be clinically based, occur through the traditional health care system, and be delivered to patients one-on-one; but more often, primary prevention efforts are community or population based (Institute of Medicine [IOM], 2010) and thus fall under the public health umbrella. Importantly, although some associate the term "public health" with a narrow focus on governmental efforts, public health encompasses a diverse group of public and private collaborators and includes the health care delivery system (IOM, 2012b). Diez Roux (2016) emphasized that the relevant definition of "public" in the term "public health" is "of or concerning the people as a whole" (p. 620).

Across the spectrum of health care, primary prevention is especially salient for children. By definition, disease prevention must occur *before* its onset, and childhood represents a time before the onset of most chronic conditions. Moreover, and as emphasized in previous chapters, health can be viewed as a cumulative process in which outcomes in one period affect outcomes in future periods. As such, childhood presents a critical window for influencing health outcomes over an individual's entire life course, and primary prevention during childhood offers a unique opportunity for minimizing the future burden of disease. Expanding on the notion of primary prevention as a form of insurance (Newhouse, 2021), new spending on public health efforts for children can be seen as a form of insurance for the nation against high future health care and non–health care costs attributable to preventable conditions.

What is more, primary prevention plays an important role in connecting people with community resources (e.g., social services, nutrition assistance programs) and is recognized as a prominent lever for reducing health disparities and achieving health equity. Thus, primary prevention activities represent an important element of the full spectrum of health care that children receive, and they are critical to children's health care system transformation (see Figure 7-1).

The committee's aim in this chapter is to describe the contours of public health spending relevant to children. While social determinants of health are

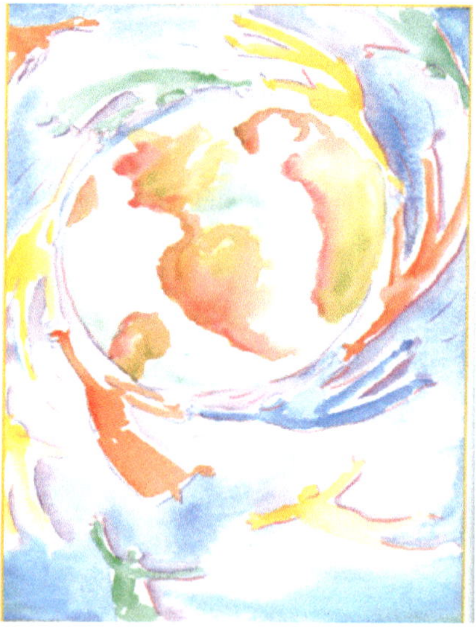

FIGURE 7-1 Connecting people, achieving health equity.
SOURCE: José Luis Bayer, Chile; © Peace Child International, used with permission.

part of the public health perspective (such as spending to reduce poverty or improve housing), this discussion is limited to public health spending that is primarily health care related, in alignment with this report's focus.

PUBLIC HEALTH

As in earlier reports (IOM, 1998, 2003a, 2012a,b,c), the committee's conception of public health is broad, involving organized community efforts aimed at preventing poor health and disease at the population level. Providing essential public health services, such as those in Box 7-1, requires interaction among government health agencies, the health care system, the private sector, community organizations, and other public–private partnerships. The work of public health has evolved to address changing societal needs. Traditionally, public health has engaged systems and policy to mitigate infectious disease and unsafe conditions (IOM, 2012c). Among others, important programs for children, youth, and families have increased the availability of vaccines, developed standards for safer foods and water, prevented childhood lead poisoning, and lessened tobacco use. Given the complex nature of health challenges in the United States today, public

BOX 7-1
Essential Public Health Services

1. Assess and monitor population health status, factors that influence health, and community needs and assets
2. Investigate, diagnose, and address health problems and hazards affecting the population
3. Communicate effectively to inform and educate people about health, factors that influence it, and how to improve it
4. Strengthen, support, and mobilize communities and partnerships to improve health
5. Create, champion, and implement policies, plans, and laws that impact health
6. Utilize legal and regulatory actions designed to improve and protect the public's health
7. Enable equitable access to the individual services and care needed to be healthy
8. Build and support a diverse and skilled public health workforce
9. Improve and innovate public health functions through ongoing evaluation, research, and continuous quality improvement
10. Build and maintain a strong organizational infrastructure for public health

SOURCE: de Beaumont Foundation and Public Health National Center for Innovations, 2024. https://debeaumont.org/10-essential-services/

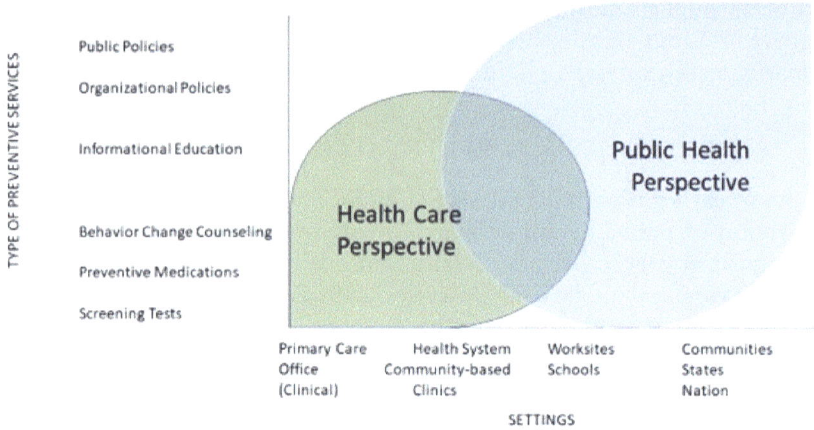

FIGURE 7-2 Public health and health care system integration.
SOURCE: Adapted from Rechel (2020) and Community Preventive Services Task Force.

health is core to fighting chronic conditions and health disparities that often have roots in childhood experiences.

Public health and health care each bring significant assets to partnerships that may improve child health outcomes. Figure 7-2 illustrates the integration of services and settings as public health and health care collaborate on primary prevention. Early experiences in several cities suggest public health–health care collaborations enhance chronic disease care, preventive service delivery, and maternal–child health. Reviews of such collaborations indicate that delineating shared goals, data structure and sharing rules, and resource constraints, as well as asset mapping, are important steps (Martin-Misener et al., 2012; McVicar et al., 2019). The goals of public health–health care collaborations require articulation and careful measurement (see Chapter 9).

A variety of models of collaboration have been developed and have evolved over time. Beginning with individual partnership models used by specific practices or groups of health care practices and public health staff, some models[1] evolved into regional networks around topic areas or disease conditions. A desired final phase of such models is an ecosystem model, whereby all the partners in both public health and health care share integrated communications, data, and performance evaluation. Since many networks studied were still in early phases of development, few networks have been observed to reach the most mature stages. Developing these models and spreading them to new sites with a greater focus on children

[1]See Derr (2023) for a history of public health community collaboration.

will require more resources (see further discussion at end of the chapter). Given that child health and primary prevention efforts include significant community components, without public health partnerships, they are not likely to improve significantly.

Important Public Health Programs for Children

This section highlights effective public health strategies, interventions, and policies that have historically and continuously benefited young people across the nation. From preventive measures to community-based programs and nationwide policies, these initiatives have had a tangible, positive impact on the lives of millions of American children and families. The selected issues below focus on improved outcomes for children across the United States. It is important to note that public policies (such as decisions that affect community environment and housing options) can have indirect negative consequences on children's health. It was beyond the scope of the committee's work to examine these.

Maternal and Infant Health

Increased attention to maternal and infant health has led to heightened efforts and resources aimed at enhancing health outcomes and reducing disparities (Hill, Artiga, & Ranji, 2022; Koppaka, 2011a; Lassi, Kumar, & Bhutta, 2016). Programs administered through the Health Resources and Services Administration (HRSA), discussed in greater depth below, provide public health leadership and financial support for maternal and child health programs nationwide. These programs focus on improving access to prenatal care and promoting healthy behaviors during pregnancy. Additional efforts—such as the Pregnancy Risk Assessment Monitoring System and the Collaborative Improvement and Innovation Network, breastfeeding support programs, and safe sleep campaigns—are meaningful strategies for identifying and combatting infant mortality risks (Centers for Disease Control and Prevention [CDC], 2013; Mehta et al., 2021).

Vaccine-Preventable Diseases

Childhood immunizations, and vaccines generally, are a notable public health success (Amanna & Slifka, 2020; CDC, 1999; Koppaka, 2011a,b). Instances of individuals suffering from preventable infectious diseases, such as measles, diphtheria, and whooping cough, have reached historic lows (CDC, n.d.a, 2020b, 2024i,n). From 2000 to 2010 alone, an estimated 2.5 million deaths were prevented yearly among children under age 5 years using measles, polio, and diphtheria-tetanus-pertussis vaccines (Koppaka, 2011a).

Several public health initiatives have contributed to increased rates of childhood immunization, helping to protect children from vaccine-preventable diseases. The Vaccines for Children (VFC) program, discussed further below, is supported through CDC's (2024a,j,q) National Center for Respiratory Diseases. National immunization awareness campaigns and community outreach efforts at the national, state, and local levels educate parents, caregivers, and health care providers about the importance of childhood vaccinations and provide information on vaccine safety and efficacy, recommended immunization schedules, and the benefits of vaccination in preventing serious illness (CDC, 2019a, 2024a; Kaufman et al., 2018; National Vaccine Advisory Committee, 2013).

While childhood vaccines have saved lives and money, vaccine hesitancy remains a persistent concern for population health (Nuwarda et al., 2022). School immunization requirements, which are implemented at the state level, mandate that children receive certain vaccines before enrolling in schools and child care facilities (Seither et al., 2023a,b). These requirements help ensure high vaccination coverage rates among school-aged children. However, a recent CDC report that used data from the 2021–2022 school year revealed that while rates of unvaccinated and undervaccinated children remain low, the share of U.S. kindergartners receiving state-required vaccines continues to decrease (Seither et al., 2023a,b). As discussed in Chapter 3, it is important to underscore the value of trust in information about vaccines from public health officials and health care providers (Funk et al., 2023).

Fluoridation of Water

Community water fluoridation programs have been implemented across the United States since the mid-20th century (Armfield, 2010; Department of Health and Human Services Federal Panel on Community Water Fluoridation, 2015). Fluoride is added to public water supplies at optimal levels to prevent tooth decay. This public health measure has been shown to benefit children and families by reducing the prevalence of dental caries (also known as cavities), promoting oral health, and improving overall wellbeing (Boehmer et al., 2023).

Tobacco Control

Tobacco use affects child health in various ways, including prenatal exposure to smoke, secondhand smoke, and smokeless tobacco products (Gould et al., 2020; Jenssen et al., 2023). Prenatal exposure can result in birth defects, preterm birth, growth restriction, and stillbirth. Postnatally, secondhand smoke exposure increases the risk of neonatal and infant death, respiratory infections, meningococcal disease, and asthma attacks (Been & Sheikh, 2018). Children and adolescents who use various tobacco products face an elevated risk of nicotine dependence and are more prone to continued tobacco use into adulthood. Since the release of the first Surgeon General's Report on tobacco in 1964, evidence-based policies and interventions at federal, state, and local levels have reduced tobacco use substantially for people of all ages (Been & Sheikh, 2018; Koppaka, 2011a). Some key initiatives include the regulation of tobacco sales to people under a certain age; tobacco taxes, which are particularly effective for reducing tobacco use among youth; tobacco advertising restrictions, which reduce children's exposure to pro-tobacco messages; and smoke-free policies, which protect nonsmokers from secondhand smoke exposure and contribute to social norms around smoking (Cruz et al., 2019; Jenssen et al., 2023).

Youth tobacco prevention programs and educational campaigns targeted at children and adolescents often use school-based interventions, community outreach, and media campaigns to deliver anti-tobacco messages and promote healthy behaviors (Flay, 2009; Jenssen et al., 2023). However, continued efforts and vigilance are necessary to address remaining challenges and prevent tobacco use initiation among youth. Youth use of e-cigarettes, vapes, and other electronic devices that contain nicotine has increased significantly over the past decade (Birdsey et al., 2023; Jones & Salzman, 2020). While regulations and flavor bans by the Food and Drug Administration have helped to restrict the sale of flavored vaping products (Li et al., 2022a), the evolving landscape of electronic smoking products and marketing tactics necessitates continued vigilance and adaptation of strategies for protecting children and adolescents from the harms of vaping.

Motor-Vehicle Safety

Like tobacco reduction, improved motor-vehicle safety is another public health effort that began in the 1960s and has resulted in significant improvements for children (CDC, 1999). Government and community recognition of the need for motor-vehicle safety prompted the initiation of programs by federal and state governments, academic institutions, community-based organizations, and private organizations. Public health initiatives aimed at improving motor-vehicle safety for children in the United States are driven by a multifaceted approach.

First, child-passenger safety laws have been established in most states (Insurance Institute for Highway Safety [IIHS], 2024). These laws mandate the use of appropriate child safety seats, booster seats, or seat belts (based on age, weight, and height), thereby increasing compliance and reducing the risk of injuries or fatalities in crashes (Bae et al., 2014; Eichelberger, Chouinard, & Jermakian, 2012; Mannix et al., 2012; Zaza et al., 2001). Currently, 49 states and the District of Columbia have implemented seat belt laws for adults, while all 50 states and the District of Columbia have enacted legislation safeguarding children in vehicles (IIHS, 2024; Koppaka, 2011a). Moreover, public health agencies advocate for legislation and improved safety standards, working alongside policy makers and industry stakeholders to promote advancements in technology and vehicle design (Fleetwood, 2017; Pollack Porter, Rutkow, & McGinty, 2018).

Education and outreach programs further raise awareness among parents and caregivers about the importance of proper restraint usage, providing guidance on installation and highlighting potential consequences of misuse (Britton et al., 2023; Penmetsa, Wang, & Nambisan, 2017; Sartin et al., 2019). Child safety seat inspection stations and other related programs, often established through public–private collaborations, offer hands-on assistance to ensure correct installation and enhance the effectiveness of restraints (O'Neil et al., 2013; Ostergaard & Guzzetta, 2021; Tessier, 2010).

Additionally, graduated driver licensing policies for teen drivers have contributed to a decrease in the number of teenage crash fatalities (Baker, Chen, & Li, 2007).

Finally, community partnerships and collaborations facilitate the dissemination of information and implementation of targeted interventions, leveraging existing networks to reach a broader audience and enhance motor-vehicle safety for children (Buttazzoni et al., 2024; Ehiri et al., 2006; Turner et al., 2005).

Government Public Health Departments

State and local health departments are critical nodes in the funding of public health programs for children, drawing not only on federal resources but also, to a variable extent across states, on revenue generated by user fines and fees as well as state government funds (including, e.g., from state cigarette taxes; IOM, 2012b,c). To provide services to communities, local health departments also rely on contributions and collaborations with businesses, media, schools, policy makers, and health care systems in the community.

Funding for public health has declined significantly across all federal, state, and local levels in the past two to three decades, compared with spending on direct health care services. While estimates of national public health spending vary, they consistently reveal underinvestment (IOM, 2012b,c). Available estimates put spending on public health activities at less than 5% of the nation's health-related spending (Farberman & Kelley, 2020; Himmelstein & Woolhandler, 2016). DeSalvo and colleagues (2019) estimate that the national investment in public health is $19/person, which leaves a $13/person gap in annual spending necessary to achieve core public health capabilities associated with the Foundational Public Health Services model.[2] As such, activities to promote population health

[2]The Foundational Public Health Services model defines a minimum set of public health capabilities and programs for communities (see https://phaboard.org/center-for-innovation/public-health-frameworks/the-foundational-public-health-services).

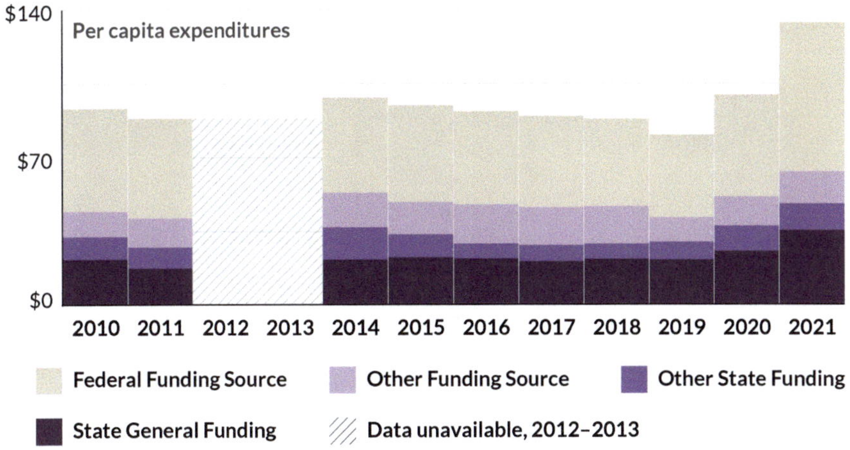

FIGURE 7-3 Amount of public health expenditures by funding source.
NOTE: Expenditures are shown by fiscal year, which is defined in the Profile Survey as July through June (e.g., Fiscal Year 2021 was from July 1, 2020 – June 30, 2021).
SOURCE: ASTHO, 2023.

and prepare for and prevent emergencies that impact the wellbeing of communities have been challenged by a shrinking workforce and insufficient funding to fulfill mission (Association of State and Tribal Health Officials [ASTHO], 2023).

States provide about 28% of overall state health department revenues and 21% of local health department revenues on average. Federal funds cover the rest of state and local health department activities (McKillop, Farberman, & Lieberman, 2023; see Figure 7-3). In fiscal year (FY) 2021, federal sources predominantly funded state health agency WIC services,[3] chronic and infectious disease initiatives, and hazard preparedness and response. The expenditure categories of injury prevention, environmental health, administrative functions, and quality of services were largely funded by state sources (ASTHO, 2023).

Over the past 10 years, the average and per capita expenditures for public health agencies have varied; most are relatively stable, although considerable variations exist across states and communities. In FY 2021, public health spending increased significantly to respond directly to the COVID-19 pandemic. Spending to address the emergency represented approximately one-third of 2021 total state public health agency expenditures (ASTHO, 2023; see Figure 7-4). Of those expenditures not related to COVID-19, about 15% went toward clinical services and consumer care and 11% supported

[3]WIC stands for Special Supplemental Nutrition Program for Women, Infants, and Children.

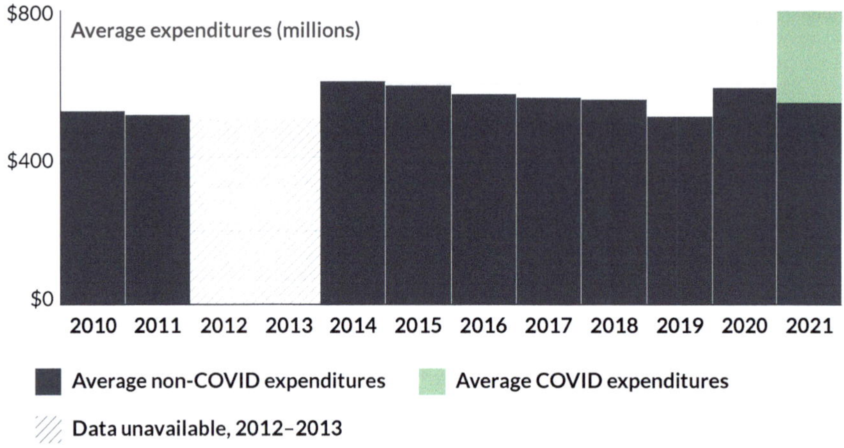

FIGURE 7-4 Average raw and per capita public health expenditures for state public health agencies, 2010–2021.
NOTES: The number of reporting agencies varies each year and by funding source. Expenditures are shown by fiscal year, which is defined in the Profile Survey as July through June (e.g., Fiscal Year 2021 was from July 1, 2020–June 30, 2021).
SOURCE: ASTHO, 2023.

WIC programs. The extra investment during the emergency has not been sustained despite the importance of prevention to child health (Martin et al., 2021, 2023; Trust for America's Health, 2023). One ongoing challenge is that federal funding for state and local public health efforts is often allocated by disease category and is thus compartmentalized, leaving little flexibility for responsiveness to local priorities or for cross-cutting capabilities (IOM, 2012b). It is noteworthy, however, that efforts to convert categorical grants into more flexible funding have been found to result in decreased funding (based on theoretical program administration cost savings and flexible funds that risk being diverted to unrelated priorities (Leider et al., 2018).

FEDERAL PROGRAMS FOR MEETING COMMUNITY NEEDS

Federal spending on children includes tax provisions and other income supports, as well as funding for direct provision of health care services and spending on social services such as nutrition, education, child care, and housing (see Figure 7-5). About half of this spending is universal, and the other half targets families with lower incomes and historically marginalized populations (Lou et al., 2023). The bulk of federal spending on children is directed to tax provisions, which are not covered in this study, but do reduce child poverty (National Academies of Sciences, Engineering, and Medicine

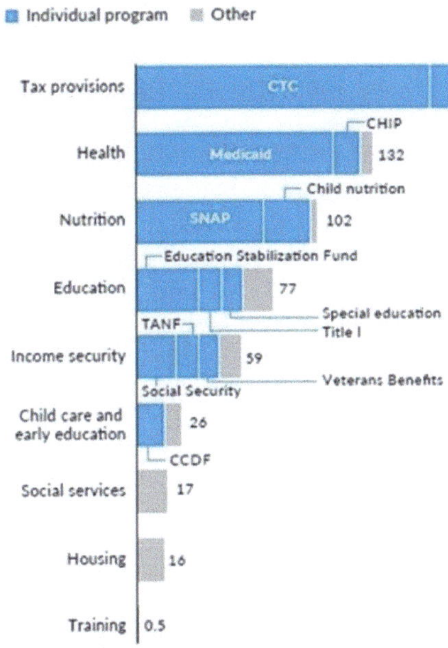

FIGURE 7-5 Federal expenditures on children by category and major programs, 2021, in billions of dollars.
NOTES: Programs that spend less than $10 billion are not shown separately but are included as part of "Other" and in the totals by category. CCDF = Child Care and Development Fund; CHIP = Children's Health Insurance Program; CTC = child tax credit; EIP = economic impact payments (pandemic response stimulus checks administered through the tax code); EITC = earned income tax credit; ESI = employer-sponsored health insurance; SNAP = Supplemental Nutrition Assistance Program; SSI = Supplemental Security Income; TANF = Temporary Assistance for Needy Families.
SOURCE: Lou et al., 2023. Authors' estimates based primarily on Office of Management and Budget, Budget of the United States Government, Fiscal Year 2023.

[National Academies], 2019a, 2023g) and have an indirect influence on health. Another significant portion of funding is for direct health care services (discussed in Chapter 6).

This section reviews federal expenditures on social services with impact on population health. Many programs are administered through the U.S. Department of Health and Human Services (HHS). Key HHS operating divisions and offices that support children's health care financially include HRSA, CDC, the Indian Health Service, the Substance Abuse and Mental Health Services Administration (SAMHSA), and the Administration for Children and Families (ACF). Other government agencies with programs aimed at improving the health, wellbeing, and future productivity of children and youth include the U.S. Department of Agriculture (USDA) and U.S. Department of Education. This review does not include all relevant current and former programs that support preventive services, and some important services and contexts are not discussed here (First Focus on Children, 2023). For example, research shows that variations in stable housing, transportation, and access to parks and green space all shape inequities for children and families that affect health and wellbeing. These areas of programs, policies, and systems are not the focus of the solutions discussed in this report and are well documented in other reports (National Academies, 2017a, 2019a,d, 2023g).

This section focuses on the programs, policies, and systems that more directly serve primary preventive care needs, aim to reduce health disparities, and improve population health. It is organized around funding for services through grants to the states for providing preventive services in community settings and promoting maternal and early child health; nutritious meals; substance use disorder prevention and treatment; and mental and behavioral health services.

The agencies discussed provide funding in various forms—including block, programmatic, and competitive grants—to state and local health departments, nongovernmental organizations, state and local education agencies, tribal nations, territory administrators, faith-based institutions, and other partners to provide health care to children. A common feature of such services is that they are often, although not exclusively, community based, allowing the interventions to be adapted to local characteristics and priorities. They can take on different forms; be universal or targeted to at-risk individuals; be delivered to individuals or to groups; or be delivered by health care systems, workplaces, the military, schools, child care centers, and state or local health departments (Community Preventive Services Task Force, 2022).

Preventive Services

Head Start and Early Head Start

ACF funds local partners to provide health and wellbeing services to children under age 5 years through the Head Start and Early Head Start programs. In addition to early learning services, Head Start supports health by engaging children in physical activity, serving nutritious meals and snacks, ensuring that children receive developmental screenings, promoting oral hygiene, promoting resilience, and providing parenting support (ACF, 2023a,b).

Created as part of President Lyndon Johnson's War on Poverty, Head Start provides comprehensive early childhood education, health, nutrition, and parent support services to low-income, preschool-age (ages 3–5 years) children and their families. Early Head Start was created in 1995 to aid pregnant women and children from birth to age 3 years (Office of Head Start, 2023a,b). Families receive services in their homes and/or Head Start centers, which are locally operated and funded directly by ACF (Office of Head Start, 2023b,c). In addition to Head Start and Early Head Start, the American Indian and Alaska Native Head Start program began in 1965 and provides grants to federally recognized American Indian and Alaska Native tribes; the Migrant and Seasonal Head Start program (started in 1969) provides services to migrant farm workers and their families.

Head Start and Early Head Start have notable direct impacts on children's health outcomes. Compared with children who are not receiving these services, children enrolled in Early Head Start are more likely to be immunized and have access to services for their disabilities (Love et al., 2002). Those in Head Start are more likely to receive dental checkups (Lee & Gortmaker, 2013) and have improved oral health knowledge, behaviors, and activities (Joufi, Claiborne, & Shuman, 2021). Children with obesity, overweight, or underweight are more likely to have a healthier body mass index by kindergarten (Lumeng et al., 2015). In addition, Head Start has been shown to improve mental health outcomes (D'Onise, Lynch, & McDermott, 2010).

Parent involvement in Head Start has indirect impacts on health outcomes, with children demonstrating significantly better socioemotional, language, and cognitive development (Love et al., 2002) when their parents are involved. Head Start graduates are less likely to be in poor health as adults and more likely to report positive parenting behaviors. The children of Head Start graduates have significantly lower odds of becoming teen parents (Barr & Gibbs, 2017; Bauer & Schanzenbach, 2016; Deming, 2009; Johnson, 2010).

The reach and impact of the Head Start program differs across states (National Academies, 2019d) and varies by community and family cultural background. Black children are shown to experience greater gains in self-esteem and socioemotional development, and Hispanic children demonstrate notable gains in educational outcomes (Bauer & Schazenbach, 2016). Although 33% of Black children living in poverty are enrolled in Head Start, compared with 23% of Asian and 27% of Hispanic children, funding per child is lower in states that enroll higher percentages of Black children. The average funding per child across the five areas with the highest percentage of Black children (Washington, DC; Georgia; Louisiana; Maryland; Mississippi) was $9,450, compared with $12,654 in the five states with the lowest percentage (Idaho, Montana, Utah, Vermont, and Wyoming), adjusting for differences in cost of living by state (Friedman-Krauss, Barnett, & Duer, 2022).

Because of insufficient funding, Head Start serves less than half of all 3- and 4-year-olds living in poverty (Barnett & Friedman-Krauss, 2016); this varies widely across states, with an estimated 56% in North Dakota and an estimated 9% in Nevada (Friedman-Krauss, Barnett, & Duer, 2022). Early Head Start reaches about 9% of all eligible children and families. Nationally, around 13% of children enrolled in Head Start and 12% in Early Head Start qualify for special education services under the Individuals with Disabilities Education Act (Friedman-Krauss, Barnett, & Duer, 2022).

The COVID-19 pandemic negatively impacted enrollment in Head Start, as nationally 287,000 fewer children attended in 2020–2021 than in 2018–2019 (the enrollment rate dropped from 41% to 30%), in spite of increased funding for COVID-19 relief. In FY 2022, Head Start and Early Head Start were appropriated $11,036,820,000, an increase of $289 million over FY 2021 (ACF, 2023b).

Centers for Disease Control and Prevention

CDC invests in health surveillance and research as well as prevention activities, which fall variably along the spectrum of direct to indirect children's health care services. Most directly relevant to primary preventive care is the funding CDC provides through the Prevention and Public Health Fund, which makes up 10% of CDC's budget, totaling $903 million in FY 2023 (McKillop & Lieberman, 2023; this fund also supports SAMHSA and ACF). By statute, the Prevention and Public Health Fund supports a range of programs, spanning disease prevention; early detection; chronic disease management; mental health and injury prevention programs; and promotion of healthy lifestyles, including increasing nutrition and physical activity and reducing tobacco use. The fund provides financial support to states and communities directly so they can address their most pressing health challenges and community needs (Trust for America's Health, 2023).

Within the Fund, programs that target the health and wellbeing of children and families most directly include the immunization program, Preventive Health and Health Services Block Grants for state-specific needs, childhood lead poisoning surveillance, maternity and breastfeeding care through hospitals, early care and education collaboratives, and suicide prevention.

The immunization program improves access to vaccination by covering the cost for uninsured children and adults, those on Medicaid, and American Indians and Alaska Natives. It also supports critical infrastructure for collecting and tracking data related to immunization, supporting safety and quality improvement. Passed into law in 1993 in response to a measles outbreak in the United States, the Vaccines for Children (VFC) program provides vaccines to children at no cost, providing critical access to those families who might not be able to pay otherwise. All vaccines recommended by CDC's Advisory Committee on Immunization Practices are eligible for coverage through VFC. An earlier study estimates that, during the first 20 years of the program, the increase in vaccination rates for children born between 1994 and 2013 has helped prevent 21 million hospitalizations and 732,000 deaths, and has resulted in an estimated net savings of $1.38 trillion in total societal costs, which includes an estimated net $295 billion in direct costs (Whitney et al., 2014). The VFC program has been cited as one of the reasons measles has not been endemic since 2000 (Orenstein, 2023).

VFC has also contributed to the narrowing of racial/ethnic and socioeconomic inequities in access to vaccination, leading to a decreased disparity in vaccination rates. An estimated 50% of children are eligible for the VFC program in the United States, with younger children more likely to be eligible and adolescents less likely (Kang et al., 2023; Lindley, Smith, & Rodewald, 2011). A majority of children served by VFC identify with a racially marginalized community (Walker et al., 2014). In FY 2022, VFC was appropriated $5.54 billion (CDC, 2024a).

From the Prevention and Public Health Fund, CDC also administers the Preventive Health and Health Services (PHHS) Block Grant to states, tribes, local health departments, and territories. In FY 2020, this totaled $149,098,135, and of that, 2.9% ($3,882,662) was allocated explicitly to maternal, infant, and child health care (CDC, 2023f). Evaluation of the impact of the PHHS Block Grants has not identified any specific child or maternal health outcomes but rather support for the broader public health infrastructure (CDC, 2023f).

In 2023, the Fund also administered $17 million to prevent childhood lead poisoning, $9.75 million for hospitals to promote breastfeeding, and $12 million for Garrett Lee Smith grants through SAMHSA for prevention and early intervention of youth suicide in a variety of settings (Trust for America's Health, 2023).

Since 1999, CDC has also funded the Racial and Ethnic Approaches to Community Health (REACH) program, focused on reducing health disparities among specific racial/ethnic groups by funding state and local health departments, tribes, universities, and community-based organizations. Grantees are instructed to use funds to build partnerships in communities with the highest burden of health inequity. While there are no child-specific requirements for use of the funding, REACH grantees have demonstrated positive impacts on child health outcomes, such as increased breastfeeding (Witt et al., 2021) and increased access to and consumption of fruits and vegetables through food prescriptions (Jones, VanWassenhove-Paetzol et al., 2020). In FY 2022, the REACH program received $43.45 million (Trust for America's Health, 2022).

The Good Health and Wellness in Indian Country (GHWIC) program is CDC's largest investment to improve health for American Indians and Alaska Natives. Similar to REACH, GHWIC aims to reinforce work already under way in communities and support culturally appropriate approaches to health. Apart from a goal to increase breastfeeding, none of GHWIC's goals are child specific. In FY 2022, the program received $22.5 million (Trust for America's Health, 2022).

Despite efforts to create a separate fund for prevention services and activities, federal priorities have diverted funding from the Prevention and Public Health Fund away from prevention activities toward direct health care services (Harkin, 2013). Even more concerning are expected cuts to programs such as VFC that deliver a significant amount of preventive care to children (Miller, 2023).

CDC also administers the National Center on Birth Defects and Developmental Disabilities (NCBDDD), which provides resources for research, awareness, public health practice, and surveillance, with a focus on child health and disability. NCBDDD's efforts have included evaluating the impact of folic acid supplementation; promoting standards of preconception care; providing resources for attention deficit and hyperactivity disorder and autism spectrum disorder, including the "Learn the Signs. Act Early" campaign for facilitating earlier diagnosis for these conditions; and creating surveillance systems for sickle cell disease and thalassemia (Boyle, Cordero, & Trevathan, 2012). NCBDDD funds the Early Hearing Detection and Intervention program, which promotes hearing screening, diagnosis, and early intervention, ensuring that infants are screened for hearing loss, that those who need it receive a full evaluation, and that those with hearing loss receive intervention services (CDC, 2024l). NCBDDD also provides resources for developing treatments for hemophilia and funds comprehensive hemophilia treatment centers. CDC studies have shown that people with hemophilia who receive care from a hemophilia treatment center are 40% less likely to be hospitalized and less likely to die because of bleeding complications (CDC, n.d.c), compared with those who do not receive this care. In FY 2022, NCBDDD (2023) received $177 million in appropriations.

Maternal and Early Child Health

HRSA Title V Maternal and Child Health Block Grant

Through the Maternal and Child Health Bureau (MCHB), HRSA (2023j) administers block grants to states for improving access to health care—including prenatal–postnatal services, preventive and primary care for children, and community-based services—focused on low-income individuals and children and youth with special health care needs. Through legislative and administrative decisions, the MCHB has evolved since its founding in 1912 as the Children's Bureau to better respond to the needs of children and families. Title V was established as part of the Social Security Act (1935 § 501) to provide "grants to states for maternal and child welfare." States are required to provide a level of matching for funds they receive in federal Title V block grant support. With the establishment of Medicaid in 1965, Title V funds have been increasingly used to fill gaps in the system of care for children and mothers (Warren & Kavanaugh, 2023).

> [For] three decades, state Title V programs have played an important role in increasing access to and use of timely prenatal care and other family health care services through outreach and coordination by (1) facilitating

> partnerships among agencies that provide direct services to pregnant women; (2) helping to ensure that maternal and child health professionals in WIC, Head Start, and other public programs provide pregnant women with accurate and current information on coverage in their state; (3) increasing access to presumptive Medicaid eligibility, which provides pregnant women with access to immediate prenatal care; and (4) increasing continuity of coverage for low-income women who become pregnant. (National Academies, 2019d, p. 333)

Title V programs have a significant history of supporting very young children, stemming back to the Children's Bureau, which among its first activities published an "Infant Care" pamphlet in 1914 and had a series of "Baby Week Campaigns" in 1917. Subsequent investments and priorities included children with special health care needs ("children who are crippled or who are suffering from conditions which lead to crippling") as part of the Social Security Act (1935 § 501) and children from low-income neighborhoods as part of Medicaid (Warren & Kavanaugh, 2023). Currently, at least 30% of federal support for state programs has been allocated for well-child programs, and at least 30% goes to programs for children with special health care needs (formerly the Crippled Children's Service; HRSA, 2019). As with women's health, state programs have helped to facilitate partnerships across key agencies; improve knowledge of the health status of children and youth in the state; and link households with other agencies, especially Medicaid and the U.S. Social Security Administration (for Supplemental Security Income coverage; National Academies, 2019d). In FY 2022, Title V maternal and child health block grants were appropriated $736 million (Black Maternal Health Caucus, 2023; HRSA, 2023g).

Maternal, Infant, and Early Childhood Home Visiting

HRSA, in partnership with ACF, administers the Maternal, Infant, and Early Childhood Home Visiting (MIECHV) program to fund states and jurisdictions. The program provides for voluntary home visits during early pregnancy and childhood to families in at-risk communities to provide parenting support and child-centered services in the home (e.g., developmental screenings; HRSA, 2023f). By law, state and territory awardees are required to implement evidence-based home visiting models. ACF created the Home Visiting Evidence of Effectiveness (HomVEE) project to conduct thorough and transparent reviews of early childhood home visiting models (HHS, n.d.).

In FY 2018, the MIECHV program provided nearly 1 million home visits and served approximately 150,000 parents and children in 76,000 families across all 50 states; Washington, DC; 5 territories; and 23 tribal and urban

American Indian and Alaska Native communities (HRSA, n.d.c). It has been reported that 40% of U.S. counties provide home visiting services, with 13 states offering home visiting in 75% of counties and 10 states providing it in 10 or fewer counties (NHVRC, 2018). The National Home Visiting Resource Center (2023) estimates that more than 22 million additional families could benefit but were not being reached. The MIECHV program was reauthorized in 2018 at a funding level of $400 million annually through 2022 (Sandstrom, 2019). The 2022 reauthorization increased funding and established new procedures through 2027 (CRS, 2023a,b).

Positive health impacts of the MIECHV program in some settings have included fewer preterm and low birth weight babies, more children adequately immunized and completing well-child visits, greater achievement of developmental milestones, fewer child emergency department visits, and better maternal physical and mental health (Sandstrom, 2019). While nurse home visiting can provide important health care services for children, mother wellbeing, and family functioning (Goldfeld et al., 2022), the evidence for their effectiveness at a population level is currently mixed. Studies reviewed by HomVEE have noted lower rates of newborn death, preterm and low-weight birth, and need for emergency or hospital care in the first year of life (Sandstrom, 2019).[4] Other studies have found that such programs do not improve birth outcomes, even for non-Hispanic Black mothers (McConnell et al., 2022; Robling et al., 2016). Findings may differ because of the implementation of different home visiting models in different settings and variation of use across the United States (see Figure 7-6).

Some of the variability shown in Figure 7-6 is due to different state decisions to support home visiting programs through a mix of funding sources, including funding from MIECHV, as well as from Medicaid, Title V, Temporary Assistance for Needy Families, Child Welfare, and Head Start. Additionally, under a recent reauthorization, MIECHV opted for a new model for distributing funds to states. In addition to investing in evidence-based interventions from a list created by HomVEE, the newer model authorizes states to use up to 25% of their grant funds to enter into public–private partnerships called pay-for-success agreements (see further discussion of this model below).

[4]HomVEE has also looked specifically at models with potential relevance for American Indian and Alaska Native families and children. Family Spirit is an example of a model designed for American Indian pregnant women and families with children younger than age 3 years; it utilizes paraprofessional home visitors from the community to support mothers' and caregivers' parenting skills. Studies have found favorable impacts on maternal health, child development, and positive parenting practices (HHS, 2022).

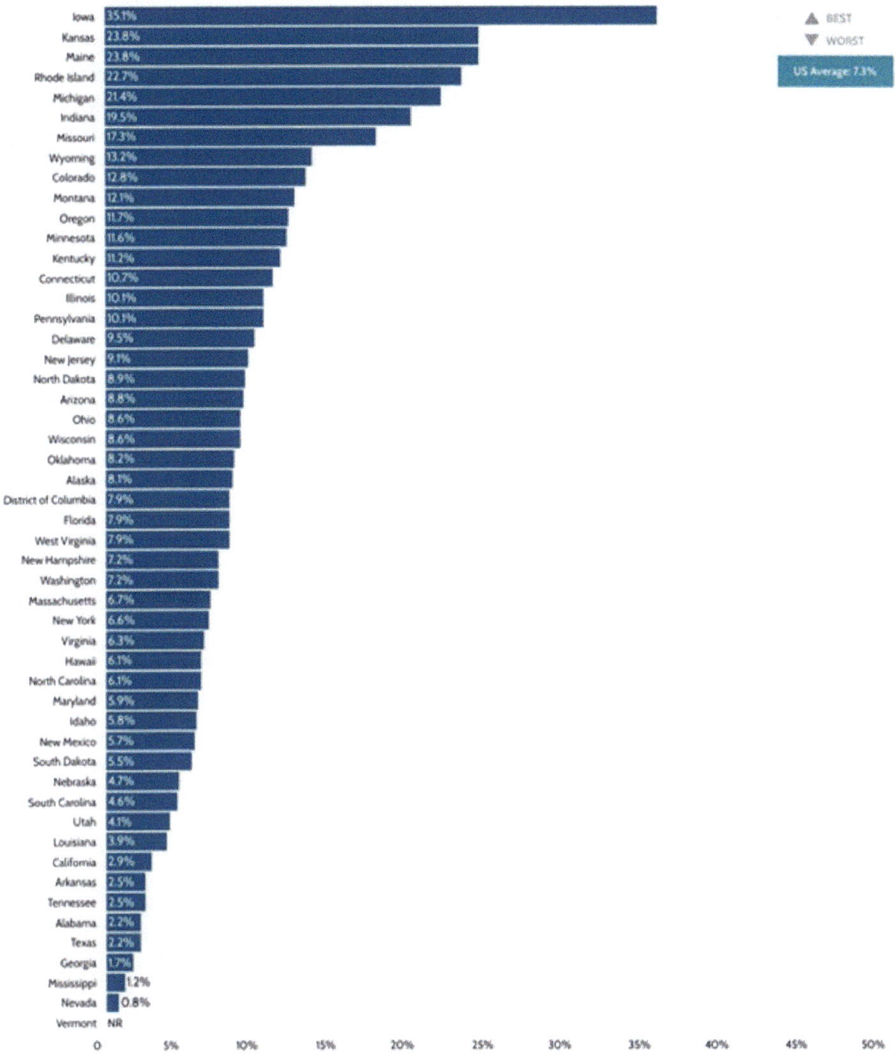

FIGURE 7-6 Variation across states in percentage of children served in evidence-based home visiting programs.
NOTES: Estimated percentage of eligible children is calculated as the percent of children under age 3 years served by home visiting programs out of all children under age 3 in families with incomes below 150% of the federal poverty level. Vermont's home visiting participation numbers were impacted by model changes during 2019 and likely not reflective of accurate participation rates. NR = not reported.
SOURCE: National Home Visiting Resource Center Yearbook (2020) and American Community Survey 1-year Public Use Microdata Sample (Census Bureau, 2018, 2019).

Nutritious Meals

USDA provides health care to children by distributing funds through programs such as WIC, the Supplemental Nutrition Assistance Program (SNAP), and the Summer Food Service Program (discussed below), as well as the National School Lunch and School Breakfast programs (discussed in Chapter 8, see also USDA, 2023a).

Special Supplemental Nutrition Program for Women, Infants, and Children

In WIC, USDA provides federal grants to states for "supplemental foods, health care referrals, and nutrition education for low-income pregnant, breastfeeding, and non-breastfeeding postpartum women, and to infants and children up to age 5 who are found to be at nutritional risk" (USDA, 2023c, para. 1). Families with incomes below 100% or 185% of the federal poverty level (depending on the state) are eligible for WIC, and the program serves half of all infants in the United States.

WIC provides assistance through breastfeeding support and education, healthy foods, nutrition education and counseling, screening referrals to other services, and vouchers to purchase fruits and vegetables from authorized farmers' markets (USDA, 2024a). WIC services are provided in many settings, including county health departments, hospitals, mobile clinics, community centers, schools, public housing sites, migrant health centers and camps, and Indian Health Service facilities (USDA, 2024a).

To be eligible to receive benefits, WIC participants need to meet four categories of requirements: categorical, residential, income, and nutrition risk (USDA, 2024a). Infants younger than age 1 year; children younger than age 5 years; and women who are pregnant, postpartum (up to 6 months), or breastfeeding meet the WIC categorical requirement. To meet the residential requirement, participants need to reside in the state or local service area in which they apply but are not required to have lived in that area for a minimum amount of time. Participants also have to earn incomes at or below income standards that are set by state agencies and fall within 100% and 185% of the federal poverty guidelines issued annually by HHS. Additionally, participants need to be determined by a health professional to have at least one medical (e.g., anemia, underweight) or dietary (e.g., poor diet) condition from a list of conditions indicating nutrition risk that is set by states (USDA, 2018).

Participation rates among eligible children decline significantly after infancy. Over 98% of eligible infants participate; however, participation rates decline among children ages 1, 2, 3, and 4 years—65%, 49%, 44%, 25%, respectively—and only 52% of eligible pregnant individuals participate (Trippe et al., 2019; USDA, 2024b). Factors contributing to decreased participation rates have been reported as concerns regarding immigration status, lack of transportation to attend in-person appointments, and administrative barriers that made it more difficult for families to enroll or stay enrolled in WIC (National Academies, 2017a; Vargas & Pirog, 2016). Participation increased during the pandemic because of the multiple waivers that existed (e.g., remote benefits issuance, physical presence, allowance of uploading electronic certification documents) that streamlined certification and increased the fruit and vegetable benefit (National Academies, 2023c).

In FY 2018, WIC served approximately 6.9 million people and cost the federal government about $5.3 billion (USDA, 2019). Numerous studies using varied methods have found evidence of improved birth outcomes for participating women (see, e.g., Figlio, Hamersma, & Roth, 2009; Fingar et al., 2017; Foster, Jiang, & Gibson-Davis, 2010; Hoynes, Page, & Stevens, 2011). These studies found reductions in the likelihood of low birth weight (Figlio, Hamersma, & Roth, 2009; Hoynes, Page, & Stevens, 2011) and reductions in infant mortality (Khanani et al., 2010). Studies generally have found that the effects of WIC on birth outcomes are stronger for women with lower education levels, those living in areas of high poverty, and those who are African American (Hoynes, Page, & Stevens, 2011; Khanani et al., 2010). The Center on Budget and Policy Priorities concluded that WIC is a "cost-effective investment that improves the nutrition and health of low-income families—leading to healthier infants, more nutritious diets, and better health care for children, and subsequently to higher academic achievement for students" (Carlson & Neuberger, 2021, p. 1). Other studies—particularly in regard to 2009 improvements in the program that promoted consumption of fruits, vegetables, whole grains, and low-fat dairy products—have found improved dietary intake, perinatal outcomes, and early children development (Guan et al., 2021; Hamad et al., 2019a,b; Schultz, Byker Shanks, & Houghtaling, 2015; Tester, Leung, & Crawford, 2016).

Supplemental Nutrition Assistance Program

SNAP "provides food benefits to low-income families to supplement their grocery budget so they can afford the nutritious food essential to health and well-being" (USDA, 2023d, para. 1). The program targets those whose incomes are less than 130% of the federal poverty level. The maximum monthly benefit for a family of four in 2023 was $939, to be used for purchasing food at participating stores. The program expects that participating households will spend about 30% of their own financial resources purchasing food.

In 2017, an estimated 42 million people benefited from SNAP (Nchako & Cai, 2018). Children represented 44% of SNAP participants and received 43% of the benefits. One in five children in the United States received SNAP benefits in 2017. Participation in SNAP is generally high for those that are eligible (82% nationally, but as low as 55% in some states).

The main barrier to SNAP utilization among children is the ineligibility of many immigrant groups. Among immigrants, only those with permanent residency and those who are refugees can access SNAP benefits. Those who are undocumented and those awaiting permanent residency are not eligible. Having parents or siblings in the latter categories affects the benefit levels of eligible children who are U.S. citizens. Of the total number of SNAP participants, 8% were children with U.S. citizen status living with noncitizen adults (Cronquist & Lauffer, 2019). Undocumented noncitizens of the United States are not eligible for SNAP, but noncitizens who have lived in the United States for at least 5 years, receive disability-related assistance, or are less than 18 years of age are eligible (if they also meet the general eligibility requirements; USDA, 2023e).

SNAP has been linked to improvements in newborn health, improved child outcomes, reduced poverty, and improved economic and health outcomes in adulthood (Almond, Hoynes, & Schanzenbach, 2011; Bailey et al., 2020; Carlson & Keith-Jennings, 2018; Hoynes & Schanzenbach, 2015; Hoynes, Miller, & Simon, 2015; Hoynes, Page, & Stevens, 2011; Hoynes, Schanzenbach, & Almond, 2016). However, SNAP does not eliminate food insecurity. SNAP benefits per meal are estimated to be 25% less than the average cost of a low-income meal and do not cover the cost of a low-income meal in 99% of U.S. counties (Waxman, Gundersen, & Thompson, 2018). Evidence supports the importance of expanding SNAP benefits during the summer months, when children lack access to free and reduced-price lunches through school (Carlson & Keith-Jennings, 2018). A report by the National Academies on reducing child poverty found that expanding SNAP benefits, accounting for the needs of adolescents, and increasing benefits during the summer months could decrease child poverty rates by as much as 2.3%, depending on how large the expansion is (National Academies, 2019a).

Summer Food Service Program

Other programs, such as the Summer Food Service Program, also extends the availability of free meals for low-income populations into the summer months when children are not in school. Several demonstrations have shown that expanding meal programs can minimize the observed spike in food insecurity during the summer (Collins & Klerman, 2017; Gundersen & Ziliak, 2015).

Before 2020, many children lacked access to a food site during the summer. According to one study, in 2018, only 43% of children lived in a census tract with a meal site; this resulted in one child participating in the summer program for every seven participating in school lunch programs (Bauer & Parsons, 2020). During the COVID-19 pandemic, Congress authorized electronic benefit transfer (EBT) payments, providing vouchers for grocery purchases instead of prepared meals during the summer. The summer EBT program was made permanent in December 2022. Thirty-five states, 5 territories, and 4 tribal governments have opted into the EBT program as of January 1, 2024. This new approach to tackling food insecurity and promoting nutrition has added flexibility and has helped address community challenges to accessing to this free service for those eligible.

Mental and Behavioral Health Services

Linking Actions for Unmet Needs in Children's Health

SAMHSA's (2023b) Linking Actions for Unmet Needs in Children's Health (Project LAUNCH; and its sister program Indigenous-Project LAUNCH, focused on American Indian and Alaska Native communities and U.S. territories and Pacific jurisdictions), provides grants to partner organizations to screen children and caregivers for mental health needs, improve the capacities of adult caregivers of young children to help support their healthy socioemotional development, prevent behavioral disorders, identify and address behavioral concerns before they develop into serious emotional disturbances, and integrate behavioral health into primary care. The goal of Project LAUNCH has been to improve outcomes along multiple dimensions through cross-sector engagement to mitigate risk factors contributing to poor child outcomes and to promote protective factors that support resilience and healthy development (see Figure 7-7). One study in Massachusetts found indicators of program success, demonstrating longitudinal improvement in social, emotional, and behavioral outcomes of children and decreased symptoms of stress and depression in caregivers. This has led the way to expanding and improving sustainability of the model (Molnár et al., 2018). Current LAUNCH models aim, for example, to expand a team-based pediatric primary care approach—partnering an early childhood mental health clinician with a family or lived experience representative—to reach additional cities (Massachusetts); add mental health consultation to existing home visiting and parent engagement initiatives (California); support cross-sector engagement among departments of public health and mental health, university child development resources, and existing public–private partnerships for children (Alabama); and strengthen a family-focused network of culturally connected health and wellness services (Confederated Salish and Kootenai Tribes, n.d.).[5] In FY 2022, $23.5 million was appropriated for Project LAUNCH (SAMHSA, 2022c).

[5]For more information and additional grantees, see https://healthysafechildren.org/project-launch-grantees

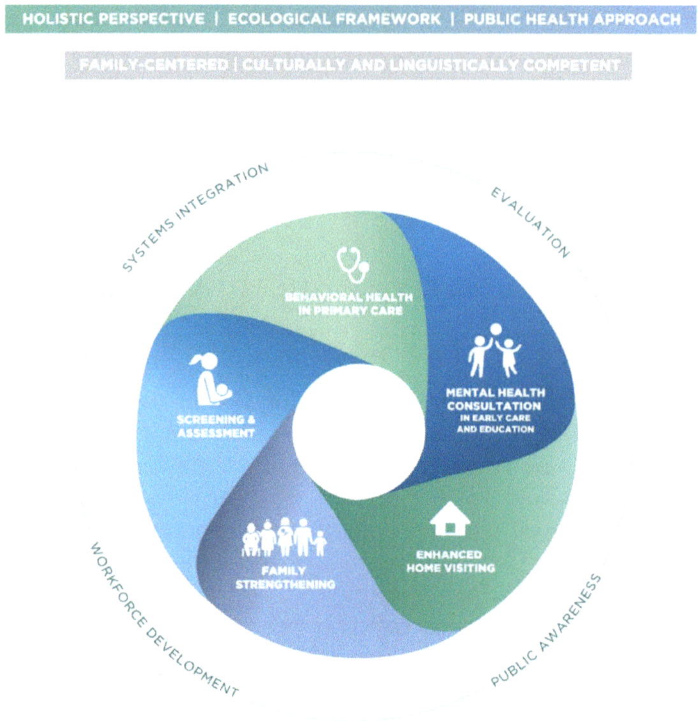

FIGURE 7-7 Project LAUNCH (Linking Actions for Unmet Needs in Children's Health).
SOURCE: American Institutes for Research, n.d.

Other Funding and Programs for Supporting Mental Health in Particular Populations

SAMHSA funds numerous prevention and treatment programs for supporting positive mental and behavioral health. The rise in the number of programs reflects a robust response to growing concern nationally and in communities on the state of mental health for children and youth, as well as growing recognition of populations most in need. Many have criticized the lack of a comprehensive mental health care system for children and families (Bringewatt & Gershoff, 2010; Cummings, Wen, & Druss, 2011). As discussed in Chapter 5, mental health services have been notably fragmented from primary preventive care, but emergent efforts are focused on integration with primary care and community settings most accessible to individuals. Access to mental health programs is particularly valuable to marginalized populations that have experienced years of disadvantage and discrimination. There is evidence that children and families from low-income and historically marginalized communities have a lower likelihood of engagement in high-quality mental health services (Hodgkinson et al., 2017; Rodgers et al., 2022) than those from other communities. As noted earlier, programs presented here do not capture all efforts in this area.

SAMHSA's Infant and Early Childhood Mental Health (IECMH) grants provide services to children from birth to age 12 years and their parents/caregivers at risk for serious emotional disturbance through multigenerational therapy and evidence-based mental health promotion, prevention, and treatment interventions (SAMHSA, 2023a). IECMH services foster socioemotional functioning, the development of positive relationships with adults and peers, and the creation of a solid sense of identity and autonomy. A strong foundation of socioemotional processes is likely to prevent the emergence of mental health problems in infancy and early childhood, as well as later in the life course (National Academies, 2023g). In addition to individual grants to provide mental health services, the program supports a consultation center. The Center of Excellence for IECMH Consultation provides technical assistance to programs, classroom staff, and families (Ash, Mackrain, & Johnston, 2013; Brinamen, Taranta, & Johnston, 2012; Duran et al., 2009). A number of studies have documented the effectiveness of the Center for reducing child behavior problems, improving teacher–child relationships and classroom climate, and lowering suspension and expulsion rates and teacher turnover (Brennan et al., 2008; Center of Excellence for IECMH Consultation, 2021; Hepburn et al., 2013; Perry et al., 2010; SAMHSA, 2014; Shivers, Faragó, & Gal-Szabo, 2022). In FY 2022, IECMH grants were appropriated $9.98 million through SAMHSA (2022a).

SAMHSA's National Child Traumatic Stress Initiative improves treatment and services for children, adolescents, and families that have experienced traumatic events. Authorized by Congress as part of the Children's Health Act (2000), the initiative created a National Child Traumatic Stress Network (NCTSN) to increase access to effective trauma- and grief-focused treatment and services and support the development of trauma-informed child-serving systems (SAMHSA, 2024). NCTSN recognizes that certain populations are at increased risk for exposure to trauma, including children dealing with substance abuse or experiencing homelessness, those with caregivers in the active military or returned home as veterans, those who identify as LGBTQ+, those who have intellectual and developmental disabilities, and those whose family is experiencing economic stress. In FY 2022, NCTSN grantees provided screening to more than 84,000 individuals and evidence-based treatment to more than 42,000 children, adolescents, and family members, with thousands more benefiting indirectly through the training and consultation provided by NCTSN grantees. In FY 2022, the initiative was appropriated $81.88 million through SAMHSA (2022c).

SAMHSA's Tribal Behavioral Health Grants provide support for mental health care for tribes and tribal organizations and are intended to prevent and reduce suicidal behavior and substance abuse and to promote positive mental health among American Indian and Alaska Native young people ages 24 years and younger. Goals for these grants include developing and implementing an array of integrated services and supports for improving outcomes by working with tribes to support strategies that have been shown to be effective or promising in Native communities. In FY 2022, the Tribal Behavioral Health Grants program was appropriated $20.73 million through SAMHSA (2022c).

EXPANDING RESOURCES TO ADVANCE COMMUNITY-LEVEL HEALTH PROMOTION AND DISEASE PREVENTION

As discussed above, the federal government provides a great deal of funding and support for direct and indirect health care through state, tribal, and local agencies. Many federal programs serve important needs in local communities, and many programs have provided assistance for decades and have evolved to address a changing society. However, the needs are great, and many programs fail to reach all eligible children, youth, and families. Furthermore, several barriers hamper efforts to achieve positive population health outcomes and health equity. Promising models need to be expanded so they can benefit more children and families in local communities. There is opportunity to further integrate programs with health care systems to identify children, youth, and families in need and monitor progress together. Important as well is adapting these models to meet the specific cultural and community needs of participant children and families. Several funding sources could become more available and widely used to address some of these needs.

Community Benefit and Reinvestment Activities

Nonprofit Hospitals

Nonprofit hospitals benefit financially from tax exemptions at the federal, state, and local levels when they invest in community benefit activities (i.e., initiatives, activities, and investments undertaken to improve health in the communities they serve; Government Accountability Office, 2023e; Hilltop Institute, n.d.). Of approximately 6,000 hospitals in the United States, about half are identified as nongovernment, nonprofit community hospitals and thus qualify for tax-exempt status (American Hospital Association [AHA], 2024). AHA (2024) estimates the total forgone federal revenue from the hospital tax exemption at $12.4 billion in 2019.

In exchange for tax exemption, hospitals engage in a variety of community benefits that they must document. Significant opportunities exist for government institutions to address gaps in coordination and oversight of these investments (Riley, Clary, & Higgins, 2019). Although these funds originate from health care systems via tax exemption, they need not be directed toward clinical care. Community benefits from nonprofit hospitals, and potentially health plans, represent potential sources of funding that can be directed toward a wide variety of activities, including community-based primary preventive health care for children and adolescents. Input from a broad set of stakeholders, including those engaged in other federal planning activities around maternal and child health, can also ensure that the investments align with other local initiatives. With local stakeholder input, hospitals can tailor their programs and practices flexibly to address their communities' specific needs and concerns (Hut, 2023).

The federal government has implemented policies for quantifying community benefits of hospitals and conducting community health needs assessments in order to increase transparency and accountability. However, community health needs assessments are not required explicitly to examine any particular priority area, such as community-based prevention, or any population, such as children. Thus, there is a disconnect between services that could benefit child health, in both the short and long terms, and the investments that are actually made under community benefit, particularly investments that go beyond direct patient care in the facility. Planning for child health promotion and prevention services through community needs assessment is promoted through many disparate channels. To illustrate, states are required by federal law to conduct comprehensive needs assessments as a condition of Title V MCHB Grant support every 5 years. At the same time, tax-exempt hospitals must report their community health needs assessments every 3 years.

A major step toward increased transparency came in 2009, when the Internal Revenue Service (IRS) published an updated version of its Form 990, including Schedule H, a special tax form for hospitals on which community benefit activities are catalogued (Evashwick & Jackson, 2020). The IRS also began requiring hospital facilities to track their community benefits spending in relation to costs incurred by, for example, bad debt or the cost of Medicare participation. Hospitals record, for example, charity care and Medicaid payment shortfalls as community benefit, along with activities that are not tied to patient care but might involve community health improvement services (Kanter et al., 2020). Following the implementation of Schedule H, the Patient Protection and Affordable Care Act (ACA, 2012 § 9007) instituted triennial community health needs assessments for nonprofit hospitals beginning in 2012 (Evashwick & Jackson, 2020; IRS, 2023). As part of these assessments, hospitals are required to solicit and consider input from health experts and may also consider input from consumer groups, community organizations, academics, local governments, and other community stakeholders (National Academy for State Health Policy, 2019). Hospital organizations with multiple facilities must conduct a community health needs assessment for each facility. Additionally, hospitals must promulgate implementation strategies for addressing their identified community health needs. However, there is no legal definition of "community benefits" and little guidance on how to integrate community experts into assessments, which leaves hospitals with considerable flexibility in implementing strategies and interventions in their communities (Riley, Morrison, & McEvoy, 2019; Santos, 2020).

In addition to calls for greater transparency and planning around community investments by hospitals, there has been considerable, ongoing policy debate around the level of community benefit investment, particularly whether hospitals are generating total benefits commensurate with the financial relief they receive through tax exemption (Congressional Research Service, 2010). One comparison of the value of community benefits and tax exemptions in nonprofit hospitals found that the amount of community benefits and charity care provided by nonprofits varied substantially across organizations and that 86% of nonprofit hospitals provided less charity work than the value of their tax exemptions (Zare, Eisenberg, & Anderson, 2022). A separate analysis found that nationally this gap amounted to a total fair-share deficit of $25.7 billion (Lown Institute, 2024).

Other studies have found that despite lower uninsured rates since the passage of the ACA, community benefits among nonprofit hospitals have not increased over time (Kanter et al., 2020), as might be expected with greater resources available to hospitals. Medicaid expansion under the ACA had a significant impact on hospital financing, reducing uncompensated care from 4.1 percentage points to 3.1 percentage points of hospital operating costs based on short-run estimates (Dranove, Garthwaite, & Ody, 2016). These reductions in uncompensated care occurred almost exclusively in states with Medicaid expansions and were larger in hospitals that had higher pre-ACA uncompensated care burdens and nonprofit hospitals. Despite the reduction in uncompensated care, there appears to be little evidence that community benefits among nonprofit hospitals increased. A separate news report revealed that seven of the ten most profitable hospitals in the country are nonprofits and found that since passage of the ACA, revenues of the most profitable hospitals have increased by 15%, while charity care has dropped by 35% (Ofri, 2020). The Medicaid expansion has had a somewhat complex impact on the accounting of community benefits, decreasing charity care, but increasing the amount counted as "unreimbursed" Medicaid expenditures, meaning aggregate payments declined relative to aggregate charges (Kanter et al., 2020). Ultimately, research does not support that insurance expansion under Medicaid increased nonprofit hospitals' spending on community-directed, preventive services.

Nonprofit hospitals are exempt not only from federal taxes, but also from state income tax, state and local sales tax, and state and local property tax. In some states, there have been more deliberate steps to direct community benefit spending than at the federal level. Eleven states have their own reporting requirements (Hilltop Institute, n.d.), while Massachusetts has established elaborate guidelines for community-benefit priority areas, reporting, and evaluation as part of its determination-of-need process for hospitals (Office of the Attorney General, 2018). Five states extend beyond reporting and explicitly require a minimum spending amount on community benefits for nonprofit hospitals. In Illinois and Utah, for example, these amounts are tied to the amount of the hospitals' property tax exemption (Atkeson & Higgins, 2021).

Tax-Exempt Health Plans

Despite policy movement around greater accountability among tax-exempt hospitals, in most cases there are no analogous community benefit requirements or reporting for tax-exempt health insurance plans. Recently, a national analysis identified 92 federally tax-exempt health plans (60 plans excluding dental plans) and examined the "profits" (i.e., total revenues less total expenses) generated by health insurance plans that are tax exempt under federal law as 501(c)(4) "social welfare organizations" (Plummer et al., 2023). This represents a missed opportunity to engage an important health stakeholder in community health planning and promotion. These tax-exempt health plans do not face similar transparency requirements to tax-exempt hospitals. One exception is Massachusetts, which established community benefits guidelines for health maintenance organizations that parallel the guidelines for nonprofit hospitals. These guidelines apply only to health maintenance organizations, not other types of insurers, such as preferred provider organizations.

Community Reinvestment Approaches

Changing community benefit requirements would target only tax-exempt hospitals and health plans. For-profit entities, on the other hand, contribute tax dollars to federal, state, and local governments, which may or may not be invested in primary preventive services for children. Reinvestment approaches could span health care entities regardless of their tax status.

A somewhat related example exists in the banking realm. Under the Community Reinvestment Act (CRA, 1977), banks are encouraged to help meet the credit needs of communities in which they do business, with a particular focus on low- and moderate-income communities. Such investments are not required but are viewed favorably in merger and other business reviews. Under the CRA, banks report performance metrics in a standardized fashion, depending on their size, and ratings are made public and searchable. There is evidence that the CRA induced small increases in bank activity in low- and middle-income areas (Brevoort, 2022).

While implementation in the health care context may be more complex, the basic principle of a reporting requirement with particular focus and benefit for disadvantaged communities has precedence in other sectors. A strict approach in the health care context might serve to tie reporting and evaluation more stringently to certificate-of-need standards where they exist, or to accreditation more broadly.

Financing Mechanisms for Supporting Community Partnerships

Increased investment in child health through population- and community-level primary prevention can be gained from cross-sector work among public health, health care, and other child-serving sectors and will require repurposing of some funds and additional resources. Several financing strategies are articulated here.

Repurposing Funds for Multisector, Child Health–Related Outcomes

Major social service programs in housing, employment, and transportation invest billions of dollars in U.S. cities and states annually. Very few of these programs are directed, advised, or evaluated in terms of child outcomes, even though they are strongly connected to child health. Large child health care systems have increasingly engaged with public agencies and private partners in focusing major projects on aspects of child health or community development in areas with child health concerns.

The Center for Community Investment[6] underscores the important role in many communities of large health care systems' political, operational, and fiscal strength in facilitating the pipeline of community development. Levels of collaboration across sectors vary, but they are similar to the collaborative activities described previously between public health and health care. Steps include (1) shared goals and accountability (easiest) in investments, (2) shared governance and collaboration on improvement (harder), (3) shared data (harder yet), and (4) shared savings (hardest). Often, these steps take advantage of the relative strengths of various partners in the activities. For example, when appropriate, public officials can make available with right of first refusals any properties with

[6]See https://centerforcommunityinvestment.org

tax delinquency or abandonment. Private developers bring construction and application experience to efforts such as the Low-Income Housing Tax Credit competition. Hospitals often have expertise in subcontracting construction, legal aspects of property acquisition, and project management. Together, these teams can be highly competitive for contested tax credit deals.

Reclassification of Community Prevention as Part of Medical Loss Ratio

The medical loss ratio (MLR) is the proportion of medical premiums paid to insurers that reimbursed provider claims in a given period (Centers for Medicare & Medicaid Services [CMS], 2010). In 2010, the ACA required that the National Association of Insurance Commissioners develop standardized regulations that provided minimum MLRs (i.e., limiting administrative costs and profit) in public-sector plans and required transparency in reporting. The MLR is critical to managed care and accountable care organizations caring for children, in that care investments that are covered in the MLR will gradually be reflected in the capitation rate they are paid. Care investments that are not counted as part of the MLR will count only as additional overhead without revenue.

Currently, community prevention is not counted in CMS guidance on actuarial calculations of the MLR, so any prevention investments made count against managed care or accountable care organizations that take the initiative with community prevention. For example, evidence-based community programs such as the Good Behavior Game for young children (Kellam et al., 2011) or Earned Income Tax Credit assistance, both of which improve long-term outcomes, are added costs when used by managed care or accountable care organizations. If they were counted as part of the MLR rules by CMS, these expenses would allow improved capitation rates for value-based purchasing contracts caring for children and adolescents.

Pay-for-Success Models

Pay-for-success models, including the program supported by the U.S. Treasury Department, offer the enticing concept of using private-sector investments to support public goods or outcomes. This model creates an avenue for private-sector partners to fund preventive health interventions and requires states to pay only if the private partner delivers improved outcomes. First trialed for prison recidivism in the United Kingdom, pay-for-success models encourage investors to bid on supporting investments that generate public savings and return the savings to investors. Pay-for-success models have generated investments in teen pregnancy prevention in South Carolina and early school intervention in Utah.

The goal of the model is clear: to monitor and improve outcomes on average; however, a number of downsides, including two main concerns, have been noted.

First, pay-for-success models have been most attractive as returns for investors when an expensive event (e.g., return to prison) is avoided *and* the savings are generated to a single public agency (such as the justice system). To identify such opportunities, a feasibility study is required before projects begin—these studies call for significant collaboration and buy-in. Kennedy-Moulton and colleagues (2022) noted that barriers identified by feasibility studies include legal and administrative complexity, community-based organization capacity, and agreeable outcome tracking. As a result, although feasibility studies have been conducted in more than 65 communities nationwide, few projects have been fully funded (Karaca-Mandic et al., 2023).

Second, pay-for-success programs that are funded have an increased incentive to engage in "risk-score gaming"—that is, to target those most likely to succeed, which has the potential to widen disparities if based on proxies for advantage or disadvantage, such as neighborhood or race (Chomilo, 2023). Prevention programs for children tend to have very long-term yields with no single event dominating savings and no single agency garnering most of the savings. As a result, pay-for-success models for children have not attracted a great deal of private investment. Instead, they have received very modest investments from mission-driven foundations and investors, which limits their scope.

Mandated Investment by Health Plans

Another option for increasing resources for child-focused prevention and health promotion involves mandated investment by health plans and possibly provider organizations. Mandated investment can come in any one of several ways:

- Health plans are taxed directly, with funds set aside by the taxing authority for prevention investments—California is currently undertaking this approach (Durham, 2023). Massachusetts had a similar plan from 2012 to 2020. As of 2023, 18 states tax their health plans, with varied uses for those funds.[7]
- Health plans are subject to a minimum investment requirement specified by state or federal regulatory authorities, as in the CRA (1977) for the banking industry.
- Health plans have incentives or capitation withheld until specific outcomes are achieved. Oregon and Ohio have instituted initiatives that do not require specific health plan investments but withhold dollars until outcome goals are met.

[7]See https://www.kff.org/other/state-indicator/states-with-an-mco-provider-tax-in-place

To date, no studies examine the effectiveness of these strategies for generating resources to invest in prevention and child health. Moreover, when funds are generated, considerable questions remain about how best to expend them to enable flexibility, rapid cycle improvement, and community-focused services. Mann and Ferguson (2020) argue that developing flexible community wellness funds provides the most opportunity to improve child health in a way that is respectful to community wishes and allows local strengths to be brought to the fore.

CONCLUSION

Primary preventive care is critical for child populations and dictates the assurance of conditions in which families and communities can be healthy and well. Many communities in the United States are challenged to provide children and families with the environments and services they need to be healthy; in these contexts, the role of public health needs to be intensified. State and local health departments, however, are woefully underfunded. Many public health efforts lack coherence and coordination. Moreover, no minimum package of public health services is ensured in each locality.

The federal government provides significant funding for preventive programs around maternal health, early child development, and nutrition. There is less funding available for mental and behavioral health services, but these programs are starting to expand. Despite the commitment to support populations in need, significant variations remain in the extent of support among states, and investments are insufficient to reach all who would be eligible for the programs. Another consideration is whether program requirements are appropriately flexible to accommodate specific community needs. This chapter presented several strategies for increasing resources and reinvestment in preventive activities aimed at improving child and community health.

Public health defined broadly goes beyond government public health departments and requires collaboration across sectors. Substantial and lasting improvements in population health can be achieved only through collaborative efforts with shared goals between the health care systems and public health efforts. Nonprofit hospitals and health care systems can focus their community benefit dollars to pursue long-term strategies for building healthier neighborhoods and advancing upstream initiatives aimed at mitigating the root causes of poor health and wellbeing, especially in low-income communities. Health care systems and government health agencies can be anchors and advocates for the equitable expansion of high-quality care and services, responsive to health-related social needs in the communities they serve.

8

Opportunities for Health Promotion and Disease Prevention in Schools

[There's] need for a robust school-based health center network to provide basic access to preventive services. Children in inner cities and poor rural areas might not have [. . .] access to a doctor.

—Comment to committee from health care consultant,
Queens, New York

Schools are an opportune setting in which to advance child and adolescent health because children spend so much of their time there. They provide a central focus and experience for children and youth—unlike any set of institutions for other age groups. By offering services in schools, the health care system can meet children, youth, and families where they are, reducing burdens many families face when navigating inequities in geographic or financial access to health care providers and care. Some schools provide substantial amounts of preventive health and treatment services for children and youth, including health and socioemotional education programs, school nursing, school-based health centers, and various counseling and mental health prevention and treatment programs. In addition, 94% of public and private schools participate in national school breakfast and lunch programs and provide nutritious meals to nearly 30 million children in the United States (U.S. Department of Agriculture [USDA], 2023b). Schools may also assist in outreach and enrollment of eligible children in public health insurance and income support programs.

In some schools, health care has been delivered in a universal manner to all children and in a targeted manner to those who have been identified by teachers, school nurses, and counselors as being at risk. Teachers may deliver curricular content around socioemotional wellness, physical fitness, nutrition, reproductive health, and substance abuse prevention. School nurses may address acute illnesses and injuries, provide medication management, implement and advance public health campaigns, and coordinate health care with families and health care professionals. And counselors (depending on the type) may deliver individualized mental health counseling, support socioemotional wellbeing through class lessons, and assist in mental health crisis response. School-based health centers may provide preventive, reproductive, and mental health care (Allison et al., 2007; Juszczak, Melinkovich, & Kaplan, 2003; School-Based Health Alliance [SBHA], 2014). The availability of these services varies greatly across schools.

Evidence shows that when schools adopt or offer these opportunities, both health and education outcomes can be improved and disparities narrowed (Community Preventive Services Task Force, 2016a,b; Connor et al., 2024; Koening et al., 2018; Ran, Chattopadhyay, & Hahn, 2016). The committee sees great promise in leveraging schools and other community resources to expand their provision of critical prevention and promotion services for young children; preparation for adolescence and learning healthy living and sexuality; substance abuse prevention; and management of low-severity acute illnesses and comanagement of chronic conditions, such as asthma, diabetes mellitus, anxiety, and depression. Furthermore, teachers and coaches are present in children's day-to-day lives and, if supported, can provide essential safe, stable relationships for children and youth with adults.

This chapter highlights the important bidirectional connections between education and health and highlights the existing role of schools in children's health. It concludes with opportunities for augmenting this role to strengthen the provision of services in schools to promote improved health and wellbeing.

CONNECTIONS BETWEEN EDUCATION AND HEALTH

Schools offer more than education. In partnership with health care and other sectors, schools seek to help children prepare to enter adulthood; to create a healthy and productive life; and to optimize their potential to meet their economic and social needs, maintain and improve their own health, and contribute to the workplace and the community. Health outcomes and educational achievement have shown to be correlated in a number of ways in the literature. Healthier students are better, more engaged learners (Basch, 2011). Educational achievement is tied to improved long-term health and economic productivity; the measure of years of completed schooling has a strong causal connection with higher earnings and other important measures of life success and wellbeing, and thus with economic mobility in adulthood (National Academies of Sciences, Engineering, and Medicine [National

Academies], 2023g). Conversely, low academic achievement is strongly associated with risk-taking behavior, compromised health status, and reduced longevity (Braveman, Ergerter, & Williams, 2011; Lande et al., 2003).[1]

However, in the United States, research shows that just 42% of children between the ages of 3 and 5 years are considered to be "healthy and ready to learn" across four domains, suggesting that most children are at risk and in need of additional supports (Ghandour et al., 2021). A range of factors impacts school-readiness results, including parent mental health status, adverse childhood experiences, and access to neighborhood amenities such as parks and libraries. Additionally, children exposed to adverse childhood experiences (39% of children ages 0–17 years) are substantially and significantly more likely to fail to be ready for school, miss 2 or more weeks of school in a year, repeat a grade in school, and lack resilience (Jackson, Testa, & Vaughn, 2021; Lipscomb et al., 2021). School absenteeism has worsened markedly since the pandemic, with an increase of chronic absenteeism (defined as missing 10% of the school year), from 15% before the pandemic to an estimated 26% of public students in most recent data (Mervosh & Paris, 2024). In high-poverty districts chronic absenteeism was 19% prepandemic, soaring to 36% more recently (Return2Learn Tracker, 2023).

Illness and chronic physical and mental health conditions are common causes of school absenteeism, influencing academic success (Centers for Disease Control and Prevention [CDC], 2021a, 2024e). Children from low-income and racially or ethnically marginalized populations in the United States are more likely to develop chronic health problems than are more affluent and non-Hispanic White children and less likely to have a usual source of medical care (Bloom, Cohen, & Freeman, 2012). Children suffering from chronic conditions may have a harder time attending and completing school, and asthma and other chronic health conditions have been linked to lower academic achievement (Agnafors, Barmark, & Sydsjö, 2021; Basch, 2011; McLeod, Uemura, & Rohrman, 2012). For example, between 2018 and 2020, a median of 37.3% of children missed days of school because of their asthma, ranging from 26.6% in New Hampshire to 53.6% of children in New York (CDC, 2023a, 2024b). One study found that student-reported and school-based health center–recorded asthma explained 14–18% of student absenteeism, even after accounting for other health and social risks (Johnson et al., 2019).

Opportunities for supporting the wellbeing of children and youth in school in collaboration with the health care system and other sectors are missed too often. The American Academy of Pediatrics has suggested opportunities for pediatric professionals to identify children who have been

[1]It is important to note that deleterious health outcomes in schools are correlated with exclusionary disciplinary practices, including expulsion and suspension (Eyllon et al., 2022).

absent and to promote school attendance and address causes of chronic absenteeism (Allison & Attisha, 2019). Interventions that may contribute to school completion, such as services and programs to address mental health, substance use, violence, pregnancy, and school climate, also have evidence for improving health outcomes (Freudenberg & Ruglis, 2007). Moreover, students who drop out of school are not able to benefit from services such as school-based health centers, which have documented benefits including reducing health care costs (Ran, Chattopadhyay, & Hahn, 2016).

Continued and additional partnerships between health and education sectors can help to address these gaps and opportunities for children. Existing recommendations in the field call for implementing evidence-based strategies for promoting family resilience and parent–child connection and for building child and youth resilience, socioemotional capabilities, and children's capacity to persist in learning and achieving goals.

Moreover, given the relationship between health and education and the promise of schools as contributing to child health and wellbeing, indicators of school readiness can be used to reflect the health of young children (Ghandour et al., 2018) and as a measure of the performance of the children's health care system in the United States. The National Academy of Medicine's Perspectives paper *Vital Signs for Pediatric Health* (Kaminski et al., 2023) calls for using measures such as school readiness, high school graduation rates, and rates of school absenteeism as child health care system performance measures, intended to be achieved jointly in collaboration with families, schools, and the community (see also Johnson et al., 2019).

THE ROLE OF SCHOOLS IN CHILDREN'S HEALTH CARE

Schools play important roles in influencing the health of students and their parents, and sometimes even the surrounding community. They can facilitate public health insurance enrollment, provide nutrition and assist in combatting child hunger, and manage chronic conditions and promote health (CDC, 2021b, 2024e; Fabina, Hernandez, & McElrath, 2023). This section briefly describes each of these roles.[2] Delivery of care through school-based health centers and mental health services is discussed in subsequent sections.

Facilitating Public Insurance Enrollment

As discussed in Chapter 6, improving access to insurance and reducing churn in enrollment is an effective way to promote child health. Children with insurance not only have better access to care but also have better

[2]The sections that follow largely refer to *public* schools in the United States. Approximately 80% of U.S. children attended public elementary or secondary schools in 2021 (Fabina, Hernandez, & McElrath, 2023).

health outcomes, as discussed in Chapter 4. Enrolling eligible students in Medicaid or the Children's Health Insurance Program (CHIP) not only improves their health, enabling them to do better in school, but can have positive budgetary implications for schools.

State health officials can coordinate with school administrators and nurses to enroll eligible children in these programs. Connecticut's health insurance exchange, for example, partners with the state's departments of Social Services and Education to identify uninsured students in the public school system and conduct targeted outreach to their families. Florida's KidCare builds and maintains partnerships with school nurses and administrators to disseminate information about CHIP to the parents of potentially eligible children. North Carolina, Virginia, Arkansas, Massachusetts, and Missouri have similar programs, partnering directly with school nurses, and Wyoming engages school counselors and psychologists to assist in monitoring insurance status and conducting CHIP outreach (National Academy for State Health Policy, 2019). The federal government can match state and local expenditures for administrative activities, including outreach and enrollment (Tsai, 2022).

Recent federal efforts aim to reduce churn in Medicaid and CHIP programs. Effective January 1, 2024, Congress enacted a federal requirement for 12-month continuous enrollment for all children enrolled in Medicaid and CHIP (previously had only been a state option). Several states have also sought Section 1115 waiver authority to provide additional continuous enrollment protections for Medicaid and CHIP enrollees, particularly for children (Mann & Daugherty, 2023).

Improving Access to Nutrition and Combatting Child Hunger

Given the prevalence of food insecurity in households across the country, especially in those with children, school meals can be an important setting for positive interventions to address child hunger (National Academies, 2023g).[3] Food insecurity during childhood is associated with worse physical health (Gundersen & Kreider, 2009; Thomas, Miller, & Morrissey, 2019) and mental health (McIntyre et al., 2013), lower academic achievement in childhood (Jyoti, Frongillo, & Jones, 2005), and worse psychological distress and physical health during adulthood (Fertig, 2019). School meals (including breakfast, lunch, and snacks) help combat child hunger and can encourage healthy eating (CDC, 2024c; Ralston et al., 2008).

[3]"Food insecurity" is defined as "a household-level economic and social condition of limited or uncertain access to adequate food" and is monitored with regular household surveys (USDA, 2022). Although household food insecurity has fallen for all groups over time, children in poverty are still twice as likely (28% vs. 14%) to live in a household that has experienced food insecurity. As compared with White children, Black children are 3.5 times more likely and Latino children almost 3 times more likely to live in a household that has experienced food insecurity (National Academies, 2023g).

USDA administers the National School Lunch Program (NSLP), the School Breakfast Program (SBP), and the Child and Adult Care Food Program (CACFP) through state agencies that operate with agreements with school authorities.[4]

National School Lunch Program

The NSLP is a federally assisted meal program operating in public and nonprofit private schools and residential child care institutions; it provides nutritionally balanced, low-cost or free lunches to children each school day.[5] The NLSP offers free lunch for children in families living below 130% of the federal poverty level (FPL) and reduced-cost lunch to children whose families live between 130% and 185% of the FPL. In fiscal year (FY) 2022, the program provided 4.95 billion free or reduced-priced lunches to school children, serving roughly 30.1 million students; 94% of schools, both public and private, chose to participate in the program (NSLP, 2024). Children may be eligible for NSLP if their families also participate in the Supplemental Nutrition Assistance Program, or based on their status as a homeless, migrant, runaway, or foster child (Food Research & Action Center, n.d.a,b). They can also qualify on the basis of household income, Medicaid eligibility, and family size (Food Research & Action Center, n.d.b; Office of the State Superintendent of Education, n.d.). Students from ethnically marginalized groups participate in NSLP at slightly higher levels than White students, and students from low-income households participate at higher rates than those from higher-income households (Ralston et al., 2008).

Children receiving free or reduced-price NSLP lunches consume fewer "empty calories" and more fiber, milk, fruit, and vegetables compared with income-eligible nonparticipants. They also are more likely to have adequate average intakes of calcium, vitamin A, and zinc. In addition, the NSLP is associated with lower rates of food insecurity among households with children (Ralston & Coleman-Jensen, 2017).

---

[4]The Summer Food Service Program (SFSP) also provides free meals to children, typically in congregate settings, when school is not in session (e.g., the summer months or unanticipated school closures during the school year) in areas where at least 50% of children qualify for free or reduced-price school meals. According to Toossi and Jones (2024): the number of meals served through SFSP, total spending on the program, and program participation were lower in FY 2023 compared with FY 2022. Participation in SFSP was 2.2 million in July 2023 (the month when participation in the program typically peaks), 20.3 percent less than in July 2022, when SFSP sites were able to be located in all areas and to serve meals for consumption in non-congregate settings. Participation was also 19.1 percent less than in July 2019, before the pandemic. Throughout FY 2023, the program served 136.1 million meals at a cost of $546.6 million. These figures were 9.8 percent and 8.9 percent lower, respectively, than the previous year. (p. 15)

[5]See https://www.fns.usda.gov/nslp

School Breakfast Program

The SBP provides reimbursement to states to operate nonprofit breakfast programs in schools and residential child care institutions.[6] The Food and Nutrition Service administers the SBP at the federal level. State education agencies administer the SBP, and local school food authorities operate the program in schools (USDA, 2023b). Utilization of the SBP is notably lower than that of the NSLP. In 2019–2020, only 58% of students who used the NSLP also received school breakfast. This has been attributed to barriers such as stigma and a lack of clarity on eligibility among parents or outreach to eligible students and caregivers (Hecht et al., 2023).

Universal Free Meals Policies

Increasingly, states are passing laws providing universal free lunches in school to all students regardless of income level or eligibility. As of 2023, eight states[7] have passed Healthy School Meals for All policies (Bylander, 2023). Other states have temporary policies in place or have introduced similar bills. One of the biggest benefits of these universal programs are that more students participate in school lunch, which decreases stigma and ensures all students are satiated and ready to learn (Bylander, 2023).

Moreover, the Community Eligibility Provision of the NSLP allows schools that are serving more than 25% (40% prior to October 26, 2023) of students to be directly certified to receive free school meals through their participation in select other means-tested programs; these schools may also provide free meals to all students (Toossi & Jones, 2024).[8] In a systematic review, universal free school meals (breakfast and lunch) were shown to improve diet and academic performance and decrease food insecurity, and showed no negative impacts on body mass index. These outcomes were found in students from both low- and high-income households (Cohen et al., 2021).

Child and Adult Care Food Program

CACFP, also operated through USDA, offers meals and snacks to eligible children and adults who are enrolled for care at participating child care centers, day care homes, and adult day care centers. CACFP also provides reimbursements for meals served to children and youth participating in afterschool care programs, children residing in emergency shelters, and adults over age 60 or living with a disability and enrolled in day care facilities.[9]

[6] See https://www.fns.usda.gov/sbp/school-breakfast-program

[7] California, Maine, Colorado, Minnesota, New Mexico, Vermont, Michigan, and Massachusetts.

[8] See https://www.fns.usda.gov/cn/cep

[9] See https://www.fns.usda.gov/cacfp

In FY 2019 (before the COVID-19 pandemic), approximately 4.7 million children and about 137,000 adults received CACFP meals and snacks on an average day. In that year, the program served a total of about 2.1 billion meals at a cost of $3.7 billion. In FY 2020, these figures dropped to approximately 4.3 million child and adult participants daily, and nearly 1.6 billion total meals served, with total program expenditures amounting to $2.8 billion. However, in 2021 and 2022, program participation, total meals served, and expenditures rebounded to prepandemic levels, with daily participation among children and adults reaching more than 4.6 million, 1.9 billion meals served, and costs hovering around $3.8 billion annually. In FY 2023, CACFP served 1.7 billion meals, 8.9% less than in FY 2022, although spending on the program was $3.9 billion, about the same as in FY 2022. Although fewer meals were served through this program in FY 2023 compared with FY 2022, the federal reimbursement rate for each meal served was higher in FY 2023 than in FY 2022 (Economic Research Service [ERS], 2023a; Toossi & Jones, 2024).

ERS (2023a) found evidence that participation in CACFP by child care providers improves food security for households with children enrolled in the centers; it also found that participation improves consumption of milk and vegetables (State of Childhood Obesity, n.d.).

Health Promotion and Screening

Schools have direct contact with more than 94% of school-aged children, making schools a crucial setting for assessment of health needs through screening and health promotion programs.[10] For example, CDC's Healthy Schools initiative provides funding for programs that improve nutrition, enhance physical activity and physical education, and help students manage chronic conditions. These programs are implemented through partnership with nongovernmental organizations, state education agencies, school administrators and staff, and parents (CDC, 2024e). In addition to delivering preventive services, this funding has been used to support data collection and health surveillance through the Youth Risk Behavior Surveillance System and School Health Profiles.[11] (Box 8-1 provides more detailed information about the CDC Healthy Schools initiative.) This section describes some common school-based screening and health promotion programs. Mental health promotion and school climate interventions are addressed later in the chapter.

[10] The National Home Education Research Institute estimates that approximately 6% of U.S. children were homeschooled in school year 2021–2022 (Ray, 2024).

[11] See https://www.cdc.gov/healthyschools/index.htm

BOX 8-1
CDC Healthy Schools Initiative

CDC's Healthy Schools initiative works with states, school systems, communities, and nonprofit organizations to prevent chronic disease and promote the health and wellbeing of children and adolescents in schools. The initiative is built on the Whole School, Whole Community, Whole Child (WSCC) framework. The WSCC is student centered and emphasizes the role of the community in supporting the school and the importance of evidence-based policies and practices. CDC Healthy Schools aims to promote healthier nutrition options and education, comprehensive physical activity programs and physical education, improved processes and better training to help students manage chronic conditions, health education that instills lifelong healthy habits and health literacy, and practices that improve school health services and links to clinical and community resources.

According to CDC Healthy Schools (n.d.d):

> Healthy Schools supports 20 cooperative agreement recipients in the implementation and evaluation of evidenced-based efforts to promote the health and well-being of school-age children and adolescents in underserved and disproportionately affected communities. Cooperative agreement recipients include state education and health agencies, universities, and a tribal nation. CDC provides them with technical assistance and develops specialized tools, recommendations, and resources to help in the work they do for school health. (para. 1)

SOURCE: CDC Healthy Schools, n.d.d. See: https://www.cdc.gov/healthyschools/about.htm

Health Screening Programs

Many states mandate school health screenings by law; these most commonly include hearing and vision, but may also include screening of dentition, blood pressure, scoliosis, height and weight, and mental health. Screening identifies potential issues in need of follow-up, requiring coordination with health organizations. These screenings are often conducted by school personnel, including school nurses, or in partnership with health organizations. For example, the Vision to Learn program partners with school districts through memoranda of understanding, seeking to identify students with vision problems and connect them with the glasses they need to participate in school effectively. In FY 2022–2023, Vision to Learn provided approximately 2.6 million children with vision screenings, 491,000 children with eye exams, and 400,000 children with glasses. The program operates in 288 school districts in 15 states and Washington, DC (Vision to Learn, 2023).

Uncorrected vision issues can lead to poor focus and other issues, such as headaches and eye pain. But accessing vision services can be challenging for many families, so providing the resource children need in school settings not only removes the burden from the family but also reduces stigma and results in students doing better in school. Research has demonstrated that students who receive eyeglasses through school-based vision program have improved academic outcomes (Neitzel et al., 2021). While Vision to Learn receives most of its funding from private sources, it is working with Medicaid and CHIP to ensure that all children who need glasses can get them, regardless of income (Vision to Learn, 2022).

Physical Activity and Nutrition Education

Research shows that physical activity has a host of positive physical and mental health benefits for youth, such as reducing symptoms of depression and anxiety and improving mood (National Research Council [NRC] & Institute of Medicine [IOM], 2013); it also indicates a positive association between physical activity and academic achievement for adolescents (Esteban-Cornejo et al., 2015; Kristjánsson, Sigfúsdóttir, & Allegrante, 2010; NRC & IOM, 2013; Rasberry et al., 2011). Physical activity in youth has also been associated with positive psychosocial traits, including self-efficacy, self-concept and self-worth, social behaviors, and goal orientation (NRC & IOM, 2013).

The U.S. Department of Health and Human Services recommends 60 minutes or more of physical activity per day every day of the week. However, less than one-quarter (24%) of children aged 6–17 years participate in 60 minutes of physical activity every day. In a study conducted in 2017, only 26.1% of high school students participated in at least 60 minutes per day of physical activity on all 7 days of the previous week, only 51.7% of high school students attended physical education classes in an average week, and only 29.9% of high school students attending physical education classes daily (Carlson et al., 2013; CDC, 2011; Subcommittee of the President's Council on Fitness, Sports, and Nutrition, 2012).

The *Physical Activity Guidelines for Americans Midcourse Report* Subcommittee of the President's Council on Fitness, Sports, and Nutrition (2012) found evidence that multicomponent physical activity interventions in schools can increase physical activity during school hours. These interventions typically combine enhanced physical education with other strategies such as health education, classroom physical activity, social marketing initiatives, active transportation to school, and physical environment improvements, among others. When combined with community- and family-based interventions, they also show strong evidence of increasing physical activity for adolescents outside of school (Subcommittee of the President's Council on Fitness, Sports, and Nutrition, 2012).

Interventions for increasing active travel to school, especially the Safe Routes to School program, increase the proportion of students who walk or bicycle to school and decrease traffic-related injuries around school neighborhoods (Community Preventive Services Task Force, 2021). While there is not a comprehensive inventory of Safe Routes to School programs in the United States, the *2019 National Assessment Program Report* identified over 400 programs in 44 states and Washington, DC (Zimmerman & Lieberman, 2020).

Healthy nutrition is also essential. Some schools have addressed healthy weight through educational curricula and cooking classes for students and families, healthy school meals, and screening programs for identifying students at risk.

Managing Asthma and Other Chronic Conditions

Certain conditions, including asthma, obesity, food allergies, and attention deficit hyperactivity disorder (ADHD), may require primary care practices to coordinate care with schools and will require ongoing monitoring of students during the school day. Students need to be healthy and safe to be ready to learn.

There are missed opportunities to improve asthma care within the context of the child's community settings, including schools (Yee, Fagnano, & Halterman, 2013). Multifaceted interventions in community settings—including provider and caregiver prompts (Goldstein et al., 2018; Halterman et al., 2018), use of school nurses or community health workers to provide education and care coordination (Jonas, Leu, & Reznik, 2020; Taras et al., 2004), and mitigation of environmental triggers and other social determinants—have been effective in improving asthma preventive care and outcomes (Federico et al., 2020; Matsui, Abramson, & Sandel, 2016). School-based asthma self-management interventions for children and adolescents reduce asthma-related emergency department visits and hospitalizations and increase self-reported asthma-related quality of life (Community Preventive Services Task Force, 2019a; Hollenbach, Simoneau, & Halterman, 2022). For example, a school-based asthma management program calls for facilitating communication among the child, family, clinicians, and school nurses; creating an asthma management plan for the school setting; and assessing the school environment and remediating school-based asthma triggers (Lemanske et al., 2016). Other programs that ensure children have their asthma medications and administer controller medications at schools have been effective in reducing asthma exacerbations and increasing school attendance (Hollenbach, Simoneau, & Halterman, 2022).

Children with Disabilities

As noted in Chapter 4, an estimated 13.9 million children under age 18 years (19%) in the United States have a special health care need (Health Resources and Services Administration, 2023c). These children are more likely to live in low-income neighborhoods and rely more on public health insurance; over half also have a co-occurring behavioral or mental health diagnosis, such as ADHD or anxiety (Kids Count Data Center, 2023a). Within this population, about 85% of children are not receiving the health care needed, mainly because of cost (despite having public health insurance, which is often inadequate) and access (e.g., lack of available appointments to address their disability; Kids Count Data Center, 2023a).

Schools provide educational programs and services for children with disabilities, guided by the Individuals with Disabilities Education Act (IDEA, 2004), Section 504 of the Rehabilitation Act (1973), and Title II of the Americans with Disabilities Act (1990). The IDEA mandates that children with disabilities, regardless of income or disability severity, receive access to special education and related disability services, such as adaptive equipment; assistive technology; one-on-one aides; accommodations; counseling; psychological services; physical, occupational, and speech therapy; and adapted materials. Each child with a disability receives an individualized education program based on their needs, which includes a statement of the special education and related services provided to the child (Center for Parent Information and Resources, 2022; National Academies, 2018). More than 7.3 million U.S. children (ages 3–21) currently receive special education related to their disability under IDEA (Office of Special Education Programs, 2022).

Built Environment

The built environment and facility conditions of schools can also impact student health, especially students with chronic health conditions (Eitland et al., 2020). This relationship became even more salient in light of the COVID-19 pandemic. The average U.S. school is 42 years old, and many have heating, ventilation, and air conditioning systems that are outdated (Environmental Protection Agency, 2022). The Government Accountability Office (2020) estimated that over half of all public school districts needed to update or replace multiple building systems or features in their schools. However, capital funding for such improvements may be limited as funding for school facilities primarily comes from local property taxes. Low-income communities with limited local tax bases depend on state support for these types of repairs and updates, but not all states provide capital funding for schools (Government Accountability Office, 2020).

DELIVERING CARE: SCHOOL-BASED HEALTH CENTERS

In addition to the functions described above, schools can also be the site of health care delivery. Some children can obtain some level of health care services while at school, often through school-based health centers

(SBHCs), which can provide students with preventive, reproductive, and mental health care (Allison et al., 2007; Juszczak, Melinkovich, & Kaplan, 2003; SBHA, 2014). School-based services—including, for example, physical therapy, occupational therapy, speech pathology or therapy services, psychological counseling, and nursing services—may be provided by personnel employed by a school or local education agency, and Medicaid-covered health services may also be delivered to students by contracted community providers or SBHCs (Medicaid and CHIP Payment and Access Commission [MACPAC], 2024b). This section discusses the delivery of care through SBHCs; the financing of other school-based services is discussed in the sections below.

Some SBHCs provide primary care services, including well-child care and health maintenance; others provide psychosocial services, hearing and vision screening, reproductive health services, mental health services (e.g., screening and counseling), and/or oral health services. Evidence shows that, compared with access to traditional outpatient clinics, access to SBHCs increases the use of primary care; reduces the use of emergency rooms; reduces hospitalizations; and expands access to and quality of care for underserved adolescents, even those without insurance (Soleimanpour et al., 2010). SBHCs are also popular among adolescents, who report feeling more comfortable using them than using primary care settings (Mason-Jones et al., 2012). The American Academy of Pediatrics (AAP; 2021b) recognizes the critical role of SBHCs in many communities, emphasizing their importance in providing accessible health care to children and adolescents, especially in underserved areas. SBHCs are integral in filling gaps in health care for many of the nation's children, focusing on health services provision and the promotion of health through population-based education programs (AAP, 2021b).

As of 2021, there were 2,584 SBHCs serving students and communities in 48 states, and in Washington, DC, and Puerto Rico. In 2022, this number increased to 3,900 (SBHA, 2023a). Of this number, nearly half served elementary schools, with 18% serving high schools, 14% serving middle schools, and 21% representing other mixed school models. Most provide in-person services, but the percentage of SBHCs that provide some telehealth services has grown (SBHA, 2023a). While there has been growth in the number of SBHCs over the past 20 years, only about 13% of U.S. students in public schools have access to one (Love et al., 2019). Among existing SBHCs, there is variability in the comprehensiveness of services, student body enrollment rates, and parental trust (Nahum et al., 2022).

SBHCs play an important role for underserved adolescents and can greatly increase access for underinsured and uninsured children and youth and others who find care hard to access, including those living in rural areas (Mason-Jones et al., 2012). SBHCs increase access to care by removing geographic or transportation barriers, addressing financial barriers for uninsured or underinsured students, and in some rural areas connecting students to providers in areas with otherwise limited or no access to medical providers (Kjolhede et al., 2021). According to the National School-Based Health Care Census (Love et al., 2019):

> On average, compared to schools without access to SBHCs, those with access had higher percentages of Black (24 percent versus 14 percent) and Hispanic (38 percent versus 22 percent) students enrolled. They also had a higher percentage of students who received free or reduced-price lunch (70 percent versus 53 percent). Furthermore, 77 percent of schools with access to SBHCs were eligible for Title I funding, compared to 67 percent of schools without access (data not shown). The Title I program provides financial assistance to schools with high percentages of children from low-income families. (p. 759)

SBHCs vary across the country in several ways. According to the SBHA (2023b), survey responses in 2023 across 33 states demonstrated differences in how SBHCs are supported, such as how they are defined, how funding is allocated, and alignment with national performance measures. In 2016–2017, 82% of the centers were traditional, 4% were school linked, 3% were mobile, and 12% were telehealth exclusive. The number of centers reporting any use of telehealth technology, regardless of delivery model, grew from 66 in 2007–2008 to 467 in 2016–2017 (Love et al., 2019). In 2016–2017, 85% employed nurse practitioners and 40% of centers employed physicians. In 2016–2017, 65% of centers had behavioral health providers as members of the provider team—a smaller percentage than in 2007–2008, when the share peaked at 81%. Forty-one percent (41%) of SBHCs had expanded care teams, defined as having primary care and behavioral health care staff, along with one or more of the following: oral health providers (dentists, dental assistants, or dental hygienists), vision specialists, nutritionists or registered dietitians, and other coordinators. The proportion of centers that employed oral health providers increased from 9% in 2001–2002 to 28% in 2016–2017 (Love et al., 2019). Figure 8-1 summarizes the characteristics of SBHCs.

Effects of SBHCs on Health Outcomes

According to Knopf and colleagues (2016),

> substantial educational benefits associated with SBHCs included reductions in rates of school suspension or high school non-completion and increases in grade point averages and grade promotion (Barnet, Duggan, & Devoe, 2003; Edwards, Steinman, & Hakanson, 1977; Foy & Hahn, 2009; Kerns

Characteristic	1998-99	2001-02	2004-05	2007-08	2010-11	2013-14	2016-17
All SBHCs	1,135[a]	1,496[a]	1,709[a]	1,909[a]	1,930[a]	2,315[a]	2,584
In the analysis	781	1,049	1,252	1,095	1,381	1,737	2,317
No. of SBHCs reporting by delivery model	781	1,049	1,251	1,095	1,364	1,736	2,317
Traditional model	743	1,005	1,226	1,047	1,287	1,633	1,894
School-linked model	28	28	—[b]	35	48	47	87
Mobile model	10	16	25	13	29	52	69
Telehealth-exclusive model	—[b]	—[b]	—[b]	—[b]	—[b]	4	267
No. of SBHCs reporting by sponsor type	781	1,036	1,250	1,094	1,341	1,734	2,305
Federally qualified health center	155	185	276	311	448	750	1,181
Hospital or medical center	295	356	414	301	354	330	464
Nonprofit or community-based organization	68	117	147	97	85	170	218
Local health department	156	174	217	167	178	136	130
School system	79	140	173	128	151	204	146
Other[c]	28	64	53	90	125	144	166
No. of SBHCs reporting by geographic location	781	1,028	1,252	1,095	1,364	1,731	2,310
Urban	461	663	735	620	740	887	1,074
Rural	206	260	342	298	379	599	823
Suburban	114	105	175	177	245	245	413
No. of SBHCs reporting by populations with access[d]	—[b]	687	1,244	1,089	1,264	871	2,313
Students from other schools	—[b]	392	407	407	638	753	1,010
Family of student users	—[b]	320	355	290	471	594	740
Out-of-school youth	—[b]	186	201	239	417	548	658
Faculty or school personnel	—[b]	317	235	296	468	537	904
Other people in the community	—[b]	119	153	167	238	314	399
Any nonstudent population	—[b]	—[b]	—[b]	—[b]	1,264	871	1,442
No. of SBHCs reporting by members of provider teams	781	1,026	1,208	1,018	1,381	1,737	2,317
Primary care provider	312	318	388	198	403	570	816
Primary care and behavioral health providers	260	428	548	437	461	440	550
Primary care and behavioral health providers with an expanded care team	172	280	255	383	517	727	951
No. of SBHcs reporting by funding for SBHCs[d]	—[b]	—[b]	926	968	1,286	1,540	2,301
State government funding	—[b]	—[b]	659	735	960	1,092	1,365
Federal funding	—[b]	—[b]	—[b]	354	687	804	1,062
Millions of dollars allocated by state government	$61.9	$71.1	$63.8	$83.1	$90.0	$85.0	$91.3
States allocating funds to SBHCs	33	27	20	20	19	18	17

FIGURE 8-1 Characteristics of school-based health centers (SBHCs).
SOURCE: Love et al., 2019, p. 760.

et al., 2011; McCord et al., 1993; Strolin-Goltzman et al., 2014; Walker et al., 2010). Health care utilization also improved, including substantial increases in recommended immunizations and other preventive services, and a small increase in the proportion of students who reported a regular source of health care (Allison et al., 2007; Federico et al., 2010; Gibson et al., 2013). There were benefits to students with asthma, including reductions in symptoms and incidents (Guo et al., 2005; Lurie, Bauer, & Brady, 2001; Webber et al., 2003). Effects on self-reported health and mental health status were small; however, the presence of SBHCs was associated with substantial reductions in ED [emergency department] visits and hospital utilization for all conditions. Associations between SBHC exposure and risk behaviors were mixed, with apparent increases in cigarette smoking but reductions in consumption of alcohol and other substances. Regarding sexual and reproductive behaviors associated with SBHCs, contraceptive use among females increased, childbirth decreased, and prenatal care improved. (p. 8)

SBHCs also have the potential to reduce health disparities by providing services to students from diverse racial and socioeconomic backgrounds, particularly underinsured or uninsured students. For example, according to Kjolhede and colleagues (2021),

> School-based mental health interventions, including the area of substance use services, offer an opportunity to reach the greatest number of affected youth who otherwise may not receive behavioral health care. A study in California comparing the mental health risk profile and health use of SBHC users and nonusers demonstrated that SBHCs play a role in identifying and addressing mental health concerns that might otherwise go unmet, especially among adolescents with public or no insurance. (p. 4)

In an economic evaluation conducted by the Community Preventive Services Task Force, the economic benefit of SBHCs exceeded the intervention operating cost. For example, use of SBHCs resulted in a net savings to Medicaid because of a reduction in emergency department use for services provided to youth with asthma (Kjolhede et al., 2021; Ran, Chattopadhyay, & Hahn, 2016). SBHCs may also reduce parental productivity losses.

Future Needs for SBHCs

Integrating with Other Health Care Providers

Communication and data sharing with health care systems and federally qualified health centers (FQHCs) is needed to provide comprehensive and coordinated care. For example, the number of SBHCs using electronic health records (EHRs) has increased; EHRs can potentially improve accessibility and coordination of medical records outside of SBHC hours of operation. EHRs have the potential for linking SBHCs and students to community pediatricians, other health care systems, health information exchanges, and other primary care providers (Kjolhede et al., 2021). Confidentiality for adolescents and health information access and transfer are additional challenges for SBHCs. The SBHA and American School Health Association have developed guidelines and recommendations related to confidentiality and HIPAA and FERPA privacy laws.[12]

To further integrate SBHCs into health care systems, the AAP makes the following recommendations (Kjolhede et al., 2021):

- Pediatricians involved with the development and management of SBHCs should recommend care coordination practices that promote patient access to a medical home, with attention to communication

[12]HIPAA stands for the Health Insurance Portability and Accountability Act of 1996, Pub. L. No. 104-191, 110 Stat. 1936, which protects the privacy and security of health information. FERPA stands for the Family Educational Rights and Privacy Act, Pub. L. No. 93-380, § 513, 88 Stat. 574, which safeguards the privacy of student education records.

between health care providers across settings. Pediatricians should share their expertise to assist not already PCMH [patient-centered medical home] accredited SBHCs to adopt practice changes in support of the medical home model.

- SBHCs and community primary care providers should be in communication to facilitate coordination of care and to avoid duplication and fragmentation of care. Use of an EHR-compatible form or a paper form, such as the American Academy of Pediatrics emergency information form for children with special health care needs, should be used, with the goal of strengthening communication (p. 7).

Financing SBHCs

An additional challenge for SBHCs is the development of a financially sustainable business model, as SBHCs generally require multiple funding sources to remain operational. Most SBHCs are funded by a range of public and private sources, from local and state funding to federal block grants (e.g., Maternal and Child Health Block Grants) and project grants, FQHCs, and school districts billing the federal Medicaid program (SBHA, 2022, n.d.; see Figure 8-2). The percentage of centers that bill Medicaid has increased, from 68% in 2001–2002 to 89% in 2013–2014. Similarly, billing of public and commercial insurers increased steadily in the same period, from 43% to 71% for CHIP, and from 45% to 69% for commercial payers. State grants support 76% of centers, followed by federal grants (53%) and local government grants (42%) in 2013–2014 (Love et al., 2019).

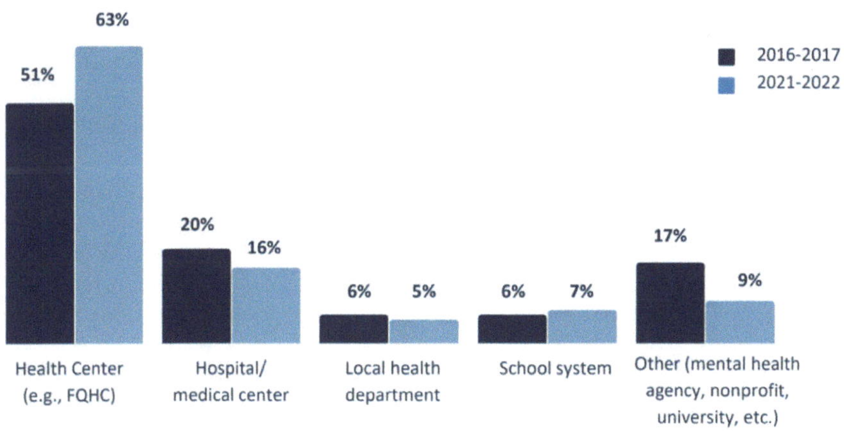

FIGURE 8-2 School-based health center sponsor types.
NOTE: FQHC = federally qualified health center.
SOURCE: Soleimanpour et al., 2023.

While there is variation across states and SBHCs, a 2017 survey of Medicaid offices across 18 states that provide dedicated funding for SBHCs identified three key policies that support their operation and success and grow SBHCs across the country (SBHA, n.d.).

First, seven states define SBHCs as a specific provider type, allowing differentiation of services provided at the SBHC from those of its sponsoring agency. This is helpful for directly attributing quality measures and improved health care outcomes.

Second, eight states waive prior authorization requirements for SBHCs, removing the burden of seeking permission from students' primary care providers to be reimbursed by Medicaid. Requiring prior authorization delays and limits care and affects the financial viability of SBHCs.

Third, state policies in Louisiana, Maryland, Michigan, and New Mexico require Medicaid managed care organizations to pay for self-referred visits by enrollees to the SBHC, even when out of network. This ensures payment to the SBHC even if it has no contract with the managed care organization.

DELIVERING CARE: MENTAL HEALTH SERVICES

School settings and resources can also be leveraged to address mental and behavioral health, as schools provide timely access to mental health screening and services in a convenient location (Hoover & Bostic, 2021; Kern et al., 2017). As discussed in Chapter 4, mental health concerns affect children and youth in every community across the country, with a notable uptick in deleterious mental health effects since the beginning of the COVID-19 pandemic (National Academies, 2022b, 2023c). Schools are increasingly recognized as an optimal setting for early intervention and prevention of child mental health problems, as they avoid many of the barriers to accessing mental health services in the community—providing a universal access point with the ability to reach more children who may not otherwise receive mental health support (Hayes et al., 2019; Hoover & Bostic, 2021; Neil & Christensen, 2009). School-based mental health programs can be universal (e.g., screening all students for mental health problems, programs that aim to build resiliency or mental health competence) or targeted (i.e., programs for children who are at risk of or are exhibiting symptoms of a mental health problem). There is great potential and evidence-based support for student educational curricula on subjects including suicide prevention (e.g., Sources of Strength), bullying prevention (e.g., STAC[13]), stress reduction and coping strategies (e.g., American Indian Life Skills), trauma, social media, conflict

[13]STAC is a bullying prevention program; the acronym stands for bystander strategies: Stealing the show, Turning it over, Accompanying others, Coaching compassion.

management, wellness, and mindfulness; some states now mandate education and screening programs (Holen et al., 2013; King, Strunk, & Sorter, 2011; Krantz et al., 2023; Midgett et al., 2020; Valido et al., 2023; Wyman et al., 2010, 2023). Peer interventions to address mental health have also shown potential for confirming the importance of youth voice and effectiveness in health promotion (e.g., Sources of Strength, Adapt for Life; Wyman et al., 2010). Teacher, school professional, and parent education in these topic areas have also proven successful in increasing support for students (e.g., Question, Persuade, Refer training, QPR Institute, n.d.). Finally, school climate and behavioral management programs (e.g., Good Behavior Game, Positive Behavioral Interventions and Supports) have demonstrated effectiveness in improving social, emotional, and behavioral outcomes and reducing exclusionary discipline and suicidal ideation (Kellam et al., 2011; Wilcox et al., 2008).

Research also shows that child mental health (including both mental health competence and difficulties) plays a critical role in shaping early learning experiences and outcomes; thus, interventions for promoting mental health among young children in educational settings can have benefits not only for their overall health and wellbeing, but also for their future academic success (O'Connor et al., 2018). In summary, evidence from systematic reviews on the impact and cost-effectiveness of school-based mental health interventions for children and youth is mixed; however, findings from countries including England and Australia suggest that a combination of universal and targeted prevention and early intervention approaches could have a significant impact if delivered in all schools (Stabile, 2023).

Guiding principles for an equitable whole child approach specify that transformative settings provide support in a tiered manner (Darling-Hammond & Cook-Harvey, 2018). The National Center for School Mental Health (2020) aims to improve the mental health and wellbeing of children and adolescents in school settings; it recommends a tiered approach to helping school districts implement mental health interventions: (1) mental health promotion services and supports; (2) early intervention; and (3) mental health treatment. In short, support needs to be provided on a timely basis for students identified with greater needs, including special education services, health and mental health services, and family supports. Box 8-2 describes a potential model for integrating mental health into school settings.

Universal Mental Health Programs and Policies

Screening

Screening for behavioral health concerns in schools is increasingly recognized as a vital component of early intervention and support for students'

BOX 8-2
Transforming Research into Action to Improve the Lives of Students (TRAILS)

The TRAILS program is built on the foundational belief that the education sector is an essential mechanism for overcoming barriers to mental health services for children and youth. Founded at the Michigan State University School of Medicine in 2013, the TRAILS nonprofit program was created to transform the landscape of youth mental health care delivery by providing school staff with the tools necessary to provide evidence-based and culturally responsible solutions to their students. The TRAILS team works in tandem with education partners to enhance mental health services available at schools by providing tailored school training, resources, assistance with implementation, and research-based preventive and mental health programs for children. This includes equipping educators, counselors, students, and communities with evidence-based mental health care approaches, such as cognitive-behavioral therapy (CBT) and mindfulness.

TRAILS is designed to provide partner schools with effective programming across three tiers of service: (1) social and emotional learning; (2) CBT and mindfulness; and (3) suicide prevention and risk management. The three-tiered TRAILS model aligns with the multitiered system of supports framework and the Positive Behavioral Interventions and Supports approach, which are evidence-based practices for providing students with academic and behavioral supports (TRAILS to Wellness, n.d.). Tier 1, social and emotional learning, trains teachers and student support staff using a five-unit curriculum focused on self-awareness, self-management, social awareness, relationship skills, and responsible decision making. Tier 2, CBT and mindfulness, trains school mental health professionals

wellbeing (Substance Abuse and Mental Health Services Administration, 2019). Using validated screening tools in education settings allows for the identification of mental health concerns at an early stage, enabling timely interventions and access to appropriate resources. It can also lead to improved academic outcomes and reduced behavioral problems. By integrating mental health screening into routine school health assessments, educators and health care professionals can help create a supportive environment that promotes the holistic wellbeing of students. While universal screening for academic concerns is typical, most school districts are not employing the same methods for behavioral health concerns (Wood & McDaniel, 2020).

One study of high school students in Pennsylvania found that youth in the universal screening group had nearly six times higher odds of being identified with depression symptoms and more than twice the odds of starting depression treatment compared with those in the targeted screening group (Guo & Jhe, 2021). Another study found that training school nurses (e.g., counselors, social workers) with seven- or ten-session manuals designed to help students cope with symptoms of depression and/or anxiety, using coping mechanisms such as mindfulness, relaxation, cognitive coping, behavioral activation, and exposure. Tier 3, suicide prevention and risk management, trains partners on the implementation of the TRAILS Student Suicide Risk Management Protocol, a clear set of steps for responding to and coordinating care for suicidality in students. This tier offers audience-specific training options for all school staff, families, and community members.

A growing body of evidence supports adoption of the TRAILS program. The seminal TRAILS study by Rodriguez-Quintana, Walker, and Lewis (2021) focused on the impact of the TRAILS Coping with COVID-19 manual, which was grounded in CBT and mindfulness. This manual offered strategies for helping students cope with pandemic-related uncertainty using a three-step model: (1) identify which portions of the situation are within one's control, (2) acknowledge and accept feelings about things beyond one's control, and (3) identify strategies to plan for or proactively address any portions of the situation that are within one's control. This resulted in increased use of CBT among school mental health professionals and significant decreases in student depression and anxiety (Rodriguez-Quintana, Walker, & Lewis, 2021). A secondary, 3-year study of 968 high school students by Smith, Almirall, and colleagues (2022) found that one-quarter of students showed a significant reduction in symptoms of depression and anxiety. TRAILS is an example of effective, school-based mental health services that can be accessed and tailored to schools across the nation. With wider adoption, this program could provide transformative care through evidence-based, sustained mental health support for students.

SOURCE: Elizabeth Koschmann, presentation to committee, June 2023.

to recognize depression allowed prompt referral of students for treatment (Law, McClanahan, & Weismuller, 2017).

Additionally, screening for eating disorders in adolescents is an important consideration because of the alarming prevalence and severe consequences associated with these conditions. Adolescence is a critical period for the development of eating disorders, with many cases emerging during this time. Early detection is critical, as eating disorders—such as anorexia nervosa, bulimia nervosa, and binge-eating disorder—can lead to numerous physical and psychological complications. Disordered eating is common, with more than one in five children and adolescents showing symptoms of disordered eating. Furthermore, eating disorders can have devastating long-term consequences, affecting not only physical health but also psychological wellbeing. Adolescents with untreated eating disorders are at heightened risk of developing comorbid mental health conditions, including depression, anxiety, and substance use disorders.

Socioemotional Learning

Consensus is growing among researchers who study child development, education, and health that socioemotional skills are essential to learning and life outcomes (National Academies, 2023c). Broadly speaking, "socioemotional learning" refers to the process through which individuals learn and apply a set of social, emotional, and related skills, attitudes, behaviors, and values that help direct their thoughts, feelings, and actions in ways that enable them to succeed in the settings where they learn and grow (e.g., Jones et al., 2017). Furthermore, research indicates that high-quality, evidence-based programs and policies that promote these skills among children can produce positive outcomes, including improved behavior, attitudes, physical and mental wellbeing, academic achievement, and college and career readiness and success (Bierman et al., 2010; Diamond & Lee, 2011; Durlak et al., 2011; Hurd & Deutsche, 2017; Jones et al., 2017; McClelland et al., 2017).

A great number of socioemotional programs are available for schools and early childhood education providers; these programs vary widely in emphasis, teaching strategies, implementation supports, and general approach. For example, some programs target emotion regulation and prosocial behavior, while others focus on executive function, growth mindsets, character traits, or other similar constructs. Some programs rely primarily on teacher modeling and whole-class discussions, while others incorporate such methods as read-alouds, games, role-playing, and music. Programs also vary substantially in their emphasis and material support for adult skill-building, school culture and climate, family and community engagement, and other components beyond direct child-focused activities or lessons.

There have been a small number of large multiprogram studies and trials of specific interventions in preschool, school, and afterschool contexts. Results from these studies are mixed. For example, large-scale, multisite, national studies show small or null effects (e.g., Social and Character Development Research Consortium, 2010), but many smaller, single-site studies report important and meaningful effects (e.g., Jones, Brown, & Lawrence Aber, 2011). Specific socioemotional learning interventions have been the subject of randomized trials; for example, a randomized trial of the RULER[14] program (see, e.g., Rivers et al., 2013) demonstrated changes in children's emotional competencies (Hagelskamp et al., 2013). The MindUp program emphasizes self- and physiological regulation and has showed positive results in children's cognitive and emotional regulatory skills (Schonert-Reichl et al., 2015).

In general, socioemotional learning programs tend to have the largest effects among students with the greatest number of risks or needs, including

[14]RULER stands for Recognizing, Understanding, Labeling, Expressing, and Regulating emotions.

those of lower socioeconomic status and those who enter school behind their peers either academically or behaviorally (e.g., Jones, Brown, & Lawrence Aber, 2011).

Schools, early childhood education settings, and out-of-school-time programs provide a unique opportunity to build students' socioemotional skills; address trauma, including that specific to pandemic experiences; and move toward educational equity. Currently, there are few evidence-based programs or interventions that successfully integrate these three areas, which can lead to unintended consequences, including focusing on student deficits rather than leveraging student assets and building on the rich experiences, knowledge, skills, and curiosity that students bring into the classroom (Ginwright, 2018; Zacarian, Alvarez-Ortiz, & Haynes, 2017).

Promoting Positive School Climate and Educator Wellbeing

Research has documented that a lack of mental health and wellbeing (e.g., depression, stress) of teachers affects their perceptions of children (Gilliam, 2005; Perry et al., 2008, 2010). Many studies on classroom climate have reported that the absence of responsive, supportive interactions with adult caregivers strongly affects young children's socioemotional functioning (Gilliam et al., 2016; Jones Harden & Slopen, 2022; Pianta & Hamre, 2009).

Mental health consultation is an approach for early childhood that focuses on adults working in classrooms with young children (Cohen & Kaufmann, 2000; Donohue, Falk, & Provet, 2000). Many of these programs are supported by school psychologists and other mental health personnel, who help teachers develop the capacity to provide socioemotional support in the classroom and address the individual mental health needs of vulnerable children (Splett et al., 2013). For example, the Center of Excellence for Infant and Early Childhood Mental Health Consultation (IECMHC) provides consultation to Head Start programs, classroom staff, and families (Ash, Mackrain, & Johnston, 2013; Brinamen, Taranta, & Johnston, 2012; Duran et al., 2009). At the program level, IECMHC consultants collaborate with administrators to develop policies and procedures (e.g., disciplinary policies, communication strategies, professional development opportunities) that promote children's socioemotional competence and a positive climate. IECMHC consultants support teachers in classrooms in the use of positive behavior supports and strategies for managing their classrooms and addressing the needs of specific children. IECMHC consultants may also collaborate with teachers and parents to create supports for children already showing challenging behavior, which may result in fewer child suspensions and expulsions.

Studies have shown that IECMHCs lead to improved socioemotional competence and reduced behavior problems among participant children (National Academies, 2023c). IECMHC is also associated with improved teacher–child relationships and classroom climate. Participating teachers have less stress and better skills in teaching socioemotional lessons. One study found that participation in an IECMHC program attenuated the association between teacher depression and child expulsion (Silver & Zinsser, 2020). At the school level, IECMHC has led to lower suspension and expulsion rates, less teacher turnover, and better staff interactions. And parents participating in IECMHC displayed better relationships with their children and missed fewer work days (Brennan et al., 2008; Center of Excellence for IECMHC, 2021; Hepburn et al., 2013; Perry et al., 2010; Substance Abuse and Mental Health Services Administration, 2014). Overall, these findings suggest that IECMHC programs can reduce disparities in mental health outcomes and the sequelae of these outcomes (e.g., suspension, expulsion; Center of Excellence for IECMHC, 2021; Shivers, Faragó, & Gal-Szabo, 2022).

Universal Cognitive-Behavioral Therapy

The Community Preventive Services Task Force recommends both universal and targeted school-based CBT programs for reducing depression and anxiety symptoms among children at risk. Universal CBT programs are delivered to all students in a school setting, regardless of their mental health status. They are geared toward helping students regulate their emotions and establish helpful coping strategies (The Community Guide, 2019a,b). Targeted interventions are provided to children who have been identified as at risk, not children who have already been given a clinical diagnosis. For the targeted programs, 29 studies show evidence that small decreases were reported for symptoms of depression and anxiety; the effect was larger when the intervention was delivered by external mental health professionals rather than trained school staff (The Community Guide, 2019b). Most important, incorporating mental health programming within school settings has been associated with improved academic outcomes, including grades, attendance, and test scores (Kase et al., 2017).

Federal Support for School-Based Mental Health Services

Federal funding for public schools to support direct mental health and socioemotional services has expanded over time. For example, in February 2023, the U.S. Department of Education (ED) announced expanded funding, through the Bipartisan Safer Communities Act (BSCA, 2022), for the School-Based Mental Health Services Grant Program, which provides funding to increase the number of school psychologists, counselors, and other mental health professionals serving students through "recruitment and retention efforts, the promotion of re-specialization and professional retraining of existing mental health providers, and through efforts to increase the diversity and cultural and linguistic competency of school-based mental health services providers" (ED, 2023, para. 9). In addition, the American Rescue Plan Act's Elementary and Secondary School Emergency Relief (2021) "provides more than $122 billion to help pre-K through grade 12 students recover from lost time in schools by supporting their mental health, as well as their social, emotional, and academic needs" (§ 2001). Allowable uses for this funding include "providing mental health services and supports, including through the implementation of evidence-based full-service community schools" (American Rescue Plan Act, 2021, § 2001).

SCHOOL-BASED HEALTH CARE WORKFORCE

School-based health providers play a role in supporting the health and wellbeing of children, youth, and families. Other providers offer different forms of health care in K–12 schools, including school psychologists, social workers, and counselors. These can play a critical role, supporting student development and success across socioemotional and academic domains. Not all schools have access to these providers. This section also briefly discusses the role of school nurses, who provide clinical services to children in schools.

It is also important to note that innovative programs at the state level have been implemented to train and credential students to work directly with their peers in school—for instance, in programs that provide suicide awareness training or knowing when to talk with a trusted adult (see, e.g., Muehlenkamp & Quinn-Lee, 2023). Two recent global systematic reviews of school-based peer-led interventions found that these interventions appear to demonstrate evidence for effectiveness, suggesting peer-led interventions may be a promising strategy for health improvement in schools, particularly for improving health-related knowledge (Dodd et al., 2022; King & Fazel, 2021). As more states and schools implement such programming, robust evaluation to understand key implementation considerations is needed.

An estimated 132,300 school nurses care for children in U.S. schools (Willgerodt, Brock, & Maughan, 2018). School nurses are frontline health care providers, serving as a bridge between the health care and education systems. They engage school communities, parents, and health care providers to promote wellness and improve health outcomes for children. School nurses can provide for the health and safety needs of students and staff or act as care coordinators for the increasing number of children with complex medical needs attending public schools. They can also provide more universal health-promoting activities, such as screenings and immunization, or organize wellness programming for students and staff. School nurses also assist students and parents with health insurance enrollment and obtaining access to health care providers (Gustafson, 2005). The National

Association of School Nurses (NASN) and the AAP recommend that school districts provide a full-time school nurse in every school building (Council on School Health et al., 2016). Box 8-3 describes the core elements of the school nursing practice framework as articulated by the NASN.

School nurses are essential for expanding access to high-quality health care for students, especially in light of the increasing number of students with complex health and social needs. Access to school nurses helps increase health care equity for students. "For many children living in or near poverty, the school nurse may be the only health care professional they regularly access" (National Academies, 2021e, p. 108).

However, only 65.7% of public schools in the United States have access to a full-time school nurse, a number that varies based on location (Willgerodt, Brock, & Tanner, 2023). Many school nurses rotate among

BOX 8-3
School Nursing Practice Framework

According to NASN (2024), four interlocking elements are present in the school nursing practice framework.

Care Coordination

- Provide direct care for emergent, episodic, and chronic mental and physical health needs.
- Connect student and family to available resources.
- Collaborate with families, school community, mental health team (including school counselors, social workers, and psychologists), and medical home.
- Develop and implement plans of care.
- Foster developmentally appropriate independence and self-advocacy.
- Provide evidence-based health counseling.
- Facilitate continuity of care with family during transitions.

Leadership

- Direct health services in school, district, or state.
- Interpret school health information and educate students, families, school staff, and policy makers.
- Advocate for district or state policies, procedures, programs, and services that promote health, reduce risk, improve equitable access, and support culturally appropriate care.
- Engage in and influence decision making within education and health systems.
- Participate in development and coordinate implementation of school emergency or disaster plans.
- Champion health and academic equity.

buildings and may have to cover two to three schools in a day or week. For example, 70% of urban schools employ a full-time nurse, whereas only 56% of rural schools employ a full-time school nurse. There are also regional differences, with the Northeast and South having the highest rate of full-time school nurses. Conversely, the West has the lowest rate at 33%, and approximately half of these work only part time (Willgerodt, Brock, & Tanner, 2023). There are also small variations in the distribution of school nurses by level of school, with high schools having slightly less coverage by either full- or part-time school nurses when compared with primary and middle schools (75% vs. 86% and 87%, respectively; Spiegelman, 2020). The current distribution of school nurses points to an equity gap across socioeconomic and geographic areas (Gratz et al., 2023). Until the workforce and funding streams support the goal of having a nurse in

- Share expertise through mentorship/preceptorship.
- Practice and model self-care.

Quality Improvement

- Participate in data collection for local, state, and national standardized data sets and initiatives.
- Transform practice and make decisions using data, technology, and standardized documentation.
- Use data to identify individual and population-level student needs, monitor student health and academic outcomes, and communicate outcomes.
- Engage in ongoing evaluation, performance appraisal, goal setting, and learning to professionalize practice.
- Identify questions in practice that may be resolved through research and evidence-based practice processes.

Community/Public Health

- Provide culturally sensitive, inclusive, holistic care.
- Conduct health screenings, surveillance, outreach, and immunization compliance activities.
- Collaborate with community partners to develop and implement plans that address the needs of school communities and diverse student populations.
- Teach health promotion, health literacy, and disease prevention.
- Provide health expertise in key roles in school, work, and community committees/councils/coalitions.
- Assess school and community for social and environmental determinants of health.

SOURCE: NASN, 2024.

every school, the current school nursing workforce needs to be allocated to target specific groups of children that concurrently lack access to pediatric primary care services. According to an NASN survey, school nurse respondents (registered nurses) stated that almost half of their time was spent on care coordination (e.g., acute and chronic condition management) and only about one-quarter of their time was spent on community and public health activities (screening, vaccination, health promotion and prevention, addressing social determinants of health; NASN, 2022). This demonstrates an opportunity to improve the ability of school nurses to support both care coordination and public health activities.

School nursing services have been shown to be a cost-beneficial investment of public money (Wang et al., 2014), warranting careful consideration by policy and decision makers when resource allocation decisions are made about school nursing positions. In a study of 78 school districts, Wang and colleagues (2014) found that

> during the 2009-2010 school year, at a cost of $79.0 million, the ESHS program prevented an estimated $20.0 million in medical care costs, $28.1 million in parents' productivity loss, and $129.1 million in teachers' productivity loss. As a result, the program generated a net benefit of $98.2 million to society. For every dollar invested in the program, society would gain $2.20. Eighty-nine percent (89%) of simulation trials resulted in a net benefit. (p. 642)

School nursing services provided in this study had a higher balance of acute and chronic care than wellness efforts, which resulted in students remaining in school rather than having to be out of school to receive treatment from a health care provider.

In the United States, funding for school nurses largely comes from ED (Wang et al., 2014; Willgerodt et al., 2024). Other funders include Medicaid, health departments, special education funds, and grants. Medicaid offers a potential sustainable revenue stream to pay for school nurses, as schools may bill for certain services performed by school nurses for Medicaid-eligible students (requirements and reimbursable services vary by state). Currently, approximately 40% of school nurses/schools bill Medicaid (Willgerodt et al., 2024).

FACILITATING AND FINANCING SCHOOL-BASED HEALTH SERVICES

While increasing school-based services is likely to have positive effects on health and education, balancing time and focus for both academic activities and health and wellness activities can be challenging. With great attention to academic outcomes, school leaders and teachers may be reticent to use valuable classroom time for activities that do not directly improve academic achievement. Improved management of physical and mental health conditions, however, may reduce absenteeism and facilitate academic achievement.

Parents and guardians of school-aged children need to understand the current and potential benefits of integrating health and education. Although they may distrust schools and health care delivery systems and have concerns about data sharing, engaging parents and communities by demonstrating the conveniences and positives of such integration will be necessary to best serve children and youth.

Regulations related to data sharing can be a barrier to integrating health care and education. FERPA (1974) protects the privacy of student education records, and HIPAA (1996) protects sensitive patient health information from being disclosed without the patient's consent or knowledge. While education and health care share the goal of improving children's health and education, different interpretations of these regulations and lack of easy data sharing can make partnership challenging. Clarifying the mechanisms and memoranda of understanding related to data sharing would further the potential of integration.

As described above, schools vary widely in services offered and the degree to which their practices are evidence based. They also differ in funding sources. Some support comes directly from Medicaid but much of the funding also stems from state and local school funds and various federal sources; each funding stream is described in turn below. These sources lead to variations that can exacerbate racial and other health disparities because of the impact of structural racism on neighborhoods and communities and on the financing of schools. In a 2022 study, only 12% of public schools reported that they could successfully deliver mental health services to all student in need (Marceno et al., 2023).

State and Local Education Funds

The structure of general funding for public education affects allocations for school-based health services. Public schools are funded by a combination of state and local education dollars, with some support from federal funding. Federal aid on average represents less than 10% of public education dollars (Gordon & Reber, 2021). By contrast, 46% of school districts' revenue emanates locally, and 47% derives from state governments—with local property taxes and state sales and income taxes as primary sources—creating wide differences across districts in resource availability. Because the education system relies so heavily on community wealth, differences in resources reflect both the prosperity and racial divide in the country.

High-poverty, majority White school districts receive about $150 less per student than the national average; however, they receive nearly $1,500 more than high-poverty, majority non-White school districts (EdBuild, 2019).

Combined, federal, state, and local government resources support the salaries of public school–employed nurses, counselors, and other staff who provide health care with some or all of their time. Schools bill Medicaid for some health care services for Medicaid-eligible students; however, the extent and scope of Medicaid billing varies widely across schools, especially across urban and rural schools, school levels, and regions of the country (Willgerodt, Brock, & Maughan, 2018).

Financing School-Based Health Services through Medicaid and CHIP

In 2014, the Centers for Medicare & Medicaid Services (CMS) began allowing schools to use Medicaid for free school-based health care services. However, uptake of this policy has been slow (CMS, 2014; Healthy Students, Promising Futures, n.d.; Wilkinson et al., 2020). As of October 2023, 25 states amended their state plans or otherwise expanded coverage to include school-based services that are not part of an individualized education program or individualized family service plan (IEP/IFSP).[15] Of those, 18 states expanded coverage for all services identified as medically necessary, while the remaining states cover a more limited set of services, often including behavioral health care. In many cases, the primary motivation for these expansions was to improve access to services, particularly behavioral health care, and to obtain Medicaid payment for services that were already being provided to students enrolled in Medicaid without an IEP/IFSP (MACPAC, 2024b; Wilkinson et al., 2020).

More recently, CMS, in consultation with ED, has issued new guidance for improving delivery of services covered by Medicaid and CHIP in school-based settings (CMS, 2023c). Both agencies strongly encourage states and schools to expand school-based services to increase access to health care and meet Early and Periodic Screening, Diagnosis, and Treatment requirements. This effort is an important part of the Biden–Harris administration's work implementing the BSCA (2022), which charged CMS

[15]Until 2014, Medicaid payment for school-based services was limited to covered services identified in a student's IEP or IFSP, in accordance with the IDEA. In 2014, CMS clarified the policy that prohibited Medicaid payment for services provided to enrolled children if those services were available without charge to the community at large. This policy change permits states to pay for medically necessary services for any Medicaid-eligible student, regardless of whether those services are identified in an IEP/IFSP or provided at no cost to other students. In states that elect this policy, schools may seek payment from Medicaid for covered services provided to Medicaid enrollees without an IEP/IFSP in addition to maintaining their obligation to provide education and related services to students with disabilities under IDEA.

with expanding access to Medicaid health care services, including behavioral health services, in schools and reducing administrative burden for states and schools.

Moreover, in February 2024, CMS issued a new notice of funding opportunity to award $50 million in grants to states to implement, expand, and enhance Medicaid and CHIP funding of school-based health services (CMS, 2024b). The grants will provide 20 states with $2.5 million in funding over 3 years, with at least 10 grants reserved for states that have not yet expanded school-based health services to all Medicaid-enrolled children, regardless of whether those children have an IEP (CMS, 2024b).[16]

In addition, the BSCA (2022) required CMS to update the 2003 *School-Based Administrative Claiming Guide*, which delineates eligibility for reimbursement of school-based services. The updated guide focuses largely on ways to decrease administrative burden on schools. Schools now have the flexibility to use a prorated monthly payment of one-twelfth of the previous year's costs, instead of a fee-for-service reimbursement model. In states that calculate the total-year cost settlement using the Random Moment Time Study (RMTS), the updated guidance decreases the number of RMTS surveys that need to be completed by school providers by a factor of 6 (Close, 2024). The new CMS guidance appears to address several barriers to Medicaid billing and the expansion of services in schools, including those related to provider qualifications for school-based health services and RMTS. It also provides new options to reduce the administrative burden associated with interim claiming.

In recent years, Medicaid-supported initiatives have provided the opportunity to develop collaborative school-based programs to increase access to primary health services in schools and to run in parallel with youth programs promoting environments that improve psychosocial, emotional, and mental health, and overall wellbeing. One example is CDC's Whole School, Whole Community, Whole Child (WSCC) model, described in Box 8-1, which integrates physical and academic education; nutrition and health education; psychological counseling; social services; and engagement of the family, school, and wider community (CDC, 2023h). The WSCC model is student centered, emphasizing the role of community in supporting school and the connections between health and academic achievement. This model not only meets the need for greater emphasis on psychosocial and physical environments within school and learning, but also focuses on engaging students as active participants in their learning and health. The focus on family and community involvement seeks to create a bidirectional link among

---

[16]These 16 states are Arizona, California, Colorado, Connecticut, Georgia, Illinois, Indiana, Kentucky, Louisiana, Massachusetts, Michigan, Nevada, New Mexico, North Carolina, Oregon, and Virginia.

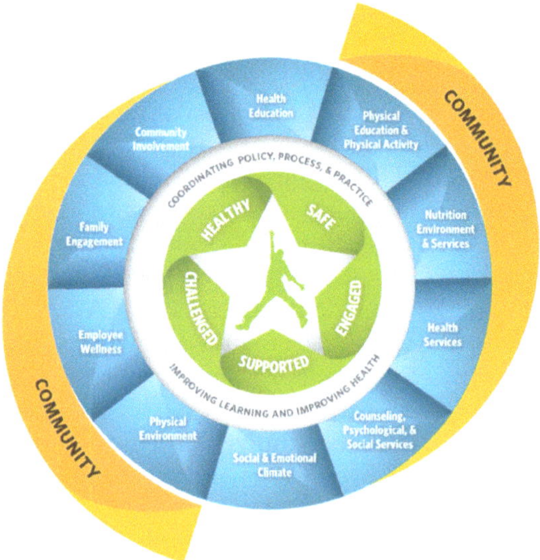

FIGURE 8-3 Whole School, Whole Community, Whole Child model.
SOURCE: CDC, 2023h.

schools, students, and families, and supports schools in contributing to the community and supports the community in contributing to student health and learning (see Figure 8-3).

This model supports innovation to increase the integration and effectiveness of school-based health services. Some of these innovations include greater telemedicine in SBHCs for expanded services (e.g., pediatric specialty consultation) with less need for lost school time. Models for increasing evidence-based practice in SBHCs and school-based mental health services are promising; these include training models from Extension for Community Healthcare Outcomes and learning health networks for measurement-based care. Further data sharing, joint governance (with health care and schools), and shared accountability for metrics can allow tracking and assessment of outcomes. Finally, embedding prevention and a developing climate of learning and wellness in schools offer promise for improving health and achievement of children and youth.

CONCLUSION

Schools can act as critical partners in advancing child, youth, and family health, as children spend a significant portion of their day in school, and schools are connected with local community groups and organizations that share the goal of seeing children and families thrive. Schools are being recognized increasingly as not just core educational institutions, but also community-based assets that can be central to building healthy and vibrant communities and transforming the health and wellbeing of children and families (National Academies, 2017a). Accordingly, schools are being incorporated into strategies for improving health care access, serving as hubs of health promotion and providers of population-based care (Maughan, 2018; National Academies, 2021c). There is an opportunity to expand and leverage the school setting for preventive care for children, health promotion and education, and the management of chronic conditions that continue to grow in incidence and complexity.

However, health services provided in schools vary significantly. The location of the school and the income level of its surrounding community, compounded by structural racism and historically biased policies, influence its effectiveness in delivering health services. There has been underinvestment in this area, and more support is needed to meet schools' potential for prevention, health promotion, and delivering health services with a focus on equity and improving services in places that need them most.

The committee highlights increasing the reach and comprehensiveness of SBHCs and increasing support for school nurses as key opportunities to leverage schools with the goal of improving children's health. There is considerable room for expansion of services within SBHCs and across schools and states, so that all children can benefit from the opportunities and health interventions that SBHCs offer. Additionally, rapid expansion over the past decade and variation in sponsorship across SBHCs warrant closer examination of quality and performance metrics, ensuring that variation in care delivery is minimized, that services are streamlined, and that the models are optimized. Reforms in current payment and incentives are also needed to facilitate expansion and ensure sustainability. (See the committee's recommendations in Chapter 10.) Moreover, recent efforts by CMS to expand coverage for all services identified as medically necessary for school-based services that are not part of an IEP/IFSP is an important step for improving access to services, particularly behavioral health care.

9

Measurement and Accountability

> *Implement performance measures that reflect "upstream" access as well as outcomes that meaningfully assess how populations experience health care delivery. Work to harmonize, or at least assure meaningful alignment, in outcome measures that are promoted by [federal programs].*
>
> —Comment to the committee by physician and medical director of integrated care, Boston, MA

To advance the vision for child health and wellbeing set forth in this report, enhanced accountability for child health and wellbeing at federal, state, and local levels is needed. Such accountability will require better and more effective measures, combined with more powerful incentives for the players involved. The United States already employs an extensive array of measurement and accountability approaches, each of which involves specifying performance goals, targets, and measures to confer rewards or withhold benefits for those being held accountable. While these efforts have resulted in some changes, taken together, existing approaches have not resulted in sufficient improvements in health care access, quality, equity, and outcomes for children and youth (Bethell, Blackwell et al., 2022; Centers for Medicare & Medicaid Services [CMS], 2024b; Lebrun-Harris et al., 2022; Schiff, Filice, & Chen, 2024).

This chapter reviews progress, gaps, and the impact of existing measurement and accountability strategies related to the child health care system, and outlines opportunities for improvement. The review considers broad characteristics of accountability measurement systems that would be needed to improve child health and wellbeing outcomes, drawing on the guiding principles detailed in Chapter 1 (see Table 9-1). In response to this review, the committee identified priority areas and opportunities for implementing an accountability measurement strategy that would support health care system transformation. These priority areas are discussed in depth after a brief summary of current strategies.

CURRENT MEASUREMENT AND ACCOUNTABILITY STRATEGIES

Health care is among the most regulated and measured of all sectors in society. In its research, the committee found that existing health care measurement and accountability strategies range from payers using quality and performance metrics to hold health care plans and providers accountable (Gardner & Kelleher, 2017; National Committee for Quality Assurance, 2023) to using metrics in licensing (Welch et al., 2017); certification (American Board of Pediatrics, n.d.; Miles, 2009); credentialing of health care professionals (National Academies of Sciences, Engineering, and Medicine [National Academies], 2017b); professional education program accreditation (Accreditation Council for Graduate Medical Education, 2023a); and accreditation of health plans, hospitals, and other health care facilities (Hussein et al., 2021; Joint Commission Resources, 2023; National Committee for Quality Assurance, 2023). Related to these strategies are efforts to report quality and performance measurement results to payers, patients, and consumers to engage market forces and drive performance improvements (Commonwealth Fund, 2022). In addition, the federal Government Performance and Results Act (1993) administered by the Office of Management and Budget (OMB) requires all federal departments and agencies to set and track performance indicators related to the achievement of strategic goals, many of which relate to child health and wellbeing (Government Accountability Office [GAO], 2023b,c; U.S. Department of Health and Human Services [HHS], 2023). Federal agencies also use performance measures to monitor many child health–related state and community programs that employ federal dollars (Bethell, Wells et al., 2023; Noorihekmat et al., 2020; Soto, Sicotte, & Motulsky, 2019)—these include Medicaid (Federal Register, 2023); Title V Block Grants (Kogan et al., 2015); community health centers (Cole et al., 2023); and home visiting (Health Resources and Services Administration [HRSA], n.d.c), early intervention (Early Childhood Technical Assistance Center, n.d.), child welfare (Administration for Children and Families [ACF], n.d.), nutrition, and early childhood education programs (U.S. Department of Agriculture, 2018, 2019, 2022). Other federal laws require nonprofit hospitals to assess and report on their efforts to provide charity care and partner with the local community to improve the health of the populations they serve, in order to maintain their tax-exempt status. Finally, numerous national, state, and local datasets and surveys of families

TABLE 9-1 Guiding Principles and the Characteristics of Accountability Measurement Systems

Guiding Principles*	Principles Applied to Measurement Strategies
Employ a Life Course Approach A life course approach requires a system-wide focus on prevention and promotion from preconception to adulthood, emphasizing upstream prevention of many health problems and promotion of healthy experiences.	Measuring the outcomes of all children and youth in a community and focusing on promoting functioning and wellbeing, rather than solely care processes or disease states, are the next steps to improve effectiveness of the health care system. Large health care systems with poor health outcomes for children in their communities cannot be said to be high-performing organizations. **Population health measures** would focus on promoting accountability for whole person and population wellbeing and allow for the assessment of health equity across various subgroups.
Partner with Families and Communities Family and community-centered care recognizes the importance of collaboration with families and communities, who are central to child health and wellbeing, in all stages of decision making.	Use of **measures salient and important to the community** is essential to ensuring that child health care systems are accountable to their communities and that communities engage fully in the coproduction of health care measures and improvements. Families and local organizations are essential partners in identifying ways to address social and relational health risks in their community (Bethell, Wells et al., 2023; Halfon, DuPlessis, & Inkelas, 2007; Palmer & Bailey, 2022; Petiwala et al., 2021). Further, measures of health care experiences and outcomes benefit from person-reported information (Arsiwala et al., 2021; Bethell, Blackwell et al., 2022; Bethell, Oppenheim et al., 2023; Co et al., 2011; Ghandour et al., 2018; Halfon, DuPlessis, & Inkelas, 2007; Office of the National Coordinator for Health Information Technology, 2023).
Prioritize and Drive Equitable Outcomes Moving toward health equity requires an intentional redistribution of focus, including resources and accountability, to families and communities that have long endured underinvestment and structural disadvantage.	Accountability for health equity needs to be featured either through parallel measures or through equity-weighted outcomes to ensure that all children are thriving (Agniel et al., 2023). Assessing disparities, discrimination, and experiences of structural racism typically requires person-reported information (Agniel et al., 2023; Calvert et al., 2022; Petkovic et al., 2017; Sisodia, Rodriguez, & Sequist, 2021). Seamless methods for collecting and integrating information and publicly sharing aggregated results will need to be created (Brands et al., 2022; Jenssen et al., 2023). **Measures that address health equity issues** of importance to community members could reflect, for example, rates of infant mortality and low birth weight, school readiness and engagement, positive mental health, and/or high school graduation.

(continued)

TABLE 9-1 Continued

Guiding Principles*	Principles Applied to Measurement Strategies
Make It Sustainable over Time Successful transformation depends on incentives and tracking performance on shared goals, ensuring transparency and open exploration of performance in partnership among health care systems, other child-serving sectors, and the families and communities they serve.	Improving population health and wellbeing outcomes for all children requires coordination within the child health care system and commitment and initiative between the health care, public health, and social services sectors. **Common goals and shared accountability measures** will be critical.

*See Chapter 1 of this report for a discussion of the committee's guiding principles in conducting research for the study report.
NOTES: The committee uses the term "population health" to refer to the health of a group of people, defined broadly. "Population" and "community" are used similarly to refer to a group of people with a shared characteristic, such as their geographic location, demographic status, health care system or provider, or even health diagnosis. The committee considers "health equity" to be the state in which everyone has the opportunity to attain their full health potential and no one is disadvantaged from achieving this potential because of social position or any other socially defined circumstance (National Academies of Sciences, Engineering, and Medicine, 2017a, 2021b). Multiple dimensions of outcomes could be considered in measuring progress toward health equity. Selection of appropriate measures will be tied to the population and improvements being considered.
SOURCE: Generated by the committee.

and youth are collected routinely and used to formally track and publicly report on child health care quality, outcomes, needs, risks, disparities, and overall system performance (Federal Interagency Forum on Child and Family Statistics [FCFS], 2022a; Jablonski & Guagliardo, 2005; Kogan et al., 2015).

Each of these measurement and accountability strategies plays an important role, with various strengths and infrastructure. Yet misalignment; limited numbers of population health and wellbeing outcomes; lack of adequate financial incentives; inefficiencies in data collection; limited data sharing; and failure to include patients, families, and communities adequately have prevented these numerous resources from being effective in achieving substantial improvements in child and youth health and wellbeing for many communities. Table 9-2 summarizes the various accountability strategies and opportunities for improvement.

Inadequacies of Current Measurement and Accountability Systems

Despite the enormous effort and resources employed to implement measurement and accountability strategies, their collective impact in improving children's quality of care and health outcomes has been slow and limited. Health care providers and systems typically report that current quality, safety, and accountability metrics are burdensome, often duplicative, and

TABLE 9-2 Overview of Existing Measurement and Accountability Strategies and Opportunities for Improvement

Existing Strategy Area	Key Opportunities for Improvement
Ensuring the quality of the workforce and health care organizations (e.g., professional licensing and certification, education, hospital and health plan accreditation, hospital community benefits standards)	Map standards used with objective performance and competence areas. Develop measures of diversity in workforce and community access.
Incentivizing high-quality care and positive outcomes (e.g., health plan and provider contracts using alternative payment models linked to measures of performance; federally required performance measures for Medicaid, community health centers, Title V, and other health-related state programs, such as home visiting and early intervention)	Focus and align performance measures across essential system collaborators, and link measures to drive shared goals for child and youth and wellbeing population outcomes.
Tracking and driving system-wide and federal agency performance (e.g., national datasets and surveys; Federal Interagency Forum on Child and Family Statistics; National Healthcare Quality and Disparities Reports (NHQDRs); tracking of federal agency strategies and performance indicators based on the Government Performance and Results Act (GPRA, 1993)	Coordinate and better disseminate annual federal *State of America's Children Report* and NHQDRs with a focus on aligned measures and child wellbeing outcomes. Coordinate across federal agency strategies and performance indicators tracked through GPRA to drive cross-agency efforts to improve child and youth wellbeing.
Engaging, activating, and partnering with consumers and patients (e.g., family engagement in systems and quality-of-care performance monitoring and improvement; public and consumer reporting of quality and performance with mechanisms for driving choice and action)	Advance family- and community-engaged governance structures; routinely collect and integrate family and community data into health care data systems; formalize use of lived experience stories; optimize use of digital health and interoperable data sharing within and among health care, public health, and community systems; and center family and youth reports of wellbeing, priorities, and quality of care.

SOURCE: Generated by the committee.

lacking incentive to focus the health care system on improving health outcomes (CMS, 2023b,f; Jacobs et al., 2023). Many prior recommendations point to feasible approaches for improvement that have yet to be widely embraced (Bass et al., 2022; Bethell, Oppenheim et al., 2023; Coker & Perrin, 2022; Garg et al., 2023; Landers et al., 2020; Institute of Medicine [IOM], 2012b; National Academies, 2019d, 2021b; Wiley & Matthews, 2017). These and other sources suggest that current approaches are inadequate for a transformed health care system in four ways.

First, the system centers largely on provider performance as a primary outcome, especially measures of care processes. Performance measures are employed mainly for compliance, accreditation, and training purposes at individual clinician, health care site, hospital, or health plan levels. The extensive focus on clinician and provider site behavior—without consideration of numerous other factors that affect child population health and without strong incentives and supports to improve on measures—limits their usefulness in improving outcomes for children and youth.

Second, quality assurance and accreditation accountability approaches engage health care systems directly in health care accountability initiatives but rarely include families or communities. Collection of data, planning efforts, data processing, and reporting efforts are centered in health care settings with little input from community members nor any consistent history of community participation or coproduction of quality planning or assessment. Reporting to patients, families, and communities on performance or child health is infrequently considered. In addition, few efforts have centered digital literacy and numeracy education for patients, families, and communities to improve their engagement. While most health care systems and accountability measurement strategies do not emphasize or effectively use person, family, and community measures of experience or outcomes (Austin et al., 2020; Bethell, Wells et al., 2023; National Health Law Program, 2021; Omoloja & Vundavalli, 2021), support for doing so is growing (CMS, 2023a,b; Schiff, Filice, & Chen, 2024).

Third, the actual measures employed in health care accountability are largely professional and site centered, as opposed to person, family, and community centered. A compliance and assurance mindset produces a clinician or health care organization orientation largely to the exclusion of community, patient, and family outcomes. In fact, such professionally oriented measures usually mean that performance is only judged among children and families that access services, while those without access are not included or reflected in denominators. Because of this, accountability results may misrepresent a best possible lens on health care performance without considering barriers to access and disparities. As an example, public and commercial payers often measure well-child visit rates and quality.[1] Yet wide gaps in both utilization and quality of well-child services persist (Bethell et al., 2004; Hirai et al., 2018; Schor & Bergman, 2021). Survey results estimate that fewer than half of children enrolled in Medicaid receive important well-child services recommended to occur in the critical first 15 months of a child's life and that performance has not improved in the past 10 years (CMS, 2022b). Similarly, only about one-third of young

[1]Measures include the proportion of all children who receive well-child services, based on the periodicity defined in the national *Bright Futures Guidelines* (American Academy of Pediatrics, 2017), which are the standard of care that health plans are required to provide through the Patient Protection and Affordable Care Act (2010), as specified in Section 2713 of the Public Health Service Act (Coverage of Preventive Health Services, 2023; HHS, 2023).

children receive screening for their development, and most families report not being asked about their concerns on their child's development (Hirai et al., 2018). Despite the existence of performance measures used to track well-visit rates, and rates of developmental screening, little progress has been made in states or local areas toward optimizing well-child services.

Fourth, measures and accountabilities among levels of the health care system and among sectors serving children are not aligned. Traditional health care accountability metrics offer little attention to coordination across sites, providers, or sectors. Even when similar performance topics are shared across programs (e.g., developmental screening, well-child visit rates), specific measures often are not aligned nor is the scoring, reporting, and dissemination of data resulting from the wide array of measures employed (Bethell, Wells et al., 2023; Boudreau et al., 2022; IOM, 2012b; National Academies, 2021b). For example, the federal government alone has numerous, often competing programs that aim to measure performance and outcomes for many, often overlapping, aspects of child health care or health, including (1) state Medicaid and Children's Health Insurance Program (CHIP) measures; (2) CMS-endorsed National Committee for Quality Assurance Healthcare Effectiveness Data and Information Set measures; (3) HRSA Community Health Centers measures; (4) Title V Block Grant National Performance and Outcomes measures; (5) ACF child welfare program measures; (6) HRSA/ACF Maternal, Infant, and Early Childhood Home Visiting measures; and (7) U.S. Department of Education Individuals with Disabilities Education Act Early Intervention program measures. A review of these programs, conducted through the Child Health and Development Project in its design of the Engagement in Action Framework (EnAct!; Bethell, Buttross et al., 2023), found that across the aforementioned programs, 309 specific performance measures were used, covering 71 unique topics; only 13 of these topics overlapped across three of more of these seven programs. Box 9-1 identifies the 13 performance measure topics that are used by three or more programs in four categories: insurance, access, and utilization; screening-related processes of care; treatment and counseling-related processes of care; and intermediate and health-related outcomes. See Appendix D for a full list of the performance measurement topics.

Other Efforts to Take Stock of Measurement Assets and Gaps

The 2004 report *Children's Health, the Nation's Wealth* was one of the first efforts to comprehensively take stock of child health measurement and data assets and gaps (National Research Council [NRC] & IOM, 2004). The report concluded that the nation is fortunate to have a wide array of data sources addressing the health of children and adolescents and health care quality for them, each providing a partial set of observations and benchmarks with which to answer questions of concern. However, it also

BOX 9-1
Key Performance Measurement Topics Used by Federal Child Health Programs

Insurance, access, and utilization

1. Adolescent well visits
2. Prenatal and postpartum care
3. Well-child visits
4. Receipt of dental care services
5. Well-woman visits

Screenings, referrals, and follow-ups

6. Early childhood developmental screening
7. Completed depression referrals
8. Tobacco, alcohol, or other drug cessation referrals/treatments for adults and/or caregivers
9. Depression screening

Care process, education, and counseling

10. Weight assessment, counseling for nutrition, physical activity

Health-related and intermediate outcomes

11. Low birth weight
12. Child and adolescent immunization status
13. Emergency department visits and injury hospitalizations

SOURCE: Generated by committee.

noted the incomplete patchwork of clinical information systems, periodic sample surveys, registries, and vital and health statistics reported by state and federal agencies and concluded that this patchwork does not facilitate the wholistic determination of either health status or health care quality for the nation's children and youth. The report's survey of existing datasets and methods reveals the need to create a national core set of salient measures; its authors suggested collecting data using these measures in every jurisdiction; using a standard approach for analysis; and making the data and analysis available in a form that will enable policy makers, health care administrators, health care systems, and the general public to evaluate progress on child health (NRC & IOM, 2004).

Box 9-2 provides an updated summary of the key national data sources important to understanding and driving improvements in child and youth wellbeing since the release of the NRC and IOM (2004) report.

BOX 9-2
Key National Sources of Data on Children's Health by Sponsor

U.S. Department of Health and Human Services

Centers for Disease Control and Prevention

- National Health and Nutrition Examination Survey
- National Vital Statistics System (NVSS)
  - Mortality (NVSS-M)
  - Natality (NVSS-N)
  - Fetal Death (NVSS-FD)
- National Health Interview Survey (NHIS)
- National Survey of Family Growth
- National Ambulatory Medical Care Survey
- Youth Risk Behavior Surveillance System
- School Health Policies and Practices Study
- Numerous online data query surveillance systems, for example:
  - WISQARS (injuries; https://wisqars.cdc.gov)
  - WONDER (mortality; https://wonder.cdc.gov)
  - NHIS Interactive Data System
- National Center for HIV/AIDS, Viral Hepatitis, STD, and Tuberculosis Prevention
- National Center for Immunization and Respiratory Diseases
- National Immunization Surveys

Health Resources and Services Administration

- Maternal and Child Health Bureau
- National Survey of Children's Health (NSCH)
- NSCH Online Interactive Data Query System (www.childhealthdata.org)

Agency for Healthcare Research and Quality

- Medical Expenditures Panel Survey and online data tools to access findings
- Kids Inpatient Database (KIDs) and online data query for hospital data
- National Consumer Assessment of Healthcare Providers and Systems Benchmarking Database

Substance Abuse and Mental Health Services Administration

- National Survey on Drug Use and Health

National Institutes of Health

- Patient-Reported Outcomes Measurement Information System

U.S. Department of Commerce

U.S. Census Bureau

- Current Population Survey and online data platform (Census Bureau, n.d.b)
- American Community Survey and online data platform (Census Bureau, n.d.a)

SOURCE: Child and Adolescent Health Measurement Initiative, 2023; analysis to update the data sources summary in *Children's Health, the Nation's Wealth* (NRC & IOM, 2004).

In addition, a growing number of online data query and dataset resources are now available to support analyses of national, state, and local measures that can inform and track the impact of health care system transformation efforts. This includes the numerous online dataset access and results query tools sponsored by the federal government (e.g., www.childhealthdata.org)[2] and an array of private-sector efforts (Brandeis University Heller School of Social Policy and Management, n.d.; KFF, n.d.; Kids Count Data Center, 2020; University of Wisconsin Population Health Institute, 2024).

The committee found evidence of progress since *Children's Health, the Nation's Wealth* (NRC & IOM, 2004) in the availability of important child health data, including the National Survey of Children's Health (Ghandour et al., 2018), data from the National Center for Education Statistics (McCoy, Cuartas, & Seiden, 2024), and new performance measurement systems (CMS, 2023a, 2024a; Kogan et al., 2015). Despite this progress, more recent efforts to evaluate the availability and effective use of measures, specifically maternal and child health measures, have arrived at similar conclusions as those in the 2004 report—population health outcomes, health equity, and community-level data and involvement, as well as alignment across child-serving systems, had all received inadequate attention in the development of measures. For example, the national, multisector, HRSA-funded Maternal and Child Health Measurement Research Network (MCH MRN), which operated between 2013 and 2021, took stock of maternal and child health measures and their use, identified gaps and strategic priorities, and took steps to create new measures and measurement resources (e.g., online searchable MCH Measurement Compendium; Child and Adolescent Health Measurement

[2]Online dataset access and results query systems that are led or sponsored by the federal government include (1) U.S. General Services Administration's Technology Transformation Services (federal independent agency)—performance.gov and data.gov; (2) CDC's National Center for Injury Prevention and Control—Web-Based Injury Statistics Query and Reporting System (https://wisqars.cdc.gov); (3) HRSA Maternal and Child Health Bureau's National Data Resource Center for Child and Adolescent Health—Child and Adolescent Health Measurement Initiative (https://childhealthdata.org); (4) CDC—Underlying Causes of Death Wide-ranging Online Data for Epidemiologic Research (https://wonder.cdc.gov); (5) Agency for Healthcare Research and Quality (AHRQ)—Healthcare Cost and Utilization Project (https://hcup-us.ahrq.gov/dataquerytools.jsp); (6) AHRQ—Online Data Tools for the Medical Expenditures Panel Survey (https://meps.ahrq.gov/mepsweb/data_stats/data_tools.jsp); (7) CDC's National Center for Health Statistics—National Health Interview Survey Interactive Data System (https://www.cdc.gov/nchs/nhis/shs.htm); (8) CMS—Medicaid Child Core Performance Measures Data and Reporting Resources (https://www.medicaid.gov/medicaid/quality-of-care/performance-measurement/adult-and-child-health-care-quality-measures/childrens-health-care-quality-measures/index.html); (9) HRSA—Title V Information System (https://mchb.tvisdata.hrsa.gov); (10) CDC—Healthy People 2030 Data (https://health.gov/healthypeople/objectives-and-data/leading-health-indicators); (11) OMB's FCFS (2023a)—*America's Children* report and data (https://www.childstats.gov/americaschildren).

Initiative [CAHMI], n.d.c).[3] These comments on overall measurement of child health do not take into account the complexity of assigning accountability to specific health care systems for children.

MEASUREMENT AND ACCOUNTABILITY STRATEGY FOR CHILD HEALTH CARE SYSTEM TRANSFORMATION

The success of any plan for a transformed health care system for children will rely on the effectiveness of the measurement and accountability methods employed. Such methods likely will need to build upon existing measurement and accountability system assets but add consideration of child population health, health equity, community engagement, and alignment with other child-serving sectors. Building on the findings outlined in the previous chapters on the science of child and youth development; the role of families, children, youth, and communities in the health care system; the strengths and challenges of the design of the current system; and the financing mechanism for the health care and public health systems, this section identifies seven priority areas for implementing an accountability measurement strategy that supports transformations in the child health care systems to improve outcomes for children and youth (see Figure 9-1):

1. Commit to population accountability measures, including health equity, for child health care systems.
2. Expedite applied research on best practices for including new measures of child and youth wellbeing in real-world settings.
3. Accelerate accountability through shared measures and improved digital health integration and data interoperability across systems and sectors.
4. Reduce accountability measurement demands to a small set of priority outcomes.
5. Provide sufficient leverage to incentivize accountability for child and youth wellbeing for health care systems and health plans.
6. Ensure engagement, transparency, and equity with patients, families, and communities.
7. Employ a data dashboard for tracking child health care system transformation goals.

---

[3]In 2018, the MCH MRN released a national strategic measurement agenda, created in partnership with families, providers, program leaders, policy makers, and experts (CAHMI, 2018). The work engaged network partners to advance the availability of measures on positive and relational health, such as child flourishing, family resilience, and connection; positive childhood experiences (Bethell, Gombojav, & Whittaker, 2019; Bethell, Jones et al., 2019); school readiness (Ghandour et al., 2018); and whole child and family measures of social determinants of health (Bruner et al., 2018). Network partners also sought to advance methods for using available data for local area estimation and to better track disparities; promote equity; and drive integrated, whole child health care systems (e.g., Integrated Child Risk Index; Bethell, Blackwell et al., 2022).

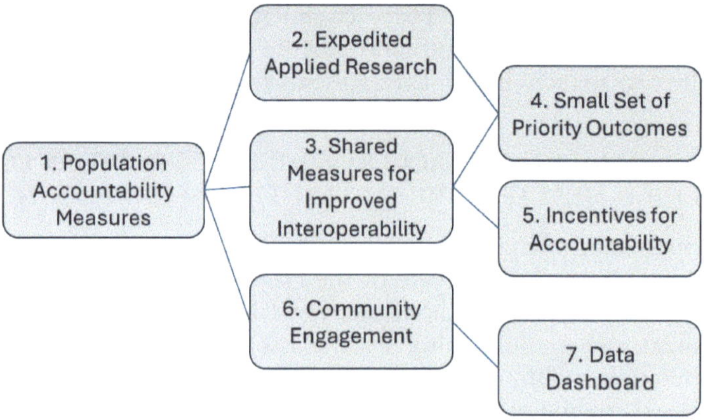
2. Expedited Applied Research
4. Small Set of Priority Outcomes
1. Population Accountability Measures
3. Shared Measures for Improved Interoperability
5. Incentives for Accountability
6. Community Engagement
7. Data Dashboard

FIGURE 9-1 Key elements of a measurement and accountability plan for a transformed child health care system.
SOURCE: Generated by the committee.

Priority Area 1: Population Accountability Measures

Accountability for health care systems has been limited mainly to persons cared for within a given system, without consideration of access barriers to health care or broader community health. In response, recommendations for including community or population measures for adults have been advanced in reports by expert panels (National Academy of Medicine [NAM], 2023; National Academies, 2023a). These reports emphasized the need for measures of whole person and whole population health to include community indicators for improving health equity and the health of the nation. "Whole health" approaches call for measures that reflect community health and functioning outside of the health care settings, especially for individuals from historically marginalized communities. Examples of whole person and whole population health measures that community stakeholders could adopt include monitoring rates of maternal or infant mortality, suicide, and educational attainment, as well as self-reported health status or patient-reported outcomes. The key to such measures is that they reflect health goals as defined by the community and that health care system metrics are reoriented to monitor community needs adequately (NAM, 2023).

Efforts to Advance Population Health Measures

The growing momentum around accountability for population health is present in the general health care system, with various plans and institutions adopting some form of population health management, either for place-based initiatives or for covered lives in insured plans. For example, Adventist Health Systems' Blue Zones initiative seeks to create healthy communities through investment in general wellbeing initiatives that have to do with built spaces, walkability, and nature (Blue Zones, 2019). In one case study, the Fort Worth, Texas, Blue Zone tracked overall community health indicators and moved from one of the least healthy to most healthy cities in a 10-year period (Blue Zones, 2019). A more modest approach focused on place-based improvement is the Community Assisted Public Goods Investment, which tracks broad community indicators of wellbeing that vary based on the goals of specific communities in their five-city effort (Nichols & Taylor, 2018). Several of the cities demonstrated improvements over the first 4 years of their investments in a focused community good.

Relatedly, non-place-based innovations have been employed by health plans across large insured populations. The advent of large-scale Medicare Advantage plans, accountable care organizations, and large Medicaid managed care contracts has sparked greater interest in population-level measures for "captured" or insured populations across different communities (Slabaugh et al., 2017). Among proposed new summary measures are total "healthy days" and more detailed measures that assess (in aggregate) disability days, self-reported quality of life, and others (Kottke et al., 2016). Unfortunately, these measures have been employed only for insured persons, not entire communities, and emphasize adult health, health behaviors, and perceptions of wellness. Similar measures to drive child health care systems to improve child and youth wellbeing are needed.

Multisector regional improvement collaboratives have also led to the inclusion of population health measures in accountability systems, and as a result, these have seen improvements in some population health indicators, such as infant mortality rate and middle school absenteeism in specific communities (Balfanz & Byrnes, 2018; Bundshuh, Ohlson, & Swanson, 2021; Cotton et al., 2019; Hirai et al., 2018; Young, Connolly Sollose, & Carey, 2020). In many of these collaboratives, health care systems provide facilitation, funding, and intervention roles in partnership with multiple non–health care sectors to identify and support shared child health goals (NAM, 2023).

As discussed in Chapter 7, collaboration between primary care and public health has particular importance for improving child health and wellbeing (Valaitis et al., 2020). Several examples of local collaborations have achieved improvements in care in both the United States and Canada (Martin-Misener et al., 2012; McVicar et al., 2019). Nevertheless, considerable barriers limit relationships between the two sectors; chief among them is the lack of shared goals or measures (Pratt et al., 2018). Successful partnerships stem from shared measures at the community level and leadership in achieving trust and commitment among partners.

Overall, a few communities, health plans, and health care systems have included community health indicators and health equity measures, but these are exceptions and not the norm. Several barriers limit incorporating community health indicators, including equity measures, into health care system accountability. First, fee-for-service payments at the clinician level remain the dominant form of payment, providing little incentive to change practice or take on new accountability (Gratale, Viveiros, & Boyer, 2022). Second, adding more accountability measures to the lengthy list of existing measures required by various payers and accreditation organizations will be met with marked resistance, along with increasing demand to simplify the number of measures (see the discussion of Priority Area 4). Third, health care systems often report being ill equipped to address community health indicators that will require them to interface with other human-service sectors to solve complex problems (Gratale et al., 2020).

Health Equity Measures

Despite the barriers, some measures will have to focus on health equity and disparities in community health if there is to be any hope of true progress in societal health for the United States (World Health Organization, 2019). The National Quality Forum (2017) notes the lack of progress in the implementation of equity measures in the United States, even though these measures will be essential to reducing inequities. This reflects in part many technical problems and a lack of consensus on methods for health care system accountability metrics for child health equity and disparities.[4] While national, state, and some local data sources are publicly available and produce data on child health equity, equity measures at the level of the health care system are also essential for improving population health indicators because of the stark differences in care provision and outcomes known to exist across systems within the same geographic area, as well as across the same systems operating across different geographies.

Efforts are under way to optimize the use of existing data and measures to provide local areas with child health equity information and to address the challenges involved in specifying separate equity measures that go beyond stratifying results of existing measures for different subgroups based on culture, race, or ethnic group. Some authors have proposed alternatives

[4]Concerns include cost of and methods for collecting data that identify specific cultural, racial, or ethnic groups; choice of specific groupings for historically marginalized populations for equity measurement; decisions about trend over time or absolute values for equity measures; and calculations about magnitude of improvement goals for equity measures that may require culturally specific interventions.

to specific equity measures, including calculating specific attributable risk scores for some neighborhoods or communities with concentrations of historically marginalized persons, in order to focus resources on areas most impacted by inequities (Dover & Belon, 2019; Martino et al., 2023). Until federal leadership emerges to shape and advance data on impactful equity measures, separate measures of child health equity are not likely to be featured in global health care system accountability, and individual health care systems will be left to create their own measures of equity for care within their walls (Hester, Nickel, & Griffin, 2020).

The new CMS Accelerating All-Payer Health Equity and Development (AHEAD) model, a 2024–2034 initiative, is an advanced set of incentives for states to engage all insurers and plans in improving measured outcomes in a coordinated fashion (CMS, 2023d). AHEAD will require new population-based performance measures that go beyond those included in traditional payer–required performance measurement sets. AHEAD and other related CMS-proposed measures move toward this whole system and whole society approach but do not appear to address child population health. Equally robust efforts to optimize child and youth health and wellbeing are needed with an enhanced focus on children's health promotion and disease prevention. The recently announced CMS-led Transforming Maternal Health model holds promise and will support states in improving care for pregnant women and their infants throughout the perinatal period, including performance measurement innovations with the full engagement of patients and communities (CMS, 2024j). More efforts like the pregnancy-focused Transforming Maternal Health model are called for to catalyze state efforts to transform the child health care system.

Unifying Population Health Measures

In response to the need for a succinct set of measures that could be employed for assessing whole system accountability in a transformed health care system, an IOM (2015) report, *Vital Signs: Core Metrics for Health and Health Care Progress*, recommended greatly simplifying the health care quality and accountability measurement landscape to focus on a few domains, with 15 total core measures to be shared by all payers, geographies, and health care systems, including four prominent measures of community health (Blumenthal & McGinnis, 2015). This report emphasized the role such "unifying" measures would play in a layered accountability system with federal and state agencies, private payers, and large systems uniting around the common core measures, including a few focused on health equity and overall population health, while other accountability measurement would continue in a streamlined fashion to focus on condition-, sector-, or patient-specific measurement (IOM, 2015). Tennessee became the first state in the country to roll out 12 core measures derived largely from the *Vital Signs* report, with modifications after public engagement during 2015 and 2016 (Tennessee Department of Health, 2015). The state now coordinates its annual *State Health Report* with these measures, provides communities recommended interventions for each of the indicators, and maintains a public record of the *Vital Signs* performance in the state (Tennessee Department of Health, 2023). California endorsed a similar project at the county level, allowing various communities latitude in modifying metrics (National Academies, 2017a).

The *Vital Signs* report acknowledged its emphasis on adult health care systems and that child health care systems would likely require a parallel set of accountability measures with a focus on indicators of community and population health for local and regional health care systems. Its authors recommended adding specific indicators of population health for child health care system accountability that could eventually include infant mortality, school readiness, middle school absenteeism, and high school graduation rates. Ohio is now engaged in incorporating at least two of these (infant mortality prevention and school absenteeism) into quality improvement work with Medicaid managed care plans across the state (see Box 9-3). Oregon has employed school readiness in a regional improvement effort with its coordinated care organizations for Medicaid for 3 years (Oregon Health Authority, n.d.).

National outcome measures used for the Title V Maternal and Child Health Services Block Grant Program, led by HRSA, also feature candidate population child health accountability measures similar to those set forth through the *Vital Signs* effort—including measures of school readiness, child flourishing, family resilience, and adverse childhood experiences—which are currently available across numerous child subgroups and states using the National Survey of Children's Health. Use of these Title V measures has been recommended in the EnAct! framework for statewide integrated early childhood health care systems, which was recently set forth as a national model for states (Bethell, Butross et al., 2023; Child and Adolescent Health Measurement Initiative, n.d.d; see Box 9-3).

While further demonstrations are needed, there is growing agreement about the value and potential impact of population-based outcomes measures. For example, several measures such as those noted above have been adopted as child population health measures by a large metropolitan county with a partner pediatric health care system for transparent board reporting and attached to executive compensation (Kemper et al., 2020; Phillips, 2020). These measures do not replace all other accountability metrics required by payers, regulators, and others, but community health indicators provide a unifying component to accountability

BOX 9-3
Focusing Measures and Ensuring Health Care System Engagement: The Ohio Department of Medicaid (ODM)

The ODM developed the Outcomes Acceleration for Kids learning network to align parties, reduce measurement burden, increase focus, and intensify incentives to markedly improve outcomes and health equity for children in Ohio. Traditionally, child health care improvement efforts were fielded separately by ODM, Ohio's children's hospitals, or pediatric accountable care organizations. In addition, these entities and the contracted Medicaid managed care plans (in which 98.3% of children receiving Medicaid benefits are enrolled) faced more than 40 pediatric quality measures for reporting and improvement for Medicaid. Because these efforts did not achieve the improvements sought, ODM proposed what it believes to be the first learning network composed of a Medicaid agency, managed care plans, children's hospitals, and accountable care organizations. The learning network, started in late 2022, includes several proposed innovations:

Increased focus with reduced measurement burden. All parties have agreed to a smaller set of measures for improvement efforts, reducing the number from more than 40 to only 6 measures. Participants agreed that such a focus would enable meaningful efforts on each measure.

Alignment of participants and incentives. Previously, ODM contracted with the managed care plans, and each plan contracted individually with each accountable care organization and hospital. Participants felt there was little alignment in penalties and incentives for quality indicators. Through its provider agreement with the Medicaid managed care plans, ODM hopes to support alignment of all incentives and penalties (without specifying amounts or specific partners) toward the specific six measures currently in use. In addition, ODM is endorsing a statewide improvement goal so that all receive their incentives, or none do.

Ensure engagement with sufficient risk. Employing the Quality Withhold component of its provider agreement with the Medicaid managed care plans, ODM will withhold 3% of all capitation payments for achievement of the child outcome goals on the six measures identified by the end of 3 years and partial achievement during the intervening years. Where the plans have contracts with pediatric accountable care organizations, these incentives will be shared for achieving improvements (or failing to do so).

Incorporate measures of community health in addition to quality of personal health care. Two measures from the National Academy of Medicine report *Child Vital Signs*—infant mortality rate and school absenteeism—are slated for inclusion in the coming years as long-term metrics for the learning network (IOM, 2015).

and could replace numerous process-oriented metrics going forward. As discussed above, at least two states (Ohio and Oregon) have launched pilot programs providing significant withholdings and incentives for Medicaid managed care plans serving children to achieve specific measures in school readiness or school absenteeism as appropriate goals for accountability and improvement efforts. Further, a majority of state

Medicaid medical directors responding to surveys or focus groups said they were committed to moving toward population health goals in their plans (Chisolm et al., 2019).

Priority Area 2: Expedited Applied Research

In addition to the population health and health equity measures, well-being measures have not been adequately captured in proposed accountability systems. Whole child measures that integrate information about a child's physical, mental, and functional health and their social and relational health, as well as family-centered measures, are available (Bethell, Blackwell et al., 2022; Bethell, Garner et al., 2022) and draw on already available national and state data. For example, the Title V Block Grant National Outcomes measures include positive health and functioning measures, such as school readiness, child flourishing, school engagement, and family resilience (Bethell, Gombojav, & Whitaker, 2019). The Title V Block Grant National Outcomes measures endorsed these concepts in efforts to include positive health and functioning measures, such as school readiness, child flourishing, school engagement, and family resilience (Bethell, Gombojav, & Whitaker, 2019). Whether these measures can be used for accountability of individual health care systems or networks will depend on the feasibility of scalable and reliable data collection and better evidence on how health care strategies influence these outcomes, including partnerships with public health, social services, and community-based resources.

Ongoing research is under way in the field to evolve new measures that may expand the options for health care accountability focused on child and youth wellbeing. For example, the Global Developmental Potential (GDP2) measurement concept suggests a wellbeing index that includes measures related to living a healthy life, having basic human needs met, being able to express and understand thoughts and feelings, engaging in lifelong learning, being able to adapt to change in a positive way, and experiencing positive relationships with and connecting with others (Halfon et al., 2022). While conceptually promising, GDP2 has not been specified clearly or normed for children and youth, nor has it been tested in sufficiently sized populations or compared with other indicators—thus its use cannot be recommended at this time.

Different from the GDP2 approach, some researchers and health care system leaders have suggested a measure of child thriving that includes a more proximal set of process and outcome measures designed to drive health care improvement over several years. This proposal features a composite measure of "thriving" at age 66 months using data easily accessible in current electronic health records (EHRs; Brown et al., 2020). This includes whether a child has up-to-date immunizations and a healthy body mass index; is free of dental pain; has normal or corrected vision and normal or corrected hearing; and is on track for communication, literacy, and socioemotional milestones. Baseline rates of thriving in one study employing this indicator were 13%, but data were missing for 50% of children, pointing to the seriousness of gaps in data from EHRs. Unless or until access, comprehensiveness, and data transparency problems for EHRs are resolved, measures that depend on health care system records alone will be missing large amounts of data (Brown et al., 2020). Approaches to integrate patient- and family-reported data into EHRs using family-engaged approaches have been tested for impact and feasibility, but they rely on digital health technologies that are in limited use in pediatric health care and generally not prioritized in the broader health care system (Brykman & Joseph, 2024; Coker et al., 2016; Jenssen et al., 2022; Office of the National Coordinator for Health Information Technology [ONC], 2023; Weinberg et al., 2021).

Another proposed community measure is the Child and Adolescent Thriving Index, an aggregate of several community child health and functioning indicators (Anderson, Hemez, & Kreider, 2022). This index includes 11 components: non–low birth weight in neonates, preschool attendance in children ages 3–4 years, reading proficiency in fourth-grade students, math proficiency in eighth-grade students, food security in children younger than age 18 years, general health status, nonobesity in high school students, nonsmoking and non–marijuana use in adolescents ages 12–17 years, high school graduation in young adults ages 18–21 years, and nonarrest in children ages 10–17 years. This is the broadest of the reviewed community indicators and may be farthest from measured influence of health care systems. In addition, it includes some functional measures, such as educational attendance and performance, but does not include positive health and wellbeing.

Priority Area 3: Shared Measures for Improved Interoperability

Many of the children with the greatest health risks and morbidity burdens in the health care system are challenged in dealing with multiple health care providers in diverse settings and are often also served by home visiting, early intervention, child welfare, juvenile justice, schools, special education, and other community-based organizations. Achieving the best results will require coordinated efforts both within the health care system and across various sectors to improve outcomes.

Improving Data Interoperability

Among health care settings, some progress has occurred in improving collaboration between different providers through data sharing and interoperability to improve health care processes.[5] Several new digital health technology innovations and data interoperability platforms and tools are emerging, although few have advanced beyond research and demonstration, and most focus on adult health care and interfacility data interoperability, rather than children or on sharing data across health care, school, public health, and social services settings (Canfell et al., 2022; ONC, 2020; Weinberg et al., 2021; Willis et al., 2022). Especially relevant to child wellbeing, current data interoperability efforts pay less attention to the integration of patient- and family-generated data (Anoshiravani et al., 2011; Bode et al., 2023; Ranade-Kharkar et al., 2018; Sinha et al., 2023). Nearly all hospitals and many physicians' offices use EHRs (National Academies, 2018). However, because of lack of data interoperability across EHRs and poor capacity to integrate information across multiple sources, devices, and organizations, EHRs are still largely unable to support the flow of essential data at the right time, to the right party, and for the right patient, even within the health care system alone. This is especially the case in child health care.

Although ONC notes the importance of pediatric health care applications, the field is characterized by slow progress and insufficient prioritization of pediatrics or child health data integration on the part of existing health care systems (Anoshiravani et al., 2011; ONC, 2020; Sinha et al., 2023). Child health data work has trailed work for adult health data for several reasons. Governance of child health data remains fraught, with child and parental rights sometimes in conflict, both because of sensitive areas of care for adolescents and because of the potential for child custody issues with child protective services and juvenile justice information sharing. The market for software development is smaller for pediatric software than for corresponding work among adults.

Work on child health data interoperability has also lagged without federal champions. For older people, Medicare has served such a role. Medicare has documented positive outcomes for the older population with long-standing programs, such as the Program of All-Inclusive Care for the Elderly, which provides comprehensive health care and social services in community and home settings and relies on effective data interoperability capacities (Arku et al., 2022). Others experiment with new technologies to serve the massive Medicare and Medicare Advantage markets. Child health care, however, relies heavily on Medicaid, with varying state rules and regulations and a more decentralized market. Although CMS (2020)

[5]A 2018 National Academies report defines "data interoperability" as the ability to deliver data seamlessly and automatically across time and space from and to multiple devices and organizations (National Academies, 2018; Pronovost et al., 2018).

continues to issue rules and supports to help state Medicaid programs implement effective data sharing and interoperability strategies and ONC (2020) similarly works to improve the collection, use, and sharing of data important for promoting health and delivering high-quality care, numerous gaps remain in uptake, leadership, and resources for children.

Health Information Exchanges and Exchange Portal

Health information exchanges in numerous regions of the country link diverse health care providers into a shared electronic record summary system for managing patients, even though none of these was designed with children in mind. They are often divided into three types: directed, query-based, and consumer-mediated exchanges (ONC, n.d.; Williams et al., 2012). Directed exchanges develop digital care coordination plans and integrated patient and provider reminders for managing health conditions. Query-based exchanges allow providers to investigate patient data for unplanned health care decision making. Consumer-mediated exchanges provide patient access directly to their own data. While individual EHR platforms almost always offer patient portals, these are not often user friendly and rarely allow an integrated view of all the community providers a patient or family might use. Nor do they usually offer two-way permission by families and patients for data sharing among various providers. Nonetheless, exchanges have reduced emergency room visits, improved medication reconciliation, and reduced diagnostic testing duplication for adults (GAO, 2023a). Health information exchanges have less impact for small and rural providers (Bloomrosen & Berner, 2023) and have not been shown to affect care for children. Exchange portals can capture a broader set of records for diverse participating providers who do not share a common EHR when most health care organizations in a region participate, and these networks could be expanded to include child health services provided in clinical, home, and community settings. For example, rural behavioral health home providers in Appalachia use a health information exchange to coordinate rapid responses to pediatric emergency room visits for children with psychiatric problems, to communicate with primary care clinicians around medications with parental permission, and to evaluate the effectiveness of their services (Zupkovich, 2022). This is especially important for children and adolescents with special needs who seek care at large pediatric health care systems, but also typically require an array of other home-, community-, and school-based services and support. Coordinating the launch of health information exchange with social risk screening and tracking of community services is also likely to lead to marked improvements in the effectiveness of social risk screening (Zupkovich, 2022).

Research Collaboratives

Additional examples for exchanging important health-related information in secure and meaningful ways are emerging from large research collaboratives such as PEDSnet (n.d.), an integrated network of large children's hospitals sharing EHRs for care improvement for 10 million children, representing approximately 10% of all U.S. children. PEDSnet has already provided highly precise estimates to improve Centers for Disease Control and Prevention (CDC) growth curves for children and enhanced estimates of care for numerous conditions. More importantly, they represent a larger portion of children with special pediatric conditions. For example, they may be providing data on most gene therapy received by children and adolescents in the United States and more than 80% of all specialty orthopedic hardware for some craniofacial conditions (PEDSnet, n.d.). Recognizing the potential to transform health care, the new strategic plan for PEDSnet calls for the development of a collaborative improvement network structure for enhancing outcomes for children with rare conditions. The coordinated governance, shared human-subjects protection, standard data protocols, and ability to conduct privacy-protected linkages with external datasets (such as child welfare or education) exemplify some of the first tools that will allow long-term health improvements in a coordinated fashion across multiple large child health care systems. Others emphasize the importance of integrating other digital health technology with EHRs, noting that

> A new, more effective EHR will transition away from simply supporting clinical transactions and documenting patient's medical record to an EHR that delivers key information to clinical and patient and other groups within or outside the health care system with a focus on improved child health. (p. 2) [. . .] EHRs as electronic hubs could act as office extenders, facilitating integration across health care settings, linking patients with community partners, and supporting direct patient engagement [. . .] (p. 5) (Jenssen et al., 2022)

Other recent reports emphasize the need for further expansion to address social factors in EHRs, especially for those children covered by Medicaid. Examples from data sharing for older people across diverse health and social service sectors already exist (Association for Community Affiliated Plans, 2020), but these required significant resources from Medicare Advantage plans for startup.

Cross-Sector Coordination

These previous examples describe mainly integration of data within various levels of the health care system, with little cross-sector work, which is a more complex effort that requires data interoperability between health care and, for example, schools, juvenile justice facilities, and foster care. Efforts such as the federal Collective Impact Project led by the Office of the Assistant Secretary for Planning and Evaluation delineate the needs, opportunities, and strategies essential to coordinate efforts for promoting the healthy development and wellbeing of children (ASPE, n.d.). Nonetheless, while many child health care and other health-related systems already share important performance measurement topics, in most cases the specifications for these measures are not the same, and shared measures related to the health of the whole child or community are missing. Use of common data platforms across diverse health care systems and child-serving agencies, with which information about children and youth can be standardized and shared, would support better measurement for accountability and help advance the integrated, team-based care needed to promote whole child wellbeing. An example of a tool that supports these goals in the area of early childhood preventive services is the Well Visit Planner, designed to enable an integrated early childhood health care system in the EnAct! framework (Child and Adolescent Health Measurement Initiative, n.d.b, n.d.d; Center for Healthcare Strategies [CHCS], 2022; Coker et al., 2016).

Several institutions have made significant inroads in collaborating with multisector data. The Ohio departments of Medicaid and of Health have developed data dashboards and virtual networks to engage clinicians and communities in efforts previously around improving child antipsychotic drug prescriptions and are developing new dashboards around infant mortality, maternal mortality, and sickle cell care (Ohio Department of Health, 2020). Some justice facilities have enabled access to hardwired, integrated EHRs for youth detained in regional facilities (Aalsma et al., 2019). Similarly, mandated foster care assessments can now be incorporated into the EHR for some patients in a large metropolitan county. Data interoperability was noted as a key success factor in cross-sector work between primary care and public health in prior initiatives, even though few of them have supported or focused on children outside of immunization efforts (McVicar et al., 2019).

While these examples are important, a broader approach is needed. The national EnAct! framework provides an option for statewide integrated early childhood health care systems with a focus on shared accountability and interoperable, family-engaged data sharing among health care, social services, education, public health programs, and family- and community-based services (see Figure 9-2 and Box 9-4 for a summary of the EnAct! framework's shared accountability approach). Drawing from similar frameworks focused on adults, such as the Framework for Aligning Sectors, led by the Robert Wood Johnson Foundation (n.d.), the EnAct! framework is specified for the unique goals, needs, measures, programs, policies, and

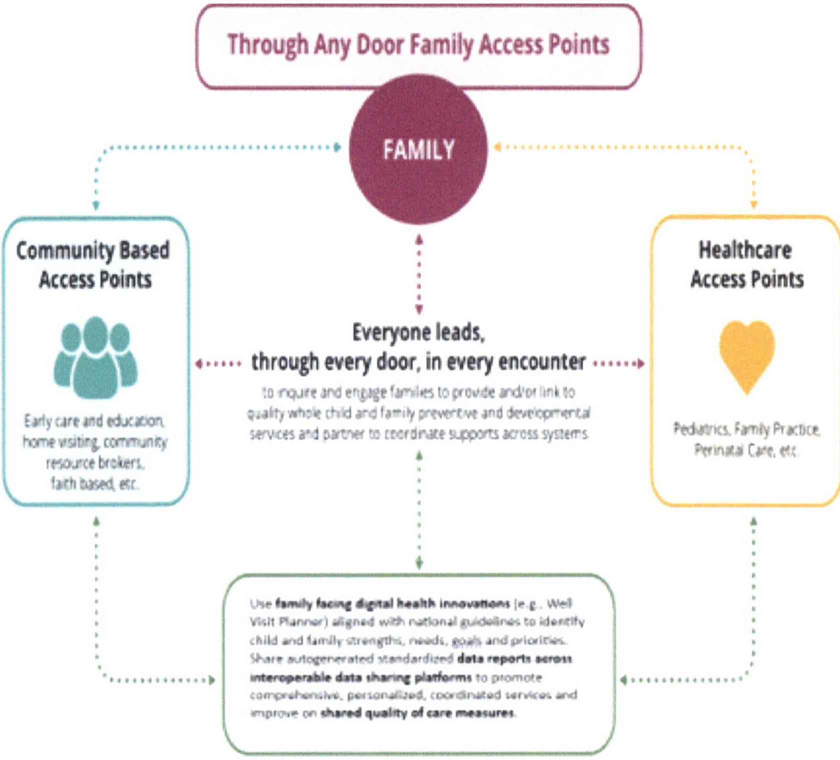

FIGURE 9-2 Catalyzing statewide integrated early childhood health care systems through shared measurement and accountability: The Engagement in Action Framework (EnAct!).
SOURCE: CAHMI, 2023.

players essential for transforming the child health care system (Bethell, Butross et al., 2023; Bethell, Oppenheim et al., 2023). Other frameworks, including the Payment for Progress model, led by the Children's Hospital Association and AcademyHealth, advance engagement across sectors with shared measurement and data interoperability to improve child and family health and wellbeing (Bethell et al., 2018).

Interoperable data sharing is widely recognized as an essential capacity in health care (CMS, 2024c; Szarfman et al., 2022), and platforms need to extend to collaborate among health care, public health, social services, and community support so as to ensure the real-time sharing of family-, child-, and youth-reported information across multiple health care providers and systems, in order to improve child health outcomes.

BOX 9-4
The Engagement in Action Framework

The 5-year Mississippi Thrive! Child Health and Development Project was charged to "yield a model for other States to utilize in improving child health and development outcomes among diverse populations" by aligning efforts between health care and other early childhood systems, including early intervention; home visiting; community-based resources and supports; child welfare; early care and education; Head Start; and the Special Supplemental Nutrition Program for Women, Infants, and Children. The model EnAct! is built on decades of work and progress in the field and is novel in its emphasis on the critical role of the child health care system in promoting the healthy development and school readiness of young children, as well as in its integration and specificity of policies, approaches to team-based care, and strategies for aligning outcome and performance measures and accountability mechanisms across system partners that focus on positive health outcomes and equity; what is more, the framework includes an implementation roadmap.

EnAct! emphasizes engagement of families "through any door" and delineates pathways for each early childhood system partner to improve on performance and accountability measures for which they are already held accountable by federal and state agencies, such as well-child visit rates, developmental and caregiver depression screening, and reductions in emergency department use and injury-related hospitalizations. The design of EnAct! was informed by data made available by the Health Resources and Services Administration to all states; these data cover school readiness; child flourishing; family resilience; children's physical, mental, developmental, social, and relational health; and systems performance and quality of care.

Anchored in principles of family engagement, EnAct! details high-leverage opportunities and specific measurement, collaboration, care design, and policy strategies that enable system partners to integrate services and ensure that all young children receive recommended well-child care services aligned with national Bright Futures guidelines. Using the Cycle of Engagement theory of change, early childhood system partners engaged in the design of EnAct! identified and set forth strategies for meeting four criteria for effective collaboration related to measurement and accountability:

Criterion 1: Use of family-engaged, integrated, and personalized whole child and family standardized assessments that can be implemented "through any door" across an array of care team members and community partners (e.g., clinicians, family support, home visiting, community health, social work professionals).

Criterion 2: Interoperable and automated scoring and reporting of whole child and family assessments, with live links to resources to support partnering with families and coordinating with community and system partners.

Criterion 3: A data sharing platform for ensuring real-time coordination of care and minimizing duplication of assessment with capacity for integration into existing electronic data platforms.

Criterion 4: Real-time capacity to assess, track, and improve quality of services using shared and valid family-centered measures aligned with national guidelines, EnAct! positive health outcomes measures (e.g., school readiness,

(continued)

BOX 9-4 Continued

child flourishing, family resilience, equity), and shared performance measures (e.g., well-child visit and developmental screening rates).

Four implementation actions and 12 associated outcomes comprise the En-Act! framework implementation roadmap. These actions address requirements for state and system leadership and infrastructure for supporting a strong coalition to drive system change, a culture that values family engagement and child wellbeing, practice-based implementation learning and technical assistance resources, and policy change. This implementation roadmap is meant as a guide; specific steps must be generated by partners and aligned to the commitment, capacity, and resources available to ensure action and progress.

SOURCE: Bethell, Butross et al., 2023.

Priority Area 4: Small Set of Priority Outcomes

Focusing on a small set of high-priority measures that align closely with the achievement of population health outcomes related to child and youth wellbeing may be more effective and efficient than a large array of measures serving different purposes. Measure reduction can allow greater attention to remaining metrics that are prioritized and reduce administrative and clinical burden. However, when local measure reduction efforts are undertaken to provide greater community input and efficiency, variation across states and communities increases and prevents accountability comparisons. Federal reduction efforts overcome this variation increase by reducing the list of prioritized measures to consider and still maintaining consistency of some metrics. National organizations such as NAM, HRSA, and CMS have a leadership role to play in reducing redundancy and measure creep.

CMS (2023d) is currently working to consolidate and standardize accountability measures to improve performance on a small set of measures for both Medicare and Medicaid. According to CMS (Jacobs et al., 2023):

> We—the leaders of many CMS centers—aim to promote high quality, safe, and equitable care. We believe aligning measures to focus provider attention and drive quality improvement and care transformation will catalyze efforts in this area. Since there is tension between measuring all important aspects of quality and reducing measure proliferation, we are proposing a move toward a building-block approach: a 'universal foundation' of quality measures that will apply to as many CMS quality-rating and value-based care programs as possible, with additional measures added on, depending on the population or setting. (p. 1)

This effort by CMS is part of a broader national quality strategy that emphasizes prevention, integrated care, and many elements of the vision set forth in this report (see Figure 9-3; CMS, 2023a, 2024b). While current measures of priority outcomes for Medicaid are not yet in place, CMS identified priority areas in which such measures are needed and detailed the types of measures envisioned for each area: (1) person-centered care; (2) equity; (3) safety; (4) affordability and efficiency; (5) chronic conditions; (6) wellness and prevention; (7) seamless care coordination; and (8) behavioral health. Person-reported data and patient and family voices are recognized as critical to these outcomes (CMS, 2023b). Ultimately, it will be critical for Medicaid to incentivize and require reporting of the Meaningful Measures initiative in contracts with the managed care organizations that provide services to over 85% of children enrolled in Medicaid in the United States.

To date, CMS reports that the launch of the Meaningful Measures initiative has reduced the number of Medicare quality measures by 18%, saving more than 3 million hours of time and a projected $128 million. It is unclear how the CMS Meaningful Measures activities will or will not translate from Medicare to Medicaid, the largest insurer of children. Preliminary priority measures (the "universal foundation") being considered by CMS for children in Medicaid include a subset of those already used in the Medicaid core set of measures that states are required to report on (Jacobs et al., 2023): (1) well-child visits (well-child visits in the first 30 months of life; child and adolescent well-care visits); (2) immunization (childhood immunization status; immunizations for adolescents); (3) weight assessment and

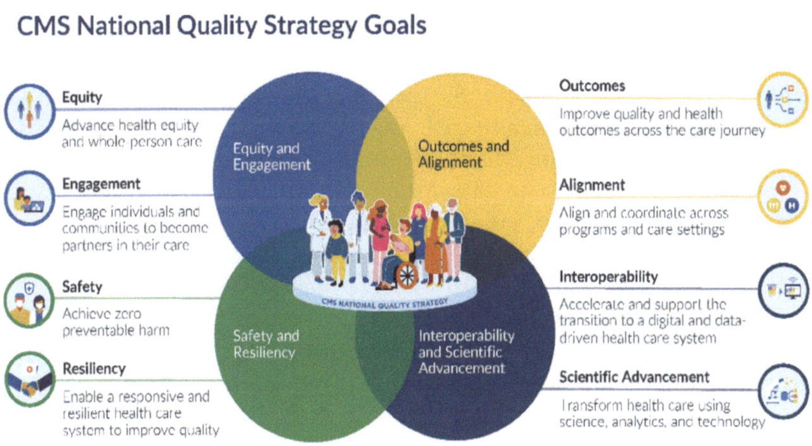
CMS National Quality Strategy Goals
Equity
Advance health equity and whole person care
Engagement
Engage individuals and communities to become partners in their care
Safety
Achieve zero preventable harm
Resiliency
Enable a responsive and resilient health care system to improve quality
Equity and Engagement
Outcomes and Alignment
Safety and Resiliency
Interoperability and Scientific Advancement
CMS NATIONAL QUALITY STRATEGY
Outcomes
Improve quality and health outcomes across the care journey
Alignment
Align and coordinate across programs and care settings
Interoperability
Accelerate and support the transition to a digital and data-driven health care system
Scientific Advancement
Transform health care using science, analytics, and technology

FIGURE 9-3 2023 Centers for Medicare & Medicaid Services (CMS) national quality strategy framework.
SOURCE: CMS, 2023a.

counseling for nutrition and physical activity for children and adolescents; (4) oral evaluation, dental services; (5) asthma medication ratio (reflects appropriate medication management of asthma); (6) screening for depression and follow-up plan; (7) follow-up after hospitalization for mental illness; (8) follow-up after emergency department visit for substance use; (9) use of first-line psychosocial care for children and adolescents on antipsychotics; (10) follow-up care for children who have been prescribed medication for attention deficit hyperactivity disorder; and (11) person-centered care.

Priority Area 5: Incentives for Accountability

Accountability systems are only successful insofar as the measures capture outcomes of importance and sufficient incentives are in place for those with agency to improve those outcomes. Health care financing strategies that link performance on priority performance measures to payment incentives are fundamentally important to drive accountability in the child health care system. Other opportunities to advance accountability include supporting managed care organization and other contracted health care organizations in implementing innovative care delivery and payment strategies with the clinicians and health professionals they employ.

State Medicaid agencies are required to develop and implement a quality strategy for contracted managed care programs to use to advance performance on quality measures and outcomes. State Medicaid agencies are held accountable for these measures and outcomes by CMS (CMS, 2024b). Such strategies are required to be developed in collaboration with stakeholders, including families. Many state Medicaid quality strategies reflect a commitment to prioritize child health through improved health promotion, prevention, and coordinated care strategies, and many emphasize engaging families as partners in care. Further, states are required to report their progress on certain child health care quality metrics each year, and for the past decade or more, state Medicaid programs have lacked improvement on most of these metrics. This calls for new approaches to achieving quality goals (CMS, 2024a; Schiff, Filice, & Chen, 2024) and suggests that incentives for managed care organizations, other health care organizations, and clinicians have been insufficient to catalyze improvement.

Current performance measurement benchmarks, incentives, and reporting strategies have not yet compelled the actions needed to establish high performance on existing child health measures or to advance the essential cross-system partnerships required to engage families and address children's physical, mental, social, and relational health needs. Numerous reports detail specific strategies Medicaid and other state child health programs can use to leverage managed care organization contracts to improve access and quality of health care services for children and youth (CMS, 2023b), and to advance integration of services between health care, community services (e.g., home visiting), social services (e.g., child welfare), and other sectors (e.g., housing, education, public safety; Bethell, Oppenheim et al., 2023; Center for Health Care Strategies, 2019b; Johnson & Bruner, 2024).

Another lever for advancing accountability for improving health care system performance for child wellbeing is Internal Revenue Service (IRS) Community Benefit Standards (Lopez, Dhodapkar, & Gross, 2021; Rozier, 2020; Soto, Sicotte, & Motulsky, 2019; see Chapter 7). Since 1954, mandatory Community Benefit Standards reporting has ostensibly held nonprofit hospitals accountable for promoting the health and wellbeing of the community. Specifically, IRS regulations include a requirement to conduct a community health needs assessment at least every 3 years and implement a strategy for meeting the community health needs identified. Numerous resources are available to support the needs assessment process, and the assessments and implementation plan are to be made widely available to the public. A recent study, however, found that only 60% of hospitals made the results of their community health needs assessment and implementation plan publicly available (Lopez, Dhodapkar, & Gross, 2021). An average score of 3.2 out of 5 on quality of these plans was assigned to those that were possible to evaluate. The authors suggested many changes to improve hospital accountability and transparency. Even among hospitals that did make their results available, many did not address specific community-identified needs, and because outcomes reporting is not required there were no assessments of interventions' effect on communities (CHCS, 2019b).

While Community Benefit Standards have not been yet documented as an effective tool for improving population health, their regulations may be an important lever for supporting the promotion of child and youth wellbeing if sufficient incentives, auditing, and performance measurement were implemented. At the same time, Community Benefit Standards only address nonprofit health care systems, and the growing number of for-profit systems do not have a similar oversight mechanism (see Chapter 7).

Priority Area 6: Community Engagement

In the mid-1990s, a large consortium of health care consumer and family organizations, representing about 88 million Americans, advanced a consumer-centered quality measurement and reporting framework and developed measures. Led by the Foundation for Accountability, this effort included collaboration with CMS, the Federal Employees Health Benefits program, numerous Fortune 500 companies and business groups on health, and community groups such as AARP and Family Voices (Skolnick, 1997). As part of this effort and sparked by expectations for the passage of legislation to establish CHIP, a new public–private collaboration, the Child and Adolescent Health Measurement Initiative (CAHMI), was launched to put families at the center of defining, measuring, and using health care performance information to drive improved quality of and outcomes for health care services (Bethell, Wells et al., 2023). Starting in 1996, CAHMI engaged and convened partners through an official national endorsing committee with representation by federal agencies (CMS, CDC, HRSA, Agency for Healthcare Research and Quality [AHRQ]), family leaders (e.g., Family Voices, National Alliance for the Mentally Ill), health care providers (e.g., American Academy of Pediatrics, American Board of Pediatrics, National Association of Children's Hospitals and Related Institutions/ Children's Hospital Association), and state programs (Medicaid, Title V). This group was charged with: (1) articulating shared goals for child health and an outcomes-based health care performance measurement framework; (2) collaborating with families, providers, payers, and government agencies to specify, validate, and support national, state, and local use of dozens of framework-aligned measures; (3) creating novel public-facing digital data query, collection, and reporting tools for use by families, providers, advocates, policy makers, the media, and researchers; and (4) generating field-building research and systems-change agendas and frameworks.

Of potential relevance today is the health outcomes–based Consumer Information Framework (Lansky & Bethell, 2001), which was defined through the CAHMI in collaboration with families. Domains of measurement based on Consumer Information Framework outcomes include: (1) the healthy development of children; (2) staying healthy; (3) getting better when acutely ill; (4) optimizing health and quality of life when living with illness; and (5) addressing changing needs, such as when children with special needs transition from child to adult health care or require longer-term services or hospice care. For each domain, families expressed the desire for information across three aspects of quality: (1) experience of care, as reported by other families (e.g., access, communication, coordination, follow-up); (2) steps to good care (e.g., screening, education, treatments, care coordination); and (3) results of good care (e.g., healthy functioning, reduced health problems, reduce use of avoidable services).

Research with families revealed that as early as 1999, families and youth were interested in using digital health data technologies to give feedback and get automated reports regarding health care. In response, the CAHMI (n.d.a) advanced technologies such as the National Data Resource Center for Child and Adolescent Health.[6] Another such technology is the Online Promoting Healthy Development Survey, which empowers families and communities to assess and receive a personalized report on

[6]See www.childhealthdata.org

the quality of preventive services for young children, using standardized, validated measures (CAHMI, n.d.b). Similar resources are available online for youth preventive care and children with special health care needs (CDC, 2020a; HRSA, n.d.a).

Early on, the Consumer Information Framework was embraced as an organizing framework for measuring and reporting on health care quality in the initial *National Health Care Quality and Disparities Report* (AHRQ, 2024; Kronick, 2016); it shaped the development of many new, validated measures for child and adolescent health that were subsequently adopted or adapted for use in National Committee for Quality Assurance and Medicaid performance measures (e.g., the Consumer Assessment for Health Providers and Plans for Children with Chronic Conditions; Bethell, Wells et al., 2023).

Despite progress, most families today lack easy access to information about the quality of the health care providers, health plans, and overall health care systems they rely on, and they are not given information in understandable and actionable ways. In addition, an infrastructure to sustain the work was lacking, and the nation currently lacks an initiative that engages public- and private-sector stakeholders in assessing, developing, and driving effective shared use of measures for accountability on outcomes families and communities value.

Overall, past efforts have not resulted in concrete mechanisms for enabling families and the community to shape or impact actions of the health care system as envisioned. Three distinct approaches to enhancing family and community engagement in health care system accountability have since emerged.

First, efforts to build community and patient digital literacy and numeracy can help prepare them to participate fully in the coproduction of health care accountability measures and improvement strategies. Health literacy educational efforts can improve individual patient outcomes and enable families to effectively participate as partners in systems governance and design efforts (Eckman et al., 2012; Sheridan et al., 2011). However, no specific studies examine how this can improve health care accountability. Moreover, as evidence grows around the benefits of self- or family-directed care models, greater engagement around accountability with families and communities is bound to emerge.

A second approach to enhancing family and community engagement is to choose health care accountability metrics that have important implications for community economic growth, such as child functioning (e.g., kindergarten readiness and high school graduation). The belief here is that business and civic leaders would engage in such initiatives more fully than those using metrics focused solely on health status. The Transforming Early Childhood Community Systems initiative (now called Data Informed

Futures; University of California, Los Angeles, n.d.) represents such a case, providing a blueprint for the effective engagement of community members, in improving child outcomes. The adoption of the same types of measures by the *Vital Signs for Health and Wellbeing of Children* (CDC, 2019d) efforts in Central Ohio grew out of strong community sentiment from business leaders and parents that such measures mattered to the entire region (Robinson & McDonald, 2023).

Finally, there has been an escalation of efforts to ensure that the child health care system engages families and communities directly with measures of performance defined by families and communities, such as the Family Engagement in Systems Assessment Tool (Dworetzky, Hoover, & Walker, 2023). Such efforts seek to activate and place families and communities as the "owners" of their health and coproducers of positive health outcomes for children. Measuring whether and how well efforts to engage with families and communities to shape the performance of the child health care system has been a long-standing priority for some national initiatives, such as Family Voices. As with the other proposals to improve engagement, real tests of change in community involvement have not occurred.

Priority Area 7: Data Dashboard

Existing federally required reports related to child health (e.g., *America's Children* [Children's Defense Fund, 2023], *National Healthcare Quality and Disparities Report* [AHRQ, 2021a]) are important, as are measurement and accountability systems led by CMS (Medicaid and CHIP), HRSA (Title V, community health centers), and others that specifically measure and promote accountability within health care systems. However, these efforts are not coordinated to provide a picture of performance across the child health care system and often define similar concepts (e.g., disability) differently. In addition, except for Title V measures, wellbeing and overall system performance are not addressed.

A dashboard of indicators specific to the goals of this report could inform existing efforts and be used across health care accountability efforts. Ideally, a national agency or cabinet-level leader would establish the dashboard and track progress on child health. Such a dashboard could enable high-level tracking of and facilitate communication on the nation's progress toward a health care system that improves child and youth outcomes in the United States; achieves health equity in those outcomes; fully engages children, youth, families, and communities; and partners with other systems and sectors to promote the health and wellbeing of the whole child, whole community, and whole society.

The design of such a dashboard may include measures that are: (1) tracking a specific outcome, whether directly or indirectly; (2) limited in number for ease of communication (e.g., at least one but no more than five measures for each goal area); (3) understandable and actionable for families, communities, and advocates as reported to the public; (4) possible to assess using existing data or short-term modifications to existing data; (5) reliant on data that are regularly available and sustained over time to ensure progress; and (6) embraced as a core management function of the lead child health agency at federal and state levels.

CONCLUSION

This chapter summarizes the landscape of measurement and accountability approaches currently used in the child health care system and identifies pathways for leveraging existing strengths and assets to establish the coordinated measurement and accountability strategies needed to support efforts to narrow gaps and inequities in children's healthy development and wellbeing at a population level. The chapter identifies and discusses seven priority areas for implementing an accountability measurement strategy that supports transformations in the child health care systems to improve outcomes for children and youth. These priority areas and key findings related to each follow:

1. Commit to population accountability measures, including health equity, for child health care systems.
   Key findings: *A growing number of initiatives is taking a whole health approach and identifying indicators of community health and health equity with promising results. However, efforts in the past decade have focused on adult health and wellbeing outcomes. Pilot measurement programs in Ohio and Oregon are focused on child health outcomes and have engaged multiple sectors, communities, and families to develop measures.*
2. Expedite applied research on best practices for including new measures of child and youth wellbeing in real-world settings.
   Key findings: *Research efforts are under way to evolve new measures, but more are needed to inform reliable data collection and integrate evidence from health care strategies that influence child health outcomes.*
3. Accelerate accountability through shared measures and improved digital health integration and data interoperability across systems and sectors.
   Key findings: *Work on data interoperability has focused on adults and the adult health care system. Given the critical links between health care, public health, and social services on child health, accelerated attention to data interoperability for the child health care system is needed.*

4. Reduce accountability measurement demands to improve priority outcomes.
   Key findings: *An array of measures for varied accountability purposes can be burdensome for health care systems and providers. CMS has launched a Meaningful Measures initiative to reduce the number of quality measures and identify a foundation of universal measures. State programs are also piloting measurement strategies around a small set of indicators for community-defined wellbeing outcomes.*
5. Provide sufficient leverage to incentivize health care systems and health plans to accelerate accountability for child and youth wellbeing.
   Key findings: *Several mechanisms for managed care and hospital benefits reporting exist that could be strengthened to drive accountability for health care services that promote child health and wellbeing and health equity.*
6. Ensure engagement, transparency, and equity with patients, families, and communities.
   Key findings: *Past research and initiatives have revealed families' expectations for quality of care and desire to be informed and part of the process of improving health care.*
7. Employ a data dashboard for tracking child health care system transformation goals.

The issues and strategies discussed in this chapter point to a fundamental need to ensure that the measures used to assess and drive accountability in the child health care system align with priority child and youth wellbeing outcomes. In addition, various public- and private-sector child health care system partners need to ensure that shared measures are developed and linked to sufficient incentives, and that implementation and the process of transformation are supported sufficiently. Finally, public reporting and transparency—and mechanisms to influence improvements when gaps in performance arise—are fundamentally important for success.

As discussed in Chapter 3, there is a need to restore the trust of families, communities, and system actors and build confidence that health care system transformation is possible. A sense of possibility and steady progress, through measurement and accountability, is essential to maintain hope and engagement of the individuals and organizations upon which transformation depends. The next chapter summarizes the committee's goals and recommendations toward advancing the importance of child health and an improved child health care system, including key actions to further develop measurement and drive accountability for child and youth wellbeing.

10

Improving the Health and Wellbeing of Children, Youth, Families, Communities, and the Nation

The mission of pediatric care should be driving the best outcomes for all *children [and] the incentives [should be] achieving this goal.*

—Comment to the committee, Pediatric Emergency Physician, Tennessee

Roughly one hundred years ago, a crisis in child health resulted in a broad social movement to improve outcomes for children (McMillan, Schumacher, & Singh, 2006; Takanishi, 1978). That movement resulted in the development of organizations and agencies that would support and organize efforts to improve health outcomes for children and adolescents, including the American Academy of Pediatrics and the Maternal and Child Health Bureau, among others. That social movement also created child labor laws, nutrition regulations, education reform, and legal protections for children that had been missing previously. Today, another transformational movement is needed, one that addresses the crisis facing America's children.

U.S. children are not well. Increasing morbidity and mortality threaten their health and wellbeing and that of the coming adult workforce. The crisis comes in the context of decades of policies that disadvantage racially and ethnically diverse and low-income communities and have resulted in inequitable opportunities for children and disparate outcomes that start in childhood and extend into adulthood. National progress to reverse this crisis and improve long-term outcomes for all Americans will come only from a dedicated and ongoing commitment to focus on children, youth, and their families. Previous and ongoing work to improve health care for Americans has had limited focus on the population under age 30. This crisis requires national recognition of the need to take the health of children and youth seriously, specifically, and differently—including changing the organization and financing of their health care and related services. Children and youth may benefit from the general developments in U.S. health organization and financing, but in many cases, child health care is excluded and children's unique needs are unmet. Without dedicated and continued focus on younger populations, the nation will continue to lag behind other industrialized countries in most indicators of child and adolescent wellbeing and lead to a young adult population that is less able to participate fully in American industry, military, and society.

Not addressing this crisis has led to serious social consequences. Today, many working-age adults have health burdens that demand public resources and limit workforce participation and military preparedness—a situation that is unlikely to change if the health care system for children is not fixed. Furthermore, with declining birth rates, the growing older population will rely on fewer employed adults for their wellbeing. Growing mortality and disability rates among U.S. working-age adults are ominous indicators of a larger epidemic of poor health in communities, outcomes of failing to provide the care that children and youth need.

The committee recognizes the many important influences on child and family health outside the health care system, especially those around poverty and income support, housing, labor markets and employment, community wellbeing, family leave and child care support, justice and education systems, and financing of these. Our recommendations focus on the health care sector, defined broadly to include public health investments in child and family health and school-based health care. While recognizing the critical role of other public, economic, and social issues on health over the life course and supporting recommendations from several previous reports by the National Academies of Sciences, Engineering, and Medicine (National Academies) on reducing child poverty and addressing the economic and social needs of children and youth, the recommendations emphasize transforming the health care system to advance child, youth, and family wellbeing.

This chapter, drawing on the findings in previous chapters, provides several calls to action for executive and legislative leadership at federal, state, territorial, and local levels. The recommendations here speak to the critical need for the nation to address health trends and the poor state of the wellbeing of America's children by strengthening policies in ways that expand opportunities for improving the health care system across states and communities. The recommendations, discussed below, focus on governmental levers for change that will allow health care systems and the pediatric workforce the flexibility to change and improve health care for children and youth. While many challenges with the current child health care system are raised in the prior chapters, the committee did not make recommendations to address all the specific challenges. In the context of implementation goals for an improved health care system, we offer a number of recommendations to establish the leadership, financing, and other resources necessary to address these challenges and support the expansion of promising innovations in health care delivery.

In Chapter 1, the committee articulated its guiding principles and vision for a transformed child and adolescent health care system. These principles were developed from a collective understanding of the challenges in the current health care system and emerging opportunities to improve the delivery of care, informed by the committee's substantial experience in health care from multiple perspectives and the large body of scientific evidence and traditional knowledge on factors promoting child and adolescent health and wellbeing.

The committee's vision recognizes the opportunities and imperative to improve population health and wellbeing by focusing health care priorities earlier in the life course. Decades of research and experience show that early life adversity and poor health lead to chronic disease and mortality in adulthood and limit individuals' capacity to participate fully in community life and the workforce. Further knowledge points to the critical influence of family and community health on child health and subsequent life course wellbeing (see Chapter 2). There is evidence of the persistence of racial inequities and injustice in access to and receipt of care and resulting health outcomes; these disparities are discussed in Chapter 3 and documented in a number of other reports (Institute of Medicine [IOM], 2003b; National Academies, 2017a; 2023c). Advancing science in social, relational, and structural determinants of health, genetics, and artificial intelligence prediction all emphasize the potential and benefits of focusing health care on prevention and earlier identification of disease.

While all of this has been well known for some time, and recognition of major disparities and discrimination in health and health care have grown during the COVID-19 pandemic, several challenges remain to refocus child health care[1] from an emphasis on treatment to an emphasis on prevention. A barrier to this shift is that growing rates of poor physical and mental conditions among children and adults can keep the emphasis on treatment as opposed to prevention. This is made more likely by current funding and financial incentives that center diagnoses and treatments and limit attention to prevention and health promotion and addressing root causes of disparities. Furthermore, there is substantial fragmentation and lack of coordination among health care systems, schools, and other community

[1]Throughout this report, the committee regards the term "child health care" to encompass maternal, prenatal, child, adolescent, family, and community health care.

resources with clear roles and interest in supporting the health and wellness of children, families, and communities.

Throughout its report, the committee aimed to document increased scientific and traditional knowledge about health and wellbeing in childhood and later adulthood, including persistent and worsening poor health among U.S. children and youth, the uneven health care system for children and youth, racism in health care and disparate outcomes, growing health problems among working-age adults, and the implications of these trends for the nation's economic productivity and prosperity. All these findings support the urgency of addressing child and adolescent health care transformation now.

In making recommendations for health care system transformation, the committee was tasked with addressing six questions (see Chapter 1, Box 1-2). These questions directed the committee to identify key levers for change that would facilitate health promotion and disease prevention; address systemic inequities and gaps in payment models; incorporate lived experiences into community- and team-based care; and enhance multisystem collaboration for improved health and wellbeing. Early in the study, the committee drew upon the questions in its charge to create a set of principles for an improved health care system (see Box 10-1); these principles guided the committee's work of developing the program and policy recommendations presented in this chapter. Adhering to these principles will enable changes in policy and practice to improve health care.

LIFE COURSE PERSPECTIVE: THE CRITICAL IMPORTANCE OF CHILD HEALTH

As discussed throughout the report, the committee takes a multigenerational, life course perspective because research has shown the inextricable link of child health to maternal and family health on one end and later adult health on the other. Substantial evidence demonstrates that health early in the life course sets the foundation for health through childhood, adolescence, and young adulthood, and for tomorrow's workforce. This science points to the importance of early life experiences and close adult relationships and to developmental origins of health and disease. The community and social environments contribute as well and help frame both typical trajectories at given times in history as well as opportunities and threats (Alwin, 2012). Early antecedents discernable in childhood contribute to adult chronic illness. For example, mental illness and substance use and addiction among most adults started with conditions in childhood and adolescence, and children with obesity are more likely than nonobese children to have obesity in adulthood. Chronic stress and allostatic load, social and structural determinants of health (especially poverty, hunger, and

BOX 10-1
Guiding Principles

1. **Employ a life course perspective.**
A transformed health care system must be rooted in the science underlying the healthy development of children and youth, recognizing the early and lifelong influences impacting healthy development and adult health, starting with preconception and prenatal periods and continuing to every stage of childhood, adolescence, and young adult life, all of which influence adult health and disease. Scientific advancements in social and structural influences, relational health, genetics, and prediction using artificial intelligence confirm the imperative potential of prevention and early intervention.

2. **Partner with families and communities, which are central to child health and wellbeing.**
Children's health care needs must be viewed in the context of family and community. Children, families, and communities serve as essential partners working together with health care providers and other care team members to drive improvements in health care.

3. **Prioritize and drive equitable outcomes through resources and accountability.**
Achieving health equity requires an intentional focus on equitable care and redistribution of resources to children living in communities that have long endured underinvestment and structural disadvantage, whose lived experience and traditional knowledge will provide ideas for a strong path forward.

4. **Make it sustainable over time.**
Sustained and successful health care system transformation relies on leaders; partners; payers; and activated communities, families, and youth that establish agreements that incentivize cross-sector partnership and prevention and track performance on shared goals.

housing insecurity), and persistent racism have oversized roles in driving the health and wellbeing of children, youth, and families. High rates of childhood adversity and poverty are associated with poorer adult physical and mental health, job opportunities, and earning potential. These adversities are most pronounced in historically marginalized communities.

Addressing family health needs and social determinants of health can improve child and family health, with strong empirical evidence linking family socioeconomic status and education level to child health outcomes. The scientific findings on the developmental origins of health and disease and the importance of the community and historical context point to the opportunity and imperative to focus population health strategies early in the life course. The connection between health and wellbeing for children and the nation's capabilities and capacity has never been clearer.

FAMILIES, COMMUNITIES, AND HEALTH CARE

Health care experiences for families seeking care vary greatly. Differential treatment, racism, discrimination, and bias are prevalent in health care service provision (see Chapters 2 and 3). The United States is one of a few resource-rich countries in the world that does not entitle young children to health care, with resulting disparities and some of the lowest rates of access to preventive care and routine services among resource-rich countries. As a result of persistent disparities in prevention and health promotion, many U.S. cities and states report high rates of infant mortality, preventable disease outbreaks, and high costs of care for many specialty conditions. Large subsets of U.S. children face barriers to positive mental and physical health and wellbeing as a result of poverty, food insecurity, unsafe or unstable housing, neighborhood segregation, insufficient access to high-quality care, and other adverse childhood experiences (see Chapter 4). This report focuses on the important opportunities the health care sector can leverage to acknowledge community needs, build care practices that better support these needs, and link families to social resources.

While some innovative programs exist, in general, U.S. health care provides only limited attention to the integration of health care for the whole family, health care across the life course, or integration of mental and behavioral health into clinical care. This report argues for collaborative and strengths-based relationships among children, families, communities, and health care professionals and systems as foundational for improving child health. Health care that centers on partnerships, strengths, and equity provides children with the greatest opportunities to receive care and resources to support their lifelong development. Community-driven solutions are necessary to address determinants of health, as families and communities are uniquely positioned to drive priorities and actions tailored to their needs.

HEALTH EQUITY

Health equity needs to be centered across all aspects of health care system transformation. Achieving health equity is an ongoing goal requiring multilevel, evidence-informed strategies and interventions at the policy, program, and system levels to distribute resources where they are needed most. Engagement and building trust in health care systems, particularly with historically marginalized populations, begins with acknowledging existing inequities and pursuing efforts to combat them in communities.

In the current system, health care institutions expose patients and families to interpersonal and structural racism throughout the care process, resulting in more expensive care and poorer patient outcomes. Racism affects which patients are accepted for appointments or how long it takes to get appointments, the location of specialty resources in pediatrics, the types of diagnoses that are offered, and the types of treatments provided (see Chapter 2). Building trust at the provider level will require ensuring that the current and future workforce is able to provide care with cultural humility and empathy and making room for dignity in care.

Child poverty remains the strongest predictor of poor health outcomes in children and youth. Poverty works against healthy living conditions and can limit access to nutritious foods, stable housing, green space, pollution-free environments, safe and nurturing relationships, and health care. Children whose families live in poverty experience worse health early in life than children growing up in higher-income families, and this disparity worsens as they age (see Chapters 2 and 4). A variety of public programs has helped decrease family poverty in several ways, including income support, underscoring the effectiveness of public investments in children (National Academies, 2019a, 2023f). Although the committee does not address the root causes of this critical determinant of health directly, it strongly supports the recommendations of prior reports by the National Academies on reducing child and intergenerational poverty (National Academies, 2019a, 2023f).

This report focuses on ways to advance child health equity through health insurance coverage and direct clinical services support (see Chapter 6) and investment in public health aimed at health promotion and disease prevention (see Chapter 7), including that delivered through schools (see Chapter 8).

SUSTAINABILITY

Sustainability includes consideration of financing, payment, trained workforce, data, and technology that will support an effective health care system. An improved child health care system, emphasizing a whole health approach (National Academies, 2023a), needs to be designed to adapt and evolve to meet the continually evolving needs of the communities and families it serves, to strategize with other sectors that share goals of child wellbeing (e.g., education, social services, justice), and to respond to an ever-changing built and natural environment. Successful health care system transformation relies on partnerships among leaders across sectors, payers, engaged families, and activated communities; such partnerships establish agreements and track performance on shared goals, ensuring transparency and open exploration of performance on population-based outcome indicators (see Chapter 9).

VISION FOR IMPROVING HEALTH AND WELLBEING OF CHILDREN AND YOUTH

The committee envisions a child and adolescent health care system a decade from now that builds from traditional knowledge in communities and empirical evidence on early life experiences, human development, and disease prevention to provide comprehensive, family-engaged, community-integrated, and equitable care focused on optimizing the healthy development and lifelong wellbeing of all children, youth, and their families. This health care system will exist within a broad, cross-sector system, notably expanding the role of schools; the envisioned health care system promotes flourishing equitably, builds on community strengths, and addresses family and community needs to create the safe, stable, and nurturing relationships and environments that all children need to thrive. Critical to a future transformed system is ensuring that the lived experiences and expressed needs of children, youth, and families set the priorities. The committee expects that the primary clinical workforce will continue to transform to a coordinated team-based care model—with physicians and nurses working alongside integrated mental and behavioral health workers, community health workers or navigators, and multisector community partners (see Chapter 5).

The committee identified five implementation goals in pursuit of this vision:

1. Elevate the importance of child and adolescent health for the nation through continuous public focus on children and youth.
2. Finance health care systems for all children, emphasizing prevention and health promotion.
3. Strengthen community-level health promotion and disease prevention.
4. Ensure co-creation and co-design of programs and structures with youth, family, and community voices and leadership.
5. Implement measurement and accountability to ensure equitable achievement of these goals.

The recommendations that follow for each of these goals attend to the compelling need for the nation to address the poor state of health and wellbeing for large numbers of America's children and youth and the major concerns regarding the nation's workforce.

Goal 1: Elevate the Importance of Child and Adolescent Health for the Nation through Continuous Public Focus on Children and Youth

Chapter 1 concludes that the nation needs sustained federal, state, and local leadership for child and family health. While many public and private organizations provide key support for children, youth, and families, no one group has clear leadership among them. Key federal agencies include the Centers for Medicare & Medicaid Services (CMS; the main health care financing program), several direct service programs, especially the Maternal and Child Health Bureau (the agency in the Health Resources and Services Administration [HRSA] charged with monitoring and improving the health of mothers and children) and the Bureau of Primary Health Care (supporting substantial numbers of community health centers across the nation), as well as the key public health efforts of the Centers for Disease Control and Prevention.

Among professional organizations, the American Academy of Pediatrics represents many but not all of the physicians and other providers who care for U.S. children and youth. Children's hospitals play an important role, but they provide inpatient services for a relatively small proportion of children. Some states have developed children's councils or boards at the cabinet level, where health is a major topic. Furthermore, the labor market and health insurers greatly influence health care payment and incentives.

The need for federal leadership on child health arises from evidence that the distinct needs of younger populations often get little attention in development of delivery models, in development of diagnostics and therapeutics, and during public health crises. Since children are not the cost drivers in health care, are only 22% of the U.S. population, and have diseases that are relatively rare, their unique needs often get lost in political and policy debates on health care. There are many examples of how child health has been deprioritized within a health care system that focuses predominantly on adults (see Chapter 1). For example, during the early period of the COVID-19 pandemic, vaccine development and availability for children were slower than for adults, and the work to ensure educational support came late and was based more on the needs of the workforce than on the needs of children and youth.

The unwinding of pandemic-related Medicaid policies provides graphic evidence of the delayed policy attention to children and youth, even despite their prominence among the Medicaid-insured population. With the unwinding, many children and youth lost critical health care coverage through preventable bureaucratic mishaps and mistakes and thus lost access to needed preventive and treatment services for long periods of time (see Chapter 6). Notably, state factors contributed to differences in children's loss of coverage. For instance, states that combine Medicaid with the Children's Health Insurance Program (CHIP) have had smooth coverage transitions, reducing loss of coverage. States with less generous CHIP income eligibility limits or with CHIP programs that have copays or premiums (26 states) have seen greater loss in coverage. Limited and late concern for children during the pandemic and other social crises exemplifies the major lapses that occur without sustained federal leadership focused on children.

National leadership must bring about coordination, facilitating communication among agencies serving children, using a child-health-in-all-policies lens, and maintaining robust data collection and review across federal agencies on the health status of all children. Previous efforts at change have floundered in part because of lack of sustained attention. The locus of leadership and coordination needs to be at the highest levels of the federal government, with clear participation across key government agencies, states, communities, and the private sector. Other nations have designated child commissioners and ombudsmen for this purpose. Creating such positions demonstrates a government's commitment to children; it ensures an entity for oversight, research, and review of public policies, as well as technical assistance for matters impacting child health (James & Wright, 2015; Kim, 2019; UNICEF, 1997). Some U.S. states have already established organizations and programs resembling children's commissions found in other countries. About half of U.S. states currently have some version of a children's cabinet, with increasing collaboration among these units (Forum for Youth Investment, 2021).

This report provides an overall guide for the types of ongoing strategy and focus on the wellbeing of children, youth, and families. Reviewing the report and implementing its recommendations would require a high-level national expert panel of families, health care leaders, and key agencies to develop a strategic framework. This prominent convening, led at the federal level, can help with reconceptualizing child health and development across sectors and elevating the importance of specific changes needed. Furthermore, such a convening could examine the strategic plans of federal government departments and agencies impacting child and youth wellbeing, including the U.S. departments of Health and Human Services, Education, Agriculture, Housing and Urban Development, Justice, and Defense, as well as the Food and Drug Administration, and advise how they could be called upon as key federal agencies serving children and families to implement changes discussed in this report. A key outcome would be a framework for change in child health coordination.

Recommendation 1-1: Federal policy makers should convene an expert panel of key stakeholders, families, community partners, and state and federal agencies to develop a framework for promoting health and wellbeing for all children and adolescents and an enduring implementation plan. The framework should strive to integrate health programs among health care, education, labor, child welfare, and justice systems and foster shared goals of improving health and wellbeing throughout the life course and advancing health equity. The framework should present options for (1) financing enhanced services, (2) monitoring coordination over time, and (3) designating key leaders and agency structures that can focus attention on the health care needs of children, youth, and families.

This convening could also identify a federal agency or federal leadership position charged with ensuring the implementation of the framework and that all policies address children and families. The agency would produce an annual report on the status of children, youth, and families, with an enduring interagency structure with key programs included. Expansion of the charge and authority of the current Interagency Working Group on Youth Programs could provide this base. The structure could include participation of adolescents and families; ensure representation from historically marginalized communities; and have advisory, coordinating, and regulatory powers for implementation and ongoing assessment. It could develop performance monitoring and quality improvement focused on whole child and family health and equity through licensing, certification, accreditation bodies, relevant programs, and agencies (see measurement and accountability in Goal 5 and Chapter 9).

Another example, within the legislative branch, might take the form of a congressional committee on life course health and wellbeing, focused on children, youth, and families (similar to the Senate Committee on Aging), to raise visibility on issues of child, youth, and family health and wellbeing and impacts on the nation's health. The committee could study relevant issues, oversee programs, and advance important causes related to launching lifelong health.

Health outcomes are highly influenced by policies, programs, and practices that shape, for example, the quality and location of health care, availability and accessibility of public transportation, land use and street connectivity, and agricultural practices (National Research Council [NRC], 2011). Health in all policies is a promising (but not novel) approach to identifying and examining a policy's health and equity impacts. The approach builds on early principles of health promotion developed in the late 1970s and 1980s, centered on concepts such as legitimacy, accountability, transparency, accessibility, participation, sustainability, and multisectoral collaboration (Pan American Health Organization, 2015; United Kingdom Department of Health and Social Care, 2020; Wernham, 2011; WHO, 1986; WHO & United Nation's Children's Fund, 1978).

A health impact assessment is a process used to support a health-in-all-policies approach to decision making (Georgia Health Policy Center, n.d.; NRC, 2011). Such a process

> uses an array of data sources and analytic methods and considers input from stakeholders to determine the potential effects of a proposed policy, plan, program, or project on the health of a population and the distribution of those effects within the population [and] provides recommendations on monitoring and managing those effects. (NRC, 2011, p. 5)

Given that social, relational, and environmental factors have strong influence on the health and wellbeing of children and youth (see Chapters 2 and 4), the committee encourages policy makers to view child health holistically and weigh a broad set of policy decisions against the consequences they will have on family and community health.

Recommendation 1-2: Federal policy makers should enact child health and health equity impact statements that include impact and cost/benefit over longer time horizons for (1) Office of Management and Budget regulations in the federal register; (2) Congressional Budget Office (CBO) scoring of legislation; and (3) all major federal programmatic and research actions involving the U.S. departments of Health and Human Services, Education, Housing and Urban Development, Agriculture, Labor, and Justice. The CBO should expand its scoring of health programs to address longer-term outcomes (including Medicare and other public health expenditures) and impacts on federal sectors beyond health care. The president's annual budget line items should also report on inclusion of children and child health and health equity impact.

Recommendation 1-3: State legislatures and agencies should implement scoring of legislation and major programmatic initiatives to inform decisions based on their impact on the health and wellbeing of children and families and on health equity.

Foundations and child and youth wellbeing advocacy organizations can play a role in elevating the importance of child health through public awareness campaigns. Activated communities and constituents can be supported and grown to hold accountable their elected representatives, other government officials, and agencies, ensuring that policies promote rather than harm the health of children, youth, families, and communities.

Recommendation 1-4: Foundations and child and youth wellbeing advocacy organizations should fund and implement a long-term, multifaceted public awareness campaign that highlights issues of child and adolescent health and describes the importance of children and adolescents for the nation's future wellbeing and economic and national security.

Several agencies carry out research programs that have greatly improved the health and wellbeing of populations of all ages; yet, here too, children and youth have been relatively neglected in the breadth and scope of this work. As part of the broader plans suggested in this report, the nation should commit to strengthen and coordinate research related to children, youth, and families, in areas of inclusion, longitudinal research addressing key transitions, and increased study of the whole family.

Recommendation 1-5: The U.S. Department of Health and Human Services—through the Agency for Healthcare Research and Quality, the Advanced Research Projects Agency for Health, the National Institutes of Health, and other research and technology funders and developers—should continue and accelerate investment in research on whole child and family health, including mothers, children, adolescents, and families. Key elements of this research follow:

- **Inclusion of children, as well as child health and equity impact evaluations, in major research and technology initiatives.**
- **Longitudinal research early and throughout the life course, assessing long-term return on investment in health and developmental/educational outcomes and across sectors.**
- **Research that includes individuals' family and community context.**
- **Research on developmental transitions and care, such as from the prenatal period to infancy and from adolescence to adulthood.**
- **Clinical trials and dissemination and implementation research, especially related to incorporating scientific and technological advances in practice and policy.**
- **Engagement of youth, families, and community in the co-creation and co-design of research.**

Goal 2: Finance Health Care Systems for All Children, Emphasizing Disease Prevention and Health Promotion

This goal and its recommendations focus on Medicaid and CHIP reform and on changing payment incentives to drive the system toward prevention and health promotion. Medicaid and CHIP, the dominant payers for health care for children and youth, ensure a major safety net for large numbers of American children who would otherwise have no insurance. Yet persistent inequities in Medicaid leave many children and youth without adequate coverage for basic services, including key preventive services. States vary in their implementation of federal Medicaid laws, which creates barriers to enrollment and differences in program eligibility and accessibility, widening the gap in insurance coverage and access to care. These barriers affect racially and ethnically marginalized populations disproportionately, contributing to place-based racial/ethnic health inequities.

The major Early and Periodic Screening, Diagnosis, and Treatment (EPSDT) benefit in Medicaid provides a strong statutory requirement for the range of services that children and youth need. A central part of Medicaid,

EPSDT has lacked updated regulations for 40 years, and the program has had little monitoring or enforcement of statutory requirements. Medicaid and CHIP reform need to strengthen an already critical program and advance it to one that invests in the best future for U.S. children and youth. See Chapter 6 for more background on Medicaid and CHIP.

A health care system that supports the health and wellbeing of all children, families, and communities—recognizing the diverse set of strengths and needs among them—requires expanded focus on disease prevention and health promotion, along with ensuring adequate insurance coverage for individuals and families and support for a range of care providers for their health care needs. The health care system needs to advance toward continuous and comprehensive health care coverage for every child and family in every community. Gaps in children's insurance coverage must be addressed so that care is uninterrupted, comprehensive, and health promoting for both children and their families.

Recommendation 2-1: Federal and state policy makers and the Centers for Medicare & Medicaid Services (CMS) should reform Medicaid and the Children's Health Insurance Program (CHIP) to ensure coverage and services for every child and parent under age 65 who lacks other insurance. Specific actions to ensure insurance coverage include

- **Providing presumptive continuous eligibility for all children through their 6th birthday and universal access to Medicaid for all those under age 26 years who lack other health insurance.**
- **Enrolling all newborns at birth in Medicaid/CHIP if not covered by another plan.**
- **Allowing undocumented children and their parents access to Medicaid/CHIP, the Health Insurance Marketplace, and other federally funded health care services.**
- **Ensuring continuous Medicaid coverage for low-income parents.**
- **Aligning the financing of child coverage in the territories with that of states through Medicaid and CHIP.**

Specific actions to improve benefits and payment include

- **Reducing state and territory variability in eligibility, enrollment, quality, and payment by raising minimum federal standards.**
- **Ensuring a national base of high-quality services by modernizing Early and Periodic Screening, Diagnosis, and Treatment (EPSDT) benefits and rules. CMS and Congress should update EPSDT regulations, and CMS and the states should implement ongoing strategies for ensuring statutory compliance.**

- **Enforcing managed care organization contracts and implementation to ensure meeting all Medicaid/CHIP standards and requirements. States should ensure transparency in managed care organization contracts and public accountability.**
- **Designing and requiring integration of Medicaid and CHIP into a single program, making CHIP permanent, establishing the same provisions as Medicaid, and eliminating differences in eligibility and benefits.**
- **Increasing transparency in provider payment rates and direct provider subsidies and raising provider payments to levels that ensure that children and adolescents have equitable access to comprehensive, team-based primary and specialty care without discrimination based on payer.**
- **CMS and the Medicaid and CHIP Payment and Access Commission should collect and analyze data that speak to the adequacy of payment for child health care services.**
- **CMS should implement a Medicaid Beneficiary Survey, modeled after the Medicare Current Beneficiary Survey, that captures beneficiaries' health and functioning; satisfaction with health care; usual source of care; and access to care, including primary care and specialty care for new and established patients.**

Although the current child health care system generally promotes wellbeing and prevention, it is hampered because of its continuing focus on disease identification and treatment reinforced by a fee-for-service payment model that pays mainly for visits and procedures. Strategies for improving population health include team-based care and community-engaged programs, combined with specific efforts at prevention and health promotion and decreasing inequities.

Current fee-for-service payment models do not allow clinicians the flexibility to work with families and communities to address health and developmental goals for children. They do not support the many well-evidenced advances in enhanced pediatric primary and subspecialty care. Furthermore, most recent efforts to change payment methods have focused on short-term cost savings among older populations with high medical expenses. Child health care offers few opportunities for major cost savings in the short term; rather, improvements are seen in long-term outcomes beyond childhood, often in education and other sectors outside of health care, as well as long-term savings in Medicare and other public health outlays. Current insurance mechanisms have not kept pace with changing demographics; environmental influences on health; major new clinical strategies; scientific breakthroughs; and technological advances, such as increased use of telehealth.

As discussed in Chapter 5, a growing literature documents the value of multidisciplinary team-based care, including nonphysician personnel, in effectively addressing the needs of children, families, and communities. The roles of nurses and community health workers have become more prominent in clinical teams, as they provide support for families in several ways—including, for example, assistance in managing chronic conditions, navigating the health care system, and accessing community resources to improve healthy living.

Chapter 2 describes the strong scientific foundation on the importance of early life experiences and how safe, stable, and nurturing relationships support health promotion and set the trajectory for lifelong health outcomes. The dramatic prominence of mental health issues among children, youth, and parents particularly calls for integrated mental and behavioral health care systems (see Chapters 4 and 5).

Taking a life course approach and reaping the benefits of improving child health requires a system-wide focus on prevention of health problems and promotion of healthy experiences, from preconception to adulthood. Achieving this goal will require implementing payment models for child health care that incentivize population health efforts in prevention and promotion, especially bringing to scale the many successful advances in pediatric care. Doing so necessitates financing for all team members; incentivizing practice transformation; and providing continuous, consistent, and comprehensive health care coverage for every child and family in every community.

Recommendation 2-2: Public and commercial payers should transition from relying predominantly on fee-for-service arrangements and explore payment incentives that emphasize prevention and health promotion services, team-based and cross-sector care, health equity, health outcomes, and longer-term return on investment. While enhancements in fee-for-service models can support needed change, related payment strategies, including direct incentives, various withholding mechanisms, and alternative payment methods, should support this transition. The Centers for Medicare & Medicaid Services (CMS) and commercial payers should use payment methods that provide direct incentives toward population health, health equity, and the health of communities. Strategies for incentivizing practice change could include tiered payments that reward high-performing pediatric care. Current payment innovations, including numerous state efforts such as per member per month or population payments, serve as key experimental steps for covering health care services for children, youth, and families.

- **CMS and commercial payers should test and implement episodic and bundled payment models that are designed for the service needs of children, youth, and families, especially those with more complex conditions.**

- **CMS, through its Center for Medicare and Medicaid Innovation (CMMI), should innovate in pediatric payment strategies and ensure inclusion of children in their programs. For example, as CMMI implements state total-cost-of-care models in the States Advancing All-Payer Health Equity Approaches and Development Model, children should be included and child health and health equity impact statements addressed.**
- **Payment should support team-based and cross-sector care, including high-performing medical homes, mental and behavioral health integration, and other innovations that support development of safe, stable, and nurturing relationships between caregivers and children; improve health equity; and build community health.**

Because of their prominence in the lives of most children and families, schools offer unique opportunities to advance child health, without parallel among institutions for adult populations (see Chapter 8). Schools can assist in outreach and enrollment of eligible children in public health insurance programs and income support programs, offer direct care through school-based health centers, and reduce food insecurity and improve dietary quality through school meals programs. Direct school health services vary widely, as do their funding sources, including some funding from Medicaid and other federal sources and local school funds. These variations can exacerbate racial and other health disparities arising from the impact of structural racism on the makeup of neighborhoods and communities and on the financing of schools. The committee calls for strengthening direct school health efforts, including efforts to grow and support school-based health centers.

Recommendation 2-3: State legislatures and Medicaid programs should adopt and enforce policies that promote equitable payment for services delivered in school-based health centers (SBHCs) and by other school providers. Policies that have been effective in several states include those that (1) define SBHCs as a specific provider type; (2) waive prior approval or authorization from primary care providers for all SBHC billing; (3) allow Medicaid managed care organization payment for "self-referred" children seen in SBHCs; and (4) incorporate clarification of laws related to data sharing, including the Health Insurance Portability and Accountability Act and the Family Educational Rights and Privacy Act. Such policies should be implemented with intent to prioritize communities that face the largest health inequities, including gaps in access to pediatric health care services, and to encourage school-based programs to leverage, support, and enhance collaborations between schools and community health centers and health care systems.

Goal 3: Strengthen Community-Level Health Promotion and Disease Prevention

While the health care system focuses on identifying and treating health conditions in individuals, public health focuses on population-level actions to promote health and prevent disease (Wiley, 2016). In the United States, far more of the investment in health flows through the health care system for medical care than through public health for primary prevention, with particular loss of benefit for the health and wellbeing of younger populations. The United Nations Children's Fund Innocenti Report Card #16 (UNICEF, 2020) found that in 2015 the United States spent just 1.3% of its gross domestic product (GDP) on families with a significant proportion of that coming through tax breaks. This is compared with an average of 2.4% GDP across wealthy nations and an average of 2.9% GDP among the three highest-ranked countries for overall child wellbeing (Netherlands, Denmark, and Norway). In a ranking of nations' child wellbeing policies, the United States ranked 28th for health care policies and last (41st) in social policies.

As discussed throughout the report, efforts to advance primary prevention are especially salient for children and youth, since childhood presents a critical window for influencing health outcomes over the life course. Public health investment focused on child populations and community-level primary prevention can protect the nation from future high costs of health care and other services to address preventable health conditions.

The committee views expansion and intensification of the nation's investment in public health as essential for strengthening population-level health promotion and disease prevention and launching lifelong health for children. Public health investment can take several forms and requires a diverse group of public and private stakeholders, including the health care system and government public health agencies, working together to contribute to the health of a community. Investment needs to extend beyond immunizations, screenings, and the like to truly address community needs. Public health efforts can be funded through and implemented in a variety of community settings: local hospitals, community health clinics, schools, and local public health departments are some discussed in this report. The key is having an entity capable of serving as a catalyst for engaging multiple stakeholders in tackling community health problems.

Effective programs shown to improve the health and wellbeing of children (see Chapter 7 for review of federal programs aimed at improving population health) need to be expanded to reach the communities most in need and reduce long-standing health disparities. The committee highlights the Child Opportunity Index or Social Vulnerability Index as a measure of geographic advantage or disadvantage to guide federal and state funding. Using these or other measures will ensure that neighborhood factors and needs drive a more equitable allocation of funding or block grants that communities receive for health and wellness services.

Furthermore, financing for the public health infrastructure, including local public health departments, needs to be strengthened. Because public health spending is highly uneven across communities,[2] the committee calls for assessing and strengthening local health departments to ensure that each has a minimum standard of core, foundational capabilities, and a strong emphasis on the health of children, families, and communities. Expanding on the notion of primary prevention as a form of insurance (Newhouse, 2021), new spending on public health initiatives for improving child health can be seen as a form of insurance for the nation against high future health care and non–health care costs attributable to preventable conditions.

Recommendation 3-1: Federal policy makers and agencies should expand funding for population-level whole child and family health promotion and disease prevention resource investments in ways that (1) provide greater and equitable support for children and families in need; (2) integrate community-level resources with child health care systems; and (3) ensure that all eligible children and families receive the highest-quality services in current public health programs. Federal programs that have particular relevance to younger populations and should be expanded to build core services for communities include

- **The Administration for Children and Families Head Start and Early Head Start programs.**
- **The U.S. Department of Agriculture Special Supplemental Nutrition Program for Women, Infants, and Children and the Supplemental Nutrition Assistance Program.**
- **The Prevention and Public Health Fund, administered through the Centers for Disease Control and Prevention, with elevated focus on younger populations.**
- **Investments in early childhood health and prevention administered through the Health Resources and Services Administration (HRSA) and the Substance Abuse and Mental Health Services Administration. Within HRSA, the Maternal and Child Health Bureau Title V block grant and targeted funding for maternal health, child health, and child development particularly merit expansion.**

[2]In its synthesis, IOM (2012b) finds that "the health departments in the poorest communities and communities that have the poorest health outcomes are among the least-well-funded" (p. 56). Mays and Smith (2009) found a more than 13-fold difference between communities with high versus low public health spending. The National Association of County and City Health Officials (NACCHO, 2020) shows a threefold difference between the 25th and 75th percentile values of annual per capita expenditures across local health departments. And Owsley, Hamer, and Mays (2020) point to the widening gap between urban and rural public health delivery systems.

Recommendation 3-2: Federal, state, and local agencies should reduce inequities in local public health department capacity and improve execution of current evidence-based support programs aimed at children to reap long-term benefits of improving child health and wellbeing.

- Federal policy makers should create a permanent Public Health Infrastructure Fund to ensure that each local health department has basic, core capabilities and technology support and to ameliorate existing inequities in public health resource availability.
- State and local agencies should evaluate existing public health capacity across communities and support coordination with other local health departments and health care systems.
- Federal and state agencies should evaluate how competitive grant-in-aid mechanisms may exacerbate resource inequities across local health departments and test alternative approaches to allocating limited resources.
- Federal and state agencies should coordinate and streamline processes and systems for ensuring strong execution of current evidence-based programs that support child health, in order to reach all who are eligible for services, using multiple points of access.

In addition to providing direct clinical services, schools engage in health promotion and disease prevention in multiple ways, including through formal and informal curriculum—which may include socioemotional learning, physical education, health class, and reproductive health education (family-life education). Teachers, counselors, and school nurses, among others, deliver these services, with a wide variety of school-based programs for improving mental health, reducing obesity, and managing chronic conditions. Many children receive meals through schools, making school meal programs a natural lever for influencing nutrition (see Chapter 8). Furthermore, teachers are present in children's day-to-day lives and, if supported, can provide safe, stable relationships for children and youth, which are essential to children's health and wellbeing (see Chapter 2). The committee identifies great promise in leveraging schools to support children's wellbeing and calls for strengthening schools' capacity around health promotion and disease prevention.

Recommendation 3-3: Federal, state, and local policy makers and agencies—in collaboration with health care systems, schools, foundations, employers, and other community partners—should expand

investment, through blended and braided funding, to support the infrastructure and resources to enhance school-based health promotion and disease prevention. Key actions include

- **Funding expansion of the Centers for Disease Control and Prevention Healthy Schools program to meet community needs.**
- **Expanding resources to meet community needs and provide nutritious meals to all eligible students through the National School Lunch Program and the School Breakfast Program.**
- **Expanding the School-Based Mental Health Services Grant Program distributed through the Bipartisan Safer Communities Act to improve the ability of communities and schools to reach all children in need.**

Several changes in tax and regulatory policy can provide substantial financing for these recommended investments. An important opportunity comes from strengthening community benefits requirements. Nonprofit hospitals benefit financially from tax exemptions at the federal, state, and local levels when they invest in community benefit activities (i.e., initiatives, activities, and investments undertaken to improve health in the communities they serve; Government Accountability Office, 2023c; The Hilltop Institute, n.d.). Of approximately 6,000 hospitals in the United States, about half are identified as nongovernment, nonprofit community hospitals, which qualify for tax-exempt status (American Hospital Association, 2024). As discussed in Chapter 7, the Internal Revenue Service requires nonprofit hospitals to assess community needs and document their community benefit activities. Efforts to strengthen this existing policy need to include retaining flexibility for hospitals to tailor their programs and practices to address the specific needs and concerns of their communities (Lucas-Judy, 2023); strengthening of these policies also needs to ensure accountability for improved health outcomes.

Beyond hospitals, community benefit strategies can be applied to nonprofit health plans with similar requirements for accountability to address local community needs. Other sources of funds for community benefit include mandating prevention investments by for-profit health plans (as California currently does) and reclassifying community prevention services as part of the medical loss ratio rather than as administrative costs (see Chapter 7). Health care for children provides substantial income for for-profit entities, especially those managed care organizations providing most Medicaid and CHIP services through state contracts. Taxation of these profits could provide substantial resources to strengthen several components of child and adolescent health care.

Recommendation 3-4: To expand investment in community-based prevention and health promotion for children, federal agencies should strengthen existing community benefit requirements and accounting mechanisms to support and incentivize health care system initiatives to advance community health.

- The Internal Revenue Service (IRS) should strengthen community benefit requirements for tax-exempt hospitals and create similar requirements for tax-exempt health plans. Reporting under the IRS Community Benefit Standards should require that nonprofit hospitals and health plans (1) use best-practice community needs assessment and improvement protocols and coordinate with existing community partnerships—or establish such partnerships—to create and implement action plans for addressing findings of community health needs assessments; (2) ensure community representation, accountability measures, and enforcement mechanisms in action plans; and (3) publicly report on progress for community-defined, cross-sector outcomes and measures for child and community health.
- The Centers for Medicare & Medicaid Services should reclassify community-based prevention programs as an allowable service, as part of the medical loss ratio.

Recommendation 3-5: State legislatures should mandate investment in community health from for-profit health care providers and managed care organizations. Such mandates should ensure that for-profit providers employ best practices for assessing community needs, engaging community representation, developing initiatives, and publicly reporting on progress for community-defined, cross-sector outcomes and measures for child and community health and health equity.

Goal 4: Ensure Co-Creation and Co-Design of Programs and Structures with Youth, Family, and Community Voices and Leadership

The perspectives of youth, family, and communities, and their lived experiences around health and the health care system, can have a critical and central role in health care and can improve outcomes (see Chapter 3). However, the impact of their voices on system change has not yet been fully realized. Health disparities and structural racism remain prominent concerns. For many families and communities in the United States, the health care system is untrustworthy. Youth, families, and communities bring critical expertise and must be partners in the co-creation and co-design of programs that will address their health and wellbeing, including health care transformation efforts, policy making, and care decisions.

The current health care system has been characterized as industry and provider centric; it needs to transform to become child, family, and community centered. Vital contributions from youth, families, and communities enables diverse voices in decision making at patient and population health levels and can inform the training of health care professionals, research activities, and quality improvement efforts (see Chapter 3). Future community partnerships will need to be supported appropriately and participants compensated.

To ensure the health and wellbeing of children and youth, engaging families of children and youth needs to be top priority. Integrating them, their perspectives, their collaboration, and their leadership, and supporting their time, are crucial at all levels, including decision making within health care systems, planning through public health agencies, and policy making and guidance at the federal and state levels.

Recommendation 4-1: Health care systems should partner with community members and leaders from historically marginalized backgrounds to co-design policies and build programs that support a more child-, family-, and community-centered health care system, supporting quality improvement, patient safety, and health equity initiatives. Such partnerships should

- **Ensure the active involvement of patients, youth, and families in the development and implementation of new science and technologies (e.g., genome sequencing, prediction models that use artificial intelligence) and models of care.**
- **Strengthen the role and diversity of patient and youth family advisory councils that reflect the communities served and address community needs.**
- **Provide education and training opportunities as well as compensation to patient, youth, and family advisors that engage in child health care system transformation initiatives and efforts.**
- **Create pathways with local community programs to involve high school and college students from marginalized communities in early mentorship and job programs, in order to promote community engagement and develop a sustained and diverse health care workforce.**
- **Provide and encourage training and volunteer opportunities for health care system employees to partner with the community to co-design, build, implement, and evaluate programs, in order to achieve excellent and equitable child health outcomes.**

Recommendation 4-2: Federal research agencies, state governments, and foundations should eliminate barriers that make it challenging

for health care entities to financially compensate patients and families for their participation in efforts to improve services or programs; they should also eliminate barriers that limit collaboration among health care, child health–related public health programs, and family- and community-based services.

Recommendation 4-3: Accrediting and certifying bodies for the training and certification of physicians, nurses, nurse practitioners, physician assistants, mental and dental health providers, and other health care workers should require training to ensure that the health care workforce is competent, diverse, team oriented, and antiracist, and able to promote relational health.

Recommendation 4-4: Hospital or health care system accrediting bodies (e.g., The Joint Commission) and recognition programs (e.g., *U.S. News & World Report* Hospital Rankings, American Nurses Association Magnet Recognition Program) should continue efforts to assess and recognize activities related to patient and family experience; diversity, equity, and inclusion; and achievement of excellent and equitable health outcomes.

Recommendation 4-5: Federal and state agencies should mandate and utilize the expertise of youth, families, and communities by generating and sustaining community representation and advisory practices that are integrated with accountability measures and enforcement mechanisms.

- Federal agencies should incorporate requirements in grants to states and territories for greater youth, family, and community engagement, including those from historically marginalized communities.
- State agencies should instruct community advisory boards to make proceedings and minutes of meetings public to ensure strong engagement.
- Federal and state agencies should support quality improvement efforts and learning health networks—with a specific focus on co-design with patients, children, youth, families, and communities—to improve outcomes tied to decreasing health disparities and quality measures that align with communities' needs.
- The Centers for Medicare & Medicaid Services should reinvigorate its Partnership for Patients program by funding capacity and capability building for children, youth, families, and community leaders to fully engage and co-lead quality improvement efforts within hospital and community innovation networks and quality improvement organizations.

Recommendation 4-6: Federal and state agencies, foundations, and other funders should provide financial support for youth-led services in local communities. This support could include

- **Research funding directed at strengthening scientific understanding of the efficacy, effectiveness, and implementation of youth-led services.**
- **Funding of youth-led services, through AmeriCorps' Healthy Futures focus area, to include training and credentialing, which should be deployed locally. The proposed expansion of funding for this program should target young people in delivering peer-led services, to massively expand their access to health promotion and mental health supports.**
- **Funding to co-create and co-design a national credential for peer-support specialists with youth-led organizations, graduate student–led national organizations, and the credentialing bodies for allied health care professionals, to expand the workforce of youth leaders. This is pivotal to providing consistency in delivery of youth-led services and to sustaining the development of the future health care workforce.**

Goal 5: Implement Measurement and Accountability to Ensure Equitable Achievement of These Goals

A transformed health care system needs to emphasize accountability for equitable, whole child, family, and community health outcomes. In Chapter 9, the committee identifies seven priority areas for implementing an accountability measurement strategy that supports improved outcomes for all children and youth: (1) commitment to child and youth population outcomes and equity measures; (2) applied research on best practices for real-world use of essential child and youth wellbeing measures; (3) shared accountability measures and improved digital health integration and data interoperability across systems and sectors; (4) reduced number of universal quality measures services to improve and track priority outcomes; (5) stronger incentives to accelerate accountability improvements; (6) engagement and transparency with patients, families, and communities on an accountability measurement framework and system performance; and (7) a national data dashboard for tracking progress on goals and recommendations for a transformed child health care system that prioritizes improving child and youth health and wellbeing.

Ongoing innovations in measurement, payment, and cross-sector services integration suggest that a child health care system that is accountable for improved child wellbeing outcomes is possible. Prior National Academies reports and other publications clearly outline the importance of community and cross-sector accountability, focused on a small set of outcome measures that are meaningful to families and communities, such as rates of infant mortality, school readiness, positive mental health, and high school graduation. Some state Medicaid programs are introducing financial incentives to managed care organizations and their provider partners to improve long-term child health. These incentives use outcome measures that capture information on not just the immediate patients of a health care system but also all children in a geographic area. Related advances include proposals for building equity into accountability metrics and forming federal agency collaborations to address federal barriers to shared accountability measures across health care, public health, and social services systems. The committee's recommendations build on this renewed commitment to greater accountability for child and adolescent health.

Recommendation 5-1: The Centers for Medicare & Medicaid Services, in collaboration with other federal agencies, should support health care systems' implementation of new and evolved accountability measurement systems that minimize overall measurement burden, have meaning for families and communities, and highlight equity. Measures should address population health, disparities, and the functioning of children, and they should promote integrated, cross-sector child health care systems of care. Key efforts include

- Providing technical support for state demonstrations on the application of an outcome-based, shared, cross-system measurement and accountability framework focused on a narrowed and integrated set of measures aimed at population health and equity using a whole child and family health approach. Such support could be coordinated with the Administration for Children and Families, the Health Resources and Services Administration, and the U.S. Department of Education.
- Partnering with other federal agencies to support state and local child health accountability-related programs, and working with the Interagency Working Group on Youth Programs and private-sector partners and experts, to develop a toolkit for best practices in engaging families, youth, and communities in the co-design and effective use of accountability measurement systems.

Recommendation 5-2: Federal research agencies tasked with improving the health and wellbeing of children and youth should continue to advance the data resources and research necessary to evolve accountability measurement systems in ways that produce robust state and local area estimates from national surveys and existing federal data

systems, support digital tools for local data collection and reporting to allow for comparable health care, public health, and policy studies, and fill key knowledge gaps in the practice of designing and using population health measures aligned with communities' needs for better health outcomes for children.

Recommendation 5-3: Federal and state governments should coordinate cross-agency efforts to monitor system performance and eliminate barriers to shared accountability across child health programs, in areas such as health care, education, child welfare, home- and community-based services, and juvenile justice. These efforts should support the development of interoperable cross-sector portals, including patient- and family-facing portals.

Recommendation 5-4: The Office of the National Coordinator for Health Information Technology should partner with the Centers for Medicare & Medicaid Services and a national committee comprising both public- and private-sector members, in order to develop a transparent reporting protocol for data submission that all payers and child-serving health care systems can use to monitor a small set of agreed-upon measures amenable to real-time (daily, weekly, monthly) electronic record submissions that include family- or patient-reported outcomes data.

CONCLUSION

This report comes at a point of national crisis in the health and wellbeing of U.S. children and youth—with graphic evidence of the effects of this crisis on the U.S. workforce, military preparedness, and burgeoning costs of adult ill health. The committee and its report take a broad view of the health care system, while recognizing the many other influences, outside of health care, that heavily affect both children and youth today and, notably, their prospects for the next decade. If child health is not elevated and efforts to improve the child health care system are not expanded, current trends point to a worsening state of health for the nation and deficits in the capacity of working-age adults.

Transforming child and adolescent health care requires an ambitious agenda. This report provides the guide and framework for that transformation. It acknowledges the national imperative for change, if the nation hopes to reverse troubling trends in the health of America's children, in racial and geographic health inequities experienced by communities, and in the current and future workforce—where rates of mortality and disability are rising, along with a growing population of older adults who will need increased support.

The nation has seen many advancements in new models of care, growing science of early childhood, new research into early identification and prevention of disease, and institutions able to support the care and system needed. The report emphasizes the strong evidence that arises from this research and how to implement needed change. Previous studies have highlighted many of these advances and opportunities, yet their implementation shows the limits of short-term changes and improvements. Few have had lasting impact, in part because of the lack of an ongoing focus on children and youth.

This report calls a national convening to consider the evidence provided and implement the blueprint the recommendations provide. This convening could help form an ongoing framework and structure for maintaining focus and progress. The report recommendations include strategies for maintaining focus on children and youth and their health care, including better assessment of the child health impact of public policies, ways to reform health care financing for children, strategies to improve public health and school health, methods of including children and families and historically marginalized communities in all aspects of program and policy, and ways to measure and ensure accountability and equity for change and outcomes. Such changes will require strong leadership and incentives at the federal and state levels.

References

Aalsma, M. C., Schwartz, K., Haight, K. A., Jarjoura, G. R., & Dir, A. L. (2019). Applying an electronic health records data quality framework across service sectors: A case study of juvenile justice system data. *eGEMs*, *7*(1), 26. https://doi.org/10.5334/egems.258

AbdulRaheem, Y. (2023). Unveiling the significance and challenges of integrating prevention levels in healthcare practice. *Journal of Primary Care & Community Health*, *14*. https://doi.org/10.1177/21501319231186500

Abràmoff, M. D., Tarver, M. E., Trujillo, S., Char, D., Obermeyer, Z., Eydelman, M. B., & Maisel, W. H. (2023). Considerations for addressing bias in artificial intelligence for health equity. *NPJ Digital Medicine*, *6*(1), 1–7. https://doi.org/10.1038/s41746-023-00913-9

Abramson, A. (2022). 2022 Trends report: Children's mental health is in crisis. *American Psychological Association*, *53*(1). https://www.apa.org/monitor/2022/01/special-childrens-mental-health

Accreditation Council for Graduate Medical Education [ACGME]. (2022). *ACGME program requirements for graduate medical education in family medicine*. https://www.acgme.org/globalassets/pfassets/programrequirements/120familymedicine2022.pdf

________. (2023a). *ACGME program requirements for graduate medical education in pediatrics*. https://www.acgme.org/globalassets/pfassets/reviewandcomment/320_pediatrics_rc_022023.pdf

________. (2023b). *Specialty and subspecialty information table*. https://www.acgme.org/globalassets/pdfs/subspecialtieslist.pdf

Acevedo-Garcia, D., Joshi, P. K., Ruskin, E., Walters, A. N., Sofer, N., & Guevara, C. A. (2021). Including children in immigrant families in policy approaches to reduce child poverty. *Academic Pediatrics*, *21*(Suppl 8), S117–S125. https://doi.org/10.1016/j.acap.2021.06.016

Acevedo-Garcia, D., McArdle, N., Hardy, E., Crisan, U., Romano, B., Norris, D., Baek, M., & Reece, J. (2014). The child opportunity index: Improving collaboration between community development and public health. *Health Affairs*, *33*, 1948–1957. https://doi.org/10.1377/hlthaff.2014.0679

Adalia, E. G., Hernández-Luengo, M., Bartolomé-Gutiérrez, R., Rodríguez-Martín, B., Jiménez-López, E., & Martínez-Andrés, M. (2021). Expectations and experiences of women in pregnancy, childbirth, and infant feeding: A qualitative research protocol. *International Journal of Qualitative Methods*, *20*. https://doi.org/10.1177/16094069211011901

Ader, J., Stille, C. J., Keller, D., Miller, B. F., Barr, M. S., & Perrin, J. M. (2015). The medical home and integrated behavioral health: Advancing the policy agenda. *Pediatrics*, *135*(5), 909–917. https://doi.org/10.1542/peds.2014-3941

Adesoye, T., Mangurian, C., Choo, E. K., Girgis, C., Sabry-Elnaggar, H., Linos, E., & Physician Moms Group Study Group. (2017). Perceived discrimination experienced by physician mothers and desired workplace changes: A cross-sectional survey. *JAMA Internal Medicine*, *177*(7), 1033–1036. https://doi.org/10.1001/jamainternmed.2017.1394

Administration for Children and Families. (n.d.). *Child welfare*. Department of Health and Human Services. https://www.acf.hhs.gov/acf_issues/child_welfare

Administration for Children and Families (ACF). (2023a). *Head Start Services*. U.S. Department of Health and Human Services, Administration for Children and Families. https://www.acf.hhs.gov/ohs/about/head-start

________. (2023b). *Head start policy and regulations*. U.S. Department of Health and Human Services. https://eclkc.ohs.acf.hhs.gov/policy/pi/acf-pi-hs-22-02

Advanced Practice Registered Nurses Joint Dialogue Group. (2008). *Consensus model for APRN regulation: Licensure, accreditation, certification & education*. https://www.ncsbn.org/public-files/Consensus_Model_for_APRN_Regulation_July_2008.pdf

Agency for Healthcare Research and Quality. (n.d.). *Interim data from national efforts to make care safer, 2010-2014*. Department of Health and Human Services. https://www.ahrq.gov/hai/pfp/interimhacrate2014.html

________. (2014). *Core functionality for pediatric electronic health records*. https://effectivehealthcare.ahrq.gov/products/pediatric-ehr/research-protocol

________. (2018). *2017 national healthcare quality and disparities report*.

________. (2020). *AHRQ's making healthcare safer reports: Shaping patient safety efforts in the 21st century*. https://www.ahrq.gov/research/findings/making-healthcare-safer/index.html

________. (2021a). *2021 national healthcare quality and disparities report* (Pub. No. 21(22)-0054-EF). U.S. Department of Health and Human Services. https://www.ahrq.gov/sites/default/files/wysiwyg/research/findings/nhqrdr/2021qdr.pdf

________. (2021b). *Cost-to-charge ratio files*. Healthcare Cost and Utilization Project (HCUP). https://hcup-us.ahrq.gov/db/ccr/costtocharge.jsp

________. (2022a). *2022 national healthcare quality and disparities report*. https://pubmed.ncbi.nlm.nih.gov/36475568

________. (2022b). *CAHPS item set for children with chronic conditions*. https://www.ahrq.gov/cahps/surveys-guidance/item-sets/children-chronic/index.html

________. (2024). *National healthcare quality and disparities reports*. U.S. Department of Health and Human Services. https://www.ahrq.gov/research/findings/nhqrdr/index.html

Agha, L., Frandsen, B., & Rebitzer, J. B. (2019). Fragmented division of labor and healthcare costs: Evidence from moves across regions. *Journal of Public Economics*, *169*, 144–159. https://doi.org/10.1016/j.jpubeco.2018.11.001

Agnafors, S., Barmark, M., & Sydsjö, G. (2021). Mental health and academic performance: A study on selection and causation effects from childhood to early adulthood. *Social Psychiatry and Psychiatric Epidemiology*, *56*(5), 857–866.

Agnew-Blais, J., & Seidman, L. J. (2013). Attention deficit/hyperactivity disorder over the life course. In K. C. Koenen, S. Rudenstine, E. Susser, & S. Galea (Eds.), *A life course approach to mental disorders*. Oxford University Press. https://doi.org/10.1093/acprof:oso/9780199657018.003.0014

Agniel, D., Cabreros, I., Damberg, C. L., Elliott, M. N., & Rogers, R. (2023). A formal framework for incorporating equity into health care quality measurement. *Health Affairs*, *42*(10), 1383–1391. https://doi.org/10.1377/hlthaff.2022.01483

Aguilar-Gaxiola, S., Ahmed, S. M., Anise, A., Azzahir, A., Baker, K. E., Cupito, A., Eder, M., Everette, T. D., Erwin, K., Felzien, M., Freeman, E., Gibbs, D., Greene-Moton, E., Hernández-Cancio, S., Hwang, A., Jones, F., Jones, G., Jones, M., Khodyakov, D., & Zaldivar, R. (2022). Assessing meaningful community engagement: A conceptual model to advance health equity through transformed systems for health. Organizing Committee for Assessing Meaningful Community Engagement in Health & Health Care Programs & Policies. *NAM Perspectives*. https://doi.org/10.31478/202202c

Aizer, A., Stroud, L., & Buka, S. (2016). Maternal stress and child outcomes: Evidence from siblings. *The Journal of Human Resources*, *51*(3), 523–555. https://doi.org/10.3386/w18422

Akers, A. Y., Davis, E. M., Jackson Foster, L. J., Morrison, P., Sucato, G., Miller, E., & Lee, M. (2014). Parental report of receipt of adolescent preventive health counseling services from pediatric providers. *Patient Education and Counseling*, *94*(2), 269–275. https://doi.org/10.1016/j.pec.2013.10.003

Al Shamsi, H., Almutairi, A. G., Al Mashrafi, S., & Al Kalbani, T. (2020). Implications of language barriers for healthcare: A systematic review. *Oman Medical Journal*, *35*(2), e122. https://doi.org/10.5001/omj.2020.40

Al-Shimari, F., Kahn, N. F., McCarty, C. A., Parker, E. O., Richardson, L. P., & Shafii, T. (2022). Provider use of time alone with adolescents: Differences by health concern. *Journal of Adolescent Health: Official Publication of the Society for Adolescent Medicine*, *71*(4), 508. https://doi.org/10.1016/j.jadohealth.2022.05.021

Alaie, I., Philipson, A., Ssegonja, R., Copeland, W. E., Ramklint, M., Bohman, H., & Jonsson, U. (2022). Adolescent depression and adult labor market marginalization: A longitudinal cohort study. *European Child & Adolescent Psychiatry*, *31*(11), 1799–1813. https://doi.org/10.1007/s00787-021-01825-3

Alaie, I., Svedberg, P., Ropponen, A., & Narusyte, J. (2023). Associations of internalizing and externalizing problems in childhood and adolescence with adult labor market marginalization. *JAMA Network Open*, *6*(6), e2317905–e2317905. https://doi.org/10.1001/jamanetworkopen.2023.17905

Alberto, C. K., Kemmick Pintor, J., Martínez-Donate, A., Tabb, L. P., Langellier, B., & Stimpson, J. P. (2021). Association of maternal-clinician ethnic concordance with Latinx youth receipt of family-centered care. *JAMA Network Open*, *4*(11), e2133857. https://doi.org/10.1001/jamanetworkopen.2021.33857

Alcusky, M. J., Mick, E. O., Allison, J. J., Kiefe, C. I., Sabatino, M. J., Eanet, F. E., & Ash, A. S. (2023). Paying for medical and social complexity in Massachusetts Medicaid. *JAMA Network Open*, *6*(9), e2332173–e2332173. https://doi.org/10.1001/jamanetworkopen.2023.32173

Alegría, M., O'Malley, I. S., Smith, R., Useche Rosania, A., Boyd, A., Cuervo-Torello, F., Williams, D. R., & Acevedo-Garcia, D. (2023). Addressing health inequities for children in immigrant families: Psychologists as leaders and links across systems. *The American Psychologist*, *78*(2), 173–185. https://doi.org/10.1037/amp0001016

Alexander, D., & Currie, J. (2017). Is it who you are or where you live? Residential segregation and racial gaps in childhood asthma. *Journal of Health Economics*, *55*, 186–200. https://doi.org/10.1016/j.jhealeco.2017.07.003

Ali, M. M., Sherman, L. J., Lynch, S., Teich, J., & Mutter, R. (2019). Differences in utilization of mental health treatment among children and adolescents with Medicaid or private insurance. *Psychiatric Services*, *70*(4). https://doi.org/10.1176/appi.ps.201800428

Alinsky, R. H., Zima, B. T., Rodean, J., Matson, P. A., Larochelle, M. R., Adger, H., Jr., Bagley, S. M., & Hadland, S. E. (2020). Receipt of addiction treatment after opioid overdose among Medicaid-enrolled adolescents and young adults. *JAMA Pediatrics*, *174*(3), e195183. https://doi.org/10.1001/jamapediatrics.2019.5183

Alker, J., & Osorio, A. (2023). Medicaid's pandemic-era continuous coverage protections helped reduce number of uninsured children. *Georgetown University McCourt School of Public Policy, Center for Children & Families*. https://ccf.georgetown.edu/2023/11/15/medicaids-pandemic-era-continuous-coverage-protections-helped-reduce-number-of-uninsured-children/

Alker, J., Miskell, S., Musumeci, M., & Rudowitz, R. (2015). *Medicaid premium assistance programs: What information is available about benefit and cost-sharing wrap-around coverage?* KFF. https://www.kff.org/report-section/medicaid-premium-assistance-programs-what-information-is-available-about-benefit-and-cost-sharing-wrap-around-coverage-introduction/

All of Us Research Program Investigators. (2019). The "All of Us" research program. *New England Journal of Medicine*, *381*(7), 668–676. https://doi.org/10.1056/NEJMsr1809937

Allen, H., Golberstein, E., & Bailey, Z. (2022). Eliminating health disparities will require looking at how much and how Medicaid pays participating providers. *Milbank Quarterly Opinion*. https://www.milbank.org/quarterly/opinions/eliminating-health-disparities-will-require-looking-at-how-much-and-how-medicaid-pays-participating-providers/

Allen, J. (2010). Improving cross-cultural care and antiracism in nursing education: A literature review. *Nurse Education Today*, *30*(4), 314–320. https://doi.org/10.1016/j.nedt.2009.08.007

Alley, D. E., Ashford, N. C., & Gavin, A. M. (2019). Payment innovations to drive improvements in pediatric care—The integrated care for kids model. *JAMA Pediatrics*, *173*(8), 717–718. https://doi.org/10.1001/jamapediatrics.2019.1703

Allison, M. A., & Attisha, E. (2019). The link between school attendance and good health. *Pediatrics*, *143*(2). https://doi.org/10.1542/peds.2018-3648

Allison, M. A., Crane, L. A., Beaty, B. L., Davidson, A. J., Melinkovich, P., & Kempe, A. (2007). School-based health centers: Improving access and quality of care for low-income adolescents. *Pediatrics*, *120*(4), e887–e894. https://doi.org/10.1542/peds.2006-2314

Almirall, D., & Chronis-Tuscano, A. (2016). Adaptive interventions in child and adolescent mental health. *Journal of Clinical Child & Adolescent Psychology*, *45*(4), 383–395. https://doi.org/10.1080/15374416.2016.1152555

Almond, D., Hoynes, H. W., & Schanzenbach, D. W. (2011). Inside the war on poverty: The impact of food stamps on birth outcomes. *Review of Economics and Statistics*, *93*(2), 387–403. https://doi.org/10.1162/REST_a_00089

Alonzo, D., Popescu, M., & Zubaroglu Ioannides, P. (2022). Mental health impact of the COVID-19 pandemic on parents in high-risk, low income communities. *International Journal of Social Psychiatry*, *68*(3), 575–581. https://doi.org/10.1177/0020764021991896

Alqahtani, J. S., Aldhahir, A. M., AlRabeeah, S. M., Alsenani, L. B., Alsharif, H. M., Alshehri, A. Y., Alenazi, M. M., Alnasser, M., Alqahtani, A. S., AlDraiwiesh, I. A., Alghamdi, S. M., Siraj, R. A., Alqahtani, H. S., Sreedharan, J. K., Alqahtani, A. S., & Alzahrani, E. M. (2022). Future acceptability of respiratory virus infection control interventions in general population to prevent respiratory infections. *Medicina*, *58*(7). https://doi.org/10.3390/medicina58070838

Alsan, M., & Wanamaker, M. (2018). Tuskegee and the health of black men. *The Quarterly Journal of Economics*, *133*(1), 407–455. https://doi.org/10.1093/qje/qjx029

Alsheikh, A. M., Elemam, M. O., & El-Bahnasawi, M. (2020). Treatment of depression with alcohol and substance dependence: A systematic review. *Cureus Journal of Medical Science*, *12*(10), e11168–e11168. https://doi.org/10.7759/cureus.11168

Alwin, D. (2012). Integrating varieties of life course concepts. *Journal of Gerontology, Series B, Psychological Sciences and Social Sciences*, *67*, 206–220.

Amanna, I. J., & Slifka, M. K. (2020). Successful vaccines. *Current Topics in Microbiology and Immunology*, *428*, 1–30. https://doi.org/10.1007/82_2018_102

American Academy of Child and Adolescent Psychiatry (AACAP). (n.d.). *Child and adolescent mental and behavioral health resolution*. https://www.apa.org/about/policy/child-adolescent-mental-behavioral-health

_______. (2023a). *Domestic violence and children.* https://www.aacap.org/AACAP/Families_and_Youth/Facts_for_Families/FFF-Guide/Helping-Children-Exposed-to-Domestic-Violence-109.aspx

_______. (2023b). *Policy statement on behavioral healthcare workforce shortage.* https://www.aacap.org/AACAP/Policy_Statements/2023/Behavioral_Healthcare_Workforce_Shortage.aspx

American Academy of Pediatrics (AAP). (n.d). *Suicide: Blueprint for youth suicide prevention.* https://www.aap.org/en/patient-care/blueprint-for-youth-suicide-prevention/

_______. (2007). *Preamble to patient-centered medical home joint principles.* https://systems.aucd.org/docs/lend/medhome/joint_principles_preamble_aap2007.pdf

_______. (2017). *Bright futures: Guidelines for health supervision of infants, children and adolescents* (4th ed.). https://www.aap.org/Bright-Futures-Guidelines-for-Health-Supervision-of-Infants-Children-and-Adolescents-4th-Edition

_______. (2021a). *AAP-AACAP-CHA declaration of a national emergency in child and adolescent mental health.* https://www.aap.org/en/advocacy/child-and-adolescent-healthy-mental-development/aap-aacap-cha-declaration-of-a-national-emergency-in-child-and-adolescent-mental-health/

_______. (2021b). *School-based health centers serve a critical role in many communities.* https://www.aap.org/en/news-room/news-releases/aap/2021/american-academy-of-pediatrics-school-based-health-centers-serve-a-critical-role-in-many-communities/

_______. (2022). *Medical home overview: What is a medical home?* National Resource Center for Patient/Family-Centered Medical Home. https://www.aap.org/en/practice-management/medical-home/medical-home-overview/what-is-medical-home/

_______. (2023). *Recommendations for preventative pediatric health care.* https://downloads.aap.org/AAP/PDF/periodicity_schedule.pdf

_______. (2024a). *Managing medical student debt.* https://www.aap.org/en/career-resources/planning-your-career/managing-medical-student-debt/

_______. (2024b). US child population characteristic trends. https://downloads.aap.org/AAP/PDF/CHT_Child%20Population%20Characteristics.pdf

American Academy of Pediatrics Ad Hoc Task Force on Definition of the Medical Home (November 1992). "The medical home". *Pediatrics, 90*(5), 774.

American Academy of Pediatrics, American Academy of Family Physicians, & American College of Physicians-American Society of Internal Medicine. (2002). A consensus statement on health care transitions for young adults with special health care needs. *Pediatrics, 110*(6 Pt 2), 1304–1306.

American Association of Nurse Practitioners. (2022). *NP fact sheet.* https://www.aanp.org/about/all-about-nps/np-fact-sheet

American Board of Pediatrics. (n.d.). *What is board certification?* https://www.abp.org/content/what-board-certification

American Cancer Society. (2024). *Can childhood cancers be prevented?* https://www.cancer.org/cancer/types/cancer-in-children/preventing-childhood-cancers.html

American College of Obstetricians and Gynecologists (ACOG). (2011). Committee opinion: Maternal-fetal intervention and fetal care centers.

_______. (2013). *Frequently asked questions. FAQ027. Pregnancy. The Rh factor: How it can affect your pregnancy.* https://www.acog.org/womens-health/faqs/the-rh-factor-how-it-can-affect-your-pregnancy

_______. (2019). Interpregnancy care. *Obstetric Care Consensus, 8.* https://www.acog.org/clinical/clinical-guidance/obstetric-care-consensus/articles/2019/01/interpregnancy-care

American Hospital Association (AHA). (2016). Trends affecting hospitals and health systems. *Trendwatch Chartbook.* https://www.aha.org/system/files/2018-01/2016-chartbook.pdf

________. (2020). *Improving health equity through medical-legal partnerships.* https://www.aha.org/system/files/media/file/2020/11/aha-medical-legal-partnerships-1120-final.pdf

________. (2021). *Perspective: Integrated health systems help enhance value, access.* https://www.aha.org/news/perspective/2021-05-21-perspective-integrated-health-systems-help-enhance-value-access

________. (2024a). *Fast facts on U.S. hospitals, 2024.* American Hospital Association. https://www.aha.org/statistics/fast-facts-us-hospitals

American Immigration Council. (2021). Immigrants in the United States. https://www.americanimmigrationcouncil.org/sites/default/files/research/immigrants_in_the_united_states_0.pdf

American Institutes for Research. (n.d.). Project LAUNCH (Linking Actions for Unmet Needs in Children's Health) framework, Figure 7-8. https://healthysafechildren.org/project-launch-framework

________. (2017). *Principles for making health care measurement patient-centered.* https://www.air.org/sites/default/files/Patient-Centered-Measurement-Principles-April-2017.pdf

American Medical Association. (n.d.). *RBRVS overview.* https://www.ama-assn.org/about/rvs-update-committee-ruc/rbrvs-overview

American Psychological Association (APA). (n.d.). *Integrated health care.* https://www.apa.org/health/integrated-health-care

________. (2023). *What do practicing psychologists do?* https://www.apa.org/topics/psychotherapy/about-psychologists

American Psychological Association Task Force on Evidence-Based Practice for Children and Adolescents. (2008). *Disseminating evidence-based practice for children and adolescents: A systems approach to enhancing care.* https://www.apa.org/practice/resources/evidence/children-report.pdf

American Public Health Association. (n.d.). *Community health workers.* https://www.apha.org/apha-communities/member-sections/community-health-workers

American Recovery and Reinvestment Act of 2009, Pub. L. No. 111-5, 123 Stat. 115 (2009). https://www.congress.gov/bill/111th-congress/house-bill/1

American Rescue Plan Act of 2021, H.R. 1319, 117th Congress, § 2001 (2021).

Americans with Disabilities Act of 1990, 42 U.S.C. § 12131 et seq. (1990). https://www.ada.gov/pubs/adastatute08.htm

AmeriCorps. (2019). *Evidence brief: Effective CNCS-funded health futures programs.* Corporation for National & Community Service. https://americorps.gov/sites/default/files/evidenceexchange/HF_Evidence_Brief_FINAL_v2_508_1.pdf

________. (2024). *Healthy futures.* https://americorps.gov/about/what-we-do/healthy-futures

Amin, S., Soliman, M., McIvor, A., Cave, A., & Cabrera, C. (2020). Understanding patient perspectives on medication adherence in asthma: A targeted review of qualitative studies. *Patient Preference and Adherence, 14,* 541–551. https://doi.org/10.2147/ppa.S234651

Anderer, S. (2024). More than half of US rural hospitals no longer offer birthing services—Here's why. *JAMA Network, 331*(10), 815–817. https://doi.org/10.1001/jama.2024.1278

Anderson, L. R., & Hemez, P. F. (2022). *Children living with at least one foreign-born parent more likely to live with two parents than children with native-born parents.* U.S. Census Bureau. https://www.census.gov/library/stories/2022/02/over-quarter-of-children-lived-with-at-least-one-foreign-born-parent.html

Anderson, L. R., Hemez, P. F., & Kreider, R. M. (2022). *Living arrangements of children: 2019.* U.S. Census Bureau. https://www.census.gov/library/publications/2022/demo/p70-174.html

Anderst, A., Hunter, K., Andersen, M., Walker, N., Coombes, J., Raman, S., Moore, M., Ryan, L., Jersky, M., Mackenzie, A., Stephensen, J., Williams, C., Timbery, L., Doyle, K., Lingam, R., Zwi, K., Sheppard-Law, S., Erskine, C., Clapham, K., & Woolfenden, S. (2022). Screening and social prescribing in healthcare and social services to address housing issues among children and families: A systematic review. *BMJ Open*, *12*(4), e054338. https://doi.org/10.1136/bmjopen-2021-054338

Andrasfay, T., & Goldman, N. (2021). Reductions in 2020 US life expectancy due to COVID-19 and the disproportionate impact on the Black and Latino populations. *Proceedings of the National Academy of Sciences*, *118*(5), e2014746118. https://doi.org/10.1073/pnas.2014746118

Andre, F. E., Booy, R., Bock, H. L., Clemens, J., Datta, S. K., John, T. J., Lee, B. W., Lolekha, S., Peltola, H., Ruff, T. A., Santosham, M., & Schmitt, H. J. (2008). Vaccination greatly reduces disease, disability, death and inequity worldwide. *Bulletin of the World Health Organization*, *86*(2), 140–146. https://doi.org/10.2471/blt.07.040089

Andrews, L., Sahama, T., & Gajanayake, R. (2014). Contextualising co-creation of value in electronic personal health records. *2014 IEEE 16th International Conference on e-Health Networking, Applications and Services*. 10.1109/HealthCom.2014.7001872

Andrilla, C. H. A., Patterson, D. G., Garberson, L. A., Coulthard, C., & Larson, E. H. (2018). Geographic variation in the supply of selected behavioral health providers. *American Journal of Preventive Medicine*, *54*(6, Suppl 3), S199–S207. https://doi.org/10.1016/j.amepre.2018.01.004

Annie E. Casey Foundation. (n.d.). *Ensuring the future of at-risk youth*. https://www.aecf.org

________. (2023a). *The impact of the high cost of child care*. https://www.aecf.org/blog/how-the-high-cost-of-child-care-hurts-families-workers-economy

________. (2023b). *One in four kids miss annual preventative dental care, up from previous years*. https://www.aecf.org/blog/over-1-in-5-kids-miss-annual-preventative-dental-care

Anoshiravani, A., Gaskin, G., Kopetsky, E., Sandborg, C., & Longhurst, C. A. (2011). Implementing an interoperable personal health record in pediatrics: Lessons learned at an academic children's hospital. *Journal of Participatory Medicine*, *3*, e30. https://www.ncbi.nlm.nih.gov/pmc/articles/PMC3156478/

Antonovics, E., Boitsios, G., & Saliba, T. (2024). Use of virtual reality in children in a broad range of medical settings: A systematic narrative review of recent meta-analyses. *Clinical and Experimental Pediatrics*, *67*(6), 274–282. https://doi.org/10.3345/cep.2023.00388

Arain, M., Haque, M., Johal, L., Mathur, P., Nel, W., Rais, A., Sandhu, R., & Sharma, S. (2013). Maturation of the adolescent brain. *Neuropsychiatric Disease and Treatment*, *9*, 449–461.

Archer, S., Cheung, N. H. Y., Williams, I., & Darzi, A. (2021). The impact of digital health interventions on the psychological outcomes of patients and families receiving pediatric palliative care: A systematic review and narrative synthesis. *Palliative Medicine*, *35*(10), 2017–2023. https://doi.org/10.1177/02692163211026523

Arenson, M., Hudson, P. J., Lee, N., & Lai, B. (2019). The evidence on school-based health centers: A review. *Global Pediatric Health*, *6*. https://doi.org/10.1177/2333794X19828745

Arias, E., Kochanek, K. D., Xu, J., & Tejada-Vera, B. (2023). Provisional life expectancy estimates for 2022. National Center for Health Statistics, Centers for Disease Control and Prevention. *Vital Statistics Rapid Release*, 031. https://www.cdc.gov/nchs/data/vsrr/vsrr031.pdf

Arias, E., & Tejada-Vera, B. (2023). Differential impact of the COVID-19 pandemic on excess mortality and life expectancy loss within the Hispanic population. *Demographic Research*, *48*(12), 339. https://doi.org/10.4054/DemRes.2023.48.12

Aris, I. M., Perng, W., Dabelea, D., Padula, A. M., Alshawabkeh, A., Vélez-Vega, C. M., Aschner, J. L., Camargo, C. A., Jr., Sussman, T. J., Dunlop, A. L., Elliott, A. J., Ferrara, A., Zhu, Y., Joseph, C. L. M., Singh, A. M., Hartert, T., Cacho, F., Karagas, M. R., North-Reid, T., . . . Oken, E. (2022). Associations of neighborhood opportunity and social vulnerability with trajectories of childhood body mass index and obesity among US children. *JAMA Network Open*, *5*(12), e2247957. https://doi.org/10.1001/jamanetworkopen.2022.47957

Aris, I. M., Rifas-Shiman, S. L., Jimenez, M. P., Li, L. J., Hivert, M. F., Oken, E., & James, P. (2021). Neighborhood child opportunity index and adolescent cardiometabolic risk. *Pediatrics*, *147*(2), e2020018903. https://doi.org/10.1542/peds.2020-018903

Arjmand, B., Larijani, B., Sheikh Hosseini, M., Payab, M., Gilany, K., Goodarzi, P., Parhizkar Roudsari, P., Amanollahi Baharvand, M., & Hoseini Mohammadi, N. S. (2020). The horizon of gene therapy in modern medicine: Advances and challenges. *Advances in Experimental Medicine and Biology*, *1247*, 33–64. https://doi.org/10.1007/5584_2019_463

Arku, D., Felix, M., Warholak, T., & Axon, D. R. (2022). Program of All-inclusive Care for the Elderly (PACE) versus other programs: A scoping review of health outcomes. *Geriatrics (Basel)*, *7*(2). https://doi.org/10.3390/geriatrics7020031

Armakolas, A., Kotsari, M., & Koskinas, J. (2023). Liquid biopsies, novel approaches and future directions. *Cancers*, *15*(5), 1579. https://doi.org/10.3390/cancers15051579

Armfield, J. M. (2010). Community effectiveness of public water fluoridation in reducing children's dental disease. *Public Health Reports*, *125*(5), 655–664. https://doi.org/10.1177/003335491012500507

Arnett, J. J. (2000). Emerging adulthood: A theory of development from the late teens through the twenties. *American Psychologist*, *55*, 469–480.

Arnold, J. L. (2002). Disaster medicine in the 21st century: Future hazards, vulnerabilities, and risk. *Prehospital and Disaster Medicine*, *17*(1), 3–11. https://doi.org/10.1017/s1049023x00000042

Arnold P. Gold Foundation. (2014, October 30–November 1). *Recommendations from a conference on advancing compassionate, person- and family-centered care through interprofessional education for collaborative practice.* Atlanta, Georgia.

Arpin, E., Gauffin, K., Kerr, M., Hjern, A., Mashford-Pringle, A., Barros, A., Rajmil, L., Choonara, I., & Spencer, N. (2021). Climate change and child health inequality: A review of reviews. *International Journal of Environmental Research and Public Health*, *18*(20). https://doi.org/10.3390/ijerph182010896

Arrojo, M. J., Bromberg, J., Walter, H. J., & Vernacchio, L. (2023). Pediatric primary-care integrated behavioral health. *Pediatric Clinics of North America*, *70*(4), 775–789. https://doi.org/10.1016/j.pcl.2023.04.004

Arsiwala, T., Afroz, N., Kordy, K., Naujoks, C., & Patalano, F. (2021). Measuring what matters for children: A systematic review of frequently used pediatric generic PRO instruments. *Therapeutic Innovation & Regulatory Science*, *55*(5), 1082–1095. https://doi.org/10.1007/s43441-021-00311-x

Artiga, S., & Diaz, D. (2019). *Health coverage and care of undocumented immigrants.* KFF. https://www.kff.org/racial-equity-and-health-policy/issue-brief/health-coverage-and-care-of-undocumented-immigrants/

Artiga, S., & Hinton, E. (2018). *Beyond health care: The role of social determinants in promoting health and health equity.* KFF. https://www.kff.org/racial-equity-and-health-policy/issue-brief/beyond-health-care-the-role-of-social-determinants-in-promoting-health-and-health-equity/

Aryee, E., Perrin, J. M., Iannuzzi, D., Kuhlthau, K. A., & Oreskovic, N. M. (2022). Association of neighborhood characteristics with pediatric asthma. *Academic Pediatrics*, *22*(5), 818–823. https://doi.org/10.1016/j.acap.2022.01.001

Asarnow, J. R. (2020). *Suicide: Pediatric mental health minute series.* American Academy of Pediatrics. https://www.aap.org/en/patient-care/mental-health-minute/suicide/

Asarnow, J. R., Rozenman, M., Wiblin, J., & Zeltzer, L. (2015). Integrated medical-behavioral care compared with usual primary care for child and adolescent behavioral health: A meta-analysis. *JAMA Pediatrics, 169*(10), 929–937. https://doi.org/10.1001/jamapediatrics.2015.1141

Ash, A. S., & Ellis, R. P. (2012). Risk-adjusted payment and performance assessment for primary care. *Medical Care, 50*(8), 643–653. https://doi.org/10.1097/MLR.0b013e3182549c74

Ash, E., Carrington, W., Heller, R., & Hwang, G. (2023). *Exploring the effects of Medicaid during childhood on the economy and the budget.* United States Congressional Budget Office. https://www.cbo.gov/publication/59819

Ash, J., Mackrain, M., & Johnston, K. (2013). Early childhood mental health consultation: Applying central tenets across diverse practice settings. *Journal of Zero to Three, 33*(5), 28–33. https://www.zerotothree.org/wp-content/uploads/2022/06/Early-Child-hood-Mental-Health-Consultation-13-May-Digital-Journal-Issue.pdf

Ashwood, J. S., Mehrotra, A., Cowling, D., & Uscher-Pines, L. (2017). Direct-to-consumer telehealth may increase access to care but does not decrease spending. *Health Affairs, 36*(3), 485–491. https://doi.org/10.1377/hlthaff.2016.1130

Assistant Secretary for Planning and Evaluation (ASPE). (n.d.). *Early childhood systems collective impact project.* https://aspe.hhs.gov/ecs-collective-impact-project[1]

_______. (2020a). *Certified community behavioral health clinics demonstration program: Report to Congress, 2020.* https://www.aspe.hhs.gov/sites/default/files/documents/1faadf771e9567b0926e33739341cb50/ccbhc-report-congress-2020.pdf

_______. (2020b). *Preliminary cost and quality findings from the national evaluation of the certified community behavioral health clinic demonstration* [Report to Congress]. U.S. Department of Health and Human Services. https://aspe.hhs.gov/reports/preliminary-cost-quality-findings-national-evaluation-certified-community-behavioral-health-clinic-0

_______. (2022a). *Access to preventive services without cost-sharing: Evidence from the Affordable Care Act* (Issue Brief No. HP-2022-01). https://aspe.hhs.gov/sites/default/files/documents/786fa55a84e7e3833961933124d70dd2/preventive-services-ib-2022.pdf

_______. (2022b). *How increased funding can advance the mission of the Indian Health Service to improve health outcomes for American Indians and Alaska Natives.* U.S. Department of Health and Human Services. https://aspe.hhs.gov/sites/default/files/documents/1b5d32824c31e113a2df43170c45ac15/aspe-ihs-funding-disparities-report.pdf

_______. (2022c). *Impact of the COVID-19 pandemic on the hospital and outpatient clinician workforce.* Office of Health Policy, U.S. Department of Health and Human Services. https://aspe.hhs.gov/sites/default/files/documents/9cc72124abd9ea25d58a22c7692dccb6/aspe-covid-workforce-report.pdf

_______. (2023a). *Children's health coverage trends: Gains in 2020–2022 reverse previous losses.* U.S. Department of Health and Human Services. https://aspe.hhs.gov/reports/childrens-health-coverage-trends

Association for Community Affiliated Plans (ACAP). (2020). *Addressing social determinants of health through dual-eligible special needs plans.* https://www.communityplans.net/research/11927

Association of American Medical Colleges. (2021). *The complexities of physician supply and demand: Projections from 2019 to 2034.* https://www.aamc.org/media/54681/download

Association of State and Territorial Health Officials (ASTHO). (2023). *ASTHO profile of state and territorial public health* (Vol. 6). http://www.astho.org/profile/

Atkeson, A., & Higgins, E. (2021). *How states can hold hospitals accountable for their community benefit expenditures.* National Academy for State Health Policy. https://nashp.org/how-states-can-hold-hospitals-accountable-for-their-community-benefit-expenditures/

Atrash, H. K., Johnson, K., Adams, M., Cordero, J. F., & Howse, J. (2006). Preconception care for improving perinatal outcomes: The time to act. *Maternal and Child Health Journal, 10*(5 Suppl), S3–S11. https://doi.org/10.1007/s10995-006-0100-4

Aubin, A. M., McAuliffe, L., Williams, K., Issah, A., Diacci, R., McAuliffe, J. E., Sabdia, S., Phung, J., Wang, C. A., & Pennell, C. E. (2023). Combined vaginal progesterone and cervical cerclage in the prevention of preterm birth: A systematic review and meta-analysis. *American Journal of Obstetrics & Gynecology MFM*, *5*(8), 101024. https://doi.org/10.1016/j.ajogmf.2023.101024

Austin, E., Lee, J. R., Amtmann, D., Bloch, R., Lawrence, S. O., McCall, D., Munson, S., & Lavallee, D. C. (2020). Use of patient-generated health data across healthcare settings: Implications for health systems. *JAMIA Open*, *3*(1), 70–76. https://doi.org/10.1093/jamiaopen/ooz065

Autism and Developmental Disabilities Monitoring Network. (2018). *Community report on autism, 2018*. Centers for Disease Control and Prevention. https://www.cdc.gov/autism/media/pdfs/addm-community-report-2018-h.pdf

Azok, J. G., O'Donnell, K. A., Long, M. E., Wang, H. C., Crook, T., Pogemiller, M. I., Momotaz, H., Knight, A. B., Burns, R. A., Harrison, V. A., Schmidt, S. M., Van Opstal, E. R., & Weinstein, A. R. (2024). Factors influencing medical students' career choice to pursue pediatrics. *Journal of Pediatrics, 265*, 113525. https://doi.org/10.1016/j.jpeds.2023.113525

Backer, C. L., Overman, D. M., Dearani, J. A., Romano, J. C., Tweddell, J. S., Kumar, S. R., Marino, B. S., Bacha, E. A., Jaquiss, R. D. B., Zaidi, A. N., Gurvitz, M., Costello, J. M., Pierick, T. A., Ravekes, W. J., Reagor, J. A., St. Louis, J. D., Spaeth, J., Mahle, W. T., Shin, A. Y., … Pasquali, S. K. (2023). Recommendations for centers performing pediatric heart surgery in the United States. *Annals of Thoracic Surgery*, *116*(5), 871–907. https://doi.org/10.1016/j.athoracsur.2023.08.016

Badger, D. (2022). The Center for Medicare and Medicaid Innovation: The case for reform. *Inquiry*, *59*, 469580221118036. https://doi.org/10.1177/00469580221118036

Bae, J. Y., Anderson, E., Silver, D., & Macinko, J. (2014). Child passenger safety laws in the United States, 1978–2010: Policy diffusion in the absence of strong federal intervention. *Social Science & Medicine*, *100*, 30–37. https://doi.org/10.1016/j.socscimed.2013.10.035

Bagley, S. M., Larochelle, M. R., Xuan, Z., Wang, N., Patel, A., Bernson, D., Silverstein, M., Hadland, S. E., Land, T., Samet, J. H., & Walley, A. Y. (2020). Characteristics and receipt of medication treatment among young adults who experience a nonfatal opioid-related overdose. *Annals of Emergency Medicine*, *75*(1), 29–38. https://doi.org/10.1016/j.annemergmed.2019.07.030

Bahl, N. K. H., Øversveen, E., Brodahl, M., Nafstad, H. E., Blakar, R. M., Landheim, A. S., & Tømmervik, K. (2023). Multiple psychological senses of community and community influences on personal recovery processes from substance use problems in later life: A collaborative and deductive reflexive thematic analysis. *International Journal of Qualitative Studies on Health and Well-being*, *18*(1), 2190200. https://doi.org/10.1080/17482631.2023.2190200

Bai, G., Herten, M. H., Landgraf, J. M., Korfage, I. J., & Raat, H. (2017). Childhood chronic conditions and health-related quality of life: Findings from a large population-based study. *PLoS One*, *12*(6), e0178539. https://doi.org/10.1371/journal.pone.0178539

Bailey, M. J., Hoynes, H. W., Rossin-Slater, M., & Walker, R. (2020). NIBERS Working Paper Series: Is the social safety net a long-term investment? Large-scale evidence from the food stamps program. *National Bureau of Economic Research*. https://www.nber.org/system/files/working_papers/w26942/w26942.pdf

Baker, S. P., Chen, L. H., & Li, G. (2007). *Nationwide review of graduated driver licensing.* AAA Foundation for Traffic Safety. https://aaafoundation.org/nationwide-review-graduated-driver-licensing/

Balanced Budget Act of 1997, Pub. L. No. 105-33, 111 Stat. 251 (1997).

Balfanz, R., & Byrnes, V. (2018). Using data and the human touch: Evaluating the NYC inter-agency campaign to reduce chronic absenteeism. *Journal of Education for Students Placed at Risk, 23*(1–2), 107–121. https://doi.org/10.1080/10824669.2018.1435283

Ballonoff Suleiman, A., Ballard, P. J., Hoyt, L. T., & Ozer, E. J. (2019). Applying a developmental lens to youth-led participatory action research: A critical examination and integration of existing evidence. *Youth & Society.* https://doi.org/10.1177/0044118X19837871

Banerjee, A. (2020). Equity and quality of health-care access: Where do we stand and the way forward? *Indian Journal of Community Medicine, 45*(1), 4–7. https://doi.org/10.4103/ijcm.IJCM_183_19

Barnert, E., Applegarth, D. M., Aggarwal, E., Bondoc, C., & Abrams, L. S. (2020). Health needs of youth in detention with limited justice involvement. *Children and Youth Services Review, 118*, 105412. https://doi.org/10.1016/j.childyouth.2020.105412

Barnet, B., Duggan, A. K., & Devoe, M. (2003). Reduced low birth weight for teenagers receiving prenatal care at a school-based health center: Effect of access and comprehensive care. *Journal of Adolescent Health, 33*(5), 349–358. https://doi.org/10.1016/s1054-139x(03)00211-8

Barnett, W. S., & Friedman-Krauss, A. (2016). *State(s) of Head Start. National Institute for Early Education Research.* https://nieer.org/research-library/states-head-start-1

Barr, A., & Gibbs, C. (2017). Breaking the cycle? Intergenerational effects of an anti-poverty program in early childhood. *Journal of Political Economy, 130*(12), 3253–3285.

Barrett, J. T., Lee, L. K., Monuteaux, M. C., Farrell, C. A., Hoffmann, J. A., & Fleegler, E. W. (2022). Association of county-level poverty and inequities with firearm-related mortality in US youth. *JAMA Pediatrics, 176*(2), e214822. https://doi.org/10.1001/jamapediatrics.2021.4822

Barth, M. C. (2010). *Healthy steps at 15: The past and future of an innovative preventive care model for children.* The Commonwealth Fund. https://www.commonwealthfund.org/publications/fund-reports/2010/dec/healthy-steps-15-past-and-future-innovative-preventive-care

Barton, A. J., Brandt, B., Dieter, C. J., & Williams, S. D. (2020). *Social determinants of health: Nursing, health professions and interprofessional education at a crossroads.* https://www.nap.edu/resource/25982/Barton%20et%al%20Commissioned%20Paper.pdf

Barton, A. J., Murray, T. A., & Spurlock, D. R., Jr. (2020). An open letter to members of the nursing education community. *Journal of Nursing Education, 59*(4), 183. https://doi.org/10.3928/01484834-20200323-01

Basch, C. E. (2011). Asthma and the achievement gap among urban minority youth. *Journal of School Health*, 81(10), 606–613. https://doi.org/10.1111/j.1746-1561.2011.00634.x

Baseman, L., & Zettle, A. (2024). Denials and appeals in Medicaid managed care: Review of recommendations and draft chapter for March report. *Medicaid and CHIP Payment and Access Commission.* https://www.macpac.gov/wp-content/uploads/2024/01/slides_denials-and-appeals_January-2024_updated.pdf

Bass, A. E., Milosevic, I., Uhl-Bien, M., & Nadkarni, S. (2022). Shared accountability in distributed leadership for improved healthcare access: A study of a US dental institution. *Leadership in Health Services.* https://doi.org/10.1108/lhs-03-2022-0019

Bastemeijer, C. M., Boosman, H., van Ewijk, H., Verweij, L. M., Voogt, L., & Hazelzet, J. A. (2019). Patient experiences: A systematic review of quality improvement interventions in a hospital setting. *Patient Related Outcome Measures, 10*, 157–169. https://doi.org/10.2147/PROM.S201737

Bastian, B., Tejada Vera, B., Arias E., et al. (2020). *Mortality trends in the United States, 1900–2018*. Centers for Disease Control and Prevention, National Center for Health Statistics. https://www.cdc.gov/nchs/data-visualization/mortality-trends/index.htm

Batalova, J. (2024). *Frequently requested statistics on immigrants and immigration in the United States*. Migration Policy Institute. https://www.migrationpolicy.org/article/frequently-requested-statistics-immigrants-and-immigration-united-states-2024

Bauer, G. R., Churchill, S. M., Mahendran, M., Walwyn, C., Lizotte, D., & Villa-Rueda, A. A. (2021a). Intersectionality in quantitative research: A systematic review of its emergence and applications of theory and methods. *SSM–Population Health*, *14*, 100798. https://doi.org/10.1016/j.ssmph.2021.100798

Bauer, K. W., Chriqui, J. F., Andreyeva, T., Kenney, E. L., Stage, V. C., Dev, D., Lessard, L., Cotwright, C. J., & Tovar, A. (2021). A safety net unraveling: Feeding young children during COVID-19. *American Journal of Public Health*, *111*(1), 116–120. https://doi.org/10.2105/ajph.2020.305980

Bauer, L., & Parsons, J. (2020). *Why extend pandemic EBT? When schools are closed, many fewer eligible children receive meals*. The Brookings Institution. https://www.brookings.edu/articles/why-extend-pandemic-ebt-when-schools-are-closed-many-fewer-eligible-children-receive-meals/

Bauer, L., & Schanzenbach, D. W. (2016). *The long-term impact of the Head Start program*. The Hamilton Project. https://www.hamiltonproject.org/assets/files/long_term_impact_of_head_start_program.pdf

Baumann, B. C., Mitra, N., Harton, J. G., Xiao, Y., Wojcieszynski, A. P., Gabriel, P. E., Zhong, H., Geng, H., Doucette, A., Wei, J., O'Dwyer, P. J., Bekelman, J. E., & Metz, J. M. (2020). Comparative effectiveness of proton vs photon therapy as part of concurrent chemoradiotherapy for locally advanced cancer. *JAMA Oncology*, *6*(2), 237–246. https://doi.org/10.1001/jamaoncol.2019.4889

Baumgartner, J. C., Collins, S. R., & Radley, D. C. (2023). *Inequities in health insurance coverage and access for Black and Hispanic adults: The impact of Medicaid expansion and the pandemic*. The Commonwealth Fund. https://www.commonwealthfund.org/publications/issue-briefs/2023/mar/inequities-coverage-access-black-hispanic-adults

Baweja, R., Soutullo, C. A., & Waxmonsky, J. G. (2021). Review of barriers and interventions to promote treatment engagement for pediatric attention deficit hyperactivity disorder care. *World Journal of Psychiatry*, *11*(12), 1206–1227. https://doi.org/10.5498/wjp.v11.i12.1206

Bayer, R., & Galea, S. (2015). Public health in the precision-medicine era. *New England Journal of Medicine*, *373*(6), 499–501. https://doi.org/10.1056/NEJMp1506241

Bazemore, A. W., Makaroff, L. A., Puffer, J. C., Parhat, P., Phillips, R. L., Xierali, I. M., & Rinaldo, J. (2012). Declining numbers of family physicians are caring for children. *Journal of the American Board of Family Medicine*, *25*(2), 139–140. https://doi.org/10.3122/jabfm.2012.02.110203

Bazzano, A. T., Mangione-Smith, R., Schonlau, M., Suttorp, M. J., & Brook, R. H. (2009). Off-label prescribing to children in the United States outpatient setting. *Academic Pediatrics*, *9*(2), 81–88. https://doi.org/10.1016/j.acap.2008.11.010

Beck, A. F., Edwards, E. M., Horbar, J. D., Howell, E. A., McCormick, M. C., & Pursley, D. M. (2020). The color of health: How racism, segregation, and inequality affect the health and well-being of preterm infants and their families. *Pediatric Research*, *87*, 227–234. https://www.nature.com/articles/s41390-019-0513-6

Beck, A. F., Henize, A. W., Qiu, T., Huang, B., Zhang, Y., Klein, M. D., Parrish, D., Fink, E. E., & Kahn, R. S. (2022). Reductions in hospitalizations among children referred to a primary care-based medical-legal partnership. *Health Affairs*, *41*(3), 341–349. https://doi.org/10.1377/hlthaff.2021.00905

Beck, A. F., Marcil, L. E., Klein, M. D., Sims, A. M., Parsons, A. A., Shah, A. N., Riley, C. L., Bignall, O. N. R. II, Henize, A. W., Kahn, R. S., & Unaka, N. I. (2021). Pediatricians contributing to poverty reduction through clinical-community partnership and collective action: A narrative review. *Academic Pediatrics*, *21*(8S), S200–S206. https://doi.org/10.1016/j.acap.2021.04.010

Beck, A. J., Page, C., Buche, J., Rittman, D., & Gaiser, M. (2018). *Estimating the distribution of the U.S. psychiatric subspecialist workforce*. https://behavioralhealthworkforce.org/wp-content/uploads/2019/02/Y3-FA2-P2-Psych-Sub_Full-Report-FINAL2.19.2019.pdf

Beech, B. M., Ford, C., Bruce, M. A., & Norris, K. C. (2021). Poverty, racism, and the public health crisis in America. *Frontiers in Public Health*, *9*. https://doi.org/10.3389/fpubh.2021.699049

Been, J. V., & Sheikh, A. (2018). Tobacco control policies in relation to child health and perinatal health outcomes. *Archives of Disease in Childhood*, *103*(9), 817–819. https://doi.org/10.1136/archdischild-2017-313680

Behr, C. L., Hull, P., Hsu, J., Newhouse, J. P., & Fung, V. (2022). Geographic access to federally qualified health centers before and after the Affordable Care Act. *BMC Health Services Research*, *22*(1), 385. https://doi.org/10.1186/s12913-022-07685-0

Belasen, A. T., Oppenlander, J., & Belasen, A. R. (2020). The relationship between provider-patient communication and HCAHPS composite measures and hospital ratings. *International Journal for Quality in Health Care: Journal of the International Society for Quality in Health Care*, *33*(1), mzaa140. https://doi.org/10.1093/intqhc/mzaa140

Bell, I. H., Nicholas, J., Broomhall, A., Bailey, E., Bendall, S., Boland, A., Robinson, J., Adams, S., McGorry, P., & Thompson, A. (2023). The impact of COVID-19 on youth mental health: A mixed methods survey. *Psychiatry Research*, *321*, 115082. https://doi.org/10.1016/j.psychres.2023.115082

Bell, O. N., Hole, M. K., Johnson, K., Marcil, L. E., Solomon, B. S., & Schickedanz, A. (2020). Medical-financial partnerships: Cross-sector collaborations between medical and financial services to improve health. *Academic Pediatrics*, *20*(2), 166–174. https://doi.org/10.1016/j.acap.2019.10.001

Bellerose, M., Collin, L., & Daw, J. R. (2022). The ACA Medicaid expansion and perinatal insurance, health care use, and health outcomes: A systematic review. *Health Affairs (Project Hope)*, *41*(1), 60–68. https://doi.org/10.1377/hlthaff.2021.01150

Bellis, M. A., Hughes, K., Ford, K., Ramos Rodriguez, G., Sethi, D., & Passmore, J. (2019). Life course health consequences and associated annual costs of adverse childhood experiences across Europe and North America: A systematic review and meta-analysis. *The Lancet Public Health*, *4*(10), e517–e528. https://doi.org/10.1016/S2468-2667(19)30145-8

Belsky, D. W., Caspi, A., Cohen, H. J., Kraus, W. E., Ramrakha, S., Poulton, R., & Moffitt, T. E. (2017). Impact of early personal-history characteristics on the pace of aging: Implications for clinical trials of therapies to slow aging and extend healthspan. *Aging Cell*, *16*(4), 644–651. https://doi.org/10.1111/acel.12591

BeLue, R., Francis, L. A., & Colaco, B. (2009). Mental health problems and overweight in a nationally representative sample of adolescents: Effects of race and ethnicity. *Pediatrics*, *123*(2), 697–702. https://doi.org/10.1542/peds.2008-0687

Benincasa, G., Napoli, C., & DeMeo, D. L. (2024). Transgenerational epigenetic inheritance of cardiovascular diseases: A network medicine perspective. *Maternal and Child Health Journal*, *28*(4), 617–630. https://doi.org/10.1007/s10995-023-03886-z

Bennett, C. M., & Friel, S. (2014). Impacts of climate change on inequities in child health. *Children (Basel)*, *1*(3), 461–473. https://doi.org/10.3390/children1030461

Benoit, S. L., & Mauldin, R. F. (2021). The "anti-vax" movement: A quantitative report on vaccine beliefs and knowledge across social media. *BMC Public Health*, *21*(1), 2106. https://doi.org/10.1186/s12889-021-12114-8

Benz, S. A., & Burney, J. A. (2021). Widespread race and class disparities in surface urban heat extremes across the United States. *Earth's Future*, *9*(7). https://doi.org/10.1029/2021EF002016

Berger, L. M., & Font, S. A. (2015). The role of the family and family-centered programs and policies. *Future Child*, *25*(1), 155–176. https://pubmed.ncbi.nlm.nih.gov/30679897/

Bergh, E., Buskmiller, C., & Johnson, A. (2021). The future of fetal surgery. *Obstetrics Gynecology Clinics of North America*, *48*(4), 745–758. https://doi.org/10.1016/j.ogc.2021.06.004

Bergman, D. A., Keller, D., Kuo, D. Z., Lerner, C., Mansour, M., Stille, C., Richardson, T., Rodean, J., & Hudak, M. (2020). Costs and use for children with medical complexity in a care management program. *Pediatrics*, *145*(4). https://doi.org/10.1542/peds.2019–2401

Berkule, S. B., Cates, C. B., Dreyer, B. P., Huberman, H. S., Arevalo, J., Burtchen, N., Weisleder, A., & Mendelsohn, A. L. (2014). Reducing maternal depressive symptoms through promotion of parenting in pediatric primary care. *Clinical Pediatrics*, *53*(5), 460–469. https://doi.org/10.1177/0009922814528033

Berry, J. G., Hall, M., Cohen, E., O'Neill, M., & Feudtner, C. (2015). Ways to identify children with medical complexity and the importance of why. *Journal of Pediatrics*, *167*(2), 229–237. https://doi.org/10.1016/j.jpeds.2015.04.068

Berry, J. G., Hall, M., Neff, J., Goodman, D., Cohen, E., Agrawal, R., Kuo, D., & Feudtner, C. (2014). Children with medical complexity and Medicaid: Spending and cost savings. *Health Affairs (Project Hope)*, *33*(12), 2199–2206. https://doi.org/10.1377/hlthaff.2014.0828

Berry, J. G., Perrin, J. M., Hoover, C., Rodean, J., Agrawal, R. K., & Kuhlthau, K. A. (2021). Health care insurance adequacy for children and youth with special health care needs. *Pediatrics*, *148*(4). https://doi.org/10.1542/peds.2020-039891

Berry, L. L., Rock, B. L., Smith Houskamp, B., Brueggeman, J., & Tucker, L. (2013). Care coordination for patients with complex health profiles in inpatient and outpatient settings. *Mayo Clinic Proceedings*, *88*(2), 184–194. https://doi.org/10.1016/j.mayocp.2012.10.016

Best Pharmaceuticals for Children Act (BPCA), Pub. L. No. 107–109, 115 Stat. 1408 (2002).

Bethell, C. D., Blackwell, C. K., Gombojav, N., Davis, M. B., Bruner, C., & Garner, A. S. (2022a). Toward measurement for a whole child health policy: Validity and national and state prevalence of the integrated child risk index. *Academic Pediatrics*, *22*(6), 952–964. https://doi.org/10.1016/j.acap.2021.12.001

Bethell, C. D., Blumberg, S. J., Stein, R. E., Strickland, B., Robertson, J., & Newacheck, P. W. (2015). Taking stock of the CSHCN screener: A review of common questions and current reflections. *Academic Pediatrics*, *15*(2), 165–176. https://doi.org/10.1016/j.acap.2014.10.003

Bethell, C., Buttross, S., Schiff, J., Bergman, D., Hanna, H., Oppenheim, S., Bailey, M., Patterson, R., Leach, B., & Cattrell, N. (2023a). *The Engagement in Action Framework: Toward an integrated early childhood health system to promote the early and lifelong health of all children and families*. Child and Adolescent Health Measurement Initiative, Johns Hopkins Bloomberg School of Public Health. https://www.cahmi.org/docs/default-source/ms-enact-documents/enact!-framework-overview-

Bethell, C. D., Garner, A. S., Gombojav, N., Blackwell, C., Heller, L., & Mendelson, T. (2022b). Social and relational health risks and common mental health problems among US children: The mitigating role of family resilience and connection to promote positive socioemotional and school-related outcomes. *Child and Adolescent Psychiatric Clinics of North America*, *31*(1), 45–70. https://doi.org/https://doi.org/https://doi.org/10.1016/j.chc.2021.08.001

Bethell, C. D., Gombojav, N., & Whitaker, R. C. (2019). Family resilience and connection promote flourishing among US children, even amid adversity. *Health Affairs*, *38*(5), 729–737. https://doi.org/10.1377/hlthaff.2018.05425

Bethell, C. D., Jones, J., Gombojav, N., Linkenbach, J., & Sege, R. (2019). Positive childhood experiences and adult mental and relational health in a statewide sample: Associations across adverse childhood experiences levels. *JAMA Pediatrics*, *173*(11), e193007-e193007. https://doi.org/10.1001/jamapediatrics.2019.3007

Bethell, C. D., Kennedy, S., Martinez-Vidal, E., & Simpson, L. (2018). Payment for progress: Investing to catalyze child and family well-being using personalized and integrated strategies to address social and emotional determinants of health. *Child and Adolescent Health Measurement Initiative, John Hopkins University, and AcademyHealth*. https://academyhealth.org/sites/default/files/payment_for_progress_fullreport_nov2018.pdf

Bethell, C. D., Newacheck, P. W., Fine, A., Strickland, B. B., Antonelli, R. C., Wilhelm, C. L., Honberg, L. E., & Wells, N. (2014). Optimizing health and health care systems for children with special health care needs using the life course perspective. *Maternal and Child Health Journal*, *18*(2), 467–477. https://doi.org/10.1007/s10995-013-1371-1

Bethell, C. D., Oppenheim, S., Hrivnak, P. E., & Woodward, K. (2023b). The Engagement in Action Framework partnership landscape analysis of relevance, roles and measures across early childhood health system partners. Child and Adolescent Health Measurement Initiative. Attachment C to *Mississippi Thrive! Summary Report*. The Child & Adolescent Health measurement Initiative; Mississippi Thrive! Child Health Development Project, Children's of Mississippi and Mississippi State University. https://cahmi.org/docs/default-source/ms-enact-documents/attachment-c_enact

Bethell, C. D., Reuland, C. H., Halfon, N., & Schor, E. L. (2004). Measuring the quality of preventive and developmental services for young children: National estimates and patterns of clinicians' performance. *Pediatrics*, *113*(Suppl 6), 1973–1983. https://pubmed.ncbi.nlm.nih.gov/15173469/

Bethell, C. D., Wells, N., Bergman, D., Reuland, C., Stumbo, S. P., Gombojav, N., & Simpson, L. A. (2023c). Scaling family voices and engagement to measure and improve systems performance and whole child health: Progress and lessons from the child and adolescent health measurement initiative. *Maternal and Child Health Journal*. https://doi.org/10.1007/s10995-023-03755-9

Bezgrebelna, M., McKenzie, K., Wells, S., Ravindran, A., Kral, M., Christensen, J., Stergiopoulos, V., Gaetz, S., & Kidd, S. A. (2021). Climate change, weather, housing precarity, and homelessness: A systematic review of reviews. *International Journal of Environmental Research and Public Health*, *18*(11). https://doi.org/10.3390/ijerph18115812

Bhattad, P. B., & Pacifico, L. (2022). Empowering patients: Promoting patient education and health literacy. *Cureus Journal of Medical Science*, *14*(7). https://doi.org/10.7759/cureus.27336

Bhide, A., & Chakraborty, K. (2020). General principles for psychotherapeutic interventions in children and adolescents. *The Indian Journal of Psychiatry*, 62(Suppl 2), S299–S318. https://doi.org/10.4103/psychiatry.IndianJPsychiatry_811_19

Bian, J., Cristaldi, K. K., Summer, A. P., Su, Z., Marsden, J., Mauldin, P. D., & McElligott, J. T. (2019). Association of a school-based, asthma-focused telehealth program with emergency department visits among children enrolled in South Carolina Medicaid. *JAMA Pediatrics*, *173*(11), 1041–1048. https://doi.org/10.1001/jamapediatrics.2019.3073

Bicer, S., Hutchinson, N., Feldhake, E., Nelson, A., Oliviero, E., Waligóra, M., & Kimmelman, J. (2023). Timing for first-in-minor clinical trials of new cancer drugs. *Journal of Pediatrics*, *263*, 113705. https://doi.org/10.1016/j.jpeds.2023.113705

Bierman, K. L., Coie, J. D., Dodge, K. A., Greenberg, M. T., Lochman, J. E., McMahon, R. J., & Pinderhughes, E. (2010). The effects of a multiyear universal social–emotional learning program: The role of student and school characteristics. *Journal of Consulting and Clinical Psychology*, *78*(2), 156. https://doi.org/10.1037/a0018607

Bipartisan Safer Communities Act (BSCA), Pub. L. No. 117-159, 136 Stat. 1313 (2022).

Birdsey, J., Cornelius, M., Jamal, A., Park-Lee, E., Cooper, M. R., Wang, J., Sawdey, M. D., Cullen, K. A., & Neff, L. (2023). Tobacco product use among U.S. middle and high school students—National Youth Tobacco Survey, 2023. *Morbidity and Mortality Weekly Report*, *72*(44), 1173–1182. https://www.cdc.gov/mmwr/volumes/72/wr/mm7244a1.htm

Bisgaier, J., & Rhodes, K. V. (2011). Auditing access to specialty care for children with public insurance. *New England Journal of Medicine*, *364*(24), 2324–2333. https://doi.org/10.1056/NEJMsa1013285

Bishop, T. F., Press, M. J., Keyhani, S., & Pincus, H. A. (2014). Acceptance of insurance by psychiatrists and the implications for access to mental health care. *JAMA Psychiatry*, *71*(2), 176–181. https://doi.org/10.1001/jamapsychiatry.2013.2862

Bitsko, R. H., Claussen, A. H., Lichstein, J., Black, L. I., Jones, S. E., Danielson, M. L., Hoenig, J. M., Davis Jack, S. P., Brody, D. J., Gyawali, S., Maenner, M. J., Warner, M., Holland, K. M., Perou, R., Crosby, A. E., Blumberg, S. J., Avenevoli, S., Kaminski, J. W., & Ghandour, R. M. (2022). Mental health surveillance among children—United States, 2013–2019. *Morbidity and Mortality Weekly Report Supplements*, *71*(2), 1–42. https://doi.org/10.15585/mmwr.su7102a1

Black, L. I., & Zablotsky, B. (2020). *Urgent care center and retail health clinic utilization among children: United States, 2019* (NCHS Data Brief No. 393). National Center for Health Statistics, Centers for Disease Control and Prevention. https://www.cdc.gov/nchs/products/databriefs/db393.htm

Black Maternal Health Caucus. (2023). *FY2023 appropriations wins*. https://blackmaternal-healthcaucus-underwood.house.gov/FY2023-appropriations-wins

Blair, I. V., Steinerc, J. F., & Havranek, E. P. (2011). Unconscious (implicit) bias and health disparities: Where do we go from here? *The Permanente Journal*, *15*(2), 71–78. https://doi.org/10.7812/tpp/11.979

Blendon, R. J., Benson, J. M., & Hero, J. O. (2014). Public trust in physicians—U.S. medicine in international perspective. *New England Journal of Medicine*, *371*(17), 1570–1572. https://doi.org/10.1056/NEJMp1407373

Bloom, B., Cohen, R. A., & Freeman, G. (2012). Summary health statistics for U.S. children: National Health Interview Survey, 2011. National Center for Health Statistics. *Vital and Health Statistics*, *10*(254). https://www.cdc.gov/nchs/data/series/sr_10/sr10_247.pdf

Bloomrosen, M., & Berner, E. S. (2023). Findings from the 2023 yearbook section on Health Information Exchange. *Yearbook of Medical Informatics*, *32*(1), 195–200. https://doi.org/10.1055/s-0043-1768755

Blue Zones. (2019). *Blue Zones Project news: Fort Worth's transformation from one of unhealthiest cities in America*. https://www.bluezones.com/2019/05/blue-zones-project-news-fort-worths-transformation-from-one-of-unhealthiest-cities-in-america/#

Blumberg, S. J., Read, D., Avila, R. M., & Bethell, C. D. (2010). Hispanic children with special health care needs from Spanish-language households. *Pediatrics*, *126*(Suppl 3), S120–128. https://doi.org/10.1542/peds.2010-1466E

Blumenthal, D., & McGinnis, J. M. (2015). Measuring *Vital signs*: An IOM report on core metrics for health and health care progress. *Journal of the American Medical Association*, *313*(19), 1901–1902. https://doi.org/10.1001/jama.2015.4862

Blumenthal-Barby, J. S., Kostick, K. M., Delgado, E. D., Volk, R. J., Kaplan, H. M., Wilhelms, L. A., McCurdy, S. A., Estep, J. D., Loebe, M., & Bruce, C. R. (2015). Assessment of patients' and caregivers' informational and decisional needs for left ventricular assist device placement: Implications for informed consent and shared decision-making. *Journal of Heart and Lung Transplantation*, *34*(9), 1182–1189. https://doi.org/10.1016/j.healun.2015.03.026

Bode, L., Mast, M., Rathert, H., Elise Study, G., Jack, T., & Wulff, A. (2023). Achieving interoperable datasets in pediatrics: A data integration approach. *Studies in Health Technology and Informatics*, *305*, 327–330. https://doi.org/10.3233/shti230496

Bodenheimer, T. (2019). Building powerful primary care teams. *Mayo Clinic Proceedings*, *94*(7), 1135–1137. https://doi.org/10.1016/j.mayocp.2019.05.017

Bodenheimer, T. S., & Smith, M. D. (2013). Primary care: Proposed solutions to the physician shortage without training more physicians. *Health Affairs (Project Hope)*, *32*(11), 1881–1886. https://doi.org/10.1377/hlthaff.2013.0234

Boehmer, T. J., Lesaja, S., Espinoza, L., & Ladva, C. N. (2023). Community water fluoridation levels to promote effectiveness and safety in oral health—United States, 2016–2021. *Morbidity and Mortality Weekly Report,* *72*(22), 593. https://doi.org/10.15585/mmwr.mm7222a1

Bogin, J. (2006). Enhancing developmental services in primary care: The Help Me Grow experience. *Journal of Developmental and Behavioral Pediatrics*, *27*(Suppl 1). https://doi.org/10.1097/00004703-200602001-00004

Bohra, N. (2023). Nearly 1.7 million Texans lose Medicaid as state nears end of "unwinding". *The Texas Tribune*. https://www.texastribune.org/2023/12/14/texas-medicaid-unwinding/

Bole, A., Bernstein, A., & White, M. J. (2024). The built environment and pediatric health. *Pediatrics, 153*(1), e2023064773. https://doi.org/10.1542/peds.2023-064773

Bolnick, H. J., Bui, A. L., Bulchis, A., Chen, C., Chapin, A., Lomsadze, L., Mokdad, A. H., Millard, F., & Dieleman, J. L. (2020). Health-care spending attributable to modifiable risk factors in the USA: An economic attribution analysis. *Lancet Public Health*, *5*(10), e525–e535. https://doi.org/10.1016/s2468-2667(20)30203-6

Bombard, Y., Baker, G. R., Orlando, E., Fancott, C., Bhatia, P., Casalino, S., Onate, K., Denis, J.-L. & Pomey, M.-P. (2018). Engaging patients to improve quality of care: A systematic review. *Implementation Science*, *13*(1), 98. https://doi.org/10.1186/s13012-018-0784-z

Bor, J., Venkataramani, A. S., Williams, D. R., & Tsai, A. C. (2018). Police killings and their spillover effects on the mental health of black Americans: A population-based, quasi-experimental study. *The Lancet*, *392*(10144), 302–310. https://doi.org/10.1016/S0140-6736(18)31130-9

Borodovsky, J. T., Krueger, R. F., Agrawal, A., & Grucza, R. A. (2020). A decline in propensity toward risk behaviors among U.S. adolescents. *Journal of Adolescent Health, 65*(6), 745–751. https://doi.org/10.1016/j.jadohealth.2019.07.001

Boston Medical Center. (2023). *StreetCred*. https://www.bmc.org/streetcred

Boudreau, A., Hamling, A., Pont, E., Pendergrass, T. W., Richerson, J., Simon, H. K., Byerley, J. S., Dodson, N. A., Horowitz, E. N., Ray, K. N., Leslie, L. K., Barone, L. F., Hackell, J. M., Abularrage, J. J., Almendarez, Y. M., Berhane, A. M., Cantrell, P. E., Kafer, L. M., Schafer, K. S., . . . Skatrud, A. (2022). Pediatric primary health care: The central role of pediatricians in maintaining children's health in evolving health care models. *Pediatrics*, *149*(2). https://doi.org/10.1542/peds.2021-055553

Boudreaux, E. D., & O'Hea, E. L. (2004). Patient satisfaction in the Emergency Department: A review of the literature and implications for practice. *The Emergency Medicine Journal*, *26*(1), 13–26. https://doi.org/10.1016/j.jemermed.2003.04.003

Boudreaux, M., Chu, J., & Lipton, B. J. (2023). School-based health centers, access to care, and income-based disparities. *JAMA Network Open*, *6*(9), e2334532. https://doi.org/10.1001/jamanetworkopen.2023.34532

Bovell-Ammon, A., McCann, N. C., Mulugeta, M., Ettinger de Cuba, S., Raifman, J., & Shafer, P. (2022). Association of the expiration of Child Tax Credit advance payments with food insufficiency in US households. *JAMA Network Open*, *5*(10), e2234438. https://doi.org/10.1001/jamanetworkopen.2022.34438

Boyce, W. T. (2016). Differential susceptibility of the developing brain to contextual adversity and stress. *Neuropsychopharmacology*, *41*(1), 142–162. https://doi.org/10.1038/npp.2015.294

Boyce, W. T., Levitt, P., Martinez, F. D., McEwen, B. S., & Shonkoff, J. P. (2021). Genes, environments, and time: The biology of adversity and resilience. *Pediatrics*, *147*(2). https://doi.org/10.1542/peds.2020-1651

Boyd, R. C., Butler, L., & Benton, T. D. (2018). Understanding adolescents' experiences with depression and behavioral health treatment. *The Journal of Behavioral Health Services & Research*, *45*(1), 105–111. https://doi.org/10.1007/s11414-017-9558-7

Boyle, C. A., Cordero, J. F., & Trevathan, E. (2012). The National Center on Birth Defects and Developmental Disabilities: Past, present, and future. *American Journal of Preventive Medicine*, *43*(6), 655–658. https://doi.org/10.1016/j.amepre.2012.08.015

Branch, B., & Conway, D. (2022). Health insurance coverage by race and Hispanic origin: 2021. U.S. Census Bureau. *American Community Survey Briefs*. https://www.census.gov/content/dam/Census/library/publications/2022/acs/acsbr-012.pdf

Brandeis University Heller School of Social Policy and Management. (n.d.). *Child opportunity index*. https://www.diversitydatakids.org/child-opportunity-index

Brands, M. R., Gouw, S. C., Beestrum, M., Cronin, R. M., Fijnvandraat, K., & Badawy, S. M. (2022). Patient-centered digital health records and their effects on health outcomes: Systematic review. *The Journal of Medical Internet Research*, *24*(12), e43086. https://doi.org/10.2196/43086

Braveman, P., Arkin, E., Orleans, T., Proctor, D., Acker, J., & Plough, A. (2018). What is health equity? *Behavioral Science & Policy*, *4*(1), 1–14. https://doi.org/10.1353/bsp.2018.0000

Braveman, P., & Barclay, C. (2009). Health disparities beginning in childhood: A life-course perspective. *Pediatrics*, *124*(Suppl 3), S163–S175. https://doi.org/10.1542/peds.2009-1100d

Braveman, P., Ergerter, S., & Williams, D. R. (2011). The social determinants of health: Coming of age. *The Annual Review of Public Health*, *32*, 381–398. https://doi.org/10.1146/annurev-publhealth-031210-101218

Brennan, E. M., Bradley, J. R., Allen, M. D., & Perry, D. F. (2008). The evidence base for mental health consultation in early childhood settings: Research synthesis addressing staff and program outcomes. *Early Education and Development*, *19*(6), 982–1022. https://doi.org/10.1080/10409280801975834

Breton, C. V., Landon, R., Kahn, L. G., Enlow, M. B., Peterson, A. K., Bastain, T., Braun, J., Comstock, S. S., Duarte, C. S., Hipwell, A., Ji, H., LaSalle, J. M., Miller, R. L., Musci, R., Posner, J., Schmidt, R., Suglia, S. F., Tung, I., Weisenberger, D., Zhu, Y., & Fry, R. (2021). Exploring the evidence for epigenetic regulation of environmental influences on child health across generations. *Communications Biology*, *4*(1), 769. https://doi.org/10.1038/s42003-021-02316-6

Brevoort, K. P. (2022). *Does giving CRA credit for loan purchases increase mortgage credit in low-to-moderate income communities?* Finance and Economics Discussion Series. Board of Governors of the Federal Reserve System. https://doi.org/10.17016/FEDS.2022.047

Breysse, P., Farr, N., Galke, W., Lanphear, B., Morley, R., & Bergofsky, L. (2004). The relationship between housing and health: Children at risk. *Environmental Health Perspectives*, *112*(15), 1583–1588. https://doi.org/10.1289/ehp.7157

Briggs, R. D., Silver, E. J., Krug, L. M., Mason, Z. S., Schrag, R. D. A., Chinitz, S., & Racine, A. D. (2014). Healthy steps as a moderator: The impact of maternal trauma on child social-emotional development. *Clinical Practice in Pediatric Psychology*, 2(2), 166–175. https://doi.org/10.1037/cpp0000060

Brignone, E., George, D. R., Sinoway, L., Katz, C., Sauder, C., Murray, A., Gladden, R., & Kraschnewski, J. L. (2020). Trends in the diagnosis of diseases of despair in the United States, 2009–2018: A retrospective cohort study. *BMJ Open*, *10*(10), e037679. https://doi.org/10.1136/bmjopen-2020-037679

Brill, A. (2023). *The overlooked decline in community health center funding*. Matrix Global Advisors and National Association of Community Health Centers. https://www.nachc.org/wp-content/uploads/2023/07/Overlooked-Decline-Community-Health-Center-Funding_2023_Full-report.pdf

Brinamen, C. F., Taranta, A. N., & Johnston, K. (2012). Expanding early childhood mental health consultation to new venues: Serving infants and young children in domestic violence and homeless shelters. *Infant Mental Health Journal*, *33*(3), 283–93. https://doi.org/10.1002/imhj.21338.

Bringewatt, E. H., & Gershoff, E. T. (2010). Falling through the cracks: Gaps and barriers in the mental health system for America's disadvantaged children. *Children and Youth Services Review*, *32*(10), 1291–1299. https://doi.org/10.1016/j.childyouth.2010.04.021

Britton, J., Jacobs, K., Haidar, T., Stolworthy, C., Armstrong, A., Merritt, N., Parry, N., Vogt, K., & Priestap, F. (2023). Child restraint systems: Understanding confidence in proper use and addressing the need for education. *Heliyon*, *9*(7), e17409. https://doi.org/10.1016/j.heliyon.2023.e17409

Broder, T., & Lessard, G. (2023). *Overview of immigrant eligibility for federal programs*. National Immigration Law Center. https://www.nilc.org/issues/economic-support/overview-immeligfedprograms/

Broder-Fingert, S., Mateo, C. M., & Zuckerman, K. E. (2020). Structural racism and autism. *Pediatrics*, *146*(3). https://doi.org/10.1542/peds.2020-015420

Bronner, K. K., & Skinner, J. (2022). *Geographic variations in spending and utilization across payer types*. Dartmouth Institute for Health Policy and Clinical Practice. https://books.google.com/books?id=DuVP0AEACAAJ

Brookman-Frazee, L., Baker-Ericzén, M., Stahmer, A., Mandell, D., Haine, R. A., & Hough, R. L. (2009). Involvement of youths with autism spectrum disorders or intellectual disabilities in multiple public service systems. *Journal of Mental Health Research in Intellectual Disabilities*, *2*(3), 201–219. https://doi.org/10.1080/19315860902741542

Brooks, T., Park, E., & Roygardner, L. (2019). *Medicaid and CHIP enrollment decline suggests the child uninsured rate may rise again*. Georgetown University Health Policy Institute, Center for Children & Families. https://ccf.georgetown.edu/wp-content/uploads/2019/06/Enrollment-Decline.pdf

Brooks, T., Roygardner, L., Artiga, S., Pham, O., & Dolan, R. (2020). *Medicaid and CHIP eligibility, enrollment, and cost sharing policies as of January 2020: Findings from a 50-state survey*. KFF. https://www.kff.org/report-section/medicaid-and-chip-eligibility-enrollment-and-cost-sharing-policies-as-of-january-2020-findings-from-a-50-state-survey-executive-summary/

Brown, C. M., Samaan, Z. M., Mansour, M. E., Glance, A., Morehous, J. F., Taylor, S., Hawke, J., & Kahn, R. S. (2020). A framework to measure and improve well-being in primary care. *Pediatrics*, *145*(1). https://doi.org/10.1542/peds.2019-1531

Brown, D. W., Anda, R. F., Tiemeier, H., Felitti, V. J., Edwards, V. J., Croft, J. B., & Giles, W. H. (2009). Adverse childhood experiences and the risk of premature mortality. *American Journal of Preventive Medicine*, *37*(5), 389–396. https://doi.org/10.1016/j.amepre.2009.06.021

Brown, D. W., Kowalski, A. E., & Lurie, I. Z. (2015). *Medicaid as an investment in children: What is the long-term impact on tax receipts?* (NBER Working Paper No. 20835). National Bureau of Economic Research. https://www.nber.org/papers/w20835

Brown, J., Breslau, J., Wishon, A., Miller, R., Kase, C., Dunbar, M., Stewart, K., Briscombe, B., Rose, T., Dehus, E., & DeWitt, K. (2022). *Implementation and impacts of the certified community behavioral health clinic demonstration: Findings from the national evaluation*. https://aspe.hhs.gov/sites/default/files/documents/60f121a777ee63b20008e43ad45518bf/ccbhc-implementation-impacts-findings.pdf

Brown, J. D., & Wissow, L. S. (2009). Discussion of sensitive health topics with youth during primary care visits: Relationship to youth perceptions of care. *Journal of Adolescent Health*, *44*(1), 48–54. https://doi.org/10.1016/j.jadohealth.2008.06.018

________. (2010). Screening to identify mental health problems in pediatric primary care: Considerations for practice. *International Journal of Psychiatry in Medicine*, *40*(1), 1–19. https://doi.org/10.2190/PM.40.1.a

Brownstein, J. N., Hirsch, G. R., Rosenthal, E. L., & Rush, C. H. (2011). Community health workers "101" for primary care providers and other stakeholders in health care systems. *Journal of Ambulatory Care Management*, *34*(3), 210–220. https://doi.org/10.1097/JAC.0b013e31821c645d

Bruen, B., & Ku, L. (2017). *Community health centers reduce the costs of children's health care*. Geiger Gibson/RCHN Community Health Foundation Research Collaborative. https://geigergibson.publichealth.gwu.edu/48-community-health-centers-reduce-costs-childrens-health-care

Brundage, S. C., & Levine, C. (2019). *The ripple effect: The impact of the opioid epidemic on children and families*. United Hospital Fund and Milbank Memorial Fund. https://addictionmedicineupdates.org/wp-content/uploads/2019/04/The-Ripple-Effect.pdf

Bruner, C., & Hayes, M. (2023). Federal health policy requires child health investment focus. *Health Affairs Forefront*. https://doi.org/10.1377/forefront.20230920.430993

Bruner, C., & Johnson, K. (2018). *Federal spending on prenatal to three: Developing a public response to improving developmental trajectories and preventing inequities*. Center for the Study of Social Policy. https://cssp.org/wp-content/uploads/2018/08/CSSP-Prenatal-to-Three.pdf

Bruner, C., Johnson, K., Bethell, C., Dworkin, P., Kotelchuck, M., Perrin, E., Shaw, J., Trefz, M. N., & Whitaker, R. (2018). *Next steps in family-focused screening to address social determinants of health for young children in pediatric primary care*. Report of the Social Determinants of Health Technical Working Group of the Maternal and Child Health Measurement Research Network. https://www.cahmi.org/docs/default-source/resources/next-steps-in-family-focused-screening-to-address-social-determinants-of-health-for-young-children-in-pediatric-primary-care-(2018).pdf?sfvrsn=8e6d882d_0

Bruner, C., & Kotelchuck, M. (2023). *From efficacy to effectiveness: Community health workers, medical homes, and the measurement systems to support them* (Working Paper No. 2023), InCK Marks Initiative. https://www.inckmarks.org/docs/11-17-2023/InCK%20Marks%20CHW%20Metrics%20Working%20Paper.pdfInCK Marks CHW Metrics Working Paper.pdf

Brykman, K., Houston, R., & Bailey, M. (2021). *Value-based payment to support children's health and wellness: Shifting the focus from short-term to life course impact*. Center for Health Care Strategies. https://www.chcs.org/resource/value-based-payment-to-support-childrens-health-and-wellness-shifting-the-focus-from-short-term-to-life-course-impact/

Brykman, K., Jacobs, L. S., & Casau, A. (2024). *Developing financially sustainable child health transformation: Lessons from primary care innovators*. Center for Health Care Strategies. https://www.chcs.org/media/Developing-Financially-Sustainable-Child-Health-Transformation.pdf

Brykman, K., & Joseph, N. (2024). *Tech-enabled solutions as a tool to address health-related social needs in Medicaid: Opportunities and policy considerations*. Center for Health Care Strategies.

Buchmueller, T., Ham, J. C., & Shore-Sheppard, L. D. (2016). The Medicaid program. In R. A. Moffitt (Ed.), *Economics of means-tested transfer programs in the United States* (Vol. 1, pp. 21–136). University of Chicago Press. http://www.nber.org/chapters/c13486

Buchmueller, T. C., Levy, H. G., & Valletta, R. G. (2019). *Medicaid expansion and the unemployed.* http://www.nber.org/papers/w26553

Bucholz, E. M., Toomey, S. L., & Schuster, M. A. (2019). Trends in pediatric hospitalizations and readmissions: 2010–2016. *Pediatrics*, *143*(2), e20181958. https://doi.org/10.1542/peds.2018-1958

Buckles, K., Guldi, M. E., & Schmidt, L. (2019). *Fertility trends in the United States, 1980–2017: The role of unintended births* (NBER Working Paper No. 25521). National Bureau of Economic Research. https://www.nber.org/papers/w25521

Buettgens, M., Nichols, A., & Dorn, S. (2023). *Ensuring continuous eligibility for Medicaid and CHIP.* Urban Institute. https://www.urban.org/research/publication/ensuring-continuous-eligibility-medicaid-and-chip-children

Buhr, T., & Blendon, R. J. (2011). Trust in government and health care institutions. In Blendon, R. J., Brodie, M., Benson, J. M., & Altman, D. E (Eds.), *American Public Opinion and Health Care.* https://doi.org/10.4135/9781452240077

Buitron de la Vega, P., Losi, S., Sprague Martinez, L., Bovell-Ammon, A., Garg, A., James, T., Ewen, A. M., Stack, M., DeCarvalho, H., Sandel, M., Mishuris, R. G., Deych, S., Pelletier, P., & Kressin, N. R. (2019). Implementing an EHR-based screening and referral system to address social determinants of health in primary care. *Medical Care*, *57*(Suppl 2), S133–S139. https://doi.org/10.1097/mlr.0000000000001029

Buka, S. L., Beers, L. S., Biel, M. G., Counts, N. Z., Hudziak, J., Parade, S. H., Paris, R., Seifer, R., & Drury, S. S. (2022). The family is the patient: Promoting early childhood mental health in pediatric care. *Pediatrics*, *149*(Suppl 5). https://doi.org/10.1542/peds.2021-053509L

Bullinger, L., & Boy, A. (2023). Association of expanded child tax credit payments with child abuse and neglect emergency department visits. *JAMA Network Open*, *6*(2), e2255639. https://doi.org/10.1001/jamanetworkopen.2022.55639

Bullinger, L., & Fong, K. (2020). Evictions and neighborhood child maltreatment reports. *Housing Policy Debate*, *31*, 1–26. https://doi.org/10.1080/10511482.2020.1822902

Bundshuh, H., Ohlson, M., & Swanson, A. (2021). Finding support & significance at school—Program evaluation of a chronic absenteeism reduction initiative. *National Youth at Risk Journal*, *5*. https://doi.org/10.20429/nyarj.2021.050104

Burak, E. W. (2018). *Promoting young children's healthy development in Medicaid and CHIP.* Georgetown University McCourt School of Public Policy, Center for Children & Families. https://ccf.georgetown.edu/2018/10/17/promoting-young-childrens-healthy-development-in-medicaid-and-the-childrens-health-insurance-program-chip/

________. (2023). *Zero to six continuous coverage proposed in Pennsylvania, approved in New Mexico.* Georgetown University McCourt School of Public Policy, Center for Children and Families. https://ccf.georgetown.edu/2023/12/21/0-6-continuous-coverage-proposed-in-pennsylvania-approved-in-new-mexico/

Bureau of Labor Statistics (BLS). (2023). *Occupational employment and wages, May 2022: 21-1094 community health workers.* https://www.bls.gov/oes/current/oes211094.htm

Burns, K., & Fox, L. (2022). *The impact of the 2021 expanded child tax credit on child poverty.* U.S. Census Bureau. https://www.census.gov/library/working-papers/2022/demo/SEHSD-wp2022-24.html

Busque, A. A., Jabbour, E., Patel, S., Couture, É., Garfinkle, J., Khairy, M., Claveau, M., & Beltempo, M. (2022). Incidence and risk factors for autism spectrum disorder among infants born <29 weeks' gestation. *Paediatrics & Child Health*, *27*(6), 346–352. https://doi.org/10.1093/pch/pxac065

Buttazzoni, A., Pham, J., Nelson Ferguson, K., Fabri, E., Clark, A., Tobin, D., Frisbee, N., & Gilliland, J. (2024). Supporting children's participation in active travel: Developing an online road safety intervention through a collaborative integrated knowledge translation approach. *International Journal of Qualitative Studies on Health and Well-being*, *19*(1), 2320183. https://doi.org/10.1080/17482631.2024.2320183

Butterfield, L., Cash, J., & Pham, K. (2015). Drug shortages and implications for pediatric patients. *The Journal of Pediatric Pharmacology and Therapeutics*, *20*(2), 149–152. https://doi.org/10.5863/1551-6776-20.2.149

Butz, M., May, E. S., Häussinger, D., & Schnitzler, A. (2013). The slowed brain: Cortical oscillatory activity in hepatic encephalopathy. *Archives of Biochemistry and Biophysics*, *536*(2), 197–203. https://doi.org/10.1016/j.abb.2013.04.004

Byhoff, E., Cohen, A. J., Hamati, M. C., Tatko, J., Davis, M. M., & Tipirneni, R. (2017). Screening for social determinants of health in Michigan health centers. *Journal of the American Board of Family Medicine*, *30*(4), 418–427. https://doi.org/10.3122/jabfm.2017.04.170079

Bylander, A. (2023). *States show us what is possible with free healthy school meals for all policies*. Food Research & Action Center. https://frac.org/blog/free-healthy-school-meals-for-all-policies

Byrd, D., Ceacal, Y. R., Felton, J., Nicholson, C., Rhaney, D. M. L., McCray, N., & Young, J. (2017). A modern doll study. *Race, Gender, & Class*, *24*(1–2), 186–202. https://www.jstor.org/stable/10.2307/26529244

Cabral, M., Kim, B., Rossin-Slater, M., Schnell, M., & Schwandt, H. (2021). *Trauma at school: The impacts of shootings on students' human capital and economic outcomes*. National Bureau of Economic Research. https://www.nber.org/papers/w28311

Cady, R. G., & Belew, J. L. (2017). Parent perspective on care coordination services for their child with medical complexity. *Children*, *4*(6). https://doi.org/10.3390/children4060045

Cainelli, E., & Bisiacchi, P. (2023). Neurodevelopmental disorders: Past, present, and future. *Children (Basel)*, *10*(1). https://doi.org/10.3390/children10010031

Cakici, J. A., Dimmock, D. P., Caylor, S. A., Gaughran, M., Clarke, C., Triplett, C., Clark, M. M., Kingsmore, S. F., & Bloss, C. S. (2020). A prospective study of parental perceptions of rapid whole-genome and -exome sequencing among seriously ill infants. *American Journal of Human Genetics*, *107*(5), 953–962. https://doi.org/10.1016/j.ajhg.2020.10.004

Calabrese, S., Lee, S., Mollica, M. A., Wiener, L., Mendley, S., Adams, L., & Blachman-Demner, D. (2022). Navigating pediatric to adult healthcare transition: A National Institutes of Health workshop. *Journal of Pediatrics*, *244*, 234–240.e231. https://doi.org/10.1016/j.jpeds.2022.01.052

California Children's Trust. (2022). *Reimagining California's approach to children's behavioral health*. https://cachildrenstrust.org

California Mental Health Services Authority. (n.d.). *Peer certification*. https://www.calmhsa.org/peer-certification/

California Pan-Ethnic Health Network. (2018). *California reducing disparities project strategic plan to reduce mental health disparities*. https://cpehn.org/publications/california-reducing-disparities-project-strategic-plan-reduce-mental-health-disparities/

California School-Based Health Alliance. (2022). *Navigating the promise of school-based health centers: A guide for health care leaders*. https://www.schoolhealthcenters.org/wp-content/uploads/2022/10/Navigating-the-Promise-of-SBHCs.pdf

Calvert, M. J., Cruz Rivera, S., Retzer, A., Hughes, S. E., Campbell, L., Molony-Oates, B., Aiyegbusi, O. L., Stover, A. M., Wilson, R., McMullan, C., Anderson, N. E., Turner, G. M., Davies, E. H., Verdi, R., Velikova, G., Kamudoni, P., Muslim, S., Gheorghe, A., O'Connor, D., . . . Denniston, A. K. (2022). Patient reported outcome assessment must be inclusive and equitable. *Nature Medicine*, *28*(6), 1120–1124. https://doi.org/10.1038/s41591-022-01781-8

Camacho, S., & Clark Henderson, S. (2022). The social determinants of adverse childhood experiences: An intersectional analysis of place, access to resources, and compounding effects. *International Journal of Environmental Research and Public Health*, *19*(17). https://doi.org/10.3390/ijerph191710670

Camenga, D. R., Hammer, L. D., the Committee on Substance Use & Prevention, & Committee on Child Health Financing. (2022). Improving substance use prevention, assessment, and treatment financing to enhance equity and improve outcomes among children, adolescents, and young adults. *Pediatrics*, *150*(1), e2022057992. https://doi.org/10.1542/peds.2022-057992

Campbell, F., Conti, G., Heckman, J. J., Moon, S. H., Pinto, R., Pungello, E., & Pan, Y. (2014). Early childhood investments substantially boost adult health. *Science*, *343*(6178), 1478–1485. https://doi.org/10.1126/science.1248429

Campbell, K. (2022). Preparing health-care systems for future pandemics. *Nature, 610,* S38–S40. https://doi.org/10.1038/d41586-022-03356-6

Canadian Pediatric Society. (2008). Ethical issues in health research in children. (2008). *Paediatrics & Child Health, 13*(8), 707–712. https://doi.org/10.1093/pch/13.8.707

Cancer Research Institute. (n.d.). *How cellular immunotherapies are changing the outlook for cancer patients.* https://www.cancerresearch.org/treatment-types/adoptive-cell-therapy

Canedo, J. R., Miller, S. T., Schlundt, D., Fadden, M. K., & Sanderson, M. (2018). Racial/ethnic disparities in diabetes quality of care: The role of healthcare access and socioeconomic status. *Journal of Racial and Ethnic Health Disparities*, *5*(1), 7–14. https://doi.org/10.1007/s40615-016-0335-8

Canfell, O. J., Littlewood, R., Burton-Jones, A., & Sullivan, C. (2022). Digital health and precision prevention: Shifting from disease-centred care to consumer-centred health. *Australian Health Review*, *46*(3), 279–283. https://doi.org/10.1071/ah21063

Canfield, C. F., Miller, E. B., Shaw, D. S., Morris, P., Alonso, A., & Mendelsohn, A. L. (2020). Beyond language: Impacts of shared reading on parenting stress and early parent-child relational health. *Developmental Psychology*, *56*(7), 1305–1315. https://doi.org/10.1037/dev0000940

Canfield, C. F., Miller, E. B., Taraban, L., Aviles, A. I., Rosas, J., Mendelsohn, A. L., Morris, P., & Shaw, D. (2023). Impacts of a tiered intervention on child internalizing and externalizing behavior in the context of maternal depression. *Development and Psychopathology*, 1–11. https://doi.org/10.1017/S0954579423001475

Canfield, C. F., Weisleder, A., Cates, C. B., Huberman, H. S., Dreyer, B. P., Legano, L. A., Johnson, S. B., Seery, A., & Mendelsohn, A. L. (2015). Primary care parenting intervention and its effects on the use of physical punishment among low-income parents of toddlers. *Journal of Developmental & Behavioral Pediatrics*, *36*(8), 586–593. https://doi.org/10.1097/DBP.0000000000000206

Cantor, J. H., McBain, R. K., Pera, M. F., Bravata, D. M., & Whaley, C. M. (2021). Who is (and is not) receiving telemedicine care during the COVID-19 pandemic. *American Journal of Preventive Medicine*, *61*(3), 434–438. https://doi.org/10.1016/j.amepre.2021.01.030

Caplan, Z. (2023). *U.S. older population grew from 2010 to 2020 at fastest rate since 1880 to 1890.* U.S. Census Bureau. https://www.census.gov/library/stories/2023/05/2020-census-united-states-older-population-grew.html

Capra, L., Tezza, G., Mazzei, F., & Boner, A. L. (2013). The origins of health and disease: The influence of maternal diseases and lifestyle during gestation. *Italian Journal of Pediatrics*, *39*, 7. https://doi.org/10.1186/1824-7288-39-7

Carabin, H. (2021). One health: A crucial approach to preventing and preparing for future pandemics. *The Conversation.* https://theconversation.com/one-health-a-crucial-approach-to-preventing-and-preparing-for-future-pandemics-173637

Carlo, A. D., Basu, A., Unützer, J., & Jordan, N. (2024). Acceptance of insurance by psychiatrists and other physicians, 2007–2016. *Psychiatric Services*, *75*(1), 25–31. https://doi.org/10.1176/appi.ps.202100669

Carlson, C. J., Farrell, M. J., Grange, Z., Han, B. A., Mollentze, N., Phelan, A. L., Rasmussen, A. L., Albery, G. F., Bett, B., Brett-Major, D. M., Cohen, L. E., Dallas, T., Eskew, E. A., Fagre, A. C., Forbes, K. M., Gibb, R., Halabi, S., Hammer, C. C., Katz, R., . . . Webala, P. W. (2021). The future of zoonotic risk prediction. *Philosophical Transactions of the Royal Society B: Biological Sciences*, *376*(1837), 20200358. https://doi.org/10.1098/rstb.2020.0358

Carlson, J. A., Sallis, J. F., Chriqui, J. F., Schneider, L., McDermid, L. C., & Agron, P. (2013). State policies about physical activity minutes in physical education or during school. *Journal of School Health*, *83*(3), 150–156. https://doi.org/10.1111/josh.12010

Carlson, S., & Keith-Jennings, B. (2018). *SNAP is linked with improved nutritional outcomes and lower health care costs.* Center on Budget and Policy Priorities. https://www.cbpp.org/research/snap-is-linked-with-improved-nutritional-outcomes-and-lower-health-care-costs

Carlson, S., & Neuberger, Z. (2021). *WIC works: Addressing the nutrition and health needs of low-income families for 40 years.* Center on Budget and Policy Priorities.

Carman, K. L., Dardess, P., Maurer, M., Sofaer, S., Adams, K., Bechtel, C., & Sweeney, J. (2013). Patient and family engagement: A framework for understanding the elements and developing interventions and policies. *Health Affairs (Project Hope)*, *32*(2), 223–231. https://doi.org/10.1377/hlthaff.2012.1133

Carmeli, C., Steen, J., Petrovic, D., Lepage, B., Delpierre, C., Kelly-Irving, M., Bochud, M., Kivimäki, M., Vineis, P., & Stringhini, S. (2020). Mechanisms of life-course socioeconomic inequalities in adult systemic inflammation: Findings from two cohort studies. *Social Science & Medicine*, *245*, 112685. https://doi.org/10.1016/j.socscimed.2019.112685

Carrilero, N., Pérez-Jover, V., Guilabert-Mora, M., & García-Altés, A. (2023). Gender bias in pediatric care: Health professionals' opinions and perceptions. *Health Science Reports*, *6*(10), e1615. https://doi.org/10.1002/hsr2.1615

Carson, J., & Boege, S. (2020). *The intersection of food availability, access, & affordability with food security and health.* Carsey School of Public Policy, University of New Hampshire. https://nhchildrenshealthfoundation.org/assets/2021/02/Carsey_Food-Insecurity-Literature-Review_Final_121720.pdf

Carter, B., Young, S., Ford, K., & Campbell, S. (2024). The concept of child-centered care in healthcare: A scoping review. *Pediatric Reports*, *16*(1), 114–134. https://doi.org/10.3390/pediatric16010012

Case, A., & Deaton, A. (2017). Mortality and morbidity in the 21st century. *Brookings Papers on Economic Activity*, 397–476. https://doi.org/10.1353/eca.2017.0005

________. (2022). The great divide: Education, despair, and death. *Annual Review of Economics*, *14*, 1–21. https://doi.org/10.1146/annurev-economics-051520-015607

Casey, B. J., Jones, R. M., Levita, L., Libby, V., Pattwell, S. S., Ruberry, E. J., Soliman, F., & Somerville, L. H. (2010). The storm and stress of adolescence: Insights from human imaging and mouse genetics. *Developmental Psychobiology*, *52*(3), 225–235. https://doi.org/10.1002/dev.20447

Casimir, G. (2019). Why children's hospitals are unique and so essential. *Frontiers in Pediatrics*, *7*, 466742. https://doi.org/10.3389/fped.2019.00305

Cassedy, A., Fairbrother, G., & Newacheck, P. W. (2008). The impact of insurance instability on children's access, utilization, and satisfaction with health care. *Ambulatory Pediatrics*, *8*(5), 321–328. https://doi.org/10.1016/j.ambp.2008.04.007

Castro, L. C., & Avina, R. L. (2002). Maternal obesity and pregnancy outcomes. *Current Opinion in Obstetrics and Gynecology, 14*(6). https://journals.lww.com/co-obgyn/fulltext/2002/12000/maternal_obesity_and_pregnancy_outcomes.5.aspx

Castro-Ramirez, F., Al-Suwaidi, M., Garcia, P., Rankin, O., Ricard, J. R., & Nock, M. K. (2021). Racism and poverty are barriers to the treatment of youth mental health concerns. *Journal of Clinical Child & Adolescent Psychology, 50*(4), 534–546. https://doi.org/10.1080/15374416.2021.1941058

Catalani, C. E., Findley, S. E., Matos, S., & Rodriguez, R. (2009). Community health worker insights on their training and certification. *Progress in Community Health Partnerships, 3*(3), 227–235. https://doi.org/10.1353/cpr.0.0082

Catalano, R. F., & Kellogg, E. (2020). Fostering healthy mental, emotional, and behavioral development in children and youth: A national agenda. *Journal of Adolescent Health, 66*(3), 265–267. https://doi.org/10.1016/j.jadohealth.2019.12.003

Catenaccio, E., Rochlin, J. M., & Simon, H. K. (2021). Differences in lifetime earning potential between pediatric and adult physicians. *Pediatrics, 148*(2). https://doi.org/10.1542/peds.2021-051194

Cates, C. B., Weisleder, A., Berkule Johnson, S., Seery, A. M., Canfield, C. F., Huberman, H., Dreyer, B. P., & Mendelsohn, A. L. (2018). Enhancing parent talk, reading, and play in primary care: Sustained impacts of the video interaction project. *Journal of Pediatrics, 199*, 49–56.e41. https://doi.org/10.1016/j.jpeds.2018.03.002

Cates, C. B., Weisleder, A., Dreyer, B. P., Berkule Johnson, S., Vlahovicova, K., Ledesma, J., & Mendelsohn, A. L. (2016). Leveraging healthcare to promote responsive parenting: Impacts of the video interaction project on parenting stress. *Journal of Child and Family Studies, 25*(3), 827–835. https://doi.org/10.1007/s10826-015-0267-7

Ceccarelli, C., Prina, E., Muneghina, O., Jordans, M., Barker, E., Miller, K., Singh, R., Acarturk, C., Sorsdhal, K., Cuijpers, P., Lund, C., Barbui, C., & Purgato, M. (2022). Adverse childhood experiences and global mental health: Avenues to reduce the burden of child and adolescent mental disorders. *Epidemiology and Psychiatric Sciences, 31*, e75. https://doi.org/10.1017/S2045796022000580

Census Bureau. (n.d.a). American Community Survey (ACS).

________. (n.d.b). Current Population Survey (CPS). https://www.census.gov/programs-surveys/cps.html

________. (1996). *Population projections of the United States by age, sex, race, and Hispanic origin: 1995–2050.* https://www.census.gov/library/publications/1996/demo/p25-1130.html

________. (2018). *2018 ACS 1-year public use microdata sample (PUMS) files.* https://acsdatacommunity.prb.org/discussion-forum/f/forum/510/2018-acs-1-year-public-use-microdata-sample-pums-files

________. (2019). *2019 ACS 1-year public use microdata sample (PUMS).* https://www2.census.gov/programs-surveys/acs/tech_docs/pums/accuracy/2019AccuracyPUMS.pdf

________. (2021). *HI-08. Health insurance coverage status and type of coverage by selected characteristics for children under 18 (all children).* Bureau of Labor Statistics. https://www.census.gov/data/tables/time-series/demo/income-poverty/cps-hi/hi-08.2015.html#list-tab-1099645920

________. (2023a). *2020 census demographic and housing characteristics file (DHC).* https://www.census.gov/programs-surveys/decennial-census/decade/2020/planning-management/release/about-2020-data-products.html

________. (2023b). *Percentage of children under the age of 19 without health insurance coverage by selected characteristics: 2021 and 2022.*

________. (2024). *National Survey of Children's Health (NSCH).* https://www.census.gov/programs-surveys/nsch.html

Center for the Advancement of Youth. (n.d.). *The developmental understanding and legal collaboration for everyone (DULCE) implementation project.* University of Mississippi Medical Center. https://umc.edu/Research/Centers-and-Institutes/Centers/Center-for-the-Advancement-of-Youth/Research/DULCE.html

Center for Behavioral Health Statistics and Quality. (2021). *Racial/ethnic differences in substance use, substance use disorders, and substance use treatment utilization among people aged 12 or older (2015–2019).* Substance Abuse and Mental Health Services Administration. https://www.samhsa.gov/data/sites/default/files/reports/rpt35326/2021NSDUHSUChartbook.pdf

Center for Children and Families. (n.d.). *Unwinding continuous coverage.* Georgetown University Health Policy Institute. https://ccf.georgetown.edu/subtopic/unwinding-phe/

Center for Evidence-Based Policy. (2022). *Payment model primer: Global payments.* https://centerforevidencebasedpolicy.org/CEbP_PaymentModelPrimer_GlobalPayments.pdf

Center for Health Care Strategies (CHCS). (2019a). *Accelerating child health transformation.* https://www.chcs.org/project/accelerating-child-health-transformation/

________. (2019b). *Exploring the impact of integrated Medicaid managed care on practice-level integration of physical and behavioral health access.* https://www.chcs.org/resource/exploring-the-impact-of-integrated-medicaid-managed-care-on-practice-level-integration-of-physical-and-behavioral-health/

________. (2022). *Value-based payment to support children's health and wellness: Shifting the focus from short-term to life course impact.* https://www.chcs.org/resource/value-based-payment-to-support-childrens-health-and-wellness-shifting-the-focus-from-short-term-to-life-course-impact/

Center for Healthcare Quality and Payment Reform. (n.d.). *Addressing the crisis in rural maternity care.* https://ruralhospitals.chqpr.org/downloads/Rural_Maternity_Care_Crisis.pdf

Center for Parents & Children. (n.d.). *PlayReadVIP.* https://cpc.pitt.edu/intervention-models/video-interaction-project/

Center for Parent Information and Resources. (2022). *All about the IEP.* https://www.parentcenterhub.org/iep

Center for the Study of Social Policy (CSSP). (n.d.a). *Developmental understanding and legal collaboration for everyone (DULCE).* https://cssp.org/our-work/project/dulce/

________. (2018). *Pediatrics supporting parents program analysis: Program and site selection process and results.* Center for the Study of Social Policy. https://cssp.org/wp-content/uploads/2018/11/Pediatrics-Supporting-Parents-Memo.pdf

Center for the Study of Social Policy & Pediatrics Supporting Parents. (2018). *Program analysis: Program and site selection process and results.* https://cssp.org/wp-content/uploads/2018/11/Pediatrics-Supporting-Parents-Memo.pdf

Center of Excellence for Infant & Early Childhood Mental Health Consultation (IECMHC). (2021). *Annotated bibliography: The evidence base for infant and early childhood mental health consultation (IECMHC).* Georgetown University Center for Child and Human Development. http://www.iecmhc.org/documents/CoE-Annotated-Bibliography.pdf

Center on the Developing Child. (2009). *Maternal depression can undermine the development of young children* (Working Paper No. 8). Harvard University. http://www.developingchild.harvard.edu/

Center for the Study of Social Policy. (n.d.b). *DULCE: Creating family-centered systems of care.* https://cssp.org/our-work/project/dulce/

Centers for Disease Control and Prevention (CDC). (n.d.a). *Advisory committee on immunization practices (ACIP).* U.S. Department of Health and Human Services. https://www.cdc.gov/vaccines/acip/index.html

________. (n.d.b.). Funded School Health Partners. U.S. Department of Health and Human Services. https://www.cdc.gov/healthyschools/fundedpartners.htm

_______. (n.d.c). *Hemophilia.* U.S. Department of Health and Human Services. https://www.cdc.gov/hemophilia/?CDC_AAref_Val=https://www.cdc.gov/ncbddd/hemophilia/documents/a-simmons_htc-brochure-508c.pdf

_______. (n.d.d). Most recent national asthma data. U.S. Department of Health and Human Services. https://www.cdc.gov/asthma/most_recent_national_asthma_data.htm

_______. (n.d.e). *Research anthology: Telehealth and telemedicine.* U.S. Department of Health and Human Services. https://www.cdc.gov/phlp/php/publications/research-anthology-telehealth-and-telemedicine.html

_______. (n.d.f). *Web-based injury statistics query and reporting system (WISQARS).* U.S. Department of Health and Human Services. https://wisqars.cdc.gov

_______. (1997). *Principles of community engagement* (1st ed.). Agency for Toxic Substances and Disease Registry, U.S. Department of Health and Human Services.

_______. (1999). Achievements in public health, 1900–1999 impact of vaccines universally recommended for children—United States, 1990–1998. *Morbidity and Mortality Weekly Report, 48*(12), 243–248. https://www.cdc.gov/mmwr/preview/mmwrhtml/00056803.htm

_______. (2011). School health guidelines to promote healthy eating and physical activity. *Morbidity and Mortality Weekly Report: Recommendations and Reports*, *60*(5), 1–76. https://www.cdc.gov/healthyschools/npao/pdf/mmwr-school-health-guidelines.pdf

_______. (2013). CDC grand rounds: Public health approaches to reducing U.S. infant mortality. *Morbidity and Mortality Weekly Report*, *62*(31), 625–628. https://www.cdc.gov/mmwr/preview/mmwrhtml/mm6231a3.htm

_______. (2018). *National health interview survey.* National Center for Health Statistics, U.S. Department of Health and Human Services. https://www.cdc.gov/nchs/nhis/shs/tables.htm

_______. (2019a). *Immunization information systems (IIS): About IIS.* U.S. Department of Health and Human Services. https://www.cdc.gov/iis/about/?CDC_AAref_Val=https://www.cdc.gov/vaccines/programs/iis/about.html

_______. (2019b). *Preventing adverse childhood experiences: Leveraging the best available evidence.* National Center for Injury Prevention and Control, Division of Violence Prevention.

_______. (2019c). *Spotlight on: Racial and ethnic differences in children identified with autism spectrum disorder (ASD).* U.S. Department of Health and Human Services. https://www.cdc.gov/ncbddd/autism/addm-community-report/differences-in-children.html

_______. (2019d). *Vital signs: Adverse childhood experiences (ACEs).* U.S. Department of Health and Human Services. https://www.cdc.gov/vitalsigns/aces/modules/VS_ACE.pdf

_______. (2020a). Health services for teens. U.S. Department of Health and Human Services. https://www.cdc.gov/healthyyouth/healthservices/index.htm

_______. (2020b). *Vaccine safety: Overview, history, and how it works.* U.S. Department of Health and Human Services. https://www.cdc.gov/vaccinesafety/ensuringsafety/history/index.html

_______. (2020c). *2020 community report on autism.* U.S. Department of Health and Human Services. https://www.cdc.gov/autism/media/pdfs/addm-community-report-2020-h.pdf

_______. (2021a). *CDC healthy schools: Chronic health conditions.* U.S. Department of Health and Human Services. https://www.cdc.gov/healthyschools/chronicconditions.htm

_______. (2021b). *CDC healthy schools: Whole school, whole community, whole child (WSCC).* U.S. Department of Health and Human Services. https://www.cdc.gov/healthyschools/wscc/index.htm

_______. (2021c). *Essentials for childhood: Creating safe, nurturing relationships and environments for all children.* U.S. Department of Health and Human Services. https://www.cdc.gov/violenceprevention/childabuseandneglect/essentials/index.html?CDC_AA_refVal=https%3A%2F%2Fwww.cdc.gov%2Fviolenceprevention%2Fchildabuseandneglect%2Fessentials.html

________. (2021d). *Most recent national asthma data.* U.S. Department of Health and Human Services. https://www.cdc.gov/asthma/most_recent_national_asthma_data.htm

________. (2021e). *National diabetes statistics report.* U.S. Department of Health and Human Services. https://www.cdc.gov/diabetes/data/statistics-report/index.html

________. (2022a). *The U.S. Public Health Service untreated syphilis study at Tuskegee: Timeline.* U.S. Department of Health and Human Services. https://www.cdc.gov/tuskegee/timeline.htm

________. (2022b). *Violence prevention: Fast facts.* U.S. Department of Health and Human Services. https://www.cdc.gov/violenceprevention/childabuseandneglect/fastfact.html

________. (2023a). *CDC-BRFSS-ACBS 18-20 child prevalence table 12.* U.S. Department of Health and Human Services. https://www.cdc.gov/brfss/acbs/2018/multiple_year/acbs_prevalence_18-20_table12.html

________. (2023b). *Data and statistics on children's mental health.* U.S. Department of Health and Human Services. https://www.cdc.gov/childrensmentalhealth/data.html

________. (2023c). *Healthcare use data 2020: Emergency department visits.* U.S. Department of Health and Human Services. https://www.cdc.gov/asthma/healthcare-use/2020/table_a.html

________. (2023d). *Healthcare use data 2020: Hospitalizations.* U.S. Department of Health and Human Services. https://www.cdc.gov/asthma/healthcare-use/2020/table_b.html

________. (2023e). *Improving access to care.* U.S. Department of Health and Human Services. https://www.cdc.gov/childrensmentalhealth/access.html

________. (2023f). *Preventive health and health services block grant evaluation report: 2022 framework measures assessment—Key findings.* U.S. Department of Health and Human Services. https://www.cdc.gov/phhs-block-grant/media/PHHS-Block-Grant-Measures-Assessment-2022-Key-Findings-Report.pdf

________. (2023g). *Spotlight on a new pattern in racial and ethnic differences emerges in autism spectrum disorder (ASD) identification among 8-year-old children.* U.S. Department of Health and Human Services. https://www.cdc.gov/ncbddd/autism/addm-community-report/spotlight-on-racial-ethnic-differences.html

________. (2023h). *Whole school, whole community, whole child (WSCC).* U.S. Department of Health and Human Services. https://www.cdc.gov/healthyschools/wscc/index.htm

________. (2023i). *Youth risk behavior survey data summary & trends report: 2011–2021.* U.S. Department of Health and Human Services. https://www.cdc.gov/healthyyouth/data/yrbs/pdf/yrbs_data-summary-trends_report2023_508.pdf

________. (2024a). *About the vaccines for children (VFC) program.* U.S. Department of Health and Human Services. https://www.cdc.gov/vaccines-for-children/about/?CDC_AAref_Val=https://www.cdc.gov/vaccines/programs/vfc/about/index.html

________. (2024b). *Asthma: Data, statistics, and surveillance.* U.S. Department of Health and Human Services. https://www.cdc.gov/asthma/asthmadata.htm#:~:text=The%20current%20asthma%20prevalence%20among,2001%20to%208.0%25%20in%202021

________. (2024c). *Benefits of healthy eating for children.* U.S. Department of Health and Human Services. https://www.cdc.gov/nutrition/php/resources/healthy-eating-benefits-for-children.html

________. (2024d). *CDC data modernization efforts accelerate nation's ability to detect and rapidly respond to health threats.* U.S. Department of Health and Human Services. https://www.cdc.gov/media/releases/2024/p0411-CDC-data-modernization.html

________. (2024e). *CDC healthy schools.* U.S. Department of Health and Human Services. https://www.cdc.gov/healthyschools/index.htm

________. (2024f). *Childhood obesity facts: Prevalence of childhood obesity in the United States.* U.S. Department of Health and Human Services. https://www.cdc.gov/obesity/php/data-research/childhood-obesity-facts.html

________. (2024g). *Child and teen BMI categories.* U.S. Department of Health and Human Services. https://www.cdc.gov/bmi/child-teen-calculator/bmi-categories.html

________. (2024h). *Developmental disability basics.* U.S. Department of Health and Human Services. https://www.cdc.gov/child-development/about/developmental-disability-basics.html

________. (2024i). *Fast facts on global immunization.* U.S. Department of Health and Human Services. https://www.cdc.gov/global-immunization/fast-facts/index.html

________. (2024j). Health and economic benefits of routine childhood immunizations in the era of the Vaccines for Children program—United States, 1994–2023. *Morbidity and Mortality Weekly Report, 73*(31), 682–685. https://www.cdc.gov/mmwr/volumes/73/wr/mm7331a2.htm

________. (2024k). *Health disparities in suicide.* U.S. Department of Health and Human Services. https://www.cdc.gov/suicide/disparities/index.html

________. (2024l). *Hearing loss in children.* U.S. Department of Health and Human Services. https://www.cdc.gov/hearing-loss-children/?CDC_AAref_Val=https://www.cdc.gov/ncbddd/hearingloss/publichealth.html

________. (2024m). *Perinatal quality collaboratives.* U.S. Department of Health and Human Services. https://www.cdc.gov/maternal-infant-health/pqc/index.html

________. (2024n). *Prevention and control of infectious diseases.* U.S. Department of Health and Human Services. https://www.cdc.gov/earlycare/infectious-diseases/index.html

________. (2024o). *Providing quality family planning services.* U.S. Department of Health and Human Services. https://www.cdc.gov/reproductive-health/hcp/contraception-guidance/quality-family-planning.html?CDC_AAref_Val=https://www.cdc.gov/reproductivehealth/contraception/qfp.htm

________. (2024p). *Vaccines for children (VFC) program information for providers.* U.S. Department of Health and Human Services. https://www.cdc.gov/vaccines/programs/vfc/providers/index.html

________. (2024q). *What is children's mental health?* U.S. Department of Health and Human Services. https://www.cdc.gov/childrensmentalhealth/basics.html

________. (2024r). *People with certain medical conditions and COVID-19 risk factors.* U.S. Department of Health & Human Services. https://www.cdc.gov/covid/risk-factors/index.html

Centers for Medicare & Medicaid Services (CMS). (n.d.a). *Children's health care quality measures, core set of children's health care quality measures.* U.S. Department of Health and Human Services. https://www.medicaid.gov/medicaid/quality-of-care/performance-measurement/adult-and-child-health-care-quality-measures/childrens-health-care-quality-measures/index.html

________. (n.d.b). *CHIP eligibility.* U.S. Department of Health and Human Services. https://www.medicaid.gov/chip/eligibility/index.html

________. (n.d.c). *Early and periodic screening, diagnostic and treatment.* U.S. Department of Health and Human Services. https://www.medicaid.gov/medicaid/benefits/early-and-periodic-screening-diagnostic-and-treatment/index.html

________. (n.d.d). *Guidance & regulations.* U.S. Department of Health and Human Services. https://www.cms.gov/medicare/payment/fee-for-service-providers/shared-savings-program-ssp-acos/guidance-regulations

________. (n.d.e). *Integrated care for kids (InCK) model.* U.S. Department of Health and Human Services. https://www.cms.gov/priorities/innovation/innovation-models/integrated-care-for-kids-model

________. (n.d.f). *Partial hospitalization programs.* U.S. Department of Health and Human Services. https://www.cms.gov/medicare-coverage-database/view/lcd.aspx?LCDId=37633

________. (n.d.g). *National health expenditure fact sheet.* U.S. Department of Health and Human Services. https://www.cms.gov/research-statistics-data-and-systems/statistics-trends-and-reports/nationalhealthexpenddata/nhe-fact-sheet.html

________. (n.d.h). Benefits. *Medicaid.gov.* U.S. Department of Health and Human Services. https://www.medicaid.gov/chip/benefits/index.html

________. (2010). Medical Loss Ratio: Getting Your Money's Worth on Health Insurance. https://www.cms.gov/cciio/resources/fact-sheets-and-faqs/medical-loss-ratio

________. (2014). *Fiscal year 2014 justification of estimates for appropriations committees.* U.S. Department of Health and Human Services. https://www.cms.gov/about-cms/agency-information/performancebudget/downloads/fy2014-cj-final.pdf

________. (2020). *CMS interoperability and patient access final rule (CMS-9115-F).* U.S. Department of Health and Human Services. https://www.cms.gov/priorities/key-initiatives/burden-reduction/policies-and-regulations/cms-interoperability-and-patient-access-final-rule-cms-9115-f

________. (2021a). *2021 Medicare parts a & b premiums and deductibles.* U.S. Department of Health and Human Services. https://www.cms.gov/newsroom/fact-sheets/2021-medicare-parts-b-premiums-and-deductibles

________. (2021b). *October 2021 healthcare common procedure coding system (HCPCS) quarterly update reminder.* U.S. Department of Health and Human Services. https://www.hhs.gov/guidance/document/october-2021-healthcare-common-procedure-coding-system-hcpcs-quarterly-update-reminder

________. (2021c). *Synthesis of evaluation results across 21 Medicare models, 2012–2020.* U.S. Department of Health and Human Services. https://www.cms.gov/priorities/innovation/data-and-reports/2022/wp-eval-synthesis-21models

________. (2022a). *About the CMS innovation center.* https://www.cms.gov/priorities/innovation/about

________. (2022b). *Synthesis of evaluation results across 21 Medicare models, 2012–2020.* U.S. Department of Health and Human Services. https://www.cms.gov/priorities/innovation/data-and-reports/2022/wp-eval-synthesis-21models

________. (2023a). *Cascade of meaningful measures.* U.S. Department of Health and Human Services. https://www.cms.gov/cascade-measures

________. (2023b). *CMS finalizes physician payment rule that advances health equity.* U.S. Department of Health and Human Services. https://www.cms.gov/newsroom/press-releases/cms-finalizes-physician-payment-rule-advances-health-equity

________. (2023c). *Delivering service in school-based settings: A comprehensive guide to Medicaid services and administrative claiming.* U.S. Department of Health and Human Services. https://www.cms.gov/newsroom/fact-sheets/delivering-service-school-based-settings-comprehensive-guide-medicaid-services-and-administrative

________. (2023d). *Meaningful measures 2.0: Moving to measure prioritization and modernization.* U.S. Department of Health and Human Services. https://www.cms.gov/medicare/quality/meaningful-measures-initiative/meaningful-measures-20

________. (2023e). *Medicaid and CHIP coverage of lawfully residing children & pregnant individuals.* U.S. Department of Health and Human Services. https://www.medicaid.gov/medicaid/enrollment-strategies/medicaid-and-chip-coverage-lawfully-residing-children-pregnant-individuals

________. (2023f). *Medicaid program; Medicaid and children's health insurance program (CHIP) managed care access, finance, and quality.* U.S. Department of Health and Human Services. https://www.federalregister.gov/documents/2023/05/03/2023-08961/medicaid-program-medicaid-and-childrens-health-insurance-program-chip-managed-care-access-finance

________. (2023g). *November 2022 Medicaid and CHIP enrollment trends snapshot.* U.S. Department of Health and Human Services. https://www.medicaid.gov/medicaid/national-medicaid-chip-program-information/downloads/november-2022-medicaid-chip-enrollment-trend-snapshot.pdf

________. (2023h). *Psychiatric residential treatment facility providers.* U.S. Department of Health and Human Services. https://www.cms.gov/medicare/health-safety-standards/certification-compliance/psychiatric-residential-treatment-facility-providers

________. (2023i). Summary of Medicaid and CHIP payment-related provisions: Ensuring access to Medicaid services (CMS 2442-P) and Medicaid and children's health insurance program (CHIP) managed care access, finance, and quality (CMS-2439-P). *Fact Sheets.* U.S. Department of Health and Human Services. https://www.cms.gov/newsroom/fact-sheets/summary-medicaid-and-chip-payment-related-provisions-ensuring-access-medicaid-services-cms-2442-p#_ftn1

________. (2023j). *Telehealth for providers: What you need to know.* U.S. Department of Health and Human Services. https://www.cms.gov/files/document/telehealth-toolkit-providers.pdf

________. (2024a). *Aligning quality measures across CMS—The universal foundation.* U.S. Department of Health and Human Services. https://www.cms.gov/medicare/quality/cms-national-quality-strategy/aligning-quality-measures-across-cms-universal-foundation

________. (2024b). *CMS announces $50 million in grants to deliver critical school-based health services to children.* U.S. Department of Health and Human Services. https://www.cms.gov/newsroom/press-releases/cms-announces-50-million-grants-deliver-critical-school-based-health-services-children

________. (2024c). *CMS interoperability and prior authorization final rule (CMS-0057-F).* U.S. Department of Health and Human Services. https://www.cms.gov/priorities/key-initiatives/burden-reduction/interoperability/policies-and-regulations/cms-interoperability-and-prior-authorization-final-rule-cms-0057-f

________. (2024d). *CMS national quality strategy.* U.S. Department of Health and Human Services. https://www.cms.gov/medicare/quality/meaningful-measures-initiative/cms-quality-strategy

________. (2024e). *Integrated care for kids (InCK) model: Second evaluation report.* U.S. Department of Health and Human Services. https://www.cms.gov/priorities/innovation/data-and-reports/2024/inck-model-second-eval-rpt

________. (2024f). Medicaid program; Ensuring access to Medicaid services. *Federal Register.* U.S. Department of Health and Human Services. https://www.federalregister.gov/documents/2024/05/10/2024-08363/medicaid-program-ensuring-access-to-medicaid-services

________. (2024g). *NHE fact sheet.* U.S. Department of Health and Human Services. https://www.cms.gov/data-research/statistics-trends-and-reports/national-health-expenditure-data/nhe-fact-sheet#:~:text=Historical%20NHE%2C%202021 %3A&text=Medicare%20spending%20grew%208.4%25%20to,28%20percent%20of% 20total%20NHE.

________. (2024h). *Quality of care for children in Medicaid and CHIP: Findings from the 2022 child core set.* U.S. Department of Health and Human Services. https://www.medicaid.gov/sites/default/files/2024-01/2022-child-chartpack.pdf

________. (2024i). *TEAM decarbonization and resilience initiative.* U.S. Department of Health and Human Services. https://www.cms.gov/team-decarbonization-and-resilience-initiative

________ (2024j). *Transforming Maternal Health (TMaH) model.* U.S. Department of Health and Human Services. https://www.cms.gov/priorities/innovation/innovation-models/transforming-maternal-health-tmah-model

Chang, A. R., & Slopen, N. (2023). Racial and ethnic disparities for unmet needs by mental health condition: 2016 to 2021. *Pediatrics, 153*(1). https://doi.org/10.1542/peds.2023-062286

Chang, C.-H., Bynum, J. P. W., & Lurie, J. D. (2019). Geographic expansion of federally qualified health centers 2007–2014. *The Journal of Rural Health*, *35*(3), 385–394. https://doi.org/10.1111/jrh.12330

Chaudhry, S. B., Armbrecht, E. S., Shin, Y., Matula, S., Caffrey, C., Varade, R., Jones, L., & Siegfried, E. (2013). Pediatric access to dermatologists: Medicaid versus private insurance. *Journal of the American Academy of Dermatology*, *68*(5), 738–748. https://doi.org/10.1016/j.jaad.2012.10.034

Cheng, H., Luo, W., Si, S., Xin, X., Peng, Z., Zhou, H., Liu, H., & Yu, Y. (2022). Global trends in total fertility rate and its relation to national wealth, life expectancy and female education. *BMC Public Health*, *22*, 1346. https://doi.org/10.1186/s12889-022-13656-1

Cheng, T. L. (2004). Primary care pediatrics: 2004 and beyond. *Pediatrics*, *113*(6), 1802–1809. https://doi.org/10.1542/peds.113.6.1802

________. (2023). Making maternal child health a population health priority in Maryland. *Pediatric Clinics of North America*, *70*(1), 53–65. https://doi.org/10.1016/j.pcl.2022.09.010

Cheng, T. L., Cohn, R. D., & Dover, G. J. (2008). The genetics revolution and primary care pediatrics. *Journal of the American Medical Association*, *299*(4). https://doi.org/10.1001/jama.299.4.451

Cheng, T. L., Goodman, E., & Committee on Pediatric Research. (2015). Race, ethnicity, and socioeconomic status in research on child health. *Pediatrics*, *135*(1), e225–e237. https://doi.org/10.1542/peds.2014-3109

Cheng, T. L., & Jenkins, R. R. (2009). Health disparities across the lifespan: Where are the children? *Journal of the American Medical Association*, *301*(23), 2491–2492. https://doi.org/10.1001/jama.2009.848

Cheng, T. L., Johnson, S. B., & Goodman, E. (2016a). Breaking the intergenerational cycle of disadvantage: The three-generation approach. *Pediatrics*, *137*(6). https://doi.org/10.1542/peds.2015-2467

Cheng, T. L., & Mistry, K. B. (2019). The uniqueness and importance of children in addressing health disparities across the life course: Implications for research. *Epidemiology*, *30*(Suppl 2), S60–S64. https://doi.org/10.1097/ede.0000000000001069

________. (2023). Clarity on disparity: Who, what, when, where, why, and how. *Pediatric Clinics of North America*, *70*(4), 639–650. https://doi.org/10.1016/j.pcl.2023.03.003

Cheng, T. L., Monteiro, N., DiMeglio, L. A., Chien, A. T., Peeples, E. S., Raetz, E., Scheindlin, B., & Denne, S. C. (2016). Seven great achievements in pediatric research in the past 40 years. *Pediatric Research*, *80*(3), 330–337. https://doi.org/10.1038/pr.2016.95

Cheng, T. L., Moon, M., & Artman, M. (2020). Shoring up the safety net for children in the COVID-19 pandemic. *Pediatric Research*, *88*(3), 349–351. https://doi.org/10.1038/s41390-020-1071-7

Cheng, T. L., & Solomon, B. S. (2014). Translating life course theory to clinical practice to address health disparities. *Maternal and Child Health Journal*, *18*(2), 389–395. https://doi.org/10.1007/s10995-013-1279-9

Chetty, R., Hendren, N., Jones, M. R., & Porter, S. R. (2019). Race and economic opportunity in the United States: An intergenerational perspective. *The Quarterly Journal of Economics*, *135*(2), 711–783. https://doi.org/10.1093/qje/qjz042

Child and Adolescent Health Measurement Initiative (CAHMI). (n.d.a). *Data resource center for child and adolescent health*. https://www.childhealthdata.org

________. (n.d.b). *Engagement in Action (EnAct!) Framework*. https://www.cahmi.org/our-work-in-action/engagement-in-action/EnAct!Framework

________. (n.d.c). *National maternal and child health measures compendium*. https://www.cahmi.org/our-work-in-action/measurement-in-action/compendium

_______. (2018). *Maternal and child health measurement research network (MCH-MRN) strategic agenda.* https://www.cahmi.org/docs/default-source/resources/maternal-and-child-health-national-strategic-measurement-agenda-full-report.pdf?sfvrsn=fe258d7c_0

_______. (2023). *Two page summary of the engagement in action framework.* https://cahmi.org/docs/default-source/ms-enact-documents/enact!-framework-two-pager

_______. (2024). *Data resource center for child and adolescent health. Analysis of the 2021-22 National Survey of Children's Health for the NASEM committee to improve child and youth well-being through children's healthcare system transformation.*

Child Enrollment Scientific Vision Working Group. (2017). *Opportunities enabled through the enrollment of children in the All of Us research program.* All of Us Research Program Advisory Panel. https://allofus.nih.gov/sites/default/files/cesvwg_1-18-18.pdf

Children's Bureau. (n.d.) *Mental health apps. Childhelp hotline.* https://www.childhelphotline.org/teen-apps/

Children's Defense Fund. (2023). *2023 state of America's children report.* https://www.childrensdefense.org/tools-and-resources/the-state-of-americas-children/soac-child-poverty/

Children's Health Act of 2000, Pub. L. No. 106-310, 114 Stat. 1101 (2000).

Children's Hospital Association (CHA). (n.d.). *How can we help*? https://www.childrenshospitals.org/contact-us

_______. (2023). *Industry impact report summary.* https://www.childrenshospitals.org/-/media/files/events/lsg-cha-industry-impact-report-summary-12-8-23.pdf

Children's National Hospital. (2023a). *AI: The "single greatest tool" for improving access to pediatric healthcare.* Innovation District. https://innovationdistrict.childrensnational.org/ai-the-single-greatest-tool-for-improving-access-to-pediatric-healthcare/

_______. (2023b). *Social work services in the Heart Institute.* https://childrensnational.org/departments/childrens-national-heart-institute/resources-for-families/social-work-heart-institute

Chilukuri, N., Cheng, T. L., Psoter, K., Mistry, K., Connor, K. A., Levy, D. J., & Upadhya, K. (2018). Effectiveness of a pediatric primary care intervention to increase maternal folate use: Results from a cluster randomized control trial. *Journal of Pediatrics*, *192*, 247–252. https://doi.org/10.1016/j.jpeds.2017.09.020

Chin, M. H., Afsar-Manesh, N., Bierman, A. S., Boyington, J. E., Cykert, S., Grumbach, K., et al. (2023). Guiding principles to address the impact of algorithm bias on racial and ethnic disparities in health and health care. *JAMA Network Open, 6*(12), e2345050. https://doi.org/10.1001/jamanetworkopen.2023.45050

Chisolm, D. J., Brook, D. L., Applegate, M. S., & Kelleher, K. J. (2019). Social determinants of health priorities of state Medicaid programs. *BMC Health Services Research*, *19*(1), 167. https://doi.org/10.1186/s12913-019-3977-5

Choi, J. H., Correia de Sousa, J., Fletcher, M., Gabutti, G., Harrington, L., Holden, M., Kim, H., Michel, J. P., Mukherjee, P., Nolan, T., Welte, T., & Maggi, S. (2022). Improving vaccination rates in older adults and at-risk groups: Focus on pertussis. *Aging Clinical and Experimental Research*, *34*(1), 1–8. https://doi.org/10.1007/s40520-021-02018-3

Chomilo, N. (2023). Can capitalism drive health equity? Considering the benefits and risks of social drivers of health bonds. *Health Affairs*, *42*(3), 392–394. https://doi.org/10.1377/hlthaff.2022.01689

Chomilo, N. T. (2022). *Health care application for certain populations* (DHS-8209A-ENG). https://edocs.dhs.state.mn.us/lfserver/Public/DHS-8209A-ENG

Chorniy, A. V., Currie, J., & Sonchak, L. (2018). *Does prenatal WIC participation improve child outcomes?* National Bureau of Economic Research. https://ideas.repec.org/p/nbr/nberwo/24691.html

Christrup, S., Hoagland, G. W., Loud, G., Werber Serafini, M., & Strong, K. (2023). *Cleaner health care: Hospital emissions mitigation*. Bipartisan Policy Center. https://bipartisanpolicy.org/report/cleaner-health-care-hospital-emissions-mitigation/

Chukmaitov, A., Dahman, B., Garland, S. L., Dow, A., Parsons, P. L., Harris, K. A., & Sheppard, V. B. (2022). Addressing social risk factors in the inpatient setting: Initial findings from a screening and referral pilot at an urban safety-net academic medical center in Virginia, USA. *Preventive Medicine Reports, 29*, 101935. https://doi.org/10.1016/j.pmedr.2022.101935

Chung, R. J., Lee, J. B., Hackell, J. M., Alderman, E. M., Committee on Adolescence, & Committee on Practice & Ambulatory Medicine. (2024). Confidentiality in the care of adolescents: Technical report. *Pediatrics, 153*(5), e2024066327. https://doi.org/10.1542/peds.2024-066327

Chung, S. T., Krenek, A., & Magge, S. N. (2023). Childhood obesity and cardiovascular disease risk. *Current Atherosclerosis Reports*, 1–11. https://doi.org/10.1007/s11883-023-01111-4

Cianconi, P., Hanife, B., Grillo, F., Betro, S., Lesmana, C. B. J., & Janiri, L. (2023). Eco-emotions and psychoterratic syndromes: Reshaping mental health assessment under climate change. *Yale Journal of Biology and Medicine*, *96*(2), 211–226. https://doi.org/10.59249/earx2427

Cisneros-Franco, J. M., Voss, P., Thomas, M. E., & de Villers-Sidani, E. (2020). Critical periods of brain development. *Handbook of Clinical Neurology*, *173*, 75–88. https://doi.org/10.1016/B978-0-444-64150-2.00009-5

Clark, H., Coll-Seck, A. M., Banerjee, A., Peterson, S., Dalglish, S. L., Ameratunga, S., Balabanova, D., Bhan, M. K., Bhutta, Z. A., Borrazzo, J., Claeson, M., Doherty, T., El-Jardali, F., George, A. S., Gichaga, A., Gram, L., Hipgrave, D. B., Kwamie, A., Meng, Q., . . . Costello, A. (2020). A future for the world's children? A WHO–UNICEF–Lancet Commission. *The Lancet*, *395*(10224), 605–658. https://doi.org/10.1016/S0140-6736(19)32540-1

Clark, K. B., & Clark, M. K. (1939). The development of consciousness of self and the emergence of racial identification in negro preschool children. *The Journal of Social Psychology*, *10*(4), 591–599. https://doi.org/10.1080/00224545.1939.9713394

Clay, A. M., & Parsh, B. (2016). Patient- and family-centered care: It's not just for pediatrics anymore. *AMA Journal of Ethics*, *18*(1), 40–44. https://doi.org/10.1001/journalofethics.2016.18.1.medu3-1601

Claypool, N., & Moore de Peralta, A. (2021). The influence of adverse childhood experiences (ACEs), including the COVID-19 pandemic, and toxic stress on development and health outcomes of Latinx children in the USA: A review of the literature. *International Journal on Child Maltreatment: Research, Policy and Practice*, *4*(3), 257–278. https://doi.org/10.1007/s42448-021-00080-y

Clayton, S., & Karazsia, B. T. (2020). Development and validation of a measure of climate change anxiety. *Journal of Environmental Psychology*, *69*, 101434. https://doi.org/10.1016/j.jenvp.2020.101434

Close, J. (2024) Medicaid reimbursement for school-based mental health services. *Pediatrics*, *153*(4), e2023064074. https://doi.org/10.1542/peds.2023-064074

Co, J. P. T., Sternberg, S. B., & Homer, C. J. (2011). Measuring Patient and Family Experiences of Health Care for Children. *Academic Pediatrics, 11*(3), S59-S67. https://doi.org/10.1016/j.acap.2011.01.009

Cochrane, B. S., Ritchie, D., Lockhard, D., Picciano, G., King, J. A., & Nelson, B. (2019). A culture of compassion: How timeless principles of kindness and empathy become powerful tools for confronting today's most pressing healthcare challenges. *Healthcare Management Forum, 32*(3), 120–127. https://doi.org/10.1177/0840470419836240

Cogburn, C. D. (2019). Culture, race, and health: Implications for racial inequities and population health. *The Milbank Quarterly*, 97(3), 736–761. https://doi.org/10.1111/1468-0009.12411

Cohen, E., Berry, J. G., Sanders, L., Schor, E. L., & Wise, P. H. (2018). Status complexicus? The emergence of pediatric complex care. *Pediatrics, 141*(Suppl 3), S202–S211. https://doi.org/10.1542/peds.2017-1284E

Cohen, E., & Kaufmann, R. (2000). *Early childhood mental health consultation* (DHHS Pub. No. CMHS-SVP0151). Center for Mental Health Services, Substance Abuse and Mental Health Services Administration.

Cohen, E., Kuo, D. Z., Agrawal, R., Berry, J. G., Bhagat, S. K., Simon, T. D., & Srivastava, R. (2011). Children with medical complexity: An emerging population for clinical and research initiatives. *Pediatrics, 127*(3), 529–538. https://doi.org/10.1542/peds.2010-0910

Cohen, E., & Patel, H. (2014). Responding to the rising number of children living with complex chronic conditions. *Canadian Medical Association Journal, 186*(16), 1199–1200. https://doi.org/10.1503/cmaj.141036

Cohen, K. A., Stiles-Shields, C., Winquist, N., & Lattie, E. G. (2021). Traditional and nontraditional mental healthcare services: Usage and preferences among adolescents and younger adults. *The Journal of Behavioral Health Services & Research, 48*(4), 537–553. https://doi.org/10.1007/s11414-020-09746-w

Cohen, R. A., & Cha, A. E. (2023). *Health insurance coverage: Early release of estimates from the national health interview survey, 2022.* U.S. Department of Health and Human Services, National Center for Health Statistics. https://www.cdc.gov/nchs/data/nhis/earlyrelease/insur202305_1.pdf

Cohen, R. A., Martinez, M. E., & Zammitti, E. P. (2015). *Health insurance coverage: Early release of estimates from the National Health Interview Survey, 2015.* National Center for Health Statistics. Retrieved from https://www.cdc.gov/nchs/data/nhis/earlyrelease/insur201905.pdf

Cohen Ross, D., Guyer, J., Lam, A., & Toups, M. (2019). *Fostering social and emotional health through pediatric primary care: A blueprint for leveraging Medicaid and CHIP to finance change.* Center for the Study of Social Policy and Manatt Health. https://www.packard.org/wp-content/uploads/2021/01/CSSP-Medicaid-Blueprint-1.pdf

Cohn, L. N., Pechlivanoglou, P., Lee, Y., Mahant, S., Orkin, J., Marson, A., & Cohen, E. (2020). Health outcomes of parents of children with chronic illness: A systematic review and meta-analysis. *Journal of Pediatrics, 218*, 166–177.e2. https://doi.org/10.1016/j.jpeds.2019.10.068

Cohodes, S., Grossman, D., Kleiner, S., & Lovenheim, M. F. (2016). The effect of child health insurance access on schooling: Evidence from public insurance expansions. *Journal of Human Resources, 51*(3), 727–759. https://doi.org/10.3368/jhr.51.3.1014-6688R1

Coker, T. R., Castor, C., Ellison, J. S., Tullius, C., Hymel, B., Patterson, K., Barkin, S. L., Dreyer, B. P., Mendelsohn, A. L., & Dreyer, B. (2023). Effectiveness of a primary care intervention integrating promotion of responsive caregiving and early childhood development. *Pediatrics, 151*(3), e2022058529. https://doi.org/10.1542/peds.2022-058529

Coker, T. R., Chacon, S., Elliott, M. N., Bruno, Y., Chavis, T., Biely, C., Bethell, C. D., Contreras, S., Mimila, N. A., Mercado, J., & Chung, P. J. (2016). A parent coach model for well-child care among low-income children: A randomized controlled trial. *Pediatrics, 137*(3), e20153013. https://doi.org/10.1542/peds.2015-3013

Coker, T. R., Elliott, M. N., Kanouse, D. E., Grunbaum, J. A., Schwebel, D. C., Gilliland, M. J., Tortolero, S. R., Peskin, M. F., & Schuster, M. A. (2009). Perceived racial/ethnic discrimination among fifth-grade students and its association with mental health. *American Journal of Public Health, 99*(5), 878–884. https://doi.org/10.2105/AJPH.2008.144329

Coker, T. R., Moreno, C., Shekelle, P. G., Schuster, M. A., & Chung, P. J. (2014). Well-child care clinical practice redesign for serving low-income children. *Pediatrics, 134*(1), e229–e239. 10.1542/peds.2013-3775

Coker, T. R., & Perrin, J. M. (2022) The NASEM report on implementing high-quality primary care—Implications for pediatrics. *JAMA Pediatrics, 176*(3), 221–222. https://10.1001/jamapediatrics.2021.4594

Coker, T. R., Rodriguez, M. A., & Flores, G. (2010). Family-centered care for US children with special health care needs: Who gets it and why? *Pediatrics, 125*(6), 1159–1167. https://doi.org/10.1542/peds.2009-1994

Coker, T. R., Thomas, T., & Chung, P. J. (2013). Does well-child care have a future in pediatrics? *Pediatrics, 131*(Suppl 2), S149–S159. https://doi.org/10.1542/peds.2013-0252f

Cole, M. B., Lee, E. K., Frogner, B. K., Wright, B. (2023). Changes in Performance Measures and Service Volume at US Federally Qualified Health Centers During the COVID-19 Pandemic. *JAMA Health Forum, 4*(4), e230351. https://doi.org/10.1001/jamahealthforum.2023.0351

Coleman-Jensen, A., Rabbitt, M. P., Gregory, C. A., & Singh, A. (2022). *Statistical supplement to household food security in the United States in 2021.* U.S. Department of Agriculture.

Colich, N. L., Rosen, M. L., Williams, E. S., & McLaughlin, K. A. (2020). Biological aging in childhood and adolescence following experiences of threat and deprivation: A systematic review and meta-analysis. *Psychological Bulletin, 2*(999). https://doi.org/10.1037/bul0000270

Colizzi, M., Lasalvia, A., & Ruggeri, M. (2020). Prevention and early intervention in youth mental health: Is it time for a multidisciplinary and trans-diagnostic model for care? *International Journal of Mental Health Systems, 14*(1), 23. https://doi.org/10.1186/s13033-020-00356-9

Collins, A. M., & Klerman, J. A. (2017). Improving nutrition by increasing Supplemental Nutrition Assistance Program benefits. *American Journal of Preventive Medicine, 52*(2S2), S179–S185. https://doi.org/10.1016/j.amepre.2016.08.032

Colmer, J., Voorheis, J., & Williams, B. (2022). *Air pollution and economic opportunity in the United States.* https://www.colorado.edu/economics/sites/default/files/attached-files/colmer.pdf

Colombo, J., Gustafson, K. M., & Carlson, S. E. (2019). Critical and sensitive periods in development and nutrition. *Annals of Nutrition and Metabolism, 75*(Suppl 1), 34–42. https://doi.org/10.1159/000508053

Committee on Adolescence, Braverman, P. K., & Murray, P. J. (2011). Health care for youth in the juvenile justice system. *Pediatrics, 128*(6), 1219–1235. https://doi.org/10.1542/peds.2011-1757

Committee on Adolescent Health Care. (2020). *Committee opinion number 803: Confidentiality in adolescent health care.* The American College of Obstetricians and Gynecologists. https://www.acog.org/clinical/clinical-guidance/committee-opinion/articles/2020/04/confidentiality-in-adolescent-health-care

Committee on Coding and Nomenclature, Andreae, M. C., Bradley, J. F., Brewer, E. D., Calabrese, J., Krug, S. E., Liechty, E. A., Linzer, J. F., Pillsbury, J. M, & Tuli, S. Y. (2014). Application of the resource-based relative value scale system to pediatrics. *Pediatrics, 133*(6), 1158–1162. https://doi.org/10.1542/peds.2014-0866

Committee on Obstetric Practice. (2017). Committee opinion No. 713: Antenatal corticosteroid therapy for fetal maturation. *Obstetrics & Gynecology, 130*(2), e102–e109. https://doi.org/10.1097/aog.0000000000002237

Commonwealth Fund. (2022). *The impact of climate change on our health and health systems.* https://www.commonwealthfund.org/publications/explainer/2022/may/impact-climate-change-our-health-and-health-systems

The Community Guide. (2019a). *Mental health: Universal school-based cognitive behavioral therapy programs to reduce depression and anxiety symptoms.* https://www.thecommunityguide.org/findings/mental-health-universal-school-based-cognitive-behavioral-therapy-programs-reduce-depression-anxiety-symptoms.html

_______. (2019b). Targeted school-based cognitive behavioral therapy programs to reduce depression and anxiety symptoms.

Community Mental Health Act of 1963, Pub. L. No. 88-164, 77 Stat. 282 (1963).

Community Preventive Services Task Force (CPSTF). (2015). *Social determinants of health: School-based health centers task force finding and rationale statement.* Community Preventive Services Task Force. https://www.thecommunityguide.org/media/pdf/SDOH-School-Based-Health-Centers-508.pdf

_______. (2016a). School-based health centers to promote health equity: Recommendation of the community preventive services task force. *American Journal of Preventive Medicine, 51*(1), 127–128.

_______. (2016b). *Social determinants of health: School-based health centers, task force finding and rationale statement.* https://www.thecommunityguide.org/media/pdf/SDOH-School-Based-Health-Centers-508.pdf

_______. (2019a). *The community guide systematic review: Asthma: School-based self-management interventions for children and adolescents with asthma.* https://www.thecommunityguide.org/findings/asthma-school-based-self-management-interventions-children-and-adolescents-asthma.html

_______. (2019b). *The community guide systematic review: Mental health: Universal school-based cognitive behavioral therapy programs to reduce depression and anxiety symptoms.* https://www.thecommunityguide.org/findings/mental-health-universal-school-based-cognitive-behavioral-therapy-programs-reduce-depression-anxiety-symptoms.html

_______. (2021). *The community guide: Physical activity: Interventions to increase active travel to school.* https://www.thecommunityguide.org/media/pdf/OnePager-Active-Transport-School-508.pdf

_______. (2022). *2022 annual report to Congress. The community guide.* https://www.thecommunityguide.org/pages/2022-annual-report-congress.html

Community Reinvestment Act of 1977, 12 U.S.C. § 2901 (1977).

Confederated Salish and Kootenai Tribes. (n.d.). *Confederated Salish and Kootenai tribes website.* https://csktribes.org/

Congressional Budget Office (CBO). (2019). *Federal subsidies for health insurance coverage for people under age 65: 2019 to 2029.* https://www.cbo.gov/publication/55085

_______. (2020). *How CBO analyzes approaches to improve health through disease prevention.* https://www.cbo.gov/publication/56345

_______. (2023). *An Update to the Budget Outlook: 2023 to 2033.* https://www.cbo.gov/publication/59096

Congressional Research Service (CRS). (2010). *501(c)(3) hospitals and the community benefit standard.* https://crsreports.congress.gov/product/pdf/RL/RL34605/10

_______. (2019). *Federal grants to state and local governments: A historical perspective on contemporary issues* (CRS Report No. 40638). https://sgp.fas.org/crs/misc/R40638.pdf

_______. (2023a). *Centers for Disease Control and Prevention (CDC) funding overview* (CRS Report No. R47207). https://crsreports.congress.gov/product/pdf/R/R47207

_______. (2023b). *Medicaid: An overview* (CRS Report No. R43357). https://crsreports.congress.gov/product/pdf/R/R43357

Conners, G. P., Kressly, S. J., Perrin, J. M., Richerson, J. E., Sankrithi, U. M., Committee on Practice and Ambulatory Medicine, Committee on Pediatric Emergency Medicine, Section on Telehealth Care, Section on Emergency Medicine, Subcommittee on Urgent Care, & Task Force on Pediatric Practice Change. (2017). Nonemergency acute care: When it's not the medical home. *Pediatrics, 139*(5), e20170629. https://doi.org/10.1542/peds.2017-0629

Connor, K. A., Spin, P., Smith, B. M., Marshall, B. R., Calderon, G. V., Prichett, L., Jones, V. C., Connor, R, Cheng, T. L., Klein, L. M., & Johnson, S. B. (2024). Effect of a comprehensive school-based health center on academic growth in K-8th grade students. *Academic Pediatrics, 24*(7), 1124–1132. https://doi.org/10.1016/j.acap.2024.03.018

Consolidated Appropriations Act, 2023, Pub. L. No. 117-328, 136 Stat. 4459 (2022).

Constantino, J. N., Abbacchi, A. M., Saulnier, C., Klaiman, C., Mandell, D. S., Zhang, Y., Hawks, Z., Bates, J., Klin, A., Shattuck, P., Molholm, S., Fitzgerald, R., Roux, A., Lowe, J. K., & Geschwind, D. H. (2020). Timing of the diagnosis of autism in African American children. *Pediatrics*, *146*(3). https://doi.org/10.1542/peds.2019-3629

Conway, D. (2020). *Health insurance coverage among young adults aged 19 to 34: 2018 and 2019*. U.S. Census Bureau, U.S. Department of Commerce. https://www.census.gov/content/dam/Census/library/publications/2020/acs/acsbr20-02.pdf

Cooley, W. C., & Sagerman, P. J. (2011). Supporting the health care transition from adolescence to adulthood in the medical home. *Pediatrics*, *128*(1), 182–200. https://doi.org/10.1542/peds.2011-0969

Corallo, B., Garfield, R., Tolbert, J., & Rudowitz, R. (2021). *Medicaid enrollment churn and implications for continuous coverage policies*. KFF. https://www.kff.org/report-section/medicaid-enrollment-churn-and-implications-for-continuous-coverage-policies-appendix/

Cornell, E. (2019). *Strengthening children's social-emotional well-being and ensuring a parent-led agenda: Transforming the pediatric well-child visit through technology*. https://helpmegrownational.org/wp-content/uploads/2021/11/Pediatrics-Supporting-Parents_Phase-1-Full-Final-Report.pdf

Cornell, E., Therriault, C., & Dworkin, P. (2021). *Strengthening children's social-emotional well-being and ensuring a parent-led agenda: Transforming the pediatric well-child visit through technology*. Pediatrics Supporting Parents and Help Me Group National Center. https://helpmegrownational.org/wp-content/uploads/2021/11/Pediatrics-Supporting-Parents_Phase-1-Full-Final-Report.pdf

Cornell, P. Y., Halladay, C. W., Ader, J., Halaszynski, J., Hogue, M., McClain, C. E., Silva, J. W., Taylor, L. D., & Rudolph, J. L. (2020). Embedding social workers in Veterans Health Administration primary care teams reduces emergency department visits. *Health Affairs (Project Hope)*, *39*(4), 603–612. https://doi.org/10.1377/hlthaff.2019.01589

Coronavirus Aid, Relief, and Economic Security Act, Pub. L. No. 116-136, 134 Stat. 281 (2020).

Cosgrove, S., Moore-Monroy, M., Jenkins, C., Castillo, S. R., Williams, C., Parris, E., Tran, J. H., Rivera, M. D., & Brownstein, J. N. (2014). Community health workers as an integral strategy in the REACH U.S. program to eliminate health inequities. *Health Promotion Practice*, *15*(6), 795–802. https://doi.org/10.1177/1524839914541442

Costain, G., Cohn, R. D., & Malkin, D. (2020). Precision child health: An emerging paradigm for paediatric quality and safety. *Current Treatment Options in Pediatrics*, 6(4), 317–324. https://doi.org/10.1007/s40746-020-00207-2

Costich, M. A., Peretz, P. J., Davis, J. A., Stockwell, M. S., & Matiz, L. A. (2019). Impact of a community health worker program to support caregivers of children with special health care needs and address social determinants of health. *Clinical Pediatrics*. https://doi.org/10.1177/0009922819851263

Cotton, Q. D., Smith, P., Ehrenthal, D. B., Green-Harris, G., & Kind, A. J. H. (2019). A case study on a university-community partnership to eliminate racial disparities in infant mortality: Effective strategies and lessons learned. *Social Work in Public Health*, *34*(8), 673–685. https://doi.org/10.1080/19371918.2019.1671933

Council for a Strong America. (2022). *Mission: Readiness members meet with Rep. Wenstrup to discuss new ineligibility data*. Council for a Strong America. https://www.strongnation.org/articles/2014-mission-readiness-members-meet-with-rep-wenstrup-to-discuss-new-ineligibility-data

________. (2023a). *77 Percent of American youth can't qualify for military service*. https://www.strongnation.org/articles/2006-77-percent-of-american-youth-can-t-qualify-for-military-service

_______. (2023b). *Mission readiness, we need . . . all that they can be.* https://www.strongnation.org/articles/2288-we-need-all-that-they-can-be

Council on Community Pediatrics, Gitterman, B. A., Flanagan, P. J., Cotton, W. H., Dilley, K. J., Duffee, J. H., Green, A. E., Keane, V. A., Krugman, S. D., Linton, J. M., McKelvey, C. D., & Nelson, J. L. (2016). Poverty and child health in the United States. *Pediatrics, 137*(4), e20160339. https://doi.org/10.1542/peds.2016-0339

Council on School Health, Holmes, B. W., Sheetz, A., Allison, M., Ancona, R., Attisha, E., Beers, N., De Pinto, C., Gorski, P., Kjolhede, C., Lerner, M., Weiss-Harrison, A., & Young, T. (2016). Role of the school nurse in providing school health services. *Pediatrics, 137*(6). https://doi.org/10.1542/peds.2016-0852

Counts, N. Z. (2022). *Behavioral health care in the United States: How it works and where it falls short (explainer).* Commonwealth Fund.

_______. (2023). *Understanding the U.S. behavioral health workforce shortage.* The Commonwealth Fund. https://www.commonwealthfund.org/publications/explainer/2023/may/understanding-us-behavioral-health-workforce-shortage

Counts, N. Z., Mistry, K. B., & Wong, C. A. (2021a). The need for new cost measures in pediatric value-based payment. *Pediatrics, 147*(2), e20194037. https://doi.org/10.1542/peds.2019-4037

Counts, N. Z., Roiland, R. A., & Halfon, N. (2021b). Proposing the ideal alternative payment model for children. *JAMA Pediatrics.* https://doi.org/10.1001/jamapediatrics.2021.0247

Coutinho, M. T., Subzwari, S. S., McQuaid, E. L., & Koinis-Mitchell, D. (2020). Community health workers' role in supporting pediatric asthma management: A review. *Clinical Practice in Pediatric Psychology, 8*(2), 195–210.

Coverage and Authorization of Service. 42 C.F.R. § 438.210(a)(2) (2024).

Coverage of Preventive Health Services, 29 C.F.R. § 2590.715-2713 (2023). https://www.law.cornell.edu/cfr/text/29/2590.715-2713

Cowling, T. E., Cecil, E. V., Soljak, M. A., Lee, J. T., Millett, C., Majeed, A., Wachter, R. M., & Harris, M. J. (2013). Access to primary care and visits to emergency departments in England: A cross-sectional, population-based study. *PLoS One, 8*(6), e66699. https://doi.org/10.1371/journal.pone.0066699

Coyne, I., Holmström, I., & Söderbäck, M. (2018). Centeredness in healthcare: A concept synthesis of family-centered care, person-centered care and child-centered care. *Journal of Pediatric Nursing, 42*, 45–56. https://doi.org/10.1016/j.pedn.2018.07.001

Creamer, J., Schrider, E. A., Burns, K., & Chen, F. (2022). Table: Poverty thresholds for 2021 by size of family and number of related children under 18 years. In J. Creamer, E. A. Shrider, K. Burns, & F. Chen, *Poverty in the United States: 2021.* U.S. Census Bureau. https://www.census.gov/library/publications/2022/demo/p60-277.html

Cree, R. A., Bitsko, R. H., Robinson, L. R., Holbrook, J. R., Danielson, M. L., Smith, C., Kaminski, J. W., Kenney, M. K., & Peacock, G. (2018). Health care, family, and community factors associated with mental, behavioral, and developmental disorders and poverty among children aged 2-8 years—United States, 2016. *Morbidity and Mortality Weekly Report, 67*(50), 1377–1383. https://doi.org/10.15585/mmwr.mm6750a1

Criado, C. (2019). *Invisible women, part IV: Going to the doctor.* Abrams Press.

Cronin, C. E., Franz, B., Choyke, K., Rodriguez, V., & Gran, B. K. (2021). For-profit hospitals have a unique opportunity to serve as anchor institutions in the U.S. *Preventive Medicine Reports, 22*, 101372. https://doi.org/10.1016/j.pmedr.2021.101372

Cronquist, K., & Lauffer, S. (2019). *Characteristics of supplemental nutrition assistance program households: Fiscal year 2017.* https://fns-prod.azureedge.net/sites/default/files/ops/Characteristics2017.pdf

Cruz, T. B., Rose, S. W., Lienemann, B. A., Byron, M. J., Meissner, H. I., Baezconde-Garbanati, L., Huang, L. L., Carroll, D. M., Soto, C., & Unger, J. B. (2019). Pro-tobacco marketing and anti-tobacco campaigns aimed at vulnerable populations: A review of the literature. *Tobacco Induced Diseases*, *17*, 68. https://doi.org/10.18332/tid/111397

Cuellar, A. E. (2022). Parity and provider networks. *Psychiatric Services*, *73*(9), 961. https://doi.org/10.1176/appi.ps.22073009

Cuellar, A. E., & Calonge, B. N. (2022). The community preventive services task force: 25 years of effectiveness, economics, and equity. *American Journal of Preventive Medicine*, *62*(6), e371–e373. https://doi.org/10.1016/j.amepre.2022.01.019

Cummings, J. R., & Druss, B. G. (2011). Racial/ethnic differences in mental health service use among adolescents with major depression. *Journal of the American Academy of Child and Adolescent Psychiatry*, *50*(2), 160–170. https://doi.org/10.1016/j.jaac.2010.11.004

Cummings, J. R., Wen, H., & Druss, B. G. (2011). Racial/ethnic differences in treatment for substance use disorders among U.S. adolescents. *Journal of the American Academy of Child and Adolescent Psychiatry*, *50*(12), 1265–1274. https://doi.org/10.1016/j.jaac.2011.09.006

Curfman, A., Hackell, J. M., Herendeen, N. E., Alexander, J. J., Marcin, J. P., Moskowitz, W. B., Bodnar, C. E. F., Simon, H. K., & McSwain, S. D. (2021a). Telehealth: Improving access to and quality of pediatric health care. *Pediatrics*, *148*(3). https://doi.org/10.1542/peds.2021-053129

Curfman, A., McSwain, S. D., Chuo, J., Olson, C. A., & Simpson, K. (2021b). An economic framework to measure value of pediatric telehealth. *Telemedicine and e-Health*, *27*(12), 1440–1442. https://doi.org/10.1089/tmj.2020.0520

Curfman, A., McSwain, S. D., Chuo, J., Yeager-McSwain, B., Schinasi, D. A., Marcin, J., Herendeen, N., Chung, S. L., Rheuban, K., & Olson, C. A. (2021c). Pediatric telehealth in the COVID-19 pandemic era and beyond. *Pediatrics*, *148*(3). https://doi.org/10.1542/peds.2020-047795

Currie, J., & Chorniy, A. (2021). Medicaid and child health insurance program improve child health and reduce poverty but face threats. *Academic Pediatrics*, *21*(Suppl 8), S146–S153. https://doi.org/10.1016/j.acap.2021.01.009

Currie, J., Decker, S., & Lin, W. (2008). Has public health insurance for older children reduced disparities in access to care and health outcomes? *Journal of Health Economics*, *27*(6), 1567–1581. https://doi.org/10.1016/j.jhealeco.2008.07.002

Currie, J., & Duque, V. (2019). Medicaid: What does it do, and can we do it better? *The Annals of the American Academy of Political and Social Science*, *686*(1), 148–179. https://doi.org/10.1177/0002716219874772

Currie, J., & Gruber, J. (1996). Saving babies: The efficacy and cost of recent changes in the Medicaid eligibility of pregnant women. *Journal of Political Economy*, *104*(6), 1263–1296. http://www.jstor.org/stable/2138939

Currie, J., & Kahn, R. (2012). Children with disabilities: Introducing the issue. *The Future of Children*, *22*(1), 3–11. http://www.jstor.org/stable/41475644

Currie, J., Ray, S. H., & Neidell, M. (2011). Quasi-experimental studies suggest that lowering air pollution levels benefits infants' and children's health. *Health Affairs (Project Hope)*, *30*(12), 2391–2399. https://doi.org/10.1377/hlthaff.2011.0212

Currie, J., & Rossin-Slater, M. (2015). Early-life origins of life-cycle well-being: Research and policy implications. *Journal of Policy Analysis and Management*, *34*(1), 208–242. https://doi.org/10.1002/pam.21805

Currie, J., & Stabile, M. (2006). Child mental health and human capital accumulation: The case of ADHD. *Journal of Health Economics*, *25*(6), 1094–1118. https://doi.org/10.1016/j.jhealeco.2006.03.001

Curtin, S. C., Heron, M., Miniñom A. M., & Warner, M. (2018). *Recent increases in injury mortality among children and adolescents aged 10–19 years in the United States: 1999–2016* (National Vital Statistics Reports). National Center for Health Statistics, Centers for Disease Control and Prevention. https://www.cdc.gov/nchs/data/nvsr/nvsr67/nvsr67_04.pdf

Curtis, E., Jones, R., Tipene-Leach, D., Walker, C., Loring, B., Paine, S.-J., & Reid, P. (2019). Why cultural safety rather than cultural competency is required to achieve health equity: A literature review and recommended definition. *International Journal for Equity in Health*, *18*(1), 174. https://doi.org/10.1186/s12939-019-1082-3

Cushing, A. M., Bucholz, E. M., Chien, A. T., Rauch, D. A., & Michelson, K. A. (2021). Availability of pediatric inpatient services in the United States. *Pediatrics*, *148*(1). https://doi.org/10.1542/peds.2020-041723

Cushing, A. M., Bucholz, E., & Michelson, K. A. (2020). Trends in regionalization of emergency care for common pediatric conditions. *Pediatrics*, *145*(4), e20192989. https://doi.org/10.1542/peds.2019–2989

Cuzzolin, L., Atzei, A., & Fanos, V. (2006). Off-label and unlicensed prescribing for newborns and children in different settings: A review of the literature and a consideration about drug safety. *Expert Opinion on Drug Safety*, *5*(5), 703–718. https://doi.org/10.1517/14740338.5.5.703

Daley, A. M., Polifroni, E. C., & Sadler, L. S. (2017). "Treat me like a normal person!" A meta-ethnography of adolescents' expectations of their health care providers. *Journal of Pediatric Nursing*, *36*, 70–83. https://doi.org/10.1016/j.pedn.2017.04.009

Dalton, E. M., Krass, P., Bouchelle, Z., Fillmore, A., Katz, T., Andrade, G., Camacho, P., Candon, M., Kane, E., & Doupnik, S. K. (2023). Characteristics, disposition, and outcomes of children hospitalized for mental health boarding at a children's hospital. *Journal of Hospital Medicine*, *18*(12), 1113–1117. https://10.1002/jhm.13228

Darling-Hammond, L., & Cook-Harvey, C. M. (2018). *Educating the whole child: Improving school climate to support student success*. L. P. Institute. https://learningpolicyinstitute.org/sites/default/files/product-files/Educating_Whole_Child_REPORT.pdf

Daugherty, E., Laurila, K., Mann, C., & Tranchina, M. T. (2024). Continuous Medicaid/CHIP eligibility for children and youth: 2024 considerations for states. https://www.jdsupra.com/legalnews/continuous-medicaid-chip-eligibility-3033759

Daw, J. R., Yekta, S., Jacobson-Davies, F. E., Patrick, S. W., & Admon, L. K. (2023). Consistency and adequacy of public and commercial health insurance for US children, 2016 to 2021. *JAMA Health Forum*, *4*(11), e234179. https://doi.org/10.1001/jamahealthforum.2023.4179

Dawes, D. E. (2020). *The political determinants of health*. Johns Hopkins University Press.

de Beaumont Foundation. (n.d.). *10 Essential Public Health Services*. https://debeaumont.org/10-essential-services/

De Genna, N., Stack, D., Serbin, L., Ledingham, J., & Schwartzman, A. (2007). Maternal and child health problems: The inter-generational consequences of early maternal aggression and withdrawal. *Social Science & Medicine*, *64*, 2417–2426. https://doi.org/10.1016/j.socscimed.2007.03.001

De Sousa, Andrichik, A., Cuellar, M., Marson, J., Prestera, E., & Rush, K. (2022). *The 2022 annual homelessness assessment report to Congress*. U.S. Department of Housing and Urban Development, Office of Community Planning and Development. https://www.huduser.gov/portal/sites/default/files/pdf/2022-ahar-part-1.pdf

DeChant, P. F., Acs, A., Rhee, K. B., Boulanger, T. S., Snowdon, J. L., Tutty, M. A., Sinsky, C. A., & Thomas Craig, K. J. (2019). Effect of organization-directed workplace interventions on physician burnout: A systematic review. *Mayo Clinic Proceedings: Innovations, Quality & Outcomes*, *3*(4), 384–408. https://doi.org/10.1016/j.mayocpiqo.2019.07.006

Declercq, E., & Zephyrin, C. L. (2021). *Severe maternal morbidity in the United States: A primer*. The Commonwealth Fund. https://www.commonwealthfund.org/publications/issue-briefs/2021/oct/severe-maternal-morbidity-united-states-primer

Defense Health Agency. (2019). *Procedural instruction: Integration of primary care behavioral health services into patient-centered medical home and other primary care service settings within the military health system*. Department of Defense. https://www.health.mil/Reference-Center/DHA-Publications/2019/10/18/DHA-PI-6025-27

Del Ponte, A., Gerber, A., & Patashnik, E. M. (2023). Polarization, the pandemic, and public trust in health system actors. *Journal of Health Politics, Policy and Law*. https://doi.org/10.1215/03616878-11075562

deMayo, R., Huang, Y., Lin, E. J., Lee, J., Heggland, A., Im, J., Grindle, C., & Chandawarkar, A. (2022). Associations of telehealth care delivery with pediatric health care provider well-being. *Applied Clinical Informatics*, *13*(2), 230–241. https://doi.org/10.1055/s-0042-1742627

Deming, D. (2009). Early childhood intervention and life-cycle skill development: Evidence from Head Start. *American Economic Journal: Applied Economics*, *1*(3), 111–134. https://doi.org/10.1257/app.1.3.111

Democracy Collaborative. (n.d.). *Anchor institutions*. http://democracycollaborative.org/democracycollaborative/anchorinstitutions/Anchor%20Institutions

Department of Agriculture (USDA). (2018). *Women, infants and children (WIC). WIC eligibility requirements*. https://www.fns.usda.gov/wic/wic-eligibility-requirements.

________. (2019). *WIC program*. https://www.ers.usda.gov/topics/food-nutrition-assistance/wic-program.

________. (2022). *Food security in the U.S.: Definitions of food security*. https://www.ers.usda.gov/topics/food-nutrition-assistance/food-security-in-the-u-s/definitions-of-food-security/.

________. (2023a). *National School Lunch Program*. https://www.fns.tripp.gov/nslp

________. (2023b). *School Breakfast Program*. https://www.fns.usda.gov/sbp/school-breakfast-program

________. (2023c). *Special Supplemental Nutrition Program For Women, Infants, and Children (WIC)*. https://www.fns.usda.gov/wic

________. (2023d). *Supplemental Nutrition Assistance Program (SNAP)*. https://www.fns.usda.gov/snap/supplemental-nutrition-assistance-program

________. (2023e). *SNAP policy on non-citizen eligibility*. https://www.fns.usda.gov/snap/eligibility/citizen/non-citizen-policy

________. (2024a). *Special Supplemental Nutrition Program For Women, Infants, and Children (WIC)*. https://www.fns.usda.gov/wic

________. (2024b). *WIC participant and program characteristics 2022*. https://www.fns.usda.gov/research/wic/participant-program-characteristics-2022

Department of Defense (DoD). (2020). *2020 Qualified Military Available (QMA) study*. https://prod-media.asvabprogram.com/CEP_PDF_Contents/Qualified_Military_Available.pdf

Department of Education (ED). (2023). *U.S. Department of Education announces more than $188 million from the Bipartisan Safer Communities Act to support mental health and student wellness*. https://www.ed.gov/news/press-releases/us-department-education-announces-more-188-million-bipartisan-safer-communities-act-support-mental-health-and-student-wellness

Department of Health and Human Services (HHS). (n.d.). *What is home visiting evidence of effectiveness?* https://homvee.acf.hhs.gov/

________. (2007). *Community health worker national workforce study*. https://bhw.hrsa.gov/sites/default/files/bureau-health-workforce/data-research/community-health-workforce.pdf

________. (2016). *Facing addiction in America: The surgeon general's report on alcohol, drugs, and health*.

________. (2022). *Home visiting evidence of effectiveness, family spirit.* https://homvee.acf.hhs.gov/effectiveness/Family%20Spirit%C2%AE/In%20Brief

________. (2023). *FY annual performance plan and report.* https://www.hhs.gov/sites/default/files/fy2024-performance-plan.pdf

________. (2024). *Women's preventive services guidelines.* Health Resources and Services Administration. https://www.hrsa.gov/womens-guidelines

Department of Health and Human Services Federal Panel on Community Water Fluoridation (2015). U.S. public health service recommendation for fluoride concentration in drinking water for the prevention of dental caries. *Public Health Reports, 130*(4), 318–331. https://doi.org/10.1177/003335491513000408

De-Regil, L. M., Fernández-Gaxiola, A. C., Dowswell, T., & Peña-Rosas, J. P. (2010). Effects and safety of periconceptional folate supplementation for preventing birth defects. *The Cochrane Database of Systematic Reviews*, (10), Cd007950. https://doi.org/10.1002/14651858.CD007950.pub2

Derr, A. (2023). *History of public health community collaboration: An infographic.* VisualNetworkLabs. https://visiblenetworklabs.com/2023/04/20/public-health-collaboration-infographic/

DeSalvo, K., Parekh, A., Hoagland, G. W., Dilley, A., Kaiman, S., Hines, M., & Levi, J. (2019). Developing a financing system to support public health infrastructure. *American Journal of Public Health*, *109*(10), 1358–1361. https://doi.org/10.2105/ajph.2019.305214

Deutsch, S. A., & Fortin, K. (2015). Physical health problems and barriers to optimal health care among children in foster care. *Current Problems in Pediatric and Adolescent Health Care*, *45*(10), 286–291. https://doi.org/10.1016/j.cppeds.2015.08.002

Deverka, P. A., Lavallee, D. C., Desai, P. J., Esmail, L. C., Ramsey, S. D., Veenstra, D. L., & Tunis, S. R. (2012). Stakeholder participation in comparative effectiveness research: Defining a framework for effective engagement. *Journal of Comparative Effectiveness Research*, *1*(2), 181–194. https://doi.org/10.2217/cer.12.7

DeVoe, J. E., Tillotson, C. J., & Wallace, L. S. (2009). Children's receipt of health care services and family health insurance patterns. *Annals of Family Medicine*, *7*(5), 406–413. https://doi.org/10.1370/afm.1040

Diamond, A., & Lee, K. (2011). Interventions shown to aid executive function development in children 4–12 years old. *Science*, *333*(6045), 959–964. https://doi.org/10.1126/science.1204529

Diaz, A., Edwards, S., Neal, W. P., Ludmer, P., Bitterman, J., & Nucci, A. T. (2004). CHIP: New opportunities in adolescent health care delivery. *Mount Sinai Journal of Medicine*, *71*(3), 186–190.

Dieleman, J. L., Cao, J., Chapin, A., Chen, C., Li, Z., Liu, A., Horst, C., Kaldjian, A., Matyasz, T., Scott, K. W., Bui, A. L., Campbell, M., Duber, H. C., Dunn, A. C., Flaxman, A. D., Fitzmaurice, C., Naghavi, M., Sadat, N., Shieh, P., . . . Murray, C. J. L. (2020). US health care spending by payer and health condition, 1996–2016. *Journal of the American Medical Association*, *323*(9), 863–884. https://doi.org/10.1001/jama.2020.0734

Dietz, W. H. (1998). Health consequences of obesity in youth: Childhood predictors of adult disease. *Pediatrics*, *101*(3 Pt 2), 518–525.

Dietz, W. H., Solomon, L. S., Pronk, N., Ziegenhorn, S. K., Standish, M., Longjohn, M. M., Fukuzawa, D. D., Eneli, I. U., Loy, L., Muth, N. D., Sanchez, E. J., Bogard, J., & Bradley, D. W. (2015). An integrated framework for the prevention and treatment of obesity and its related chronic diseases. *Health Affairs (Project Hope)*, *34*(9), 1456–1463. https://doi.org/10.1377/hlthaff.2015.0371

Diez Roux, A. V. (2016). Neighborhoods and health: What do we know? What should we do? *American Journal of Public Health*, *106*(3), 430–431. https://doi.org/10.2105/ajph.2016.303064

Dimmock, D., Caylor, S., Waldman, B., Benson, W., Ashburner, C., Carmichael, J. L., Carroll, J., Cham, E., Chowdhury, S., Cleary, J., D'Harlingue, A., Doshi, A., Ellsworth, K., Galarreta, C. I., Hobbs, C., Houtchens, K., Hunt, J., Joe, P., Joseph, M., . . . Farnaes, L. (2021). Project Baby Bear: Rapid precision care incorporating rWGS in 5 California children's hospitals demonstrates improved clinical outcomes and reduced costs of care. *American Journal of Human Genetics*, *108*(7), 1231–1238. https://doi.org/10.1016/j.ajhg.2021.05.008

Doan, Q., Piteau, S., Sheps, S., Singer, J., Wong, H., Johnson, D., & Kissoon, N. (2013). The role of physician assistants in pediatric emergency medicine: The physician's view. *Canadian Journal of Emergency Medicine, 15*(6), 321–329.

Doan, Q., Sabhaney, V., Kissoon, N., Johnson, D., Sheps, S., Wong, H., & Singer, J. (2012). The role of physician assistants in a pediatric emergency department: A center review and survey. *Emergency Care*, *28*(8), 783–788.

Dodd, S., Widnall, E., Russell, A. E., Curtin, E. L., Simmonds, R., Limmer, M., & Kidger, J. (2022). School-based peer education interventions to improve health: A global systematic review of effectiveness. *BMC Public Health*, 22, 2247. https://doi.org/10.1186/s12889-022-14688-3

Domecq, J. P., Prutsky, G., Elraiyah, T., Wang, Z., Nabhan, M., Shippee, N., Brito, J. P., Boehmer, K., Hasan, R., Firwana, B., Erwin, P., Eton, D., Sloan, J., Montori, V., Asi, N., Abu Dabrh, A. M., & Murad, M. H. (2014). Patient engagement in research: A systematic review. *BMC Health Services Research*, *14*, 89. https://doi.org/10.1186/1472-6963-14-89

Domino, M. E. (2021). Unpacking the patient-centered medical home. *Health Services Research*, *56*(3), 350–351. https://doi.org/10.1111/1475-6773.13661

Donohue, P., Falk, B., & Provet, A. G. (2000). *Mental health consultation in early childhood.* Paul H. Brookes Publishing.

D'Onise, K., Lynch, J. W., & McDermott, R. A. (2010). Does an early childhood intervention affect the mental health of participants? A systematic review. *Public Health*, *124*(9), 513–521. https://doi.org/10.1016/j.puhe.2010.03.001

Dorsey, B. F., Kamimura, A., Cook, L. J., Kadish, H. A., Cook, H. K., Kang, A., Nguyen, J. B. T., & Holsti, M. (2022). Communication gaps between providers and caregivers of patients in a pediatric emergency department. *Journal of Patient Experience*, *9*. https://doi.org/10.1177/23743735221112223

Dougherty, G. B., Golden, S. H., Gross, A. L., Colantuoni, E., & Dean, L. T. (2020). Measuring structural racism and its association with BMI. *American Journal of Preventive Medicine*, *59*(4), 530–537. https://doi.org/10.1016/j.amepre.2020.05.019

Doupnik, S. K., Rodean, J., Feinstein, J., Gay, J. C., Simmons, J., Bettenhausen, J. L., Markham, J. L., Hall, M., Zima, B. T., & Berry, J. G. (2020). Health care utilization and spending for children with mental health conditions in Medicaid. *Academic Pediatrics*, *20*(5), 678–686. https://doi.org/10.1016/j.acap.2020.01.013

Douthit, N., Kiv, S., Dwolatzky, T., & Biswas, S. (2015). Exposing some important barriers to health care access in the rural USA. *Public Health, 129*(6), 611–620. https://doi.org/10.1016/j.puhe.2015.04.001

Dover, D. C., & Belon, A. P. (2019). The health equity measurement framework: A comprehensive model to measure social inequities in health. *International Journal for Equity in Health*, *18*. https://doi.org/10.1186/s12939-019-0935-0

Downing, K. F., Espinoza, L., Oster, M. E., & Farr, S. L. (2022). Preventive dental care and oral health of children and adolescents with and without heart conditions—United States, 2016–2019. *Morbidity and Mortality Weekly Report*, *71*(6), 189–195.

Drake, P., Tolbert, J., Rudowitz, R., & Damico, A. (2024). *How many uninsured are in the coverage gap and how many could be eligible if all states adopted the Medicaid expansion?* KFF. https://www.kff.org/medicaid/issue-brief/how-many-uninsured-are-in-the-coverage-gap-and-how-many-could-be-eligible-if-all-states-adopted-the-medicaid-expansion/

Dranove, D., Garthwaite, C., & Ody, C. (2016). Uncompensated care decreased at hospitals in Medicaid expansion states but not at hospitals in nonexpansion states. *Health Affairs*, *35*(8), 1471–1479. https://doi.org/10.1377/hlthaff.2015.1344

Drmic, I. E., Szatmari, P., & Volkmar, F. (2017). Life course health development in autism spectrum disorders. In N. Halfon, C. Forrest, R. Lerner, & E. Faustman, E. (Eds.), *Handbook of life course health development*. Springer. https://doi.org/10.1007/978-3-319-47143-3_11

DuBard, C. A., & Gizlice, Z. (2008). Language spoken and differences in health status, access to care, and receipt of preventive services among US Hispanics. *American Journal of Public Health*, *98*(11), 2021–2028. https://doi.org/10.2105/ajph.2007.119008

Dube, S. R., Felitti, V. J., Dong, M., Giles, W. H., & Anda, R. F. (2003). The impact of adverse childhood experiences on health problems: Evidence from four birth cohorts dating back to 1900. *Preventive Medicine*, *37*(3), 268–277. https://doi.org/10.1016/s0091-7435(03)00123-3

DuBois, S. G., Corson, L. B., Stegmaier, K., & Janeway, K. A. (2019). Ushering in the next generation of precision trials for pediatric cancer. *Science*, *363*(6432), 1175–1181. https://doi.org/10.1126/science.aaw4153

Dufendach, K. R., Eichenberger, J. A., McPheeters, M. L., Temple, M. W., Bhatia, H. L., Alrifai, M. W., Potter, S. A., Weinberg, S. T., Johnson, K. B., & Lehmann, C. U. (2015). *Core functionality in pediatric electronic health records* (Technical Brief No. 20). Agency for Healthcare Research and Quality. https://www.ncbi.nlm.nih.gov/books/NBK299021/

Duran, F., Hepburn, K., Irvine, M., Kaufmann, R., Anthony, B., Horen, N., & Perry, D. (2009). *What works? A study of effective early childhood mental health consultation programs*. Georgetown University Center for Child and Human Development. https://www.aecf.org/resources/what-works-a-study-of-effective-early-childhood-mental-health-consultation

Durbin, M. D., Fairman, K., Helvaty, L. R., Huang, M., Li, M., Abreu, D., Geddes, G. C., Helm, B. M., Landis, B. J., McEntire, A., Mitchell, D. K., & Ware, S. M. (2023). Genetic testing guidelines impact care in newborns with congenital heart defects. *Journal of Pediatrics*, *260*, 113495. https://doi.org/10.1016/j.jpeds.2023.113495

Durham, D. (2023). *All plan letter 22-029 (revised)*. California Department of Health Care Services. https://www.dhcs.ca.gov/formsandpubs/Documents/MMCDAPLsandPolicyLetters/APL2022/APL22-029.pdf

Durlak, J. A., Weissberg, R. P., Dymnicki, A. B., Taylor, R. D., & Schellinger, K. B. (2011). The impact of enhancing students' social and emotional learning: A meta-analysis of school-based universal interventions. *Child Development*, *82*, 405–432. https://doi. org/10.1111/j.1467-8624.2010.01564.x

Durrah, H. (2023a, May). *Accelerating child health transformation project* [Presentation]. Center for Health Care Strategies. Washington, D.C.

________. (2023b, September 7–8). *Building capacity for equitable patient, family, & community partnerships to support health system transformation.* [Presentation] Committee on Improving the Health and Wellbeing of Children and Youth through Health Care System Transformation. National Academy of Sciences, Engineering and Medicine. Washington, D.C.

________. (2023c, October). *Engaging patients and families to accelerate pediatric practice transformation* [Presentation]. American Academy of Pediatrics, National Conference and Exhibition. Washington, D.C.

Dworetzky, B., Hoover, C. G., & Walker, D. K. (2023). Family engagement at the systems level: A framework for action. *Maternal and Child Health Journal*, *27*(6), 969–977. https://doi.org/10.1007/s10995-023-03619-2

Dworkin, P., & Kelly, D. (2022). *Investments that help children start strong and benefit society*. The Institute for Child Success. https://www.instituteforchildsuccess.org/sc-is-home-to-innovative-investments-that-help-children-start-strong/

Dyer, Z., Alcusky, M. J., Galea, S., & Ash, A. (2023). Measuring the enduring imprint of structural racism on American neighborhoods. *Health Affairs (Project Hope)*, *42*(10), 1374–1382. https://doi.org/10.1377/hlthaff.2023.00659

Dyrbye, L. N., Satele, D., & West, C. P. (2021). Association of characteristics of the learning environment and US medical student burnout, empathy, and career regret. *JAMA Network Open*, *4*(8), e2119110. https://doi.org/10.1001/jamanetworkopen.2021.19110

Early and Periodic Screening, Diagnosis, and Treatment (EPSDT), Pub. L. No. 90-248, § 503, 81 Stat. 821, 834 (1968).

Early Childhood Technical Assistance Center. (n.d.). *Part C national program data*. https://ectacenter.org/partc/partcdata.asp

Ebbeling, C. B., Pawlak, D. B., & Ludwig, D. S. (2002). Childhood obesity: Public-health crisis, common sense cure. *Lancet*, *360*(9331), 473–482. https://doi.org/10.1016/s0140-6736(02)09678-2

Ebi, K. L., Vanos, J., Baldwin, J. W., Bell, J. E., Hondula, D. M., Errett, N. A., Hayes, K., Reid, C. E., Saha, S., Spector, J., & Berry, P. (2021). Extreme weather and climate change: Population health and health system implications. *Annual Review of Public Health*, *42*, 293–315. https://doi.org/10.1146/annurev-publhealth-012420-105026

Eby, D. (2023). *Collaborative programs to support children's health and wellbeing*. https://www.nationalacademies.org/event/06-15-2023/improving-the-health-and-wellbeing-of-children-and-youth-through-health-care-system-transformation-committee-meeting-3

Economic Research Service (ERS). (2023a). *Child and adult care food program*. U.S. Department of Agriculture. https://www.ers.usda.gov/topics/food-nutrition-assistance/child-nutrition-programs/child-and-adult-care-food-program/

________. (2023b). *Measurement*. U.S. Department of Agriculture. https://www.ers.usda.gov/topics/food-nutrition-assistance/food-security-in-the-u-s/measurement

Eckman, M. H., Wise, R., Leonard, A. C., Dixon, E., Burrows, C., Khan, F., & Warm, E. (2012). Impact of health literacy on outcomes and effectiveness of an educational intervention in patients with chronic diseases. *Patient Education and Counseling*, *87*(2), 143–151. https://doi.org/10.1016/j.pec.2011.07.020

EdBuild. (2019). *$23 billion*. https://edbuild.org/content/23-billion/full-report.pdf

Eden, A. R., Morgan, Z. J., Jetty, A., & Peterson, L. E. (2020). Proportion of family physicians caring for children is declining. *Journal of the American Board of Family Medicine*, *33*(6), 830–831. https://doi.org/10.3122/jabfm.2020.06.200089

Edwards, L. E., Steinman, M. E., & Hakanson, E. Y. (1977). An experimental comprehensive high school clinic. *American Journal of Public Health*, *67*(8), 765–766.

Ehiri, J. E., Ejere, H. O., Magnussen, L., Emusu, D., King, W., & Osberg, J. S. (2006). Interventions for promoting booster seat use in four- to eight-year-olds traveling in motor vehicles. *The Cochrane Database of Systematic Reviews*, *2006*(1), Cd004334. https://doi.org/10.1002/14651858.CD004334.pub2

Eichelberger, A. H., Chouinard, A. O., & Jermakian, J. S. (2012). Effects of booster seat laws on injury risk among children in crashes. *Traffic Injury Prevention*, *13*(6), 631–639.

Eitland, E., Klingensmith, L., MacNaughton, P., Laurent, J. C., Spengler, J., Bernstein, A., & Allen, J. G. (2020). *Foundations for student success: How school buildings influence student health, thinking, and performance.* Harvard T. H. Chan School of Public Health. https://schools.forhealth.org/wp-content/uploads/2020/02/Schools_ForHealth_UpdatedJan21.pdf

Elderkin-Thompson, V., Silver, R. C., & Waitzkin, H. (2001). When nurses double as interpreters: A study of Spanish-speaking patients in a US primary care setting. *Social Science & Medicine*, *52*(9), 1343–1358. https://doi.org/10.1016/s0277-9536(00)00234-3

Elflein, J. (2023). Percentage of children aged 0-17 years with asthma who had an asthma attack in the past 12 months in the United States from 2001 to 2021 [Graph]. *Statista.* https://www.statista.com/statistics/1128555/children-with-asthma-attacks-past-year-us/

Elisseeff, J., Badylak, S. F., & Boeke, J. D. (2021). Immune and genome engineering as the future of transplantable tissue. *New England Journal of Medicine*, *385*(26), 2451–2462. https://doi.org/10.1056/NEJMra1913421

Elmore, A. L., & Crouch, E. (2020). The association of adverse childhood experiences with anxiety and depression for children and youth, 8 to 17 years of age. *Academic Pediatrics*, *20*(5), 600–608. https://doi.org/10.1016/j.acap.2020.02.012

Elwell, S., Krichten, A. E., & Mattocks, S. (2015). Are you a leader? *Journal of Trauma Nursing*, *22*(6), 293. https://doi.org/10.1097/JTN.0000000000000160

Ely, D. M., & Driscoll, A. K. (2022). *Infant mortality in the United States: Provisional data from the 2022 period linked birth/infant death file* (NVSS Vital Statistics Rapid Release Report No. 33). Centers for Disease Control and Prevention. https://www.cdc.gov/nchs/data/vsrr/vsrr033.pdf

Environmental Protection Agency (EPA). (2012). *Coordinated federal action plan to reduce racial and ethnic asthma disparities.* https://ptfcehs.niehs.nih.gov/sites/niehs-ptfceh/files/activities/assets/files/coordinated_federal_action_plan_to_reduce_racial_and_ethnic_asthma_disparities_508.pdf (accessed September 29, 2023).

________. (2022). *Take action to improve indoor air quality in schools.* https://www.epa.gov/iaq-schools/take-action-improve-indoor-air-quality-schools

Erard, M. (2001). Stutter, memory. *Lingua Franca*, *11*(8), 40–45.

Escarce. J. J., & Kapur, K. (2006). *Hispanics and the future of America.* The National Academies Press. https://www.ncbi.nlm.nih.gov/books/NBK19910/

Estabrooks, P. A., & Shetterly, S. (2007). The prevalence and health care use of overweight children in an integrated health care system. *Archives of Pediatrics & Adolescent Medicine*, *161*(3), 222–227. https://doi.org/10.1001/archpedi.161.3.222

Esteban-Cornejo, I., Tejero-Gonzalez, C. M., Sallis, J. F., & Veiga, O. L. (2015). Physical activity and cognition in adolescents: A systematic review. *Journal of Science and Medicine in Sport*, *18*(5), 534–539.

European Pediatric Regulation (EC) No. 1901/2006 of the European Parliament (2007).

Evashwick, C. J., & Jackson, P. (2020). The evolution of community benefit: Perspective on progress toward purpose. *Frontiers in Public Health*, *8*, 27. https://doi.org/10.3389/fpubh.2020.00027

Everytown Research & Policy. (2022). *The rise of firearm suicide among young Americans.* Everytown Research & Policy. https://everytownresearch.org/report/the-rise-of-firearm-suicide-among-young-americans/

Eyllon, M., Salhi, C., Griffith, J. L., & Lincoln, A. K. (2022). Exclusionary school discipline policies and mental health in a national sample of adolescents without histories of suspension or expulsion. *Youth & Society*, *54*(1), 84–103.

Fabina, J., Hernandez, E. L., & McElrath, K. (2023). *School enrollment in the United States: 2021.* American Community Survey Reports. https://www.census.gov/content/dam/Census/library/publications/2023/acs/acs-55.pdf

Fadus, M. C., Squeglia, L. M., Valadez, E. A., Tomko, R. L., Bryant, B. E., & Gray, K. M. (2019). Adolescent substance use disorder treatment: An update on evidence-based strategies. *Current Psychiatry Reports*, *21*(10), 96–96. https://doi.org/10.1007/s11920-019-1086-0

Falbe, J., Cadiz, A. A., Tantoco, N. K., Thompson, H. R., & Madsen, K. A. (2015). Active and healthy families: A randomized controlled trial of a culturally tailored obesity intervention for Latino children. *Academic Pediatrics*, *15*(4), 386–395. https://doi.org/10.1016/j.acap.2015.02.004

Families First Coronavirus Response Act, Pub. L. No. 116-127, 134 Stat. 178 (2020).

Family Educational Rights and Privacy Act, 20 U.S.C. § 1232g. (1974).

Family Voices. (n.d.). *Assessing family engagement: Family engagement in systems tools.* Family Voices. https://familyvoices.org/fesat/

Fanta, M., Ladzekpo, D., & Unaka, N. (2021). Racism and pediatric health outcomes. *Current Problems in Pediatric and Adolescent Health Care*, *51*(10), 101087. https://doi.org/10.1016/j.cppeds.2021.101087

Farberman, R., & Kelley, B. (2020). The impact of chronic underfunding on America's public health system: Trends, risks, and recommendations, 2020. *Trust for America's Health.* https://www.tfah.org/report-details/publichealthfunding2020/

Farid, M. (2020). *The impact of federally qualified health centers on youth outcomes.* https://scholar.harvard.edu/files/mfarid/files/farid_jmp.pdf

Farley, J. P., & Kim-Spoon, J. (2014). The development of adolescent self-regulation: Reviewing the role of parent, peer, friend, and romantic relationships. *Journal of Adolescence*, *37*(4), 433–440. https://doi.org/10.1016/j.adolescence.2014.03.009

Farmer, S. A., Shalowitz, J., George, M., McStay, F., Patel, K., Perrin, J., Moghtaderi, A., & McClellan, M. (2016). Fully capitated payment breakeven rate for a mid-size pediatric practice. *Pediatrics*, *138*(2). https://doi.org/10.1542/peds.2015-4367

Fearon, A., Marsh, A., Kim, J., & Treadwell, M. (2019). Pediatric residents' perceived barriers to opioid use in sickle cell disease pain management. *Pediatric Blood Cancer*, *66*(2), e27535. https://doi.org/10.1002/pbc.27535

Federal Communications Commission (FCC). (n.d.). *Telehealth, telemedicine, and telecare: What's what?* https://www.fcc.gov/general/telehealth-telemedicine-and-telecare-whats-whatv

Federal Interagency Forum on Child and Family Statistics (FCFS). (n.d.). America's children: Key national indicators of well-being, 2023. https://www.childstats.gov/americaschildren/health8.asp

________. (2022a). *America's children in brief: Key national indicators of well-being, 2022.* Washington, DC: U.S. Government Printing Office.

________. (2022b). *Child population: Number of children (in millions) ages 0–17 in the United States by age, 1950–2022 and projected 2023–2050.* https://www.childstats.gov/americaschildren/tables/pop1.asp

________. (2023a). *America's children: Key national indicators of well-being, 2022.* https://www.childstats.gov/americaschildren

________. (2023b). *ChildStats: Food security.* https://www.childstats.gov/americaschildren/eco4.asp

Federal Register. (2023). *Medicaid program and CHIP; Mandatory Medicaid and Children's Health Insurance Program (CHIP) core set reporting.* https://www.federalregister.gov/documents/2023/08/31/2023-18669/medicaid-program-and-chip-mandatory-medicaid-and-childrens-health-insurance-program-chip-core-set

Federation of State Medical Boards. (2023). *U.S. states and territories modifying requirements for telehealth in response to COVID-19.* https://www.fsmb.org/siteassets/advocacy/pdf/states-waiving-licensure-requirements-for-telehealth-in-response-to-covid-19.pdf

Federico, M. J., McFarlane, A. E., II, Szefler, S. J., & Abrams, E. M. (2020). The impact of social determinants of health on children with asthma. *The Journal of Allergy and Clinical Immunology: In Practice*, *8*(6), 1808–1814. https://doi.org/10.1016/j.jaip.2020.03.028

Federico, S. G., Abrams, L., Everhart, R. M., Melinkovich, P., & Hambidge, S. J. (2010). Addressing adolescent immunization disparities: A retrospective analysis of school-based health center immunization delivery. *American Journal of Public Health, 100*(9), 1630–1634.

Fein, R. (2015). The early days of Medicare and Medicaid: A personal reflection. In A. B. Cohen, D. C. Colby, K. A. Wailoo, & J. E. Zelizer (Eds.), *Medicare and Medicaid at 50*. Oxford University Press.

Feinberg, M. E., Fang, S., Fosco, G. M., Sloan, C. J., Mogle, J., & Spoth, R. L. (2022). Long-term effects of adolescent substance use prevention on participants, partners, and their children: Resiliency and outcomes 15 years later during the COVID-19 pandemic. *Prevention Science*, *23*(7), 1264–1275. https://doi.org/10.1007/s11121-022-01384-2

Felitti, V. J., Anda, R. F., Nordenberg, D., Williamson, D. F., Spitz, A. M., Edwards, V., Koss, M. P., & Marks, J. S. (1998). Relationship of childhood abuse and household dysfunction to many of the leading causes of death in adults. *American Journal of Preventive Medicine*, *14*(4), 245–258. https://doi.org/10.1016/s0749-3797(98)00017-8

Fendian, C. (2021). Mental healthcare for immigrants and first-generation families: Erasing the stigma and creating solutions. *Journal Health Care Law and Policy*, *24*(1). https://digitalcommons.law.umaryland.edu/cgi/viewcontent.cgi?article=1399&context=jhclp

Ferraro, K. F., Thorpe, R. J., Jr., & Wilkinson, J. A. (2003). The life course of severe obesity: Does childhood overweight matter? *The Journals of Gerontology: Series B*, *58*(2), S110–S119. https://doi.org/10.1093/geronb/58.2.S110

Fertig, A. (2019). *The long-term health consequences of childhood food insecurity* (Discussion Paper Series No. 2019-03). University of Kentucky Center for Poverty Research. http://ukcpr.org/research

Feuer, V., Mooneyham, G. C., Malas, N. M., & Pediatric Boarding Consensus Guidelines Panel. (2023). Addressing the pediatric mental health crisis in emergency departments in the US: Findings of a national pediatric boarding consensus panel. *Journal of the Academy of Consultation-Liaison Psychiatry, 64*(6), 501–511. https://doi.org/10.1016/j.jaclp.2023.06.003

Fierman, A. H., Beck, A. F., Chung, E. K., Tschudy, M. M., Coker, T. R., Mistry, K. B., Siegel, B., Chamberlain, L. J., Conroy, K., Federico, S. G., Flanagan, P. J., Garg, A., Gitterman, B. A., Grace, A. M., Gross, R. S., Hole, M. K., Klass, P., Kraft, C., Kuo, A., . . . Cox, J. (2016). Redesigning health care practices to address childhood poverty. *Academic Pediatrics*, *16*(Suppl 3), S136–S146. https://doi.org/10.1016/j.acap.2016.01.004

Figlio, D., Hamersma, S., & Roth, J. (2009). Does prenatal WIC participation improve birth outcomes? New evidence from Florida. *Journal of Public Economics, 93*(1–2), 235–245.

Filene, J. H., Kaminski, J. W., Valle, L. A., & Cachat, P. (2013). Components associated with home visiting program outcomes: A meta-analysis. *Pediatrics*, *132*(2), S100. https://doi.org/10.1542/peds.2013-1021H

Fingar, K. R., Lob, S. H., Dove, M. S., Gradziel, P., & Curtis, M. P. (2017). Reassessing the association between WIC and birth outcomes using a fetuses-at-risk approach. *Maternal and Child Health Journal*, *21*(4), 825–835.

Finkelhor, D., Turner, H. A., Ormrod, R. K., Hamby, S., & Kracke, K. (2009). *Children's exposure to violence: A comprehensive national survey.* Office of Juvenile Justice and Delinquency Prevention. https://www.ojp.gov/pdffiles1/ojjdp/227744.pdf

Finkelstein, E. A., Graham, W. C. K., & Malhotra, R. (2014). Lifetime direct medical costs of childhood obesity. *Pediatrics*, *133*(5), 854–862. https://doi.org/10.1542/peds.2014-0063

First Focus on Children. (2023). *Children's Budget 2023*. https://firstfocus.org/wp-content/uploads/2024/03/First-Focus-on-Children-Childrens-Budget-2023_WEB.pdf

Fish, J., Uink, B., Wiglesworth, A., Tsethlikai, M., Him, D. A., & O'Keefe, V. (2023). For the next seven generations: An Indigenous strengths-based developmental science. *PsyArXiv Preprints*. https://doi.org/10.31234/osf.io/hr28s

FitzGerald, C., & Hurst, S. (2017). Implicit bias in healthcare professionals: A systematic review. *BMC Medical Ethics*, *18*(1), 19. https://doi.org/10.1186/s12910-017-0179-8

Fitzpatrick, A. M., Gillespie, S. E., Mauger, D. T., Phillips, B. R., Bleecker, E. R., Israel, E., Meyers, D. A., Moore, W. C., Sorkness, R. L., Wenzel, S. E., Bacharier, L. B., Castro, M., Denlinger, L. C., Erzurum, S. C., Fahy, J. V., Gaston, B. M., Jarjour, N. N., Larkin, A., Levy, B. D., . . . Teague, W. G. (2019). Racial disparities in asthma-related health care use in the National Heart, Lung, and Blood Institute's Severe Asthma Research Program. *Journal of Allergy and Clinical Immunology*, *143*(6), 2052–2061. https://doi.org/10.1016/j.jaci.2018.11.022

Flagg, A. M., Lin, B., Crnic, K. A., Gonzales, N. A., & Luecken, L. J. (2023). Intergenerational consequences of maternal childhood maltreatment on infant health concerns. *Maternal and Child Health Journal*, *27*(11), 1981–1989. https://doi.org/10.1007/s10995-023-03717-1

Flanagan, P., Tigue, P. M., & Perrin, J. (2019). The value proposition for pediatric care. *JAMA Pediatrics*, *173*(12), 1125. https://doi.org/10.1001/jamapediatrics.2019.3486

Flay, B. R. (2009). School-based smoking prevention programs with the promise of long-term effects. *Tobacco Induced Diseases*, *5*(1), 6. https://doi.org/10.1186/1617-9625-5-6

Fleetwood, J. (2017). Public health, ethics, and autonomous vehicles. *American Journal of Public Health*, *107*(4), 532–537. https://doi.org/10.2105/ajph.2016.303628

Fleischman, A., Hourigan, S. E., Lyon, H. N., Landry, M. G., Reynolds, J., Steltz, S. K., Robinson, L., Keating, S., Feldman, H. A., Antonelli, R. C., Ludwig, D. S., & Ebbeling, C. B. (2016). Creating an integrated care model for childhood obesity: A randomized pilot study utilizing telehealth in a community primary care setting. *Clinical Obesity*, *6*(6), 380–388. https://doi.org/10.1111/cob.12166

Fleszar, L. G., Bryant, A. S., Johnson, C. O., Blacker, B. F., Aravkin, A., Baumann, M., Dwyer-Lindgren, L., Kelly, Y. O., Maass, K., Zheng, P., & Roth, G. A. (2023). Trends in state-level maternal mortality by racial and ethnic group in the United States. *Journal of the American Medical Association*, *330*(1), 52–61. https://doi.org/10.1001/jama.2023.9043

Fletcher, J., & Wolfe, B. (2008). Child mental health and human capital accumulation: The case of ADHD revisited. *Journal of Health Economics*, *27*(3), 794–800. https://doi.org/10.1016/j.jhealeco.2007.10.010

_______. (2009). Long–term consequences of childhood ADHD on criminal activities. *Journal of Mental Health Policy and Economics*, *12*(3), 119–138.

Flores, G., Abreu, M., Schwartz, I., & Hill, M. (2000). The importance of language and culture in pediatric care: Case studies from the Latino community. *Journal of Pediatrics*, *137*(6), 842–848. https://doi.org/10.1067/mpd.2000.109150

Food and Drug Administration (FDA). (2022). *Ethical considerations for clinical investigations of medical products involving children: Guidance for industry, sponsors, and IRBs*. https://www.fda.gov/media/161740/download

_______. (2023). *Augmented reality and virtual reality in medical devices*. https://www.fda.gov/medical-devices/digital-health-center-excellence/augmented-reality-and-virtual-reality-medical-devices

Food Research & Action Center. (n.d.a). *National School Lunch Program*. https://frac.org/programs/national-school-lunch-program

________. (n.d.b). *School meal eligibility and reimbursements.* https://frac.org/school-meal-eligibility-reimbursements

Ford, C., English, A., & Sigman, G. (2004). Confidential health care for adolescents: Position paper for the society for adolescent medicine. *Journal of Adolescent Health: Official Publication of the Society for Adolescent Medicine*, *35*(2), 160–167.

Ford, T. N., & Michener, J. (2022). Medicaid reimbursement rates are a racial justice issue. https://www.commonwealthfund.org/blog/2022/medicaid-reimbursement-rates-are-racial-justice-issue

Forde, A. T., Crookes, D. M., Suglia, S. F., & Demmer, R. T. (2019). The weathering hypothesis as an explanation for racial disparities in health: A systematic review. *Annals of Epidemiology*, *33*, 1–18.e13. https://doi.org/10.1016/j.annepidem.2019.02.011

Foronda, C., Baptiste, D. L., Reinholdt, M. M., & Ousman, K. (2016). Cultural humility: A concept analysis. *Journal of Transcultural Nursing*, *27*(3), 210–217. https://doi.org/10.1177/1043659615592677

Foronda, C., Liu, S., & Bauman, E. B. (2013). Evaluation of simulation in undergraduate nurse education: An integrative review. *Clinical Simulation in Nursing*, *9*(10), e409–e416. https://doi.org/10.1016/j.ecns.2012.11.003

Forouzanfar, M. H., Alexander, L., Anderson, H. R., Bachman, V. F., Biryukov, S., Brauer, M., Burnett, R., Casey, D., Coates, M. M., Cohen, A., Delwiche, K., Estep, K., Frostad, J. J., Astha, K. C., Kyu, H. H., Moradi-Lakeh, M., Ng, M., Slepak, E. L., Thomas, B. A., . . . Murray, C. J. (2015). Global, regional, and national comparative risk assessment of 79 behavioural, environmental and occupational, and metabolic risks or clusters of risks in 188 countries, 1990–2013: A systematic analysis for the Global Burden of Disease Study 2013. *Lancet*, *386*(10010), 2287–2323. https://doi.org/10.1016/s0140-6736(15)00128-2

Forrest, C. B., Chen, C. P., Perrin, E. M., Stille, C. J., Cooper, R., Harris, K., Luo, Q., Maltenfort, M. G., & Parlett, L. E. (2024). Pediatric medical subspecialist use in outpatient settings. *JAMA Network Open*, *7*(1), e2350379. https://doi.org/10.1001/jamanetworkopen.2023.50379

Forrest, C. B., Simpson, L., & Clancy, C. (1997). Child health services research. Challenges and opportunities. *Journal of the American Medical Association*, *277*(22), 1787–1793.

Forte, A., Orri, M., Galera, C., Pompili, M., Turecki, G., Boivin, M., Tremblay, R. E., & Côté, S. M. (2020). Developmental trajectories of childhood symptoms of hyperactivity/inattention and suicidal behavior during adolescence. *European Child & Adolescent Psychiatry*, *29*(2), 145–151. https://doi.org/10.1007/s00787-019-01338-0

Forum for Youth Investment. (2021). *2020 State policy survey: Child & youth policy coordinating bodies in the United States.* https://forumfyi.org/knowledge-center/2020-state-policy-survey-child-youth-policy-coordinating-bodies-in-the-united-states/

Forum on Promoting Children's Cognitive, Affective, and Behavioral Health; Board on Children, Youth, and Families; Institute of Medicine; National Research Council. (2014). *Strategies for scaling effective family-focused preventive interventions to promote children's cognitive, affective, and behavioral health: Workshop summary.* National Academies Press. https://www.ncbi.nlm.nih.gov/books/NBK269355/

Foster, C., Schinasi, D., Kan, K., Macy, M., Wheeler, D., & Curfman, A. (2022). Remote monitoring of patient- and family-generated health data in pediatrics. *Pediatrics*, *149*(2). https://doi.org/10.1542/peds.2021-054137

Foster, C. C., Chorniy, A., Kwon, S., Kan, K., Heard-Garris, N., & Davis, M. M. (2021). Children with special health care needs and forgone family employment. *Pediatrics, 148*(3), e2020035378. https://doi.org/10.1542/peds.2020-035378

Foster, E. M., Jiang, M., & Gibson-Davis, C. M. (2010). The effect of the WIC program on the health of newborns. *Health Services Research, 45*(4), 1083–1104.

Fowler, T., Garr, D., Pietro Mager, N. D., & Stanley, J. (2020). Enhancing primary care and preventive services through interprofessional practice and education. *Israel Journal of Health Policy Research*, *9*. https://doi.org/10.1186/s13584-020-00371-8

Fox, H. B., McManus, M. A., & Yurkiewicz, S. M. (2010). *Adolescents' experiences and views on health care.* The National Alliance to Advance Adolescent Health. https://static1.squarespace.com/static/5871c0e9db29d687bc4726f2/t/5969384359cc683483dfd74e/1500067908187/Report3.+Parents%27+Perspectives+on+Health+Care+for+Adolescents.pdf

Fox, P., Porter, P. G., Lob, S. H., Boer, J. H., Rocha, D. A., & Adelson, J. W. (2007). Improving asthma-related health outcomes among low-income, multiethnic, school-aged children: Results of a demonstration project that combined continuous quality improvement and community health worker strategies. *Pediatrics*, *120*(4), e902–911. https://doi.org/10.1542/peds.2006-1805

Foy, J. E., & Hahn, K. (2009). School-based health centers: A four year experience, with a focus on reducing student exclusion rates. *Osteopathic Medicine and Primary Care*, *3*, 3. https://doi.org/10.1186/1750-4732-3-3

Frakt, A. (2020). *Bad medicine: The harm that comes from racism.* https://www.nytimes.com/2020/01/13/upshot/bad-medicine-the-harm-that-comes-from-racism.html

Franco, M. A. (2020). *Public health and social services emergency fund (provider relief fund).* Holland & Knight. https://www.hklaw.com/en/insights/publications/2020/04/public-health-and-social-services-emergency-fund

Franz, B., Cronin, C. E., Rodriguez, V., Choyke, K., Simon, J. E., & Hall, M. T. (2021). For-profit hospitals as anchor institutions in the United States: A study of organizational stability. *BMC Health Services Research*, *21*(1), 1326. https://doi.org/10.1186/s12913-021-07307-1

Frazer, K. A., & Schork, N. J. (2023). The human pangenome reference anticipates equitable and fundamental genomic insights. *Cell Genomics*, *3*(7), 100360. https://doi.org/10.1016/j.xgen.2023.100360

Frederick, T. J., Chwalek, M., Hughes, J., Karabanow, J., & Kidd, S. (2014). How stable is stable? Defining and measuring housing stability. *Journal of Community Psychology*, *42*(8), 964–979. https://doi.org/10.1002/jcop.21665

Freed, B., Segalowitz, N., & Dewey, D. (2004). Context of learning and second language fluency in French—Comparing regular classroom, study abroad, and intensive domestic immersion programs. *Studies in Second Language Acquisition*, *26*. https://doi.org/10.1017/S0272263104262064

Freed, G. L., Dunham, K. M., Gebremariam, A., & Wheeler, J. R. (2010). Which pediatricians are providing care to America's children? An update on the trends and changes during the past 26 years. *Journal of Pediatrics*, *157*(1), 148–152.e141. https://doi.org/10.1016/j.jpeds.2010.01.003

Freed, G. L., Dunham, K. M., Loveland-Cherry, C., Martyn, K. K., & Moote, M. J. (2011). Nurse practitioners and physician assistants employed by general and subspecialty pediatricians. *Pediatrics*, *128*(4), 665–672. https://doi.org/10.1542/peds.2011-0329

Freedman, M. (2020). *Health screening milestones for school-aged children.* HealthGrades. https://www.healthgrades.com/right-care/childrens-health/health-screening-milestones-for-school-aged-children

Freeman, W. M., Walker, S. J., & Vrana, K. E. (1999). Quantitative RT-PCR: Pitfalls and potential. *Biotechniques*, *26*(1), 112–122, 124–115. https://doi.org/10.2144/99261rv01

Frenier, C., & McIntyre, A. (2023). Insurance coverage transitions after disenrollment from Medicaid in Minnesota. *JAMA Network Open*, *6*(4), e239379. https://doi.org/10.1001/jamanetworkopen.2023.9379

Frenk, J., Chen, L. C., Chandran, L., Groff, E. O. H., King, R., Meleis, A., & Fineberg, H. V. (2022). Challenges and opportunities for educating health professionals after the COVID-19 pandemic. *Lancet*, *400*(10362), 1539–1556. https://doi.org/10.1016/S0140-6736(22)02092-X

Freudenberg, N., & Ruglis, J. (2007). Reframing school dropout as a public health issue. *Preventing Chronic Disease*, *4*(4), A107.

Friedman-Krauss, A. H., Barnett, W. S., & Duer, J. K. (2022). *The state(s) of Head Start and Early Head Start: Looking at equity.* https://nieer.org/research-library/states-head-start-early-head-start

Fritz, C. Q., Thomas, J., Gambino, J., Torok, M., & Brittan, M. S. (2020). Prevalence of social risks on inpatient screening and their impact on pediatric care use. *Hospital Pediatrics*, *10*(10), 859–866. https://doi.org/10.1542/hpeds.2020-0094

Froehlich, T. E., & Brinkman, W. B. (2018). Multimodal treatment of the school-aged child with attention-deficit/hyperactivity disorder. *JAMA Pediatrics*, *172*(2), 109–110. https://doi.org/10.1001/jamapediatrics.2017.4023

Frounfelker, R. L., Miconi, D., Farrar, J., Brooks, M. A., Rousseau, C., & Betancourt, T. S. (2020). Mental health of refugee children and youth: Epidemiology, interventions, and future directions. *Annual Review of Public Health*, *41*, 159–176. https://doi.org/10.1146/annurev-publhealth-040119-

Fryar, C. D., Carroll, M. D., & Afful, J. (2020). *Prevalence of overweight, obesity, and severe obesity among adults aged 20 and over: United States, 1960–1962 through 2017–2018.* NCHS Health E-Stats. https://www.cdc.gov/nchs/data/hestat/obesity-adult-17-18/obesity-adult.htm#Citation

Fulbright-Anderson, K., Auspos, P., & Anderson, A. (2001). *Community involvement in partnerships with educational institutions, medical centers, and utility companies.* Annie E. Casey Foundation and the Aspen Institute. https://www.aspeninstitute.org/wp-content/uploads/files/content/docs/CommInvolveINSTITUTIONS.PDF

Funk, C., & Lopez, M. H. (2022). *Hispanic Americans' experiences with health care.* Pew Research Center. https://www.pewresearch.org/science/2022/06/14/hispanic-americans-experiences-with-health-care/

Funk, C., Tyson, A., Kennedy, B., & Pasquini, G. (2023). *Americans' largely positive views of childhood vaccines hold steady.* Pew Research Center. https://www.pewresearch.org/science/2023/05/16/americans-largely-positive-views-of-childhood-vaccines-hold-steady/

Gage-Bouchard, E. A. (2017). Social support, flexible resources, and health care navigation. *Social Science & Medicine*, *190*, 111. https://doi.org/10.1016/j.socscimed.2017.08.015

Gajarawala, S. N., & Pelkowski, J. N. (2021). Telehealth benefits and barriers. *The Journal for Nurse Practitioners*, *17*(2), 218–221. https://doi.org/10.1016/j.nurpra.2020.09.013

Galbraith, A. A., Grossman, D. C., Koepsell, T. D., Heagerty, P. J., & Christakis, D. A. (2005). Medicaid acceptance and availability of timely follow-up for newborns with Medicaid. *Pediatrics*, *116*(5), 1148–1154. https://doi.org/10.1542/peds.2004-2584

Galbraith, A. A., Price, J., Abraham, C., Giardino, A. P., & Committee on Child Health Financing. (2023). Principles of child health care financing. *Pediatrics, 152*(3), e2023063283

Galbraith, A. A., Ross-Degnan, D., Soumerai, S. B., Abrams, A. M., Kleinman, K., Rosenthal, M. B., Wharam, J. F., Adams, A. S., Miroshnik, I., & Lieu, T. A. (2010). Use of well-child visits in high-deductible health plans. *American Journal of Managed Care*, *16*(11), 833–840.

Galbraith, A. A., Ross-Degnan, D., Soumerai, S. B., Miroshnik, I., Wharam, J. F., Kleinman, K., & Lieu, T. A. (2009). High-deductible health plans: Are vulnerable families enrolled? *Pediatrics*, *123*(4), e589–594. https://doi.org/10.1542/peds.2008-1738

Galbraith, A. A., Ross-Degnan, D., Soumerai, S. B., Rosenthal, M. B., Gay, C., & Lieu, T. A. (2011). Nearly half of families in high-deductible health plans whose members have chronic conditions face substantial financial burden. *Health Affairs (Project Hope)*, *30*(2), 322–331. https://doi.org/10.1377/hlthaff.2010.0584

Gallagher, R. W., & Polanin, J. R. (2015). A meta-analysis of educational interventions designed to enhance cultural competence in professional nurses and nursing students. *Nurse Education Today*, *35*(2), 333–340. https://doi.org/10.1016/j.nedt.2014.10.021

Gamble, V. N. (1997). Under the shadow of Tuskegee: African Americans and health care. *American Journal of Public Health*, *87*(11), 1773–1778. https://doi.org/10.2105/ajph.87.11.1773

Ganguli, I., Lee, T. H., & Mehrotra, A. (2019). Evidence and implications behind a national decline in primary care visits. *Journal of General Internal Medicine*, *34*(10), 2260–2263. https://doi.org/10.1007/s11606-019-05104-5

Garbe, A., Bode, A. A., Dunsmore, J. C., Keim-Malpass, J., & Zeanah, P. D. (2023). The Effect of Exposure to Reach Out and Read on Shared Reading Behaviors. *Academic Pediatrics*, *23*(8), 1405–1411. https://doi.org/10.1016/j.acap.2023.06.030

Garbutt, J. M., Mandrell, K. M., Allen, M., Sterkel, R., Epstein, J., Kreusser, K., O'Neil, J., Sayre, B., Sitrin, H., Stahl, K., & Strunk, R. C. (2013). Parents' experiences with pediatric care at retail clinics. *JAMA Pediatrics*, *167*(9), 845–850. https://doi.org/10.1001/jamapediatrics.2013.352

Gardner, W., & Kelleher, K. J. (2017). Core quality and outcome measures for pediatric health. *JAMA Pediatrics*, *171*(9), 827–828. https://doi.org/10.1001/jamapediatrics.2017.1685

Garfinkel, I., Sariscsany, L., Ananat, E., Collyer, S. M., Hartley, R. P., Wang, B., & Wimer, C. (2022). *The benefits and costs of a U.S. child allowance* (NBER Working Paper No. 29854). National Bureau of Economic Research.

Garg, A., Brochier, A., Tripodis, Y., Messmer, E., & Drainoni, M.-L. (2023). A social care system implemented in pediatric primary care: A cluster RCT. *Pediatrics*, *152*(2), e2023061513. https://doi.org/10.1542/peds.2023-061513

Garg, A., Toy, S., Tripodis, Y., Silverstein, M., & Freeman, E. (2015). Addressing social determinants of health at well child care visits: A cluster RCT. *Pediatrics*, *135*(2), e296–e304. https://doi.org/10.1542/peds.2014-2888

Garner, A. S., & Yogman, M. (2021a). Preventing childhood toxic stress: Partnering with families and communities to promote relational health. *Pediatrics*, *148*(2), e2021052582. https://doi.org/10.1542/peds.2021-052582

________. (2021b). Supporting healthy emotional development in young children: The role of the pediatrician. *Pediatrics*, *147*(2), e2021050861. https://doi.org/10.1542/peds.2021-050861

Gaudette, E., Pauley, G. C., & Zissimopoulos, J. (2016). *Long-term individual and population consequences of early-life access to health insurance* (Working Paper No. 2016-355). University of Michigan Retirement Research Center.

Gayle, T., Law, A., Stokes, S., Page, A., Neal, W., & Bhansali, P. (2023). Parent preferences on screening for social determinants of health in hospitalized children. *Hospital Pediatrics*, *13*(7), 623–635. https://doi.org/10.1542/hpeds.2022-006718

Gears, H., Casau, A., Buck. L., & Yard, R. (2021). *Accelerating child health care transformation: Key opportunities for improving pediatric care*. Center for Health Care Strategies. https://www.chcs.org/media/Report-Accelerating-Child-Health-Care-Transformation-Key-Opportunities-for-Improving-Pediatric-Care_8.24.21.pdf

George Washington University School of Business. (2020). *What should hospitals do to prepare for pandemics?* George Washington University School of Business. https://healthcaremba.gwu.edu/blog/what-should-hospitals-do-to-prepare-for-pandemics

Georgetown University Center for Children and Families. (2024). *Series: Improving access in Medicaid and CHIP*. https://ccf.georgetown.edu/2024/05/13/series-improving-access-in-medicaid-and-chip/

Georgia Health Policy Center. (n.d.). *Health impact assessment*. Georgia State University. https://ghpc.gsu.edu/tools-frameworks/health-impact-assessment/

Geronimus, A. T. (1996). Black/white differences in the relationship of maternal age to birthweight: A population-based test of the weathering hypothesis. *Social Science & Medicine*, *42*(4), 589–597. https://doi.org/10.1016/0277-9536(95)00159-x

Gerrity, M. (2016). *Integrating primary care into behavioral health settings: What works for individuals with serious mental illness*. https://www.milbank.org/wp-content/uploads/2016/04/Integrating-Primary-Care-Report.pdf

Ghandakly, E. C., & Fabi, R. (2021). Sterilization in US immigration and customs enforcement's (ICE's) detention: Ethical failures and systemic injustice. *American Journal of Public Health*, *111*(5), 832–834. https://doi.org/10.2105/ajph.2021.306186

Ghandour, R. M., Hirai, A. H., Moore, K. A., Robinson, L. R., Kaminski, J. W., Murphy, K., Lu, M. C., & Kogan, M. D. (2021). Healthy and ready to learn: Prevalence and correlates of school readiness among United States preschoolers. *Academic Pediatrics*, *21*(5), 818–829. https://doi.org/10.1016/j.acap.2021.02.019

Ghandour, R. M., Jones, J. R., Lebrun-Harris, L. A., Minnaert, J., Blumberg, S. J., Fields, J., Bethell, C., & Kogan, M. D. (2018). The design and implementation of the 2016 National Survey of Children's Health. *Maternal and Child Health Journal*, *22*(8), 1093–1102. https://doi.org/10.1007/s10995-018-2526-x

Gibson, E. J., Santelli, J. S., Minguez, M., Lord, A., & Schuyler, A. C. (2013). Measuring school health center impact on access to and quality of primary care. *Journal of Adolescent Health*, *53*(6), 696–705.

Gigli, K. H., Beauchesne, M. A., Dirks, M. S., & Peck, J. L. (2019). White paper: Critical shortage of pediatric nurse practitioners predicted. *The Journal of Pediatric Health Care*, *33*(3), 347–355. https://doi.org/10.1016/j.pedhc.2019.02.008

Gigli, K. H., Davis, B. S., Martsolf, G. R., & Kahn, J. M. (2021). Advanced practice provider-inclusive staffing models and patient outcomes in pediatric critical care. *Medical Care*, *59*(7), 597–603. https://doi.org/10.1097/mlr.0000000000001531

Gilbert, K. L., Shaw, M., Siddiqi, A., & Goodman, M. S. (2023). Achieving the health equity agenda through transformative community-engaged strategies. *Preventing Chronic Disease, 20*, E77. https://doi.org/10.5888/pcd20.230077

Gilliam, W. S. (2005). *Prekindergarteners left behind: Expulsion rates in state prekindergarten systems*. Foundation for Child Development. https://www.fcd-us.org/wp-content/uploads/2016/04/ExpulsionPolicyBrief.pdf

Gilliam, W. S., Maupin, A. N., Reyes, C. R., Accavitti, M., & Shic, F. (2016). *Do early educators' implicit biases regarding sex and race relate to behavior expectations and recommendations of preschool expulsions and suspensions?* Yale University Child Study Center.

Gilliland, F. D., Berhane, K., Islam, T., McConnell, R., Gauderman, W. J., Gilliland, S. S., Avol, E., & Peters, J. M. (2003). Obesity and the risk of newly diagnosed asthma in school-age children. *American Journal of Epidemiology*, *158*(5), 406–415. https://doi.org/10.1093/aje/kwg175

Ginsburg, K. R., Forke, C. M., Cnaan, A., & Slap, G. B. (2002). Important health provider characteristics: The perspective of urban ninth graders. *Journal of Developmental & Behavioral Pediatrics*, *23*(4), 237–243. https://doi.org/10.1097/00004703-200208000-00008

Ginsburg, K. R., Menapace, A. S., & Slap, G. B. (1997). Factors affecting the decision to seek health care: The voice of adolescents. *Pediatrics*, *100*(6), 922–930. https://doi.org/10.1542/peds.100.6.922

Ginwright, S. (2018). The future of healing: Shifting from trauma informed care to healing centered engagement. *Occasional Paper*, *25*, 25–32.

Gluckman, P. D., Hanson, M. A., Cooper, C., & Thornburg, K. L. (2008). Effect of in utero and early-life conditions on adult health and disease. *New England Journal of Medicine*, *359*(1), 61–73. https://doi.org/10.1056/NEJMra0708473

Golberstein, E., Gonzales, G., & Meara, E. (2019). How do economic downturns affect the mental health of children? Evidence from the National Health Interview Survey. *Health Economics*, *28*(8), 955–970. https://doi.org/10.1002/hec.3885

Goldfeld, S., Bryson, H., Mensah, F., Price, A., Gold, L., Orsini, F., Kenny, B., Perlen, S., Bohingamu Mudiyanselage, S., Dakin, P., Bruce, T., Harris, D., & Kemp, L. (2022). Nurse home visiting to improve child and maternal outcomes: 5-year follow-up of an Australian randomised controlled trial. *PLoS One*, *17*(11), e0277773. https://doi.org/10.1371/journal.pone.0277773

Goldstein, J. T., Hartman, S. G., Meunier, M. R., Panchal, B., Pecci, C. C., Zink, N. M., & Shields, S. G. (2018). Supporting family physician maternity care providers. *Family Medicine*, *50*(9), 662–671. https://doi.org/10.22454/FamMed.2018.325322

Goldstick, J. E., Cunningham, R. M., & Carter, P. M. (2022). Current causes of death in children and adolescents in the United States. *New England Journal of Medicine*, *386*(20), 1955–1956. https://doi.org/10.1056/NEJMc2201761

Gonçalves, M. I. R., Mendes, D. A., Caldeira, S., Jesus, E., & Nunes, E. (2022). Nurse-led care management models for patients with multimorbidity in hospital settings: A scoping review. *Journal of Nursing Management*, *30*(6), 1960–1973. https://doi.org/10.1111/jonm.13621

Gonzales, D., Haley, J. M., & Kenney, G. M. (2023). *One in six adults in immigrant families with children avoided public programs in 2022 because of green card concerns.* Urban Institute. https://www.urban.org/research/publication/one-six-adults-immigrant-families-children-avoided-public-programs-2022

Gonzalez, S. B., Morton, M., Patel, S., & Samuels, B. (2021). *Youth of color disproportionately impacted by housing instability.* Chapin Hall at the University of Chicago. https://www.chapinhall.org/research/youth-of-color-disproportionately-impacted-by-housing-instability/

Gonzalez-Mantilla, P. J., Hu, Y., Myers, S. M., Finucane, B. M., Ledbetter, D. H., Martin, C. L., & Moreno-De-Luca, A. (2023). Diagnostic yield of exome sequencing in cerebral palsy and implications for genetic testing guidelines: A systematic review and meta-analysis. *JAMA Pediatrics*, *177*(5), 472–478. https://doi.org/10.1001/jamapediatrics.2023.0008

Goodman, A., Joyce, R., & Smith, J. P. (2011). The long shadow cast by childhood physical and mental problems on adult life. *Proceedings of the National Academy of Sciences*, *108*(15), 6032–6037. https://doi.org/10.1073/pnas.1016970108

Goodman, R. A, Posner, S. F., Huang, E. S., Parekh, A. K., & Koh, H. K. (2013). Defining and measuring chronic conditions: Imperatives for research, policy, program, and practice. *Preventing Chronic Disease*, *10*, E66. https://doi.org/10.5888/pcd10.120239

Goodman, S. H., & Garber, J. (2017). Evidence-based interventions for depressed mothers and their young children. *Child Development*, *88*(2), 368–377. https://doi.org/10.1111/cdev.12732

Goodwin, J., Levinson, Z., & Hulver, S. (2023). *The estimated value of tax exemption for nonprofit hospitals was about $28 billion in 2020.* KFF. https://www.kff.org/health-costs/issue-brief/the-estimated-value-of-tax-exemption-for-nonprofit-hospitals-was-about-28-billion-in-2020/

Gordon, N., & Reber, S. (2021). *Addressing inequities in the US K–12 education system.* Aspen Institute Press. https://www.economicstrategygroup.org/publication/gordon-reber

Gorin, S. S., Haggstrom, D., Han, P. K. J., Fairfield, K. M., Krebs, P., & Clauser, S. B. (2017). Cancer care coordination: A systematic review and meta-analysis of over 30 years of empirical studies. *Annals of Behavioral Medicine*, *51*(4), 532–546. https://doi.org/10.1007/s12160-017-9876-2

Gottlieb, K. (2013). The Nuka system of care: Improving health through ownership and relationships. *International Journal of Circumpolar Health, 72*. https://doi.org/10.3402/ijch.v72i0.21118

Gould, G. S., Havard, A., Lim, L. L., the PSANZ Smoking in Pregnancy Expert Group, & Kumar, R. (2020). Exposure to tobacco, environmental tobacco smoke and nicotine in pregnancy: A pragmatic overview of reviews of maternal and child outcomes, effectiveness of interventions and barriers and facilitators to quitting. *International Journal of Environmental Research and Public Health, 17*(6). https://doi.org/10.3390/ijerph17062034

Government Accountability Office (GAO). (2018). *Working children: Federal injury data and compliance strategies could be strengthened*. https://www.gao.gov/assets/gao-19-26.pdf

________. (2020). *K-12 education: School districts frequently identified multiple building systems needing updates or replacement* (Report No. GAO-20-494). https://www.gao.gov/products/gao-20-494

________. (2021). *Firearm injuries: Health care service needs and costs*. https://www.gao.gov/assets/gao-21-515.pdf

________. (2023a). *Electronic health information exchange: Use has increased, but is lower for small and rural providers* (Report No. GAO-23-105540). https://www.gao.gov/products/gao-23-105540

________. (2023b). *Enhanced oversight and transparency*. https://www.gao.gov/assets/d24106202.pdf

________. (2023c). *Government performance management: Leading practices to enhance interagency collaboration and address crosscutting challenges*. https://www.gao.gov/products/gao-23-105520

________. (2023d). *Medicaid managed care: Rapid spending growth in state directed payments needs enhanced oversight and transparency* (Report No. GAO-24-106202). https://www.gao.gov/assets/d24106202.pdf

________. (2023e). *Public health preparedness: Building and maintaining infrastructure beyond the COVID-19 pandemic*. https://www.gao.gov/products/gao-24-105891

________. (2024). *Managed care plans' prior authorization decisions for children need additional oversight* (Report No. GAO-24-106532). https://www.gao.gov/products/GAO-24-106532

Government Performance and Results Act (GPRA) of 1993, Pub. L. No. 103-62, 107 Stat. 285 (1993).

Goyal, M. K., Johnson, T. J., Chamberlain, J. M., Cook, L., Webb, M., Drendel, A. L., Alessandrini, E., Bajaj, L., Lorch, S., Grundmeier, R. W., & Alpern, E. R. (2020). Racial and ethnic differences in emergency department pain management of children with fractures. *Pediatrics, 145*(5). https://doi.org/10.1542/peds.2019-3370

Goyal, M. K., Kuppermann, N., Cleary, S. D., Teach, S. J., & Chamberlain, J. M. (2015). Racial disparities in pain management of children with appendicitis in emergency departments. *JAMA Pediatrics, 169*(11), 996–1002. https://doi.org/10.1001/jamapediatrics.2015.1915

Granström, E., Wannheden, C., Brommels, M., Hvitfeldt, H., & Nyström, M. (2020). Digital tools as promoters for person-centered care practices in chronic care? Healthcare professionals' experiences from rheumatology care. *Journal of Medical Internet Research, 22*(12), e23145. https://doi.org/10.2196/23145

Gratale, D., Viveiros, J., & Boyer, K. (2022). Paediatric alternative payment models: Emerging elements. *Current Opinion in Pediatrics, 34*(1), 19–26. https://doi.org/10.1097/mop.0000000000001090

Gratale, D. J., Counts, N. Z., Hogan, L., Hewitt, A., Chang, D. I., Wong, C. A., Davis, M. B., Schoessow, G., McCabe, M. A., Johnson, K., Goldfinger, J., & Gionfriddo, P. (2020). Accountable communities for health for children and families: Approaches for catalyzing and accelerating success [Discussion Paper]. *National Academy of Medicine Perspectives*. https://doi.org/10.31478/202001b

Gratz, T., Goldhaber, D., Willgerodt, M., & Brown, N. (2023). The frontline health care workers in schools: Health equity, the distribution of school nurses, and student access. *The Journal of School Nursing*, *39*(5), 357–367. https://doi.org/10.1177/10598405211024277

Green, E. D., Gunter, C., Biesecker, L. G., Di Francesco, V., Easter, C. L., Feingold, E. A., Felsenfeld, A. L., Kaufman, D. J., Ostrander, E. A., Pavan, W. J., Phillippy, A. M., Wise, A. L., Dayal, J. G., Kish, B. J., Mandich, A., Wellington, C. R., Wetterstrand, K. A., Bates, S. A., Leja, D., . . . Manolio, T. A. (2020). Strategic vision for improving human health at the forefront of genomics. *Nature*, *586*(7831), 683–692. https://doi.org/10.1038/s41586-020-2817-4

Greenwood, B. N., Hardeman, R. R., Huang, L., & Sojourner, A. (2020). Physician–patient racial concordance and disparities in birthing mortality for newborns. *Proceedings of the National Academy of Sciences*, *117*(35), 21194–21200. https://doi.org/10.1073/pnas.1913405117

Griffith, D. M., Bergner, E. M., Fair, A. S., & Wilkins, C. H. (2021). Using mistrust, distrust, and low trust precisely in medical care and medical research advances health equity. *American Journal of Preventive Medicine*, *60*(3), 442–445. https://doi.org/10.1016/j.amepre.2020.08.019

Grimm, C. A. (2023). *High rates of prior authorization denials by some plans and limited state oversight raise concerns about access to care in Medicaid managed care*. Office of Inspector General, Department of Health and Human Services. https://oig.hhs.gov/oei/reports/OEI-09-19-00350.pdf

Groenman, A. P., Janssen, T. W. P., & Oosterlaan, J. (2017). Childhood psychiatric disorders as risk factor for subsequent substance abuse: A meta-analysis. *Journal of the American Academy of Child and Adolescent Psychiatry*, *56*(7), 556–569. https://doi.org/10.1016/j.jaac.2017.05.004

Gromada, A., Rees, G., Chzhen, Y., Carraro, A., Little, C., & Anthony, D. (2020). *Worlds of influence: Understanding what shapes child well-being in rich countries*. https://www.unicef-irc.org/publications/pdf/Report-Card-16-Worlds-of-Influence-child-wellbeing.pdf

Groves, L. H. (2020). Still "saving babies"? The impact of child Medicaid expansions on high school completion rates. *Contemporary Economic Policy*, *38*, 109–126. https://doi.org/10.1111/coep.12431

Grumbach, K., Bainbridge, E., & Bodenheimer, T. (2012). Facilitating improvement in primary care: The promise of practice coaching. *Issue Brief (Commonwealth Fund)*, *15*, 1–14.

Grummitt, L. R., Kreski, N. T., Kim, S. G., Platt, J., Keyes, K. M., & McLaughlin, K. A. (2021). Association of childhood adversity with morbidity and mortality in US adults: A systematic review. *JAMA Pediatrics*, *175*(12), 1269–1278. https://doi.org/10.1001/jamapediatrics.2021.2320

Gu, W., Zhao, Q., Yuan, C., Yi, Z., Zhao, M., & Wang, Z. (2022). Impact of adverse childhood experiences on the symptom severity of different mental disorders: A cross-diagnostic study. *General Psychiatry*, *35*(2), e100741. https://doi.org/10.1136/gpsych-2021-100741

Guan, A., Hamad, R., Batra, A., Bush, N. R., Tylavsky, F. A., & LeWinn, K. Z. (2021). The revised WIC food package and child development: A quasi-experimental study. *Pediatrics*, *147*(2), e20201853. https://doi.org/10.1542/peds.2020-1853

Guevara, J. P., Aysola, J., Wade, R., Nfonoyim, B., Qiu, M., Reece, M., & Carroll, K. N. (2023). Diversity in the pediatric research workforce: A scoping review of the literature. *Pediatric Research*, 1–11. https://doi.org/10.1038/s41390-023-02603-4

Guidi, C., & Traversa, C. (2021). Empathy in patient care: From 'clinical empathy' to 'empathic concern'. *Medicine, Health Care and Philosophy*, *24*(4), 573–585. https://doi.org/10.1007/s11019-021-10033-4

Guldi, M., & Hamersma, S. (2023). The effects of pregnancy-related Medicaid expansions on maternal, infant, and child health. *Journal of Health Economics*, *87*, 102695. https://doi.org/10.1016/j.jhealeco.2022.102695

Gulliver, A., Griffiths, K. M., & Christensen, H. (2010). Perceived barriers and facilitators to mental health help-seeking in young people: A systematic review. *BMC Psychiatry*, *10*, 113–113. https://doi.org/10.1186/1471-244X-10-113

Gundersen, C., & Kreider, B. (2009). Bounding the effects of food insecurity on children's health outcomes. *Journal of Health Economics*, *28*(5), 971–983. https://doi.org/10.1016/j.jhealeco.2009.06.012

Gundersen, C., & Ziliak, J. P. (2015). Food insecurity and health outcomes. *Health Affairs (Project Hope)*, *34*(11), 1830–1839. https://doi.org/10.1377/hlthaff.2015.0645

Guo, J. J., Jang, R., Keller, K. N., McCracken, A. L., & Cluxton, R. J. (2005). Impact of school-based health centers on children with asthma. *Journal of Adolescent Health*, *37*(4), 266–274.

Guo, S., & Jhe, G. B. (2021). Universal depression screening in schools—promises and challenges in addressing adolescent mental health need. *JAMA Network Open*, *4*(11), e2132858. https://doi.org/10.1001/jamanetworkopen.2021.32858

Gurovich, Y., Hanani, Y., Bar, O., Nadav, G., Fleischer, N., Gelbman, D., Basel-Salmon, L., Krawitz, P. M., Kamphausen, S. B., Zenker, M., Bird, L. M., & Gripp, K. W. (2019). Identifying facial phenotypes of genetic disorders using deep learning. *Nature Medicine*, *25*(1), 60–64. https://doi.org/10.1038/s41591-018-0279-0

Gusmano, M. K., & Thompson, F. J. (2018). Medicaid delivery system reform incentive payments: Where do we stand? *Health Affairs Blog*. http://dx.doi.org/10.1377/hblog20180920.103967

Gustafson, E. M. (2005). History and overview of school-based health centers in the US. *Nursing Clinics of North America*, *40*(4), 595–606. https://doi.org/10.1016/j.cnur.2005.08.001.

Guthrie, J. D., & Snyder, J. A. (2023). Improving access to care for underserved communities through telemedicine. *JAAPA: Official Journal of the American Academy of Physician Assistants*, *36*(9), 41–44. https://doi.org/10.1097/01.JAA.0000947040.98500.2e

Hacke, R., & Deane, K. G. (2017). *Improving community health by strengthening community investment: Roles for hospitals and health systems*. Center for Community Investment. https://www.rwjf.org/en/insights/our-research/2017/03/improving-community-health-by-strengthening-community-investment.html

Hagelskamp, C., Brackett, M. A., Rivers, S. E., & Salovey, P. (2013). Improving classroom quality with the RULER approach to social and emotional learning: Proximal and distal outcomes. *American Journal of Community Psychology*, *51*(3), 530–543.

Hager, B., Hasselberg, M., Arzubi, E., Betlinski, J., Duncan, M., Richman, J., & Raney, L. E. (2018). Leveraging behavioral health expertise: Practices and potential of the Project ECHO approach to virtually integrating care in underserved areas. *Psychiatric Services*, *69*(4), 366–369. https://doi.org/10.1176/appi.ps.201700211

Haggerty, R. (1975). *Child health and the community*. Wiley Interscience Publication.

Haider, A. (2021). *The basic facts about children in poverty*. The Center for American Progress. https://www.americanprogress.org/article/basic-facts-children-poverty/

Haines, A., Perkins, E., Evans, E. A., & McCabe, R. (2018). Multidisciplinary team functioning and decision making within forensic mental health. *Mental Health Review*, *23*(3), 185–196. https://doi.org/10.1108/mhrj-01-2018-0001

Hajat, A., Nurius, P., & Song, C. (2020). Differing trajectories of adversity over the life course: Implications for adult health and well-being. *Child Abuse & Neglect*, *102*, 104392. https://doi.org/10.1016/j.chiabu.2020.104392

Hakim, R. B., Boben, P. J., & Bonney, J. B. (2000). Medicaid and the health of children. *Health Care Financing Review*, *22*(1), 133–140.

Haldane, V., Jung, A. S., Foo, C. D., Bonk, M., Jamieson, M., Wu, S., Verma, M., Abdalla, S. M., Singh, S., Nordström, A., & Legido-Quigley, H. (2021). Strengthening the basics: Public health responses to prevent the next pandemic. *BMJ*, *375*, e067510. https://doi.org/10.1136/bmj-2021-067510

Haldar, S., & Hinton, E. (2023). *State policies for expanding Medicaid coverage of community health worker (CHW) services.* KFF. https://www.kff.org/medicaid/issue-brief/state-policies-for-expanding-medicaid-coverage-of-community-health-worker-chw-services

Hales, C. M., Carroll, M. D., Fryar, C. D., & Ogden, C. L. (2020). *Prevalence of obesity and severe obesity among adults: United States, 2017–2018* (NCHS Data Brief No. 360). National Center for Health Statistics, Centers for Disease Control and Prevention. https://www.cdc.gov/nchs/products/databriefs/db360.htm

Haley, J., McMorrow, S., Long, J., Kenney, G. M., Johnston, E. M., Willis, C., & Brown, K. (2023). *Assessing health care access among Medicaid/CHIP-enrolled children: A national chartbook, 2016–19.* Urban Institute. https://www.urban.org/sites/default/files/2023-04/Assessing%20Health%20Care%20Access%20among%20Medicaid-CHIP-Enrolled%20Children.pdf

Haley, J. M., Kenney, G. M., Bernstein, H., & Gonzalez, D. (2020). *One in five adults in immigrant families with children reported chilling effects on public benefit receipt in 2019.* The Urban Institute.

Haley, M. (2021). *Introducing the seventh generation principle—to promote true sustainability.* The Seventh Generation. https://theseventhgeneration.org/blog-the-seventh-generation-principle/

Halfon, N., Chandra, A., Cannon, J. S., Gardner, W., & Forrest, C. B. (2022). The Gross Developmental Potential (GDP2): A new approach for measuring human potential and wellbeing. *BMC Public Health*, *22*(1), 1626. https://doi.org/10.1186/s12889-022-14030-x

Halfon, N., DuPlessis, H., & Inkelas, M. (2007). Transforming the U.S. child health system. *Health Affairs (Project Hope)*, *26*(2), 315–330. https://doi.org/10.1377/hlthaff.26.2.315

Halfon, N., Forrest, C. B., Lerner, R. M., & Faustman, E. M. (Eds.) (2018). *Handbook of Life Course Health Development.* Springer Cham. https://doi.org/10.1007/978-3-319-47143-3

Halfon, N., & Hochstein, M. (2002). Life course health development: An integrated framework for developing health, policy, and research. *The Milbank Quarterly*, *80*(3), 433–479. https://doi.org/10.1111/1468-0009.00019

Halfon, N., Houtrow, A., Larson, K., & Newacheck, P. W. (2012). The changing landscape of disability in childhood. *Future Child*, *22*(1), 13–42. https://doi.org/10.1353/foc.2012.0004

Hall, C., Rudowitz, R., & Gifford, K. (2019). *Medicaid in the territories: Program features, challenges, and changes.* KFF. https://www.healthmanagement.com/wp-content/uploads/Issue-Brief-Medicaid-in-the-Territories-Programs-Features-Challenges-and-Changes.pdf

Hall, J. A., Roter, D. L., & Rand, C. S. (1981). Communication of affect between patient and physician. *Journal of Health and Social Behavior*, *22*(1), 18–30.

Hall, W. J., Chapman, M. V., Lee, K. M., Merino, Y. M., Thomas, T. W., Payne, B. K., Eng, E., Day, S. H., & Coyne-Beasley, T. (2015). Implicit racial/ethnic bias among health care professionals and its influence on health care outcomes: A systematic review. *American Journal of Public Health*, *105*(12), e60–76. https://doi.org/10.2105/ajph.2015.302903

Halley, M. C., Rustagi, A. S., Torres, J. S., Linos, E., Plaut, V., Mangurian, C., Choo, E., & Linos, E. (2018). Physician mothers' experience of workplace discrimination: A qualitative analysis. *BMJ*, *363*, k4926. https://doi.org/10.1136/bmj.k4926

Halterman, J. S., Fagnano, M., Tajon, R. S., Tremblay, P., Wang, H., Butz, A., Perry, T. T., & McConnochie, K. M. (2018). Effect of the school-based telemedicine enhanced asthma management (SB-TEAM) program on asthma morbidity: A randomized clinical trial. *JAMA Pediatrics*, *172*(3), e174938. https://doi.org/10.1001/jamapediatrics.2017.4938

Hamad, R., Batra, A., Karasek, D., LeWinn, K. Z., Bush, N. R., & Davis, R. L. (2019a). The impact of the revised WIC food package on maternal nutrition during pregnancy and postpartum. *American Journal of Epidemiology, 188*(8), 1493–1502. https://doi.org/10.1093/aje/kwz098

Hamad, R., Collin, D. F., Baer, R. J., & Jelliffe-Pawlowski, L. L. (2019b). Association of revised WIC food package with perinatal and birth outcomes: A quasi-experimental study. *JAMA Pediatrics, 173*(9), 845–852. https://doi.org/10.1001/jamapediatrics.2019.1706

Hamersma, S., Kim, M., & Timpe, B. (2019). The effect of parental Medicaid expansions on children's health insurance coverage. *Contemporary Economic Policy, 37*(2), 297–311. https://doi.org/10.1111/coep.12392

Hamilton, B. E., Martin, J. A., & Osterman, M. J. K. (2023). *Births: Provisional data for 2022* (National Vital Statistics Reports No. 28). https://www.cdc.gov/nchs/data/vsrr/vsrr028.pdf

Hammitt, L. L., Dagan, R., Yuan, Y., Baca Cots, M., Bosheva, M., Madhi, S. A., Muller, W. J., Zar, H. J., Brooks, D., Grenham, A., Wählby Hamrén, U., Mankad, V. S., Ren, P., Takas, T., Abram, M. E., Leach, A., Griffin, M. P., & Villafana, T. (2022). Nirsevimab for prevention of RSV in healthy late-preterm and term infants. *New England Journal of Medicine, 386*(9), 837–846. https://doi.org/10.1056/NEJMoa2110275

Hamosh, A., Amberger, J. S., Bocchini, C., Scott, A. F., & Rasmussen, S. A. (2021). Online Mendelian Inheritance in Man (OMIM®): Victor McKusick's magnum opus. *American Journal of Medical Genetics. Part A, 185*(11), 3259–3265. https://doi.org/10.1002/ajmg.a.62407

Hamp, A., Stamm, K., Lin, L., & Christidis, P. (2016). *2015 APA survey of psychology health service providers*. American Psychological Association. https://www.apa.org/workforce/publications/15-health-service-providers

Hampl, S. E., Hassink, S. G., Skinner, A. C., Armstrong, S. C., Barlow, S. E., Bolling, C. F., Avila Edwards, K. C., Eneli, I., Hamre, R., Joseph, M. M., Lunsford, D., Mendonca, E., Michalsky, M. P., Mirza, N., Ochoa, E. R., Sharifi, M., Staiano, A. E., Weedn, A. E., Flinn, S. K., . . . Okechukwu, K. (2023). Clinical practice guideline for the evaluation and treatment of children and adolescents with obesity. *Pediatrics, 151*(2). https://doi.org/10.1542/peds.2022-060640

Hanson, M. A., & Gluckman, P. D. (2014). Early developmental conditioning of later health and disease: Physiology or pathophysiology? *Physiological Reviews, 94*(4), 1027–1076. https://doi.org/10.1152/physrev.00029.2013

Hardin, H. K., Bender, A. E., Hermann, C. P., & Speck, B. J. (2021). An integrative review of adolescent trust in the healthcare provider relationship. *Journal of Advanced Nursing, 77*(4), 1645. https://doi.org/10.1111/jan.14674

Hardy, C. (2022). Empathy and calm as social resources in clinical practice. *AMA Journal of Ethics, 24*(12), e1135–1140. https://doi.org/10.1001/amajethics.2022.1135

Harkavy, I., Hartley M., Hodges R. A., Sorrentino A., & Weeks, J. (2014). Effective governance of a university as an anchor institution: University of Pennsylvania as a case study. *Leadership and Governance in Higher Education*, 2. https://www.nettercenter.upenn.edu/sites/default/files/Effective_Governance_of_a_University_as_an_Anchor_Institution-Raabe_Publishers.pdf

Harkin, T. (2013). *Statement by Senator Tom Harkin on the importance of the prevention fund to save lives and money* [Press Release]. U.S. Senate Committee on Health, Education, Labor, & Pensions. https://www.help.senate.gov/ranking/newsroom/press/statement-by-senator-tom-harkin-on-the-importance-of-the-prevention-fund-to-save-lives-and-money

Harrington, R., Washington, D. Paliani, S., Thompson, K., Rouse, L., & Anderson, A. C. (2021). A new effort to address racial and ethnic disparities in care through quality measurement. *Health Affairs*. https://www.healthaffairs.org/content/forefront/new-effort-address-racial-and-ethnic-disparities-care-through-quality-measurement

Harrison, E., Haley, C., & Shattuck, P. (2023). *Medicaid policy options: Innovative approaches to support the reduction of harmful greenhouse gas emissions from the health system*. Mathematica. https://www.mathematica.org/publications/medicaid-policy-options-innovative-approaches-to-support-the-reduction-of-harmful-greenhouse-gas

Harrison, L., Carducci, B., Klein, J. D., & Bhutta, Z. A. (2022). Indirect effects of COVID-19 on child and adolescent mental health: An overview of systematic reviews. *BMJ Global Health*, *7*(12). https://doi.org/10.1136/bmjgh-2022-010713

Hartley, K., Perazzo, J., Brokamp, C., Gillespie, G. L., Cecil, K. M., LeMasters, G., Yolton, K., & Ryan, P. (2021). Residential surrounding greenness and self-reported symptoms of anxiety and depression in adolescents. *Environmental Research*, *194*, 110628. https://doi.org/10.1016/j.envres.2020.110628

Hasan, S., Miller, A., Higginbotham, D., Saleh, E. S., & McCarty, S. (2023). Virtual and augmented reality in spine surgery: An era of immersive healthcare. *Cureus Journal of Medical Science*, *15*(8), e43964. https://doi.org/10.7759/cureus.43964

Hassen, N., Lofters, A., Michael, S., Mall, A., Pinto, A. D., & Rackal, J. (2021). Implementing anti-racism interventions in healthcare settings: A scoping review. *International Journal of Environmental Research and Public Health, 18(6)*, 2993. https://doi.org/10.3390/ijerph18062993

Hayes, D., Moore, A., Stapley, E. Humphrey, N., Mansfield, R., Santos, J., Ashworth, E., Patalay, P., Bonin, E.-M., Moltrecht, B., Boehnke, J. R., & Deighton, J. (2019). Promoting mental health and wellbeing in schools: Examining mindfulness, relaxation and strategies for safety and wellbeing in English primary and secondary schools: Study protocol for a multi-school, cluster randomised controlled trial (INSPIRE). *Trials*, *20*(640). https://doi.org/10.1186/s13063-019-3762-0

Hayhoe, B., Verma, G., Scott, K., Awolu, A., Majeed, A., Esmail, A., & Gallagher, R. (2018). Utilization of community health workers to identify and treat undernutrition in Marasmus and Kwashiorkor in children under 5 years of age in sub-Saharan Africa: A systematic review. *Global Health Action*, *11*(1), 1–11. https://doi.org/10.1080/16549716.2018.1524028

Healey, G. K. (2017). *What if our health care systems embodied the values of our communities? A reflection from Nunavut*. The Artic Institute. https://www.thearcticinstitute.org/health-care-systems-values-communities-nunavut/

Health Care PRICE Transparency Act. H.R. 3029, 117th Congress (2021–2022).

Health Insurance Marketplace. (n.d.) *Coverage for lawfully present immigrants*. U.S. Centers for Medicare & Medicaid Services. https://www.healthcare.gov/immigrants/lawfully-present-immigrants/

Health Insurance Portability and Accountability Act (HIPAA), Pub. L. No. 104–191, 110 Stat. 1936. (1996).

Health Resources and Services Administration (HRSA). (n.d.a). *Division of services for children with special health needs (DSCSHN)*. U.S. Department of Health and Human Services. https://mchb.hrsa.gov/about-us/our-offices-divisions/division-services-children-special-health-needs-dscshn

________. (n.d.b). *Children and youth with special health care needs (CYSHCN)*. Maternal and Child Health Bureau. U.S. Department of Health and Human Services. https://mchb.hrsa.gov/programs-impact/focus-areas/children-youth-special-health-care-needs-cyshcn

________. (n.d.c). *MIECHV data & continuous quality improvement*. Maternal and Child Health Bureau. U.S. Department of Health and Human Services. https://mchb.hrsa.gov/programs-impact/programs/home-visiting/miechv-data-continuous-quality-improvement

________. (n.d.d). *Who we are, Provider Relief Bureau*. U.S. Health Resources and Services Administration. U.S. Department of Health and Human Services. https://www.hrsa.gov/provider-relief#phase1

_______. (2019). *Children and youth with special health care needs (CYSHCN).* U.S. Department of Health and Human Services. https://mchb.hrsa.gov/programs-impact/focus-areas/children-youth-special-health-care-needs-cyshcn
_______. (2021). *Early childhood comprehensive systems health integration prenatal-to-three (ECCS) program awards.* U.S. Department of Health and Human Services. https://mchb.hrsa.gov/early-childhood-comprehensive-systems-health-integration-prenatal-three-eccs-program-awards
_______. (2022a). *Health center program service expansion: School-based service sites awards.* U.S. Department of Health and Human Services. https://bphc.hrsa.gov/funding/funding-opportunities/school-based-service-expansion/fy-2021-awards
_______. (2022b). *How to become a health center.* U.S. Department of Health and Human Services. https://bphc.hrsa.gov/about-health-centers/how-become-health-center
_______. (2023a). *Allied health workforce projections, 2016–2030: Community health workers.* U.S. Department of Health and Human Services. https://bhw.hrsa.gov/sites/default/files/bureau-health-workforce/data-research/community-health-workers-2016-2030.pdf
_______. (2023b). *Behavioral health workforce, 2023.* National Center for Health Workforce Analysis. U.S. Department of Health and Human Services. https://bhw.hrsa.gov/sites/default/files/bureau-health-workforce/Behavioral-Health-Workforce-Brief-2023.pdf
_______. (2023c). *Children and youth with special health care needs (CYSHCN).* U.S. Department of Health and Human Services. https://mchb.hrsa.gov/programs-impact/focus-areas/children-youth-special-health-care-needs-cyshcn
_______. (2023d). *Definition of family.* U.S. Department of Health and Human Services. https://www.hrsa.gov/get-health-care/affordable/hill-burton/family
_______. (2023e). *Health center program: Impact and growth.* U.S. Department of Health and Human Services. https://bphc.hrsa.gov/about-health-centers/health-center-program-impact-growth
_______. (2023f). *Maternal, infant, and early childhood home visiting (MIECHV) program.* U.S. Department of Health and Human Services. https://mchb.hrsa.gov/programs-impact/programs/home-visiting/maternal-infant-early-childhood-home-visiting-miechv-program
_______. (2023g). *Title V maternal and child health (MCH) block grant.* U.S. Department of Health and Human Services. https://mchb.hrsa.gov/programs-impact/title-v-maternal-child-health-mch-block-grant
_______. (2024). *Bright futures.* U.S. Department of Health and Human Services. https://mchb.hrsa.gov/programs-impact/bright-futures
HealthySteps. (n.d.a). *About HealthySteps.* https://www.healthysteps.org/
_______. (n.d.b). *Health equity.* https://www.healthysteps.org/our-impact/health-equity/bright-futures/
_______. (n.d.c). *HealthySteps: What we do, our model, tiers and core components.* https://www.healthysteps.org/what-we-do/our-model/tiers-and-core-components/
_______. (2022). *HealthySteps evidence summary.* https://dyadiccare.ucsf.edu/assets/g-file/HealthySteps_Evidence_Summary_2022_FINAL.pdf
_______. (2024). *Evidence summary.* file:///C:/Users/AAllen/Downloads/HS_Evidence-Summary-2024_FINAL.pdf
Healthy Students, Promising Futures. (n.d.). *Map: School Medicaid programs.* https://healthystudentspromisingfutures.org/map-school-medicaid-programs/
Heberlein, M. (2023). *Data update: Unwinding the continuous coverage requirements.* Medicaid and CHIP Payment and Access Commission. https://www.macpac.gov/wp-content/uploads/2023/12/05_December-Slides_Data-Update-Unwinding-the-Continuous-Coverage-Requirements.pdf

Hecht, A. A., Olarte, D. A., McLoughlin, G. M., & Cohen, J. F. W. (2023). Strategies to increase student participation in school meals in the United States: A systematic review. *Journal of the Academy of Nutrition and Dietetics*, *123*(7), 1075–1096. https://doi.org/10.1016/j.jand.2023.02.016

Heckman, J. J. (2006). Skill formation and the economics of investing in disadvantaged children. *Science*, *312*(5782), 1900–1902. https://doi.org/10.1126/science.1128898

Heckman, J. J., & Masterov, D. V. (2007). The productivity argument for investing in young children. *Review of Agricultural Economics*, *29(3)*, 446–493. https://doi.org/10.1111/j.1467-9353.2007.00359.x

Heckman, J. J., Moon, S. H., Pinto, R., Savelyev, P. A., & Yavitz, A. (2010). The rate of return to the High/Scope Perry Preschool Program. *Journal of Public Economics*, *94*(1–2), 114–128. https://doi.org/10.1016/j.jpubeco.2009.11.001

Heisler, E. (2017). *Federal health centers: An overview*. Congressional Research Service. https://sgp.fas.org/crs/misc/R43937.pdf

Heisler E. J., & McClanahan, K. P. (2020). *Advance appropriations for the Indian Health Service: Issues and options for Congress*. Congressional Research Service. https://crsreports.congress.gov/product/pdf/R/R46265

Help Me Grow (HMG) National Center. (2023). *HMG evidence base resources: The Help Me Grow model, a selection of evidence*. https://helpmegrownational.org/resources/hmg-evidence-base-resources/

________. (n.d.). *HMG models*. https://helpmegrowpc.org/hmg-model/

Hemsing, N., Greaves, L., & Poole, N. (2017). Preconception health care interventions: A scoping review. *Sexual & Reproductive Healthcare*, *14*, 24–32. https://doi.org/10.1016/j.srhc.2017.08.004

Hendren, N., & Sprung-Keyser, B. (2020). A unified welfare analysis of government policies. *Quarterly Journal of Economics*, *135*(3), 1209–1318. https://academic.oup.com/qje/article/135/3/1209/5781614

Heneghan, J. A., Goodman, D. M., & Ramgopal, S. (2023). Hospitalizations at United States children's hospitals and severity of illness by neighborhood child opportunity index. *Journal of Pediatrics*, *254*, 83–90. https://doi.org/10.1016/j.jpeds.2022.10.018

Hepburn, K. S., Perry, D. F., Shivers, M. E., & Gilliam, W. S. (2013). Early childhood mental health consultation as an evidence-based practice. *Journal of Zero to Three, 33*(5), 10–19. https://www.zerotothree.org/wp-content/uploads/2022/06/Early-Childhood-Mental-Health-Consultation-13-May-Digital-Journal-Issue.pdf

Hergenroeder, A., Wiemann, C., & Cohen, M. (2015). Current issues in transitioning from pediatric to adult-based care for youth with chronic health care needs. *Journal of Pediatrics*, *167*. 10.1016/j.jpeds.2015.08.005.

Herndon, J. H., & Pollick, K. J. (2002). Continuing concerns, new challenges, and next steps in physician-patient communication. *Journal of Bone and Joint Surgery*, *84*(2), 309–315. https://doi.org/10.2106/00004623-200202000-00019

Hero, J. O., Gidengil, C. A., Qureshi, S. N., Tanielian, T., & Farmer, C. M. (2021). *Access to health care among TRICARE-covered children*. RAND Corporation. https://www.rand.org/content/dam/rand/pubs/research_reports/RRA400/RRA472-1/RAND_RRA472-1.pdf

Herval, Á. M., Oliveira, D. P., Gomes, V. E., & Vargas, A. M. D. (2019). Health education strategies targeting maternal and child health: A scoping review of educational methodologies. *Medicine*, *98*(26).10.1097/MD.0000000000016174

Hester, G., Nickel, A. J., & Griffin, K. H. (2020). Accountability through measurement: Using a dashboard to address pediatric health disparities. *Pediatrics*, *146*(6). https://doi.org/10.1542/peds.2020-024448

Hetherington, Mc. J. (2005). *Why trust matters: Declining political trust and the demise of American liberalism*. Princeton University Press.

Heun-Johnson, H., & Levitt, P. (2018). Differential impact of Met receptor gene interaction with early-life stress on neuronal morphology and behavior in mice. *Neurobiology of Stress*, *8*, 10–20. https://doi.org/10.1016/j.ynstr.2017.11.003

Hickman, C., Marks, E., Pihkala, P., Clayton, S., Lewandowski, R. E., Mayall, E. E., Wray, B., Mellor, C., & van Susteren, L. (2021a). Climate anxiety in children and young people and their beliefs about government responses to climate change: A global survey. *The Lancet Planetary Health*, *5*(12), E863–873. https://doi.org/10.1016/S2542-5196(21)00278-3

_______. (2021b). Young people's voices on climate anxiety, government betrayal and moral injury: A global phenomenon. *SSRN Electronic Journal*. https://doi.org/10.2139/ssrn.3918955

High, P. C., LaGasse, L., Becker, S., Ahlgren, I., & Gardner, A. (2000). Literacy promotion in primary care pediatrics: Can we make a difference? *Pediatrics*, *105*(Suppl 3), 927–934. https://doi.org/10.1542/peds.105.S3.927

Hilario, C., Louie-Poon, S., Taylor, M., Gill, G. K., & Kennedy, M. (2023). Racism in health services for adolescents: A scoping review. *International Journal of Social Determinants of Health and Health Services*, *53*(3), 343–353. https://doi.org/10.1177/27551938231162560

Hill, C., Knafl, K., & Santacroce, S. (2017). Family-centered care from the perspective of parents of children cared for in a pediatric intensive care unit: An integrative review. *Journal of Pediatric Nursing*, *41*, 10–19. https://doi.org/10.1016/j.pedn.2017.11.007

Hill, K., & Hill, B. (2018). Help Me Grow Utah and the impact on family protective factors development. *Journal of Children's Services*, *13*(1), 33–43. https://doi.org/10.1108/JCS-05-2017-0016

Hill, L., Artiga, S., & Damico, A. (2024). *Health coverage by race and ethnicity, 2010–2022*. KFF. https://www.kff.org/racial-equity-and-health-policy/issue-brief/health-coverage-by-race-and-ethnicity/

Hill, L., Artiga, S., & Ranji, U. (2022). *Racial disparities in maternal and infant health: Current status and efforts to address them*. KFF. https://www.kff.org/racial-equity-and-health-policy/issue-brief/racial-disparities-in-maternal-and-infant-health-current-status-and-efforts-to-address-them/

Hillis, S. D., Blenkinsop, A., Villaveces, A., Annor, F. B., Liburd, L., Massetti, G. M., Demissie, Z., Mercy, J. A., Nelson III, C. A., Cluver, L., Flaxman, S., Sherr, L., Donnelly, C. A., Ratmann, O., & Unwin, H. J. T. (2021). COVID-19-associated orphanhood and caregiver death in the United States. *Pediatrics*, *148*(6). https://doi.org/10.1542/peds.2021-053760

The Hilltop Institute. (n.d.). *Hospital community benefit*. University of Maryland. https://www.hilltopinstitute.org/our-work/hospital-community-benefit/

Himmelstein, D. U., & Woolhandler, S. (2016). Public health's falling share of US health spending. *American Journal of Public Health*, *106*(1), 56–57. https://doi.org/10.2105/AJPH.2015.302908

Hine, J. F., Grennan, A. Q., Menousek, K. M., Robertson, G., Valleley, R. J., & Evans, J. H. (2017). Physician satisfaction with integrated behavioral health in pediatric primary care. *Journal of Primary Care & Community Health*, *8*(2), 89–93. https://doi.org/10.1177/2150131916668115

Hing, E., Decker, S. L., & Jamoom, E. (2015). *Acceptance of new patients with public and private insurance by office-based physicians: United States, 2013* (NCHS Data Brief, No. 195). National Center for Health Statistics, Center for Disease Control and Prevention, U.S. Department of Health and Human Services. https://www.cdc.gov/nchs/data/databriefs/db195.pdf

Hinton, E., & Raphael, J. (2023). *10 things to know about Medicaid managed care. Issue Brief*. KFF. https://www.kff.org/medicaid/issue-brief/10-things-to-know-about-medicaid-managed-care/

Hirai, A. H., Kogan, M. D., Kandasamy, V., Reuland, C., & Bethell, C. (2018). Prevalence and variation of developmental screening and surveillance in early childhood. *JAMA Pediatrics*, *172*(9), 857–866. https://doi.org/10.1001/jamapediatrics.2018.1524

Hoagwood, K., Burns, B. J., Kiser, L., Ringeisen, H., & Schoenwald, S. K. (2001). Evidence-based practice in child and adolescent mental health services. *Psychiatric Services*, *52*(9), 1179–1189. https://doi.org/10.1176/appi.ps.52.9.1179

Hodgkinson, S., Godoy, L., Beers, L. S., & Lewin, A. (2017). Improving mental health access for low-income children and families in the primary care setting. *Pediatrics*, *139*(1), e20151175. https://doi.org/10.1542/peds.2015-1175

Hoffman, J. (2020). Mistrust of a coronavirus vaccine could imperil widespread immunity. *The New York Times*. https://www.nytimes.com/2020/07/18/health/coronavirus-anti-vaccine.html

Hoffmann, J. A., Alegría, M., Alvarez, K., Anosike, A., Shah, P. P., Simon, K. M., & Lee, L. K. (2022). Disparities in pediatric mental and behavioral health conditions. *Pediatrics*, *150*(4). https://doi.org/10.1542/peds.2022-058227

Hogan, J. M., Gabrielsen, K. R., Luna, & N., Grothaus, D. (2003). *Substance abuse prevention: The intersection of science and practice*. Pearson Education.

Hogue, A., Becker, S. J., Wenzel, K., Henderson, C. E., Bobek, M., Levy, S., & Fishman, M. (2021). Family involvement in treatment and recovery for substance use disorders among transition-age youth: Research bedrocks and opportunities. *Journal of Substance Abuse Treatment*, *129*, 108402. https://doi.org/10.1016/j.jsat.2021.108402

Hojat, M. (2007). *Empathy in patient care: Antecedents, development, measurement, and outcomes*. Springer.

Holen, S., Waaktaar, T., Lervåg, A., & Ystgaard, M. (2013). Implementing a universal stress management program for young school children: Are there classroom climate or academic effects? *Scandinavian Journal of Educational Research*, *57*(4), 420–444. https://doi.org/10.1080/00313831.2012.656320

Holgash, K., & Heberlein, M. (2019). *Physician acceptance of new Medicaid patients*. Medicaid and CHIP Payment and Access Commission. https://www.macpac.gov/wp-content/uploads/2019/01/Physician-Acceptance-of-New-MedicaidPatients.pdf

Holguin, M., Schickedanz, A., Olson, A., & Robinson, H. (2023, November 14). Personal communication.

Holland, M., Hawks, J., Morelli, L. C., & Khan, Z. (2021). Risk assessment and crisis intervention for youth in a time of telehealth. *Contemporary School Psychology*, *25*(1), 12–26. https://doi.org/10.1007/s40688-020-00341-6

Hollenbach, J. P., Simoneau, T., & Halterman, J. S. (2022). The promise of school-based asthma interventions. *Academic Pediatrics*, *22*(3), 385–386. https://doi.org/10.1016/j.acap.2021.11.006

Holm, J., Pagán, J. A., & Silver, D. (2024). The impact of Medicaid accountable care organizations on health care utilization, quality measures, health outcomes and costs from 2012 to 2023: A scoping review. *Medical Care Research and Review*. https://doi.org/10.1177/10775587241241984

Hong, Y. R., Huo, J., & Desai, R. (2023). Trends in pediatric primary care visits during the COVID-19 pandemic. *Family Medicine*, *55*(10), 1234–1242. https://doi.org/10.22454/FamMed.2023.0421hem

Hoon, D., Taylor, M. T., Kapadia, P., Gerhard, T., Strom, B. L., & Horton, D. B. (2019). Trends in off-label drug use in ambulatory settings: 2006–2015. *Pediatrics*, *144*(4). https://doi.org/10.1542/peds.2019-0896

Hoover, S., & Bostic, J. (2021). Schools as a vital component of the child and adolescent mental health system. *Psychiatric Services*, *72*(1), 37–48. https://doi.org/10.1176/appi.ps.201900575

Horn, I. B., Cora-Bramble, D., Cheng, T. L., Jenkins, R., Pachter, L., Joseph, J., & DC Baltimore Research Center on Child Health Disparities Writing Group. (2009). Starting early: A life-course perspective on child health disparities—Research recommendations. *Pediatrics, 124*(Suppl 3), S257–S261. https://doi.org/10.1542/peds.2009-1100O

Horvath, S., & Raj, K. (2018). DNA methylation-based biomarkers and the epigenetic clock theory of ageing. *Nature Reviews Genetics, 19*(6), 371–384. https://doi.org/10.1038/s41576-018-0004-3

Hospital for Special Surgery. (2023). *Lerner Children's Pavilion: Pediatric social work/case management services*. https://www.hss.edu/pediatric-social-work.asp

Houtrow, A. J., Carle, A., Perrin, J. M., & Stein, R. E. K. (2020). Children with special health care needs on supplemental security income for disability have more health impacts and needs than other children with special health care needs on Medicaid. *Academic Pediatrics, 20*(2), 258–266. https://doi.org/10.1016/j.acap.2019.10.014

Howard-Jones, A. R., Bowen, A. C., Danchin, M., Koirala, A., Sharma, K., Yeoh, D. K., Burgner, D. P., Crawford, N. W., Goeman, E., Gray, P. E., Hsu, P., Kuek, S., McMullan, B. J., Tosif, S., Wurzel, D., & Britton, P. N. (2022). COVID-19 in children: Epidemiology, prevention and indirect impacts. *Journal of Paediatrics and Child Health, 58*(1), 39–45. https://doi.org/10.1111/jpc.15791

Howell, E. M. (2001). The impact of the Medicaid expansions for pregnant women: A synthesis of the evidence. *Medical Care Research and Review, 58*(1), 3–30. https://doi.org/10.1177/107755870105800101

Howse, J. L. (2008). Marching forward: Action steps to optimize the health of women and babies. *Women's Health Issues, 18*(Suppl 6), S10–12. https://doi.org/10.1016/j.whi.2008.08.006

Hoyert, D. L. (2021). *Maternal mortality rates in the United States, 2021*. National Center for Health Statistics, Center for Disease Control and Prevention, U.S. Department of Health and Human Services. https://www.cdc.gov/nchs/data/hestat/maternal-mortality/2021/maternal-mortality-rates-2021.htm

Hoynes, H. Miller, D., & Simon, D. (2015). *Income, the earned income tax credit, and infant health*. American Economic Association. https://www.aeaweb.org/articles?id=10.1257/pol.20120179

Hoynes, H., Page, M., & Stevens, A. H. (2011). Can targeted transfers improve birth outcomes? Evidence from the introduction of the WIC program. *Journal of Public Economics, 95*(7–8), 813–827.

Hoynes, H., & Schanzenbach, D. W. (2015). *U.S. food and nutrition programs* (NBER Working Paper No. 21057). National Bureau of Economic Research. https://doi.org/10.3386/w21057

Hoynes, H., Schanzenbach, D. W., & Almond, D. (2016). Long-run impacts of childhood access to the safety net. *American Economic Review, 106*(4), 903–934.

Hsiung, H., Patel, K., Hundal, H., Baccouche, B. M., & Tsao, K. W. (2022). Preventing substance abuse in adolescents: A review of high-impact strategies. *Cureus Journal of Medical Science, 14*(7), e27361–e27361. https://doi.org/10.7759/cureus.27361

Hsu, C., Gray, M. F., Murray, L., Abraham, M., Nickel, W., Sweeney, J. M., Frosch, D. L., Mroz, T. M., Ehrlich, K., Johnson, B., & Reid, R. J. (2019). Actions and processes that patients, family members, and physicians associate with patient- and family-centered care. *BMC Family Practice, 20*(1), 35. https://doi.org/10.1186/s12875-019-0918-7

Hsu, H., Green, A. E., Wu, Y. P., & Lantos, J. D. (2023). Telehealth: Improving access to and quality of pediatric health care. *Pediatrics, 148*(3), e2021053129. https://doi.org/10.1542/peds.2021-053129

Hudson, J. L., & Moriya, A. S. (2017). Medicaid expansion for adults had measurable 'welcome mat' effects on their children. *Health Affairs, 36*(9), 1643–1651. https://doi.org/10.1377/hlthaff.2017.0347

Huecker, M. R., King, K. C., Jordan, G. A., & Smock, W. (2024). *Domestic violence*. StatPearls Publishing.

Hughes, K., Ford, K., Bellis, M. A., Glendinning, F., Harrison, E., & Passmore, J. (2021). Health and financial costs of adverse childhood experiences in 28 European countries: A systematic review and meta-analysis. *The Lancet Public Health*, *6*(11), e848–e857. https://doi.org/10.1016/S2468-2667(21)00232-2

Hughes, M., Joslyn, A., Mojton, M., O'Reilly, M., & Dworkin, P. (2016). Connecting vulnerable children and families to community-based programs strengthens parents' perceptions of protective factors. *Infants & Young Children*, *29*(2), 116–129. https://helpmegrownational.org/wp-content/uploads/2023/03/IYC_ProtectiveFactors-MHughes.pdf

Huhndorf, S. (2017). Native wisdom is revolutionizing health care. *Stanford Social Innovation Review*, *15*(3), 18–23. https://doi.org/10.48558/QE6T-WD62

Hulsey, E. G., Li, Y., Hacker, K., Williams, K., Collins, K., & Dalton, E. (2020). Potential emerging risks among children following parental opioid-related overdose death. *JAMA Pediatrics*, *174*(5), 503–504. https://doi.org/10.1001/jamapediatrics.2020.0613

Hurd, N., & Deutsch, N. (2017). SEL-focused after-school programs. *Future of Children*, *27*(1), 95–115. https://eric.ed.gov/?id=EJ1145092

Huss, G., Barak, S., Reali, L., Magendie, C., Carrasco-Sanz, A., Somekh, E., Cohen, R., Levy, C., Namazova-Baranova, L., Vural, M., & Pettoello-Mantovani, M. (2023). Drug shortages in pediatrics in Europe: The position of the European Pediatric Societies. *Journal of Pediatrics*, *261*, 113472. https://doi.org/10.1016/j.jpeds.2023.113472

Hussein, M., Pavlova, M., Ghalwash, M., & Groot, W. (2021). The impact of hospital accreditation on the quality of healthcare: A systematic literature review. *BMC Health Services Research*, *21*(1), 1057. https://doi.org/10.1186/s12913-021-07097-6

Hut, M. (2023). How hospitals improve health equity through community-centered innovation. *NEJM Catalyst*, *4*(2). https://doi.org/10.1056/CAT.22.0329

Hutchins, H. J., Barry, C. M., Wanga, V., Bacon, S., Njai, R., Claussen, A. H., Ghandour, R. M., Lebrun-Harris, L. A., Perkins, K., & Robinson, L. R. (2022). Perceived racial/ethnic discrimination, physical and mental health conditions in childhood, and the relative role of other adverse experiences. *Adversity and Resilience Science*, *3*(2), 181–194. https://doi.org/10.1007/s42844-022-00063-z

Hwang, T. J., Orenstein, L., DuBois, S. G., Janeway, K. A., & Bourgeois, F. T. (2020). Pediatric trials for cancer therapies with targets potentially relevant to pediatric cancers. *Journal of the National Cancer Institute*, *112*(3), 224–228. https://doi.org/10.1093/jnci/djz207

Iacopetta, D., Catalano, A., Ceramella, J., Pellegrino, M., Marra, M., Scali, E., Sinicropi, M. S., & Aquaro, S. (2024). The ongoing impact of COVID-19 on pediatric obesity. *Pediatric Reports*, *16*(1), 135–150. https://doi.org/10.3390/pediatric16010013

Ibeziako, P., Kaufman, K., Campbell, E., Zou, B., Samsel, C., Qayyum, Z., Caracansi, A., & Ray, A. (2024). Reducing pediatric mental health boarding and increasing acute care access. *Journal of the Academy of Consultation-Liaison Psychiatry*. https://doi.org/10.1016/j.jaclp.2024.04.001

Ibeziako, P., Kaufman, K., Scheer, K. N., & Sideridis, G. (2022). Pediatric mental health presentations and boarding: First year of the COVID-19 pandemic. *Hospital Pediatrics*, *12*(9), 751–760. https://doi.org/10.1542/hpeds.2022-006555

Ickes, A. (2023). *Top 10 lowest-paid physician specialties*. Becker's Physician Leadership. https://www.beckersphysicianleadership.com/physician-workforce/top-10-lowest-paid-physician-specialities.html

InCK Marks. (2018). *A sourcebook on Medicaid's role in early childhood: Advancing high performing medical homes and improving lifelong health*. https://www.inckmarks.org/docs/pdfs_for_Medicaid_and_EPSDT_page/SourcebookMEDICAIDYOUNGCHILDRENALL.pdf

________. (2020). *Young child health transformation: What practice tells us*. https://inckmarks.herokuapp.com/webinars/InCKMarksPracticeTransformationComponentfinalpdf.pdf

________. (2024). Exemplary and evidenced-based healthy parenting in primary care programs, practices, and systems change initiatives: Descriptions and summary from the NASEM healthy parenting in primary care scoping review. https://www.inckmarks.org/docs/7-15-2024/inck%20marks%20descriptions%20and%20summary%20for%20nasem%20scoping%20review.pdf

Indian Health Service (IHS). (n.d.a). *About IHS.* https://www.ihs.gov/aboutihs/

________. (n.d.b). *Anchorage service area.* https://www.ihs.gov/sites/alaska/themes/responsive2017/display_objects/documents/hf/asu.pdf

________. (2005). *Office of Urban Indian health programs 2022–2026 strategic plan.* https://www.ihs.gov/sites/newsroom/themes/responsive2017/display_objects/documents/2022_Letters/DTLL-DUIOLL-enclosure_04272022.pdf

________. (2020a). *IHS profile.* https://www.ihs.gov/newsroom/factsheets/ihsprofile/

________. (2020b). *National uniform data system summary report—2020.* https://www.ihs.gov/sites/urban/themes/responsive2017/display_objects/documents/2020_UIO_UDS_Summary_Report_Final.pdf

Individuals with Disabilities Education Act (IDEA), 20 U.S.C. § 1400 et seq. (2004).

Ingraham, C. (2014, October 29). Child poverty in the U.S. is among the worst in the developed world. *The Washington Post.* https://www.washingtonpost.com/news/wonk/wp/2014/10/29/child-poverty-in-the-u-s-is-among-the-worst-in-the-developed-world/

Initiative for a Competitive Inner City (ICIC). (2011). Inner city, anchor institutions and urban economic development: From community benefit to shared value. *Inner City Highlights, 1*(2). http://community-wealth.org/content/inner-city-anchor-institutions-and-urban-economic-development-community-benefit-shared-value

Institute of Medicine (IOM). (1993). *Emergency medical services for children.* National Academy Press. https://doi.org/10.17226/2137.

________. (1998). *America's children: Health insurance and access to care.* National Academy Press. https://doi.org/10.17226/6168

________. (2000). *To err is human: Building a safer health system.* National Academy Press.

________. (2003a). *The future of the public's health in the 21st century.* The National Academies Press. https://doi.org/10.17226/10548.

________. (2003b). *Unequal treatment: Confronting racial and ethnic disparities in health care.* The National Academies Press. https://doi.org/10.17226/12875

________. (2004). *In the nation's compelling interest: Ensuring diversity in the health-care workforce.* The National Academies Press. https://doi.org/10.17226/10885.

________. (2007a). *Emergency care for children: Growing pains.* The National Academies Press. https://doi.org/10.17226/11655.

________. (2007b). *The future of disability in America.* The National Academies Press. https://doi.org/10.17226/11898.

________. (2010). *The healthcare imperative: Lowering costs and improving outcomes* [Workshop Series Summary]. The National Academies Press. https://doi.org/10.17226/12750

________. (2011). *The future of nursing: Leading change, advancing health.* The National Academies Press.

________. (2012a). *Adverse effects of vaccines: Evidence and causality.* The National Academies Press. https://doi.org/10.17226/13164

________. (2012b). *For the public's health: Investing in a healthier future.* The National Academies Press. https://doi.org/10.17226/13268

________. (2012c). *Primary care and public health: Exploring integration to improve population health.* The National Academies Press. https://doi.org/10.17226/13381

________. (2015). *Vital signs: Core metrics for health and health care progress.* The National Academies Press. https://doi.org/10.17226/19402.

Institute for Patient- and Family-Centered Care (IPFCC). (n.d.). *Patient- and family-centered care*. https://www.ipfcc.org/about/pfcc.html

Institute of Human Development and Social Change. (n.d.). *SMART Beginnings*. New York University. https://steinhardt.nyu.edu/ihdsc/projects/smart

Insurance Institute for Highway Safety (IIHS). (2024). *Child safety*. https://www.iihs.org/topics/child-safety

Internal Revenue Service (IRS). (2023). *Community health needs assessment for charitable hospital organizations—Section 501(r)(3)*. Internal Revenue Service. https://www.irs.gov/charities-non-profits/community-health-needs-assessment-for-charitable-hospital-organizations-section-501r3

International Council of Nurses (ICN). (2022). *Nursing definitions*. https://www.icn.ch/nursing-policy/nursing-definitions

Isaacs, M. R., Huang, L. N., Hernandez, M., & Echo-Hawk, H. (2005). *The road to evidence: The intersection of evidence-based practices and cultural competence in children's mental health*. National Alliance of Multi-Ethnic Behavioral Health Associations. https://www.multiculturalmentalhealth.ca/wp-content/uploads/2013/10/Isaacs-RoadtoEvidence-93006.pdf

Isen, A., Rossin-Slater, M., & Walker, W. R. (2017). Every breath you take—Every dollar you'll make: The long-term consequences of the Clean Air Act of 1970. *Journal of Political Economy*, *125*(3), 848–902. https://doi.org/10.1086/691465

Israel, B. A., Schulz, A. J., Parker, E. A., & Becker, A. B. (1998). Review of community-based research: Assessing partnership approaches to improve public health. *Annual Review of Public Health*, *19*, 173–202. https://doi.org/10.1146/annurev.publhealth.19.1.173

Iton, A., Ross, R. K., & Tamber, P. S. (2022). Building community power to dismantle policy-based structural inequity in population health. *Health Affairs*, *41*(12), 1763–1771. https://doi.org/10.1377/hlthaff.2022.00540

Iverson, I. A., Cook, N. E., & Iverson, G. L. (2024). Adverse childhood experiences are associated with perceived cognitive difficulties among high school students in the United States [Brief Research Report]. *Frontiers in Psychology*, *15*. https://doi.org/10.3389/fpsyg.2024.1293013

Jablonski, K. A., & Guagliardo, M. F. (2005). Pediatric appendicitis rupture rate: A national indicator of disparities in healthcare access. *Population Health Metrics*, *3*(1). https://doi.org/10.1186/1478-7954-3-4

Jack, B. W., Atrash, H., Coonrod, D. V., Moos, M. K., O'Donnell, J., & Johnson, K. (2008). The clinical content of preconception care: An overview and preparation of this supplement. *American Journal of Obstetrics and Gynecology*, *199*(6, Suppl 2), S266–S279. https://doi.org/10.1016/j.ajog.2008.07.067

Jackson, D. B., Testa, A., & Vaughn, M. G. (2021). Adverse childhood experiences and school readiness among preschool-aged children. *Journal of Pediatrics*, *230*, 191–197.e195. https://doi.org/10.1016/j.jpeds.2020.11.023

Jacob, V., Chattopadhyay, S. K., Thota, A. B., Proia, K. K., Njie, G., Hopkins, D. P., Finnie, R. K. C., Pronk, N. P., & Kottke, T. E. (2015). Economics of team-based care in controlling blood pressure: A community guide systematic review. *American Journal of Preventive Medicine*, *49*(5), 772–783. https://doi.org/10.1016/j.amepre.2015.04.003

Jacobs, D. B., Schreiber, M., Seshamani, M., Tsai, D., Fowler, E., & Fleisher, L. A. (2023). Aligning quality measures across CMS—The Universal Foundation. *New England Journal of Medicine*, *388*(9), 776–779. https://doi.org/10.1056/NEJMp2215539

James, B., & Wright, E. (2015). *Children's commissioners and ombudsman offices*. First Focus on Children. https://firstfocus.org/resource/childrens-commissioners-and-ombudsman-offices/

James, G., Kasper, E., Wong, C. A., Anderson, D. M., Allin, S., Steiner, M. J., Flower, K. B., Kimberg, D., & Cholera, R. (2023). Investing in child health through alternative payment models: Lessons from North Carolina integrated care for kids. *Medical Care Research and Review*. https://doi.org/10.1177/10775587231217178

Jenkins, M. G., Ford, J. B., Morris, J. M., & Roberts, C. L. (2014). Women's expectations and experiences of maternity care in NSW—What women highlight as most important. *Women Birth*, *27*(3), 214–219. https://doi.org/10.1016/j.wombi.2014.03.002

Jenkins, P. C., Lin, A., Ames, S. G., Newgard, C. D., Lang, B., Winslow, J. E., Marin, J. R., Cook, J. N. B., Goldhaber-Fiebert, J. D., Papa, L., Zonfrillo, M. R., Hansen, M., Wall, S. P., Malveau, S., Kuppermann, N., & Pediatric Readiness Study Group. (2023). Emergency department pediatric readiness and disparities in mortality based on race and ethnicity. *JAMA Network Open*, *6*(9), e2332160. https://doi.org/10.1001/jamanetworkopen.2023.32160

Jenssen, B. P., Thayer, J., Nekrasova, E., Grundmeier, R. W., & Fiks, A. G. (2022). Innovation in the pediatric electronic health record to realize a more effective platform. *Current Problems in Pediatric and Adolescent Health Care*, *52*(1), 101109. https://doi.org/10.1016/j.cppeds.2021.101109

Jenssen, B. P., Walley, S. C., Boykan, R., Little Caldwell, A., & Camenga, D. (2023). Protecting children and adolescents from tobacco and nicotine. *Pediatrics*, *151*(5). https://doi.org/10.1542/peds.2023-061804

Jetty, A., Romano, M. J., Jabbarpour, Y., Petterson, S., & Bazemore, A. (2021). A cross-sectional study of factors associated with pediatric scope of care in family medicine. *Journal of the American Board of Family Medicine*, *34*(1), 196–207. https://doi.org/10.3122/jabfm.2021.01.200300

Jeyaraman, M., Balaji, S., Jeyaraman, N., & Yadav, S. (2023). Unraveling the Ethical Enigma: Artificial Intelligence in Healthcare. *Cureus, 15*(8), e43262. https://doi.org/10.7759/cureus.43262

Jimenez, M. E., Uthirasamy, N., Hemler, J. R., Bator, A., Malke, K., Lima, D., Strickland, P. O., Ramachandran, U., Crabtree, B. F., Hudson, S. V., Mackie, T. I., & Mendelsohn, A. L. (2023). Maximizing the impact of reach out and read literacy promotion: Anticipatory guidance and modeling. *Pediatric Research*. https://doi.org/10.1038/s41390-023-02945-z

Jo, A., Larson, S., Carek, P., Peabody, M. R., Peterson, L. E., & Mainous, A. G. (2019). Prevalence and practice for rare diseases in primary care: A national cross-sectional study in the USA. *BMJ Open*, *9*(4), e027248. https://doi.org/10.1136/bmjopen-2018-027248

Jobs and Growth Tax Relief Reconciliation Act of 2003, Pub. L. No. 108-27, 117 Stat. 752 (2003). https://www.congress.gov/108/plaws/publ27/PLAW-108publ27.pdf

Johns, M., & Rosenthal, J. (2022). *How investing in public health will strengthen America's health*. Center for American Progress. https://www.americanprogress.org/article/how-investing-in-public-health-will-strengthen-americas-health/

Johns Hopkins Medicine. (2023). *Johns Hopkins Children's Center: Social work*. https://www.hopkinsmedicine.org/johns-hopkins-childrens-center/patients-and-families/our-services/social-work

Johnson, K., & Bruner, C. (2018). *A sourcebook on Medicaid's role in early childhood advancing high performing medical homes and improving lifelong health*. Child & Family Policy Center. https://www.inckmarks.org/docs/pdfs_for_Medicaid_and_EPSDT_page/SourcebookMEDICAIDYOUNGCHILDRENALL.pdf

Johnson, K., Posner, S. F., Biermann, J., Cordero, J. F., Atrash, H. K., Parker, C. S., Boulee, S., & Curtis, M. G. (2006). Recommendations to improve preconception health and health care. *Morbidity and Mortality Weekly Report, 55*(RR06), 1–23. https://www.cdc.gov/mmwr/preview/mmwrhtml/rr5506a1.htm

Johnson, K., Willis, D., & Doyle, S. (2020). *Guide to leveraging opportunities between Title V and Medicaid for promoting social-emotional development.* Center for the Study of Social Policy. https://cssp.org/wp-content/uploads/2020/12/CSSP-Leveraging-TitlveV-FULL-REPORT.pdf

Johnson, M. L., Butts-Dion, S., Menon, M., Edwards, K., & Berns, S. D. (2021). Promoting social emotional development during the paediatric well-child visit: A demonstration project. *BMJ Open Quality*, *10*(2). https://doi.org/10.1136/bmjoq-2021-001392

Johnson, R. C. (2010). The health returns of education policies from preschool to high school and beyond. *American Economic Review: Papers & Proceedings* (pp. 188–194). https://www.aeaweb.org/articles?id=10.1257/aer.100.2.188

Johnson, S., Kasparian, N. A., Cullum, A. S., Flanagan, T., Ponting, C., Kowalewski, L., & Main, E. K. (2023). Addressing adverse childhood and adult experiences during prenatal care. *Obstetrics & Gynecology*, *141*(6), 1072–1087. https://doi.org/10.1097/aog.0000000000005199

Johnson, S. B., Spin, P., Connolly, F., Stein, M., Cheng, T. L., & Connor, K. (2019). Asthma and attendance in urban schools. *Preventing Chronic Disease*, *16*, 190074. http://dx.doi.org/10.5888/pcd16.190074

Johnson, T. J., Weaver, M. D., Borrero, S., Davis, E. M., Myaskovsky, L., Zuckerbraun, N. S., & Kraemer, K. L. (2013). Association of race and ethnicity with management of abdominal pain in the emergency department. *Pediatrics*, *132*(4), e851–858. https://doi.org/10.1542/peds.2012-3127

Johnson, T. J., Winger, D. G., Hickey, R. W., Switzer, G. E., Miller, E., Nguyen, M. B., Saladino, R. A., & Hausmann, L. R. (2017). Comparison of physician implicit racial bias toward adults versus children. *Academic Pediatrics*, *17*(2), 120–126. https://doi.org/10.1016/j.acap.2016.08.010

Joint Commission Resources. (2023). *High reliability health care maturity model*. https://www.jcrinc.com/what-we-offer/high-reliability/

Jolly, S., Griffith, K. A., DeCastro, R., Stewart, A., Ubel, P., & Jagsi, R. (2014). Gender differences in time spent on parenting and domestic responsibilities by high-achieving young physician-researchers. *Annals of Internal Medicine*, *160*(5), 344–353. https://doi.org/10.7326/m13-0974

Jonas, J. A., Leu, C. S., & Reznik, M. (2020). A randomized controlled trial of a community health worker delivered home-based asthma intervention to improve pediatric asthma outcomes. *Journal of Asthma*, *59*(2), 395–406. https://doi.org/10.1080/02770903.2020.1846746

Jones, B., Currin-Mcculloch, J., Pelletier, W., Sardi-Brown, V., Brown, P., & Wiener, L. (2018). Psychosocial standards of care for children with cancer and their families: A national survey of pediatric oncology social workers. *Social Work in Health Care*, *57*(4), 221–249. https://doi.org/10.1080/00981389.2018.1441212

Jones, C. M., Merrick, M. T., & Houry, D. E. (2020a). Identifying and preventing adverse childhood experiences: Implications for clinical practice. *Journal of the American Medical Association*, *323*(1), 25–26. https://doi.org/10.1001/jama.2019.18499

Jones, C. P. (2000). Levels of racism: A theoretic framework and a gardener's tale. *American Journal of Public Health*, *90*(8), 1212–1215. https://doi.org/10.2105/ajph.90.8.1212

Jones, C. P., Jones, C. Y., Perry, G. S., Barclay, G., & Jones, C. A. (2009). Addressing the social determinants of children's health: A cliff analogy. *Journal of Health Care for the Poor and Underserved*, *20*(Suppl 4), 1–12. https://doi.org/10.1353/hpu.0.0228

Jones, E. B., & Lucienne, T. M. (2023). The integrated care for kids model: Addressing fragmented care for pediatric Medicaid enrollees in seven communities. *Journal of Health Care for the Poor and Underserved*, *34*(1), 503–509. https://doi.org/10.1353/hpu.2023.0034

Jones, K., & Salzman, G. A. (2020). The vaping epidemic in adolescents. *Missouri Medicine*, *117*(1), 56–58.

Jones, L. J., VanWassenhove-Paetzold, J., Thomas, K., Bancroft, C., Ziatyk, E. Q., Kim, L. S., Shirley, A., Warren, A. C., Hamilton, L., George, C. V., Begay, M. G., Wilmot, T., Tsosie, M., Ellis, E., Selig, S. M., Gall, G., & Shin, S. S. (2020b). Impact of a fruit and vegetable prescription program on health outcomes and behaviors in young Navajo children. *Current Developments in Nutrition*, *4*(8), nzaa109.

Jones, N. (2022). *How an Ohio children's hospital built trust, fulfilled promises—and improved housing and health in its communities*. American Hospital Association. https://www.aha.org/news/healthcareinnovation-Thursday-blog/2022-03-17-how-ohio-childrens-hospital-built-trust

Jones, S. M., Barnes, S. P., Bailey, R., & Doolittle, E. J. (2017). Promoting social and emotional competencies in elementary school. *Future of Children*, *27*(1), 49–72. https://eric. ed.gov/?id=EJ1144815

Jones, S. M., Brown, J. L., & Lawrence Aber, J. (2011). Two-year impacts of a universal school-based social-emotional and literacy intervention: An experiment in translational developmental research. *Child Development*, *82*(2), 533–554.

Jones Harden, B., & Slopen, N. (2022). *Opportunity gaps in the social-emotional development, wellbeing, and mental health of children*. The National Academies Press.

Jongen, C., McCalman, J., & Bainbridge, R. (2018). Health workforce cultural competency interventions: A systematic scoping review. *BMC Health Services Research*, *18*. https://doi.org/10.1186/s12913-018-3001-5

Joo, J. Y., & Huber, D. L. (2017). Barriers in case managers' roles: A qualitative systematic review. *Western Journal of Nursing Research*, *40*(10), 1522–1542. https://doi.org/10.1177/0193945917728689

Jordan, A., Mathis, M. L., & Isom, J. (2020). Achieving mental health equity: Addictions. *Psychiatric Clinics of North America*, *43*(3), 487–500. https://doi.org/10.1016/j.psc.2020.05.007

Jordan, P., & Hernandez-Reif, M. (2009). Reexamination of young children's racial attitudes and skin tone preferences. *Journal of Black Psychology*, *35*(3), 388–403. https://doi.org/10.1177/0095798409333621

Joseph, A. M., Davis, B. S., & Kahn, J. M. (2023). Association between hospital consolidation and loss of pediatric inpatient services. *JAMA Pediatrics*, *177*(8), 859–860. https://doi.org/10.1001/jamapediatrics.2023.1747

Joseph, K. S., Boutin, A., Lisonkova, S., Muraca, G. M., Razaz, N., John, S., Mehrabadi, A., Sabr, Y., Ananth, C. V., & Schisterman, E. (2021). Maternal mortality in the United States: Recent trends, current status, and future considerations. *Obstetrics & Gynecology*, *137*(5), 763–771. https://doi.org/10.1097/aog.0000000000004361

Joseph, K. S., & Kramer, M. S. (1996). Review of the evidence on fetal and early childhood antecedents of adult chronic disease. *Epidemiologic Reviews*, *18*(2), 158–174. https://doi.org/10.1093/oxfordjournals.epirev.a017923

Joufi, A. I., Claiborne, D. M., & Shuman, D. (2021). Oral health education and promotion activities by Early Head Start programs in the United States: A systematic review. *Journal of Dental Hygiene*, *95*(5), 14–21.

Juszczak, L., Melinkovich, P., & Kaplan, D. (2003). Use of health and mental health services by adolescents across multiple delivery sites. *Journal of Adolescent Health*, *32*(6), 108–118.

Jyoti, D. F., Frongillo, E. A., & Jones, S. J. (2005). Food insecurity affects school children's academic performance, weight gain, and social skills. *Journal of Nutrition*, *135*(12), 2831–2839. https://doi.org/10.1093/jn/135.12.2831

Kaiser, J. (2024). Major budget cuts to two high-profile NIH efforts leave researchers reeling. *Science Insider*. https://www.science.org/content/article/major-budget-cuts-two-high-profile-nih-programs-leave-researchers-reeling

Kakani, P., Chandra, A., Mullainathan, S., & Obermeyer, Z. (2020). Allocation of COVID-19 relief funding to disproportionately Black counties. *Journal of the American Medical Association*, *324*(10), 1000–1003. https://doi.org/10.1001/jama.2020.14978

Kalil, A. (2013). Effects of the great recession on child development. *The Annals of the American Academy of Political and Social Science*, *650*(1), 232–250. https://doi.org/10.1177/0002716213500453

Kalmin, M. M., Cantor, J. H., Bravata, D. M., Ho, P., Whaley, C., & McBain, R. K. (2023). Utilization and spending on mental health services among children and youths with commercial insurance. *JAMA Network Open*, 6(10), e2336979. https://doi.org/10.1001/jamanetworkopen.2023.36979

Kaminski, J. W., Barrueco, S., Kelleher, K. J., K., H., Edwards, A., & Fox, E. G. (2023). Vital signs for pediatric health: School readiness [Discussion Paper]. *National Academy of Medicine Perspectives*.

Kaminski, J. W., & Claussen, A. H. (2017). Evidence base update for psychosocial treatments for disruptive behaviors in children. *Journal of Clinical Child & Adolescent Psychology*, *46*(4), 477–499. https://doi.org/10.1080/15374416.2017.1310044

Kampmann, B., Madhi, S. A., Munjal, I., Simões, E. A. F., Pahud, B. A., Llapur, C., Baker, J., Pérez Marc, G., Radley, D., Shittu, E., Glanternik, J., Snaggs, H., Baber, J., Zachariah, P., Barnabas, S. L., Fausett, M., Adam, T., Perreras, N., Van Houten, M. A., . . . Gurtman, A. (2023). Bivalent prefusion F vaccine in pregnancy to prevent RSV illness in infants. *New England Journal of Medicine*, *388*(16), 1451–1464. https://doi.org/10.1056/NEJMoa2216480

Kan Yeung, A. W., Torkamani, A., Butte, A. J., Glicksberg, B. S., Schuller, B., Rodriguez, B., W. Ting, D. S., Bates, D., Schaden, E., Peng, H., Willschke, H., Car, J., Rahimi, K., Celi, L. A., Banach, M., Kletecka-Pulker, M., Kimberger, O., Eils, R., Shariful Islam, S. M., . . . Atanasov, A. G. (2023). The promise of digital healthcare technologies. *Frontiers in Public Health*, *11*. https://doi.org/10.3389/fpubh.2023.1196596

Kandasamy, V., Hirai, A. H., Ghandour, R. M., & Kogan, M. D. (2018). Parental perception of flourishing in school-aged children: 2011-2012 National Survey of Children's Health. *Journal of Developmental and Behavioral Pediatrics*, *39*(6), 497–507. https://doi.org/10.1097/DBP.0000000000000559

Kang, Y., Zhang, F., Chatham-Stephens, K., Carter, R. J., & Vogt, T. (2023). Vaccines for chil dren provider practices in the COVID-19 vaccination program: Barriers to participation, intentions to offer COVID-19 vaccination to children aged <5 years, and vaccination promotion, United States, March 2022. *Clinical Pediatrics*, *62*(12), 1479–1488.

Kangovi, S., Mitra, N., Grande, D., Long, J. A., & Asch, D. A. (2020). Evidence-based community health worker program addresses unmet social needs and generates positive return on investment. *Health Affairs*, *39*(2), 207–213. https://doi.org/10.1377/hlthaff.2019.00981

Kanter, G. P., Nabet, B., Matone, M., & Rubin, D. M. (2020). Association of state Medicaid expansion with hospital community benefit spending. *JAMA Network Open*, *3*(5), e205529–e205529. https://doi.org/10.1001/jamanetworkopen.2020.5529

Kaplan, S. H., Greenfield, S., & Ware, J. E., Jr. (1989). Assessing the effects of physician-patient interactions on the outcomes of chronic disease. *Medical Care*, 27(Suppl 3), S110–S127. https://doi.org/10.1097/00005650-198903001-00010

Karaca-Mandic, P., Nikpay, S., Gibbons, S., Haynes, D., 2nd, Koranne, R., & Thakor, R. (2023). Proposing an innovative bond to increase investments in social drivers of health interventions in Medicaid managed care. *Health Affairs*, *42*(3), 383–391. https://doi.org/10.1377/hlthaff.2022.00821

Karamlou, T., Johnston, D. R., Backer, C. L., Roselli, E. E., Welke, K. F., Caldarone, C. A., & Svensson, L. G. (2020). Access or excess? Examining the argument for regionalized cardiac care. *The Journal of Thoracic and Cardiovascular Surgery*, *160*(1), 30465–30467. https://doi.org/10.1016/j.jtcvs.2020.03.065

Karron, R. A. (2023). RSV illness in the young and the old—The beginning of the end? *New England Journal of Medicine*, *388*(16), 1522–1524. https://doi.org/10.1056/NEJMe2302646

Kase, C., Hoover, S., Boyd, G., West, K. D., Dubenitz, J., Trivedi, P. A., Peterson, H. J., & Stein, B. D. (2017). Educational outcomes associated with school behavioral health interventions: A review of the literature. *Journal of School Health*, *87*(7), 554–562. https://doi.org/10.1111/josh.12524

Katkin, J. P., Kressly, S. J., Edwards, A. R., Perrin, J. M., Kraft, C. A., Richerson, J. E., Tieder, J. S., & Wall, L. (2017). Guiding principles for team-based pediatric care. *Pediatrics*, *140*(2). https://doi.org/10.1542/peds.2017-1489

Kaufman, J., Ryan, R., Walsh, L., Horey, D., Leask, J., Robinson, P., & Hill, S. (2018). Face-to-face interventions for informing or educating parents about early childhood vaccination. *The Cochrane Database of Systematic Reviews*, *5*(5), Cd010038. https://doi.org/10.1002/14651858.CD010038.pub3

Kearney, M. S. & Levine, P. B. (2023). The causes and consequences of declining US fertility. In Aspen Economic Strategy Group (Ed.), *Economic policy in a more uncertain world*. Aspen Institute. https://www.economicstrategygroup.org/wp-content/uploads/2022/08/Kearney_Levine_081222.pdf

Keehan, S. P., Fiore, J. A., Poisal, J. A., Cuckler, G. A., Sisko, A. M., Smith, S. D., Madison, A. J., & Rennie, K. E. (2023). National health expenditure projections, 2022–31: Growth to stabilize once the COVID-19 public health emergency ends. *Health Affairs*, *42*(7), 886–898. https://doi.org/10.1377/hlthaff.2023.00403

Keeton, V., Soleimanpour, S., & Brindis, C. D. (2012). School-based health centers in an era of health care reform: Building on history. *Current Problems in Pediatric and Adolescent Health Care*, *42*(4), 132–156. https://doi.org/10.1016/j.cppeds.2012.03.002

Keikha, M., Jahanfar, S., & Hemati, Z. (2022). A neglected critical time to prevent maternal and offspring's adverse outcomes: The preconception period. *International Journal of Reproductive Biomedicine*, *20*(1), 65–67. https://doi.org/10.18502/ijrm.v20i1.10237

Keisler-Starkey, K., & Bunch, L. N. (2022). *Health insurance coverage in the United States: 2021*. U.S. Census Bureau. https://www.census.gov/content/dam/Census/library/publications/2022/demo/p60-278.pdf

Keisler-Starkey, K., Bunch, L. N., & U.S. Census Bureau. (2020). Health insurance coverage in the United States: 2019. *Current Population Reports*. U.S. Government Publishing Office.

Kellam, S. G., Mackenzie, A. C., Brown, C. H., Poduska, J. M., Wang, W., Petras, H., & Wilcox, H. C. (2011). The good behavior game and the future of prevention and treatment. *Addiction Science & Clinical Practice*, *6*(1), 73–84.

Kellerman, R., & Kirk, L. (2007). Principles of the patient-centered medical home. *American Family Physician*, *76*(6), 774–775.

Kelly, E., Ivers, N., Zawi, R., Barnieh, L., Manns, B., Lorenzetti, D. L., Nicholas, D., Tonelli, M., Hemmelgarn, B., Lewanczuk, R., Edwards, A., Braun, T., & McBrien, K. A. (2015). Patient navigators for people with chronic disease: Protocol for a systematic review and meta-analysis. *Systematic Reviews*, *4*, 28. https://doi.org/10.1186/s13643-015-0019-1

Kemper, A. R., Kelleher, K. J., Allen, S., Sander, C., & Brilli, R. J. (2020). Improving the health of all children in our community: The nationwide children's hospital and Franklin County, Ohio, Pediatric Vital Signs Project. *Journal of Pediatrics*, *222*, 227–230. https://doi.org/10.1016/j.jpeds.2020.03.049

Kemper, A. R., Uren, R. L., & Clark, S. J. (2006). Adoption of electronic health records in primary care pediatric practices. *Pediatrics*, *118*(1), e20–e24. https://doi.org/10.1542/peds.2005-3000

Kennedy-Moulton, K., Miller, S., Persson, P., Rossin-Slater, M., Wherry, L., & Aldana, G. (2022). *Maternal and infant health inequality: New evidence from linked administrative data*. National Bureau of Economic Research. https://www.nber.org/papers/w30693

Kepple, N. J. (2018). Does parental substance use always engender risk for children? Comparing incidence rate ratios of abusive and neglectful behaviors across substance use behavior patterns. *Child Abuse & Neglect*, *76*, 44–55. https://doi.org/10.1016/j.chiabu.2017.10.004

Kerasidou, A., Bærøe, K., Berger, Z., & Caruso Brown, A. E. (2020). The need for empathetic healthcare systems. *Journal of Medical Ethics*, *47*(12), e27. https://doi.org/10.1136/medethics-2019-105921

Kern, L., Mathur, S., Albrecht, S., Poland, S., Rozalski, M., & Skiba, R. (2017). The need for school-based mental health services and recommendations for implementation. *School Mental Health*, *9*, 1–13. https://doi.org/10.1007/s12310-017-9216-5

Kerns, S. E. U., Pullman, M. D., Walker, S. C., Lyon, A. R., Cosgrove, T. J., & Brungs, E. J. (2011). Adolescent use of school-based health centers and high school dropout. *Archives of Pediatrics & Adolescent Medicine*, *165*(7), 617–623. https://doi.org/10.1001/archpediatrics.2011.76

Kessler, R. C., Adler, L., Barkley, R., Biederman, J., Conners, C. K., Demler, O., Faraone, S. V., Greenhill, L. L., Howes, M. J., Secnik, K., Spencer, T., Ustun, T. B., Walters, E. E., & Zaslavsky, A. M. (2006). The prevalence and correlates of adult ADHD in the United States: Results from the national comorbidity survey replication. *American Journal of Psychiatry*, *163*(4), 716–723. https://doi.org/10.1176/ajp.2006.163.4.716

Key, J., Burnett, D., Babu, J. R., & Geetha, T. (2023). The effects of food environment on obesity in children: A systematic review. *Children*, *10*(1). https://doi.org/10.3390/children10010098

Key, J., Washington, E., & Hulsey, T. (2002). Reduced emergency department utilization associated with school-based clinic enrollment. *Journal of Adolescent Health, 30*(4), 273–278. https://doi.org/10.1016/S1054-139X(01)00390-1

KFF. (n.d.). *State health facts*. https://www.kff.org/statedata/

________. (2016). *Michigan's Medicaid section 1115 waiver to address effects of lead exposure in Flint*. https://www.kff.org/medicaid/fact-sheet/michigans-medicaid-section-1115-waiver-to-address-effects-of-lead-exposure-in-flint/

________. (2019). *Medicaid and CHIP eligibility, enrollment, and cost sharing policies as of January 2019: Findings from a 50-state survey*. https://www.kff.org/medicaid/report/medicaid-and-chip-eligibility-enrollment-and-cost-sharing-policies-as-of-january-2019-findings-from-a-50-state-survey/

________. (2021). *2021 Employer health benefits survey*. https://www.kff.org/report-section/ehbs-2021-section-3-employee-coverage-eligibility-and-participation/

________. (2023a). *Key facts on health coverage of immigrants*. https://www.kff.org/racial-equity-and-health-policy/fact-sheet/key-facts-on-health-coverage-of-immigrants/

________. (2023b). *Medicaid/CHIP coverage of lawfully-residing immigrant children and pregnant women*. https://www.kff.org/affordable-care-act/state-indicator/medicaid-chip-coverage-of-lawfully-residing-immigrant-children-and-pregnant-women/?currentTimeframe=0&sortModel=%7B%22colId%22:%22Location%22,%22sort%22:%22asc%22%7D

________. (2023c). *States that reported accountable care organizations in place*. https://www.kff.org/medicaid/state-indicator/states-that-reported-accountable-care-organizations-in-place/?currentTimeframe=0&sortModel=%7B%22colId%22:%22Location%22,%22sort%22:%22asc%22%7D

________. (2024). *Status of state Medicaid expansion decisions: Interactive map*. https://www.kff.org/affordable-care-act/state-indicator/state-activity-around-expanding-medicaid-under-the-affordable-care-act/?currentTimeframe=0&sortModel=%7B%22colId%22:%22Location%22,%22sort%22:%22asc%22%7D

Khadka, A., Fink, G., Gromis, A., & McConnell, M. (2020). In utero exposure to threat of evictions and preterm birth: Evidence from the United States. *Health Services Research, 55*(Suppl 2), 823–832. https://doi.org/10.1111/1475-6773.13551

Khan, A., Ramotar, M., & Landrigan, C. (2019). *Does a patient- and family-centered hospital communications program reduce medical errors?* Patient-Centered Outcomes Research Institute. https://doi.org/10.25302/8.2019.CDR.130603556

Khanani, I., Elam, J., Hearn, R., Jones, C., & Maseru, N. (2010). The impact of prenatal WIC participation on infant mortality and racial disparities. *American Journal of Public Health, 100*(Suppl 1), S204–S209.

Khekade, H., Potdukhe, A., Taksande, A. B., Wanjari, M. B., & Yelne, S. (2023). Preconception care: A strategic intervention for the prevention of neonatal and birth disorders. *Cureus Journal of Medical Science, 15*(6). https://doi.org/10.7759/cureus.41141

Khera, A. V., Chaffin, M., Wade, K. H., Zahid, S., Brancale, J., Xia, R., Distefano, M., Senol-Cosar, O., Haas, M. E., Bick, A., Aragam, K. G., Lander, E. S., Smith, G. D., Mason-Suares, H., Fornage, M., Lebo, M., Timpson, N. J., Kaplan, L. M., & Kathiresan, S. (2019). Polygenic prediction of weight and obesity trajectories from birth to adulthood. *Cell, 177*(3), 587–596.e589. https://doi.org/10.1016/j.cell.2019.03.028

Kids Count Data Center. (2020). *Kids count data center.* https://datacenter.aecf.org/

________. (2023a). *Children below 200% poverty in the United States.* Annie E. Casey Foundation. https://datacenter.aecf.org/data/tables/47-children-below-200-poverty#detailed/1/any/false/1095,2048,1729,37,871,870,573,869,36,868/any/329,330

________. (2023b). *Total population by child and adult populations.* Annie E. Casey Foundation. https://datacenter.aecf.org/data?location=USA#USA/1/0/char/0

________. (2023c). *Children in immigrant families in the United States.* Annie E. Casey Foundation. https://datacenter.aecf.org/data/tables/115-children-in-immigrant-families#detailed/1/any/false/1095,2048,1729,37,871,870,573,869,36,868/any/445,446

Kim, J., Cai, Z. R., Chen, M. L., Simard, J. F., & Linos, E. (2023). Assessing biases in medical decisions via clinician and AI chatbot responses to patient vignettes. *JAMA Network Open*, *6*(10), e2338050. doi:10.1001/jamanetworkopen.2023.38050

Kim, J., Yon, M., Lee, Y., Moon, I., Hong, J., & Hyun, T. (2017). Preconceptional use of folic acid and knowledge about folic acid among low-income pregnant women in Korea. *Nutrition Research and Practice*, *11*(3), 240–246. https://doi.org/10.4162/nrp.2017.11.3.240

Kim, O. (2019). Establishing a children's commissioner: Lessons from Australia on creating an oversight body for children's issues. *First Focus on Children.* https://firstfocus.org/resource/establishing-a-childrens-commissioner-lessons-from-australia-on-creating-an-oversight-body-for-childrens-issues/

King, C. A., Beetham, T., Smith, N., Englander, H., Button, D., Brown, P. C. M., Hadland, S. E., Bagley, S. M., Wright, O. R., Korthuis, P. T., & Cook, R. (2024). Adolescent residential addiction treatment in the US: Uneven access, waitlists, and high costs. *Health Affairs*, *43*(1), 64–71. https://doi.org/10.1377/hlthaff.2023.00777

King, K. A., Strunk, C. M., & Sorter, M. T. (2011). Preliminary effectiveness of surviving the Teens® Suicide Prevention and Depression Awareness Program on adolescents' suicidality and self-efficacy in performing help-seeking behaviors. *Journal of School Health*, *81*(9), 581–590. https://doi.org/10.1111/j.1746-1561.2011.00630.x

King, T., & Fazel, M. (2021). Examining the mental health outcomes of school-based peer-led interventions on young people: A scoping review of range and a systematic review of effectiveness. *PLoS One*, *16*(4), e0249553. https://doi.org/10.1371/journal.pone.0249553

Kingsmore, S. F., & Cole, F. S. (2022). The role of genome sequencing in neonatal intensive care units. *Annual Review of Genomics and Human Genetics*, *23*, 427–448. https://doi.org/10.1146/annurev-genom-120921-103442

Kioumourtzoglou, M. A., Coull, B. A., O'Reilly, É. J., Ascherio, A., & Weisskopf, M. G. (2018). Association of exposure to diethylstilbestrol during pregnancy with multigenerational neurodevelopmental deficits. *JAMA Pediatrics*, *172*(7), 670–677. https://doi.org/10.1001/jamapediatrics.2018.0727

Kirby, T., Connell, R., & Linneman, T. (2021). Assessment of the impact of an opioid-specific education series on rates of medication-assisted treatment for opioid use disorder in veterans. *American Journal of Health-System Pharmacy*, *78*(4), 301–309. https://doi.org/10.1093/ajhp/zxaa386

Kirkbride, J. B., Anglin, D. M., Colman, I., Dykxhoorn, J., Jones, P. B., Patalay, P., Pitman, A., Soneson, E., Steare, T., Wright, T., & Griffiths, S. L. (2024). The social determinants of mental health and disorder: Evidence, prevention and recommendations. *World Psychiatry, 23*(1), 58. https://doi.org/10.1002/wps.21160

Kjolhede, C., Lee, A. C., De Pinto, C. D., O'Leary, S. C., Baum, M., Beers, N. S., Bode, S. M., Gibson, E. J., Gorski, P., Jacob, V., Larkin, M., Christopher, R., Schumacher, H., & Council on School Health. (2021). School-based health centers and pediatric practice. *Pediatrics*, *148*(4), e2021053758. https://doi.org/10.1542/peds.2021-053758

Klass, P., Dreyer, B. P., & Mendelsohn, A. L. (2009). Reach out and read: Literacy promotion in pediatric primary care. *Advances in Pediatrics*, *56*, 11–27. https://doi.org/10.1016/j.yapd.2009.08.009

Klein, J. D., & Wilson, K. M. (2002). Delivering quality care: Adolescents' discussion of health risks with their providers. *Journal of Adolescent Health*, *30*(3), 190–195. https://doi.org/10.1016/s1054-139x(01)00342-1

Kleinman, J. C., Pierre, M. B., Jr., Madans, J. H., Land, G. H., & Schramm, W. F. (1988). The effects of maternal smoking on fetal and infant mortality. *American Journal of Epidemiology*, *127*(2), 274–282. https://doi.org/10.1093/oxfordjournals.aje.a114803

Klitzman, R. L., & Kelmenson, A. M. (2020). Experiment on identical siblings separated at birth: Ethical implications for researchers, universities, and archives today. *Journal of Medical Ethics*, *47*, 657–661.

Klonsky, E. D. (2007). The functions of deliberate self-injury: A review of the evidence. *Clinical Psychology Review*, *27*(2), 226–239. https://doi.org/10.1016/j.cpr.2006.08.002

Klonsky, E. D., Victor, S. E., & Saffer, B. Y. (2014). Nonsuicidal self-injury: What we know, and what we need to know. *Canadian Journal of Psychiatry*, *59*(11), 565–568. https://doi.org/10.1177/070674371405901101

Klugman, D., Melton, K., Maynord, P. O., Dawson, A., Madhavan, G., Montgomery, V. L., Nock, M., Lee, A., & Lyren, A. (2020). Assessment of an unplanned extubation bundle to reduce unplanned extubations in critically ill neonates, infants, and children. *JAMA Pediatrics*, *174*(6), e200268. https://doi.org/10.1001/jamapediatrics.2020.0268

Knifton, L., & Inglis, G. (2020). Poverty and mental health: Policy, practice and research implications. *BJPsych Bulletin*, *44*(5), 193–196. https://doi.org/10.1192/bjb.2020.78

Knopf, A. (2013). School-based telehealth brings psychiatry to rural Georgia. *Behavioral Healthcare*, *33*(1), 47–48.

Knopf, J. A., Finnie, R. K. C., Peng, Y., Hahn, R. A., Truman, B. I., Vernon-Smiley, M., Johnson, V. C., Johnson, R. L., Fielding, J. E., Muntaner, C., Hunt, P. C., Phyllis Jones, C., Fullilove, M. T., & Community Preventive Services Task Force. (2016). School-based health centers to advance health equity: A community guide systematic review. *American Journal of Preventive Medicine*, *51*(1), 114–126. https://doi.org/10.1016/j.amepre.2016.01.009

Knudsen, E. I. (2004). Sensitive periods in the development of the brain and behavior. *Journal of Cognitive Neuroscience*, *16*(8), 1412–1425. https://doi.org/10.1162/0898929042304796

Kodros, J. K., Bell, M. L., Dominici, F., L'Orange, C., Godri Pollitt, K. J., Weichenthal, S., Wu, X., & Volckens, J. (2022). Unequal airborne exposure to toxic metals associated with race, ethnicity, and segregation in the USA. *Nature Communications*, *13*(1), 6329. https://doi.org/10.1038/s41467-022-33372-z

Koening, K. T., Ramos, M. M., Fowler, T. T., Oreskovich, K., McGrath, J., & Fairbrother, G. A. (2018). Statewide profile of frequent users of school-based health centers: Implications for adolescent health care. *Journal of School Health*, *86*(4), 250–257.

Kogan, M. D., Dykton, C., Hirai, A. H., Strickland, B. B., Bethell, C. D., Naqvi, I., Cano, C. E., Downing-Futrell, S. L., & Lu, M. C. (2015). A new performance measurement system for maternal and child health in the United States. *Maternal and Child Health Journal*, *19*(5), 945–957. https://doi.org/10.1007/s10995-015-1739-5

Kogan, M. D., Newacheck, P. W., Blumberg, S. J., Ghandour, R. M., Singh, G. K., Strickland, B. B., & van Dyck, P. C. (2010). Underinsurance among children in the United States. *New England Journal of Medicine*, *363*(9), 841–851. https://doi.org/10.1056/NEJMsa0909994

Koh, H. K., Bantham, A., Geller, A. C., Rukavina, M. A., Emmons, K. M., Yatsko, P., & Restuccia, R. (2020). Anchor institutions: Best practices to address social needs and social determinants of health. *American Journal of Public Health*, *110*(3), 309–316. https://doi.org/10.2105/ajph.2019.305472

Kolko, D. J., & Perrin, E. (2014). The integration of behavioral health interventions in children's health care: Services, science, and suggestions. *Journal of Clinical Child & Adolescent Psychology*, *43*(2), 216–228. https://doi.org/10.1080/15374416.2013.862804

Kompaniyets, L., Pennington, A. F., Goodman, A. B., Rosenblum, H. G., Belay, B., Ko, J. Y., Chevinsky, J. R., Schieber, L. Z., Summers, A. D., Lavery, A. M., Preston, L. E., Danielson, M. L., Cui, Z., Namulanda, G., Yusuf, H, MacKenzie, W. R., Wong, K. K., Baggs, J., Boehmer, T. K., & Gundlapalli, A. V. (2021). Underlying medical conditions and severe illness among 540,667 adults hospitalized with COVID-19, March 2020–March 2021. *Preventing Chronic Disease*, *18*, 210123. http://dx.doi.org/10.5888/pcd18.210123

Koppaka, R. (2011a). Ten great public health achievements—United States, 2001–2010. *Morbidity and Mortality Weekly Report*, *60*(19), 619–623. Centers for Disease Control and Prevention. https://www.cdc.gov/mmwr/preview/mmwrhtml/mm6019a5.htmhttps://www.cdc.gov/mmwr/preview/mmwrhtml/mm6019a5.htm?s_cid=mm6019a5_w

_______. (2011b). Ten great public health achievements—Worldwide, 2001–2010. *Morbidity and Mortality Weekly Report*, *60*(24), 814–818. Centers for Disease Control and Prevention. https://www.cdc.gov/mmwr/preview/mmwrhtml/mm6024a4.htmhttps://stacks.cdc.gov/view/cdc/107650

Koskinen, J. S., Kytö, V., Juonala, M., Viikari, J. S. A., Nevalainen, J., Kähönen, M., Lehtimäki, T., Laitinen, T. P., Tossavainen, P., Jokinen, E., Magnussen, C. G., & Raitakari, O. T. (2023). Childhood dyslipidemia and carotid atherosclerotic plaque in adulthood: The cardiovascular risk in young Finns study. *Journal of the American Heart Association: Cardiovascular and Cerebrovascular Disease*, *12*(7). https://doi.org/10.1161/JAHA.122.027586

Kottke, T. E., Gallagher, J. M., Rauri, S., Tillema, J. O., Pronk, N. P., & Knudson, S. M. (2016). New summary measures of population health and well-being for implementation by health plans and accountable care organizations. *Preventing Chronic Disease*, *13*, E89. https://doi.org/10.5888/pcd13.160224

Kraft, D. (2023). *Scientific advancements and the future of health care delivery*. National Academies of Sciences, Engineering, and Medicine. https://www.nationalacademies.org/event/09-07-2023/improving-the-health-and-wellbeing-of-children-and-youth-through-health-care-system-transformation-committee-meeting-4

Krantz, L. M., Stanko-Lopp, D., Kuntz, M. J., & Wilcox, H. C. P. (2023). A guide for schools on student-directed suicide prevention programs eligible for implementation under the STANDUP Act, a rapid review and evidence synthesis. *Archives of Suicide Research*, 1–23. https://doi.org/10.1080/13811118.2023.2247033

Krieger, J., & Higgins, D. L. (2002). Housing and health: Time again for public health action. *American Journal of Public Health*, *92*(5), 758–768. https://doi.org/10.2105/ajph.92.5.758

Kristjánsson, L. Á., Sigfúsdóttir, D. I., & Allegrante, J. P. (2010). Health behavior and academic achievement among adolescents: The relative contribution of dietary habits, physical activity, body mass index, and self-esteem. *Health Education & Behavior*, *37*(1), 51–64.

Kronick, R. (2016). AHRQ's role in improving quality, safety, and health system performance. *Public Health Reports*, *131*(2), 229–232. https://doi.org/10.1177/003335491613100205

Krugman, S. (1986). The Willowbrook hepatitis studies revisited: Ethical aspects. *Reviews of Infectious Diseases*, *8*(1), 157–162. https://doi.org/10.1093/clinids/8.1.157

Krugman, S., Hodo, L. N., Morgan, Z. J., & Eden, A. R. (2023). Challenges meeting training requirements in the care of children in family medicine residency programs: A CERA study. *Family Medicine*, *55*(4), 238–244. https://doi.org/10.22454/FamMed.2023.761754

Kubb, C., & Foran, H. M. (2020). Online health information seeking by parents for their children: Systematic review and agenda for further research. *Journal of Medical Internet Research*, *22*(8), e19985. https://doi.org/10.2196/19985

Kugelmass, H. (2016). "Sorry, I'm not accepting new patients": An audit study of access to mental health care. *Journal of Health and Social Behavior*, *57*(2), 168–183. https://doi.org/10.1177/0022146516647098

Kuhlthau, K. A., Ames, S. G., Ware, A., Hoover, C. G., Wells, N., & Shelton, C. (2022). Research on family health and children and youth with special health care needs. *Academic Pediatrics*, *22*(2), S22–S27. https://doi.org/10.1016/j.acap.2021.07.019

Kuhlthau, K. A., Bloom, S., Van Cleave, J., Knapp, A. A., Romm, D., Klatka, K., Homer, C. J., Newacheck, P. W., & Perrin, J. M. (2011). Evidence for family-centered care for children with special health care needs: A systematic review. *Academic Pediatrics*, *11*(2), 136–143. https://doi.org/10.1016/j.acap.2010.12.014

Kuhlthau, K. A., & Perrin, J. M. (2001). Child health status and parental employment. *Archives of Pediatrics & Adolescent Medicine*, *155*(12), 1346–1350. https://doi.org/10.1001/archpedi.155.12.1346

Kullgren, J. T., Galbraith, A. A., Hinrichsen, V. L., Miroshnik, I., Penfold, R. B., Rosenthal, M. B., Landon, B. E., & Lieu, T. A. (2010). Health care use and decision making among lower-income families in high-deductible health plans. *Archives of Internal Medicine*, *170*(21), 1918–1925. https://doi.org/10.1001/archinternmed.2010.428

Kuo, D. Z., Cohen, E., Agrawal, R., Berry, J. G., & Casey, P. H. (2011). A national profile of caregiver challenges among more medically complex children with special health care needs. *Archives of Pediatrics & Adolescent Medicine*, *165*(11), 1020–1026. https://doi.org/10.1001/archpediatrics.2011.172

Kuo, D. Z., Houtrow, A. J., Arango, P., Kuhlthau, K. A., Simmons, J. M., & Neff, J. M. (2012). Family-centered care: Current applications and future directions in pediatric health care. *Maternal and Child Health Journal*, *16*(2), 297–305. https://doi.org/10.1007/s10995-011-0751-7

Kushel, M. B., Gupta, R., Gee, L., & Haas, J. S. (2006). Housing instability and food insecurity as barriers to health care among low-income Americans. *Journal of General Internal Medicine*, *21*(1), 71–77. https://doi.org/10.1111/j.1525-1497.2005.00278.x

Kusma, J., & Davis, M. M. (2021). Questioning the value of high-deductible health plans for children with chronic conditions. *JAMA Pediatrics*, *175*(8), 778–781. https://doi.org/10.1001/jamapediatrics.2021.0752

Kwong, M. W. (2024). *Tool: Telehealth policy finder.* Public Health Institute. https://www.phi.org/thought-leadership/state-telehealth-laws-and-reimbursement-program-policies/

La Charite, J., Khan, M., Dudovitz, R., Nuckols, T., Sastry, N., Huang, C., Lei, Y., & Schickedanz, A. (2023). Specific domains of positive childhood experiences (PCEs) associated with improved adult health: A nationally representative study. *SSM- Population Health*, *24*. https://doi.org/10.1016/j.ssmph.2023.101558

Lalloo, C., Diskin, C., Ho, M., Orkin, J., Cohen, E., Osei-Twum, J., Hundert, A., Jiwan, A., Sivarajah, S., Gumapac, A., & Stinson, J. N. (2020). Pediatric Project ECHO: Implementation of a virtual medical education program to support community management of children with medical complexity. *Hospital Pediatrics*, *10*(12), 1044–1052. https://doi.org/10.1542/hpeds.2020-0067

Lande, M., Kczorowski, J., Auinger, P., Scwartz, G., & Weitzman, M. (2003). Elevated blood pressure and decreased cognitive function among school-age children and adolescents in the United States. *Journal of Pediatrics*, *143*(6), 720–724.

Landers, G. M., Minyard, K. J., Lanford, D., & Heishman, H. (2020). A theory of change for aligning health care, public health, and social services in the time of COVID-19. *American Journal of Public Health*, *110*(S2), S178–S180. https://doi.org/10.2105/ajph.2020.305821

Lange, S. J., Kompaniyets, L., Freedman, D. S., Kraus, E. M., Porter, R., DNP3, Blanck, H. M., & Goodman, A.B. (2021). Longitudinal trends in body mass index before and during the COVID-19 pandemic among persons aged 2-19 years—United States, 2018-2020. *Morbidity and Mortality Weekly Report*, *70*(37), 1278–1283. https://doi.org/10.15585/mmwr.mm7037a3

Lansky, D., & Bethell, C. (2001). Empowering consumers to make informed choices. In D. B. Nash, *Connecting with the new healthcare consumer* (pp. 265–286). McGraw-Hill. https://www.cahmi.org/docs/default-source/default-document-library/_consumer-engagement-and-information-framework-book-chapter.pdf?sfvrsn=885c2f3b_0

Larcher, V. (2005). ABC of adolescence: Consent, competence, and confidentiality. *BMJ: British Medical Journal*, *330*(7487), 353–356. https://doi.org/10.1136/bmj.330.7487.353

Larsen, B., & Luna, B. (2018). Adolescence as a neurobiological critical period for the development of higher-order cognition. *Neuroscience and Biobehavioral Reviews*, *94*, 179–195. https://doi.org/10.1016/j.neubiorev.2018.09.005

Larson, K., Gottschlich, E. A., Cull, W. L., & Olson, L. M. (2021). High-deductible health plans for US children: Trends, health service use, and financial barriers to care. *Academic Pediatrics*, *21*(8), 1345–1354. https://doi.org/10.1016/j.acap.2021.03.001

Laspro, M., Groysman, L., Verzella, A. N., Kimberly, L. L., & Flores, R. L. (2023). The use of virtual reality in surgical training: Implications for education, patient safety, and global health equity. *Surgeries*, *4*(4), 635–646. https://doi.org/10.3390/surgeries4040061

Lassaletta, Á., Morales, J. S., Valenzuela, P. L., Esteso, B., Kahalley, L. S., Mabbott, D. J., Unnikrishnan, S., Panizo, E., & Calvo, F. (2023). Neurocognitive outcomes in pediatric brain tumors after treatment with proton versus photon radiation: A systematic review and meta-analysis. *World Journal of Pediatrics*, *19*(8), 727–740. https://doi.org/10.1007/s12519-023-00726-6

Lassi, Z. S., Kumar, R., & Bhutta, Z. A. (2016). Community-based care to improve maternal, newborn, and child health. *The International Bank for Reconstruction and Development and The World Bank*. https://www.ncbi.nlm.nih.gov/books/NBK361898/

Laurant, M., van der Biezen, M., Wijers, N., Watananirun, K., Kontopantelis, E., & van Vught, A. J. (2018). Nurses as substitutes for doctors in primary care. *The Cochrane Database of Systematic Reviews*, *7*(7), Cd001271. https://doi.org/10.1002/14651858.CD001271.pub3

Lavarreda, S. A., Brown, E. R., & Bolduc, C. D. (2011). Underinsurance in the United States: An interaction of costs to consumers, benefit design, and access to care. *Annual Review of Public Health*, *32*, 471–482. https://doi.org/10.1146/annurev.publhealth.012809.103655

LaVeist, T. A., Gaskin, D., & Richard, P. (2011). Estimating the economic burden of racial health inequalities in the United States. *International Journal of Health Services*, *41*(2), 231–238. https://doi.org/10.2190/hs.41.2.c

Law, W. C., McClanahan, R., & Weismuller, P. C. (2017). Depression screening in the school setting: Identification of the depressed adolescent. *NASN School Nurse*, *32*(6), 364–370. https://doi.org/10.1177/1942602X17726095

Lawrence, J. (2000). The Indian Health Service and the sterilization of Native American women. *American Indian Quarterly*, *24*(3), 400–419. http://www.jstor.org/stable/1185911

Laws, M. B., Lee, Y., Rogers, W. H., Beach, M. C., Saha, S., Korthuis, P. T., Sharp, V., Cohn, J., Moore, R., & Wilson, I. B. (2014). Provider-patient communication about adherence to anti-retroviral regimens differs by patient race and ethnicity. *AIDS and Behavior*, *18*(7), 1279–1287. https://doi.org/10.1007/s10461-014-0697-z

Lê Cook, B., Trinh, N. H., Li, Z., Hou, S. S. Y., & Progovac, A. M. (2019). Trends in racial/ethnic disparities in mental health care among US adolescents, 2004–2014. *JAMA Pediatrics*, *173*(4), 329–336. https://doi.org/10.1001/jamapediatrics.2018.5439

Leach-Kemon, K., Sirull, R., & Glenn, S. (2023). On gun violence, the United States is an outlier. *Institute for Health Metrics and Evaluation*. https://www.healthdata.org/news-events/insights-blog/acting-data/gun-violence-united-states-outlier

Learning to Give. (n.d.). *Learning to give*. https://www.learningtogive.org

Lebrun-Harris, L. A., Ghandour, R. M., Kogan, M. D., & Warren, M. D. (2022). Five-year trends in US children's health and well-being, 2016–2020. *JAMA Pediatrics*, *176*(7), e220056–e220056. https://doi.org/10.1001/jamapediatrics.2022.0056

Lee, L., Upadhya, K. K., Matson, P., Adger, H., & Trent, M. E. (2016). The status of adolescent medicine: Building a global adolescent workforce. *International Journal of Adolescent Medicine and Health*, *28*(3), 233. https://doi.org/10.1515/ijamh-2016-5003

Lee, M. A., & Gortmaker, S. L. (2013). Health disparities in Head Start children's dental access and oral health status. *American Journal of Public Health*, *103*(S1), S488–S493. https://doi.org/10.2105/AJPH.2013.301726

Lee, P., Bubeck, S., & Petro, J. (2023). Benefits, limits, and risks of GPT-4 as an AI chatbot for medicine. *New England Journal of Medicine*, *388*(13), 1233–1239. https://doi.org/10.1056/NEJMsr2214184

Lee, S. S., Humphreys, K. L., Flory, K., Liu, R., & Glass, K. (2011). Prospective association of childhood attention-deficit/hyperactivity disorder (ADHD) and substance use and abuse/dependence: A meta-analytic review. *Clinical Psychology Review*, *31*(3), 328–341. https://doi.org/10.1016/j.cpr.2011.01.006

Lehmann, C., O'Connor, K., Shorte, V., & Johnson, T. (2014). Use of electronic health record systems by office-based pediatricians. *Pediatrics*, *135*. https://doi.org/10.1542/peds.2014-1115

Leider, J. P., Resnick, B., Bishai, D., & Scutchfield, F. D. (2018). How much do we spend? Creating historical estimates of public health expenditures in the United States at the federal, state, and local levels. *Health Management and Policy Faculty Publications*. https://uknowledge.uky.edu/hsm_facpub/11?utm_source=uknowledge.uky.edu%2Fhsm_facpub%2F11&utm_medium=PDF&utm_campaign=PDFCoverPages

Lemanske, R. F., Kakumanu, S., Shanovich, K., Antos, N., Cloutier, M. M., Mazyck, D., Phipatanakul, W., Schantz, S., Szefler, S., Vandlik, R., & Williams, P. (2016). Creation and implementation of SAMPRO™: A school-based asthma management program. *Journal of Allergy and Clinical Immunology*, *138*(3).

Lemke, M., Kappel, R., McCarter, R., D'Angelo, L., & Tuchman, L. K. (2018). Perceptions of health care transition care coordination in patients with chronic illness. *Pediatrics*, *141*(5). https://doi.org/10.1542/peds.2017-3168

Lenahan, A., Mietzsch, U., Wood, T. R., Callahan, K. P., Weiss, E. M., Miller, D. E., German, K., Natarajan, N., Puia-Dumitrescu, M., Esposito, V., Kolnik, S., & Law, J. B. (2023). Characteristics, genetic testing, and diagnoses of infants with neonatal encephalopathy not due to hypoxic ischemic encephalopathy: A cohort study. *The Journal of Pediatrics*, *260*, 113533. https://doi.org/10.1016/j.jpeds.2023.113533

Levesque, J. F., Harris, M. F., & Russell, G. (2013). Patient-centred access to health care: Conceptualising access at the interface of health systems and populations. *International Journal for Equity in Health*, *12*(1), 18. https://doi.org/10.1186/1475-9276-12-18

Levin, J. S., Komanduri, S., & Whaley, C. (2023). Association between hospital-physician vertical integration and medication adherence rates. *Health Services Research*, *58*(2), 356–364. https://doi.org/10.1111/1475-6773.14090

Levine, D. (2023). Health providers are working with local and regional partners to meet increased demand for mental and behavioral health services. *U.S. News & World Report*.

Levins, H. (2023). *Hospital consolidation continues to boost costs, narrow access, and impact care quality.* University of Pennsylvania, Leonard Davis Institute of Health Economics. https://ldi.upenn.edu/our-work/research-updates/hospital-consolidation-continues-to-boost-costs-narrow-access-and-impact-care-quality/

Lewandowski, W., & Adamle, K. (2009). Substantive areas of clinical nurse specialist practice: A comprehensive review of the literature. *Clinical Nurse Specialist*, *23*(2), 73–90. https://doi.org/10.1097/NUR.0b013e31819971d0

Lewin, S., Munabi-Babigumira, S., Glenton, C., Daniels, K., Bosch-Capblanch, X., van Wyk, B. E., Odgaard-Jensen, J., Johansen, M., Aja, G. N., Zwarenstein, M., & Scheel, I. B. (2010). Lay health workers in primary and community health care for maternal and child health and the management of infectious diseases. *The Cochrane Database of Systematic Reviews*, *2010*(3), CD004015. https://doi.org/10.1002/14651858.CD004015.pub3

Leyenaar, J. K., Freyleue, S. D., Arakelyan, M., Goodman, D. C., & O'Malley, A. J. (2023). Pediatric hospitalizations at rural and urban teaching and nonteaching hospitals in the US, 2009–2019. *JAMA Network Open*, *6*(9), e2331807. https://doi.org/10.1001/jamanetworkopen.2023.31807

Leyenaar, J. K., Ralston, S. L., Shieh, M. S., Pekow, P. S., Mangione-Smith, R., & Lindenauer, P. K. (2016). Epidemiology of pediatric hospitalizations at general hospitals and free-standing children's hospitals in the United States. *Journal of Hospital Medicine*, *11*(11), 743–749. https://doi.org/10.1002/jhm.2624

Li, D., Ossip, D. J., Bansal-Travers, M., & Xie, Z. (2022a). Impact of the FDA flavour enforcement policy on flavoured electronic cigarette use behaviour changes. *Tobacco Control*, 31(Suppl 3), S176–S183. https://doi.org/10.1136/tc-2022-057492

Li, Q., Li, Y., Liu, B., Chen, Q., Xing, X., Xu, G., & Yang, W. (2022b). Prevalence of autism spectrum disorder among children and adolescents in the United States from 2019 to 2020. *JAMA Pediatrics*, *176*(9), 943–945. https://doi.org/10.1001/jamapediatrics.2022.1846

Liao, J. M., Lavizzo-Mourey, R. J., & Navathe, A. S. (2021). A national goal to advance health equity through value-based payment. *Journal of the American Medical Association*, *325*(24), 2439. https://doi.org/10.1001/jama.2021.8562

Likhar, A., & Patil, M. S. (2022). Importance of maternal nutrition in the first 1,000 days of life and its effects on child development: A narrative review. *Cureus Journal of Medical Science*, *14*(10), e30083. https://doi.org/10.7759/cureus.30083

Liljenquist, K., & Coker, T. R. (2021). Transforming well-child care to meet the needs of families at the intersection of racism and poverty. *Academic Pediatrics*, *21*(8S), S102–S107. https://doi.org/10.1016/j.acap.2021.08.004

Lin, L., & Stamm, K. (2020). The child and adolescent behavioral health workforce. https://www.behavioralhealthworkforce.org/project/supply-of-child-and-adolescent-behavioral-health-providers/

Lindley, M. C., Smith, P. J., & Rodewald, L. E. (2011). Vaccination coverage among U.S. adolescents aged 13-17 years eligible for the Vaccines for Children program, 2009. *Public Health Reports*, *126*(Suppl 2), 124–134.

Lindsey, M. A., Sheftall, A. H., Xiao, Y., & Joe, S. (2019). Trends of suicidal behaviors among high school students in the United States: 1991–2017. *Pediatrics*, *144*(5), e20191187. https://doi.org/10.1542/peds.2019-1187

Lindstrom Johnson, S. R., Blum, R. W., & Cheng, T. L. (2014). Future orientation: A construct with implications for adolescent health and wellbeing. *International Journal of Adolescent Medicine and Health*, *26*(4), 459–468. https://doi.org/10.1515/ijamh-2013-0333

Lindstrom Johnson, S., Jones, V., & Cheng, T. L. (2015). Promoting "Healthy Futures" to reduce risk behaviors in urban youth: A randomized controlled trial. *American Journal of Community Psychology*, *56*(1–2), 36–45. https://doi.org/10.1007/s10464-015-9734-y

Ling, J., Chen, S., Zahry, N. R., & Kao, T. A. (2023). Economic burden of childhood overweight and obesity: A systematic review and meta-analysis. *Obesity Reviews*, *24*(2), e13535. https://doi.org/10.1111/obr.13535

Linton, N. M., DeBolt, C., Newman, L. P., Tasslimi, A., & Matheson, J. (2020). Mortality rate and causes of death among refugees resettled in Washington state, 2006–2016. *Journal of Immigrant and Minority Health*, *22*(1), 3–9. https://doi.org/10.1007/s10903-019-00949-8

Lipscomb, S. T., Hatfield, B., Lewis, H., Goka-Dubose, E., & Abshire, C. (2021). Adverse childhood experiences and children's development in early care and education programs. *Journal of Applied Developmental Psychology*, 72, 101218. https://doi.org/10.1016/j.appdev.2020.101218

Lipson, D. J., Libersky, J., Bradley, K., Lewis, C., Siegwarth, A. W., & Lester, R. (2017). *Promoting access in Medicaid and CHIP managed care: A toolkit for ensuring provider network adequacy and service availability*. Centers for Medicare & Medicaid Services. U.S. Department of Health and Human Services. https://www.medicaid.gov/sites/default/files/2020-02/adequacy-and-access-toolkit.pdf

Lloyd, J., Moses, K., & Davis, R. (2020). *Recognizing and sustaining the value of community health workers and promotores*. Center for Health Care Strategies. https://www.chcs.org/media/CHCS-CHCF-CHWP-Brief_010920_FINAL.pdf

Lobach, D. F., Kawamoto, K., Anstrom, K. J., Kooy, K. R., Eisenstein, E. L., Silvey, G. M., Willis, J. M., Johnson, F., & Simo, J. (2007). Proactive population health management in the context of a regional health information exchange using standards-based decision support. *AMIA Annual Symposium Proceedings*, *2007*, 473–477.

Loew, P. (2014). *Seventh generation earth ethics: Native voices of Wisconsin*. Wisconsin Historical Society Press.

Lofthouse, J. (2022). *Improving accountability and performance in the Indian Health Service*. Mercatus Policy Brief Series. http://dx.doi.org/10.2139/ssrn.4061211

Lollar, D. (2010). *Launching into adulthood*. Paul H. Brookes Publishing Co.

Lopez, E., Neuman, T., Jacobson, G., & Levitt, L. (2020). *How much more than Medicare do private insurers pay? A review of the literature.* KFF. https://www.kff.org/medicare/issue-brief/how-much-more-than-medicare-do-private-insurers-pay-a-review-of-the-literature/

Lopez, K., Magaña, S., Morales, M., & Iland, E. (2019). Parents taking action: Reducing disparities through a culturally informed intervention for Latinx parents of children with autism. *Journal of Ethnic & Cultural Diversity in Social Work*, *28*, 1–19. https://doi.org/10.1080/15313204.2019.1570890

Lopez, L., III, Dhodapkar, M., & Gross, C. P. (2021). US nonprofit hospitals' community health needs assessments and implementation strategies in the era of the patient protection and affordable care act. *JAMA Network Open*, *4*(8), e2122237. https://doi.org/10.1001/jamanetworkopen.2021.22237

Lorch, S. A., Myers, S., & Carr, B. (2010). The regionalization of pediatric health care. *Pediatrics*, *126*(6), 1182–1190. https://doi.org/10.1542/peds.2010-1119

Lorig, K. R., & Holman, H. R. (2003). Self-management education: History, definition, outcomes, and mechanisms. *Annals of Behavioral Medicine*, *26*(1), 1–7. https://doi.org/10.1207/S15324796ABM2601_01

Lou, C., Hahn, H., Maag. E., Daly, H. S., Casas, M., & Steuerle, C. E. (2023). *Kids' share 2023: Report on federal expenditures on children through 2022 and future projections.* Urban Institute. https://www.urban.org/research/publication/kids-share-2023

Lou, C., & Lei, S. (2019). *Part of us: A data-driven look at children of immigrants.* Urban Institute. https://www.urban.org/features/part-us-data-driven-look-children-immigrants

Love, H. E., Schlitt, J., Soleimanpour, S., Panchal, N., & Behr, C. (2019). Twenty years of school-based health care growth and expansion. *Health Affairs*, *38*(5), 755–764. https://doi.org/10.1377/hlthaff.2018.05472

Love, J. M., Kisker, E. E., Ross, C. M., Schochet, P. Z., Brooks-Gunn, J., Paulsell, D., Boller, K., Constantine, J., Vogel, C., Sidle Fuligni, A., & Brady-Smith, C. (2002). *Making a difference in the lives of infants and toddlers and their families: The impacts of early Head Start. Volumes I-III: Final technical report and appendixes and local contributions to understanding the programs and their impacts.* U.S. Department of Health and Human Services, Administration for Children and Families, Office of Planning, Research and Evaluation.

Lown Institute. (2024). *Hospital community benefit spending: Improving transparency and accountability around standards for tax-exempt hospitals.* https://lownhospitalsindex.org/wp-content/uploads/2024/03/lown-institute-fair-share-policy-brief-20240321.pdf

Lucas-Judy, J. (2023, April). *Tax administration, IRS oversight of hospitals' tax-exempt status.* [Testimony before the Subcommittee on Oversight, Committee on Ways and Means, House of Representatives]. https://www.gao.gov/assets/820/819569.pdf

Lucy, C. A., Wojtaszek, J., LaLonde, L., Bruni, T. P., Ham, H. L., Sunde, E., Lancaster, B., & Maragakis, A. (2023). Pediatrician burnout before and after the COVID-19 pandemic. *Journal of Primary Care & Community Health*, *14*, 21501319231194148. https://doi.org/10.1177/21501319231194148

Ludomirsky, A. B., Schpero, W. L., Wallace, J., Lollo, A., Bernheim, S., Ross, J. S., & Ndumele, C. D. (2022). In Medicaid managed care networks, care is highly concentrated among a small percentage of physicians. *Health Affairs (Project Hope)*, *41*(5), 760–768. https://doi.org/10.1377/hlthaff.2021.01747

Lui, L. (2023). *Census Bureau releases small area income and poverty estimates for states, counties and school districts* https://www.census.gov/newsroom/press-releases/2023/saipe.html

Lumeng, J. C., Kaciroti, N., Sturza, J., Krusky, A. M., Miller, A. L., Peterson, K. E., Lipton, R., & Reischl, T. M. (2015). Changes in body mass index associated with Head Start participation. *Pediatrics*, *135*(2), e449–e456. https://doi.org/10.1542/peds.2014-1725

Luppino, F. S., de Wit, L. M., Bouvy, P. F., Stijnen, T., Cuijpers, P., Penninx, B. W., & Zitman, F. G. (2010). Overweight, obesity, and depression: A systematic review and meta-analysis of longitudinal studies. *Archives of General Psychiatry*, *67*(3), 220–229. https://doi.org/10.1001/archgenpsychiatry.2010.2

Lurie, N., Bauer, E. J., & Brady, C. (2001). Asthma outcomes at an inner-city school-based health center. *Journal of School Health*, *71*(1), 9–16.

Lyles, C. R., Lunn, M. R., Obedin-Maliver, J., & Bibbins-Domingo, K. (2018). The new era of precision population health: Insights for the All of Us Research Program and beyond. *Journal of Translational Medicine*, *16*(1), 211. https://doi.org/10.1186/s12967-018-1585-5

Lynch, J., & Smith, G. D. (2005). A life course approach to chronic disease epidemiology. *Annual Review of Public Health*, *26*, 1–35. https://doi.org/10.1146/annurev.publhealth.26.021304.144505

Lyren, A., Brilli, R. J., Zieker, K., Marino, M., Muething, S., & Sharek, P. J. (2017). Children's hospitals' solutions for patient safety collaborative impact on hospital-acquired harm. *Pediatrics*, *140*(3), e20163494. https://doi.org/10.1542/peds.2016-3494

Lyren, A., Haines, E., Fanta, M., Gutzeit, M., Staubach, K., Chundi, P., Ward, V., Srinivasan, L., Mackey, M., Vonderhaar, M., Sisson, P., Sheffield-Bradshaw, U., Fryzlewicz, B., Coffey, M., Cowden, J. D., & PHARE Cohort Study Group. (2024). Racial and ethnic disparities in common inpatient safety outcomes in a children's hospital cohort. *BMJ Quality & Safety*, *33*(2), 86–97. https://doi.org/10.1136/bmjqs-2022-015786

Lyubarova, R., Salman, L., & Rittenberg, E. (2023). Gender differences in physician burnout: Driving factors and potential solutions. *The Permanente Journal*, *27*(2), 130–136. https://doi.org/10.7812/tpp/23.023

Maag, E., Lou, C., Casas, M., Daly, H., Garriga, G., & Hunter, L. (2023). The return on investing in children: Helping children thrive. *Tax Policy Center*. https://www.taxpolicycenter.org/sites/default/files/publication/165470/the_return_on_investing_in_children.pdf

MacArthur, N. S., & Blewett, L. A. (2023). Contributions of key components of a medical home on child health outcomes. *Maternal and Child Health Journal*, *27*(3), 476–486. https://doi.org/10.1007/s10995-022-03539-7

MacDonald, A., McGill, P., & Murphy, G. (2018). An evaluation of staff training in positive behavioural support. *Journal of Applied Research in Intellectual Disabilities*, *31*(1), 124–135. https://doi.org/10.1111/jar.12460

Maenner, M. J., Warren, Z., Williams, A. R., Amoakohene, E., Bakian, A. V., Bilder, D. A., Durkin, M. S., Fitzgerald, R. T., Furnier, S. M., Hughes, M. M., Ladd-Acosta, C. M., McArthur, D., Pas, E. T., Salinas, A., Vehorn, A., Williams, S., Esler, A., Grzybowski, A., Hall-Lande, J., ... Shaw, K. A. (2023). Prevalence and characteristics of autism spectrum disorder among children aged 8 years—autism and developmental disabilities monitoring network, 11 sites, United States, 2020. *MMWR Surveillance Summaries*, *72*(2), 1–14. https://doi.org/10.15585/mmwr.ss7202a1

Magaña, S., Heydarian, N., & Vanegas, S. (2022). *Disparities in healthcare access and outcomes among racial and ethnic minoritized people with intellectual and developmental disabilities*. Oxford University Press.

Mahant, S., & Guttmann, A. (2023). Shifts in the hospital care of children in the US—A health equity challenge. *JAMA Network Open*, *6*(9), e2331763. https://doi.org/10.1001/jamanetworkopen.2023.31763

Malak, N., Rahman, M. M. & Yip, T. A. (2019). Baby bonus, anyone? Examining heterogeneous responses to a pro-natalist policy. *Journal of Population Economics*, *32*, 1205–1246.

Malcarney, M. B., Pittman, P., Quigley, L., Horton, K., & Seiler, N. (2017). The changing roles of community health workers. *Health Services Research*, *52*(Suppl 1), 360–382. https://doi.org/10.1111/hesr.12624

Malik-Soni, N., Shaker, A., Luck, H., Mullin, A. E., Wiley, R. E., Lewis, M. E. S., Fuentes, J., & Frazier, T. W. (2022). Tackling healthcare access barriers for individuals with autism from diagnosis to adulthood. *Pediatric Research*, *91*(5), 1028–1035. https://doi.org/10.1038/s41390-021-01465-y

Manatt, P., & Phillips, LLP. (2022). *COVID-19 state resource guide: Leveraging federal and state authorities to ensure access to long-term services and supports for high-risk individuals.* https://www.manatt.com/Manatt/media/Documents/Articles/LTSS-State-Resource-Guide-Update_c.pdf

Manis, D. R., Bielska, I. A., Cimek, K., & Costa, A. P. (2022). Community-informed, integrated, and coordinated care through a community-level model: A narrative synthesis on community hubs. *Healthcare Management Forum*, *35*(2), 105–111. https://doi.org/10.1177/08404704211046604

Mann, C., & Daugherty, E. (2023). *States are adopting new policies to help children stay enrolled in Medicaid and CHIP*. The Commonwealth Fund. https://www.commonwealthfund.org/blog/2023/states-are-adopting-new-policies-help-children-stay-enrolled-medicaid-and-chip

Mann, C., & Ferguson, M. (2020). Caring for the whole child: A new way to finance initiatives to improve children's health. *Insight*. https://www.manatt.com/insights/white-papers/2020/caring-for-the-whole-child-a-new-way-to-finance-in

Mannix, R., Fleegler, E., Meehan, W. P. III, Schutzman, S. A., Hennelly, K., Nigrovic, L., & Lee, L. K. (2012). Booster seat laws and fatalities in children 4 to 7 years of age. *Pediatrics*, *130*(6), 996–1002. https://doi.org/10.1542/peds.2012-1054

Marazziti, D., Cianconi, P., Mucci, F., Foresi, L., Chiarantini, I., & Della Vecchia, A. (2021). Climate change, environment pollution, COVID-19 pandemic and mental health. *Science of the Total Environment*, *773*, 145182. https://doi.org/10.1016/j.scitotenv.2021.145182

Marcal, K. E. (2018). The impact of housing instability on child maltreatment: A causal investigation. *Journal of Family Social Work*, *21*(4–5), 331–347. https://doi.org/10.1080/10522158.2018.1469563

Marceno, L., Patel, P., Lambert, E., & Steel King, M. (2023). *Improving access to school-based behavioral health services through Medicaid.* The Commonwealth Fund. https://www.commonwealthfund.org/blog/2023/improving-access-school-based-behavioral-health-services-through-medicaid

Margolius, D., Wong, J., Goldman, M. L., Rouse-Iniguez, J., & Bodenheimer, T. (2012). Delegating responsibility from clinicians to nonprofessional personnel: The example of hypertension control. *Journal of the American Board of Family Medicine*, *25*(2), 209–215. https://doi.org/10.3122/jabfm.2012.02.100279

Mariño-Ramírez, L., Jordan, I. K., Nápoles, A. M., & Pérez-Stable, E. J. (2022). Comparison of US firearm-related deaths among children and adolescents by race and ethnicity, 1999–2020. *Journal of the American Medical Association*, *328*(23), 2359–2360. https://doi.org/10.1001/jama.2022.19508

Maron, J. L., Kingsmore, S., Gelb, B. D., Vockley, J., Wigby, K., Bragg, J., Stroustrup, A., Poindexter, B., Suhrie, K., Kim, J. H., Diacovo, T., Powell, C. M., Trembath, A., Guidugli, L., Ellsworth, K. A., Reed, D., Kurfiss, A., Breeze, J. L., Trinquart, L., & Davis, J. M. (2023). Rapid whole-genomic sequencing and a targeted neonatal gene panel in infants with a suspected genetic disorder. *Journal of the American Medical Association*, *330*(2), 161–169. https://doi.org/10.1001/jama.2023.9350

Marrast, L., Himmelstein, D. U., & Woolhandler, S. (2016). Racial and ethnic disparities in mental health care for children and young adults: A national study. *International Journal of Health Services*, *46*(4), 810–824. https://doi.org/10.1177/0020731416662736

Marshall, A. N., Chuang, R. J., Chow, J., Ranjit, N., Dave, J. M., Mathur, M., Markham, C., & Sharma, S. V. (2022). Food insecurity among low-income households with children participating in a school-based fruit and vegetable co-op. *Children (Basel)*, *9*(8). https://doi.org/10.3390/children9081250

Martin, A. B., Hartman, M., Benson, J., Catlin, A., & The National Health Expenditure Accounts Team. (2023). National health care spending in 2021: Decline in federal spending outweighs greater use of health care. *Health Affairs*, *42*(1), 6–17. https://doi.org/10.1377/hlthaff.2022.01397

Martin, A. B., Hartman, M., Lassman, D., & Catlin, A. (2021). National health care spending in 2019: Steady growth for the fourth consecutive year. *Health Affairs*, *40*(1), 14–24. https://doi.org/10.1377/hlthaff.2020.02022

Martin, L., Smith, H., & Phillips, W. (2005). Bridging 'town & gown' through innovative university-community partnerships. *The Innovation Journal: The Public Sector Innovation Journal*, *10*.

Martin-Misener, R., Valaitis, R., Wong, S. T., Macdonald, M., Meagher-Stewart, D., Kaczorowski, J., O'Mara, L., Savage, R., & Austin, P. (2012). A scoping literature review of collaboration between primary care and public health. *Primary Health Care Research & Development*, *13*(4), 327–346. https://doi.org/10.1017/s1463423611000491

Martini, R., Hilt, R., Marx, L., Chenven, M., Naylor, M., Sarvet, B., Committee on Collaboration with Medical Professionals, & Kroeger Ptakowski, K. (2012). *Best principles for integration of child psychiatry into the pediatric health home*. American Academy of Child & Adolescent Psychiatry. https://www.aacap.org/App_Themes/AACAP/docs/clinical_practice_center/systems_of_care/best_principles_for_integration_of_child_psychiatry_into_the_pediatric_health_home_2012.pdf

Martino, S. C., Mathews, M., Beckett, M. K., Agniel, D., Hambarsoomian, K., Scholle, S. H., Collins, S., Quigley, D. D., Darabidian, B., & Elliott, M. N. (2023). Development of a Medicare plan dashboard to promote health equity. *American Journal of Managed Care*, *29*(3), e91–e95. https://doi.org/10.37765/ajmc.2023.89335

Mascia, A. E., Daugherty, E. C., Zhang, Y., Lee, E., Xiao, Z., Sertorio, M., Woo, J., Backus, L. R., McDonald, J. M., McCann, C., Russell, K., Levine, L., Sharma, R. A., Khuntia, D., Bradley, J. D., Simone, C. B., 2nd, Perentesis, J. P., & Breneman, J. C. (2023). Proton FLASH radiotherapy for the treatment of symptomatic bone metastases: The FAST-01 nonrandomized trial. *JAMA Oncology*, *9*(1), 62–69. https://doi.org/10.1001/jamaoncol.2022.5843

Mason-Jones, A. J., Crisp, C., Momberg, M., Koech, J., Koker, P. D., & Mathews, C. (2012). A systematic review of the role of school-based healthcare in adolescent sexual, reproductive, and mental health. *Systematic Reviews*, *1*(1), 49. https://doi.org/10.1186/2046-4053-1-49

MassHealth. (2022). *Fact sheet: MassHealth's newly approved 1115 demonstration extension supports accountable care and advances health equity*. https://www.mass.gov/doc/1115-waiver-extensionfact-sheet/download

Masten, A. S., & Barnes, A. J. (2018). Resilience in children: Developmental perspectives. *Children (Basel)*, *5*(7). https://doi.org/10.3390/children5070098

Mather, M. & Scommegna, P. (2024). *Fact sheet: Aging in the United States*. Population Reference Bureau. https://www.prb.org/resources/fact-sheet-aging-in-the-united-states/

Mathur, M., Rampersad, A., Howard, K., Goldman, G. M. (2005). Physician assistants as physician extenders in the pediatric intensive care unit setting—A 5-year experience. *Pediatric Critical Care Medicine*, *6*(1), 14–19. https://doi.org/10.1097/01.PCC.0000149133.50687.A1

Matsui, E. C., Abramson, S. L., & Sandel, M. T. (2016). Indoor environmental control practices and asthma management. *Pediatrics*, *138*(5). https://doi.org/10.1542/peds.2016-2589

Matthews, K., Morgan, I., Davis, K., Estriplet, T., Perez, S., & Crear-Perry, J. A. (2021). Pathways to equitable and antiracist maternal mental health care: Insights from Black women stakeholders. *Health Affairs*, *40*(10), 1597–1604. https://doi.org/10.1377/hlthaff.2021.00808

Maughan, E. D. (2018). School nurses: An investment in student achievement. *Phi Delta Kappan*, *99*(7), 8–14. https://doi.org/10.1177/0031721718767853

Mauro, P. M., Gutkind, S., Annunziato, E. M., & Samples, H. (2022). Use of medication for opioid use disorder among US adolescents and adults with need for opioid treatment, 2019. *JAMA Network Open*, *5*(3), e223821. https://doi.org/10.1001/jamanetworkopen.2022.3821

Mays, G. P., & Smith, S. A. (2009). Geographic variation in public health spending: Correlates and consequences. *Health Services Research*, *44*(5 Pt 2), 1796–1817. https://doi.org/10.1111/j.1475-6773.2009.01014.x

Mazurek, M. O., Brown, R., Curran, A., & Sohl, K. (2017). ECHO autism: A new model for training primary care providers in best-practice care for children with autism. *Clinical Pediatrics*, *56*(3), 247–256. https://doi.org/10.1177/0009922816648288

McClafferty, H. H., Hubbard, D. K., Foradori, D., Brown, M. L., Profit, J., & Tawfik, D. S. (2022). Physician health and wellness. *Pediatrics*, *150*(5). https://doi.org/10.1542/peds.2022-059665

McClain, M. B., Shahidullah, J. D., Mezher, K. R., Haverkamp, C. R., Benallie, K. J., & Schwartz, S. E. (2020). School-clinic care coordination for youth with ASD: A national survey of school psychologists. *Journal of Autism and Developmental Disorders*, *50*(9), 3081–3091. https://doi.org/10.1007/s10803-019-03985-3

McClelland, M. M., Tominey, S. L., Schmitt, S. A., & Duncan, R. (2017). SEL interventions in early childhood. *Future of Children*, *27*(1).

McConnell, M. A., Rokicki, S., Ayers, S., Allouch, F., Perreault, N., Gourevitch, R. A., Martin, M. W., Zhou, R. A., Zera, C., Hacker, M. R., Chien, A., Bates, M. A., & Baicker, K. (2022). Effect of an intensive nurse home visiting program on adverse birth outcomes in a Medicaid-eligible population: A randomized clinical trial. *Journal of the American Medical Association*, *328*(1), 27–37. https://doi.org/10.1001/jama.2022.9703

McConnochie, K. M., Ronis, S. D., Wood, N. E., & Ng, P. K. (2015). Effectiveness and safety of acute care telemedicine for children with regular and special healthcare needs. *Telemedicine and e-Health*, *21*(8), 611–621. https://doi.org/10.1089/tmj.2014.0175

McCord, M., Fierman, A., Sisco, S., Canfield, C., Manjunath, S., Cohen, N., Havens, J., Wilcox, W., Tomopoulos, S., Stein Albert, M., Abraham, T., Charney, A., Acri, M., & Piwnica-Worms, K. (2024). A two-generation, early childhood advanced primary care model. *Pediatrics*, *153*(4), e2023062567. https://doi.org/10.1542/peds.2023-062567

McCord, M. T., Klein, J. D., Foy, J. M., & Fothergill, K. (1993). School-based clinic use and school performance. *Journal of Adolescent Health*, *14*(2), 91–98.

McCoy, D. C., Cuartas, J., & Seiden, J. (2024). Country-level improvements in nurturing care and child development. *JAMA Pediatrics*, *178*(1), 84–86. https://doi.org/10.1001/jamapediatrics.2023.4615

McCrae, J. S., Robinson, J. A. L., Spain, A. K., Brickhouse, T. H., Goff, S. L., Greiner, M. V., & Guevara, J. P. (2021). The Mitigating Toxic Stress study design: Approaches to developmental evaluation of pediatric health care innovations addressing social determinants of health and toxic stress. *BMC Health Services Research*, *21*(1), 1–13. https://doi.org/10.1186/s12913-021-06057-4

McCurley, J. L., Gutierrez, A. P., & Gallo, L. C. (2017). Diabetes prevention in U.S. Hispanic adults: A systematic review of culturally tailored interventions. *American Journal of Preventive Medicine*, *52*(4), 519–529. https://doi.org/10.1016/j.amepre.2016.10.028

McGinnis, J. M., & Foege, W. H. (2004). The immediate vs the important. *Journal of the American Medical Association*, *291*(10), 1263–1264. https://doi.org/10.1001/jama.291.10.1263
McGough, M., Claxton, G., Amin, K., & Cox, C. (2024). *How do health expenditures vary across the population?* Peterson-KFF Health System Tracker. https://www.healthsystemtracker.org/chart-collection/health-expenditures-vary-across-population/#Share%20of%20total%20population%20and%20total%20health%20spending,%20by%20age%20group,%202021
McIntyre, L., Williams, J. V., Lavorato, D. H., & Patten, S. (2013). Depression and suicide ideation in late adolescence and early adulthood are an outcome of child hunger. *Journal of Affective Disorders*, *150*(1), 123–129. https://doi.org/10.1016/j.jad.2012.11.029
McIntyre, P. (2002). *Adolescent friendly health services: An agenda for change*. https://www.who.int/publications-detail-redirect/WHO-FCH-CAH-02.14
McKay, S. & Parente, V. (2019). Health disparities in the hospitalized child. *Hospital Pediatrics*, *9*(5), 317–325. https://doi.org/10.1542/hpeds.2018-0223
McKee, M. D., Rubin, S. E., & Campos, G. (2011). Challenges of providing confidential care to adolescents in urban primary care: Clinician perspectives. *Annals of Family Medicine*, *9*(1), 37–43. https://doi.org/10.1370/afm.1186
McKillop, M., Farberman, R. K., & Lieberman, D. A. (2023). *Ready or not: Protecting the public's health from disease, disaster, and bioterrorism. Special selection on the intersection of health equity and emergency preparedness*. Trust for America's Health. https://www.tfah.org/wp-content/uploads/2023/03/2023-ReadyOrNot-FINALc.pdf
McKillop, M., & Lieberman, D. A. (2023). The impact of chronic underfunding on America's public health system: Trends, risks, and recommendations 2023. *Trust for America's Health*. https://www.tfah.org/wp-content/uploads/2023/06/TFAH-2023-PublicHealthFundingFINALc.pdfT
McLaughlin, M., & Rank, M. R. (2018). Estimating the economic cost of childhood poverty in the United States. *Social Work Research*, *42*(2), 73–83. https://doi.org/10.1093/swr/svy007
McLeod, J. D., Uemura, R., & Rohrman, S. (2012). Adolescent mental health, behavior problems, and academic achievement. *Journal of Health and Social Behavior*, *53*(4), 482–497.
McLeod, S. (2023). *Robbers cave experiment: Realistic conflict theory*. SimplyPsychology https://www.simplypsychology.org/robbers-cave.html
McMillan, J. H., Schumacher, S., & Singh, J. (2006). *Research in education: Evidence-based inquiry*. Pearson Education.
McMorrow, S., Kenney, G. M., Long, S. K., & Anderson, N. (2015). Uninsurance among young adults continues to decline, particularly in Medicaid expansion states. *Health Affairs (Project Hope)*, *34*(4), 616–620. https://doi.org/10.1377/hlthaff.2015.0044
McPherson, M., Arango, P., Fox, H., Lauver, C., McManus, M., Newacheck, P. W., Perrin, J. M., Shonkoff, J. P., & Strickland, B. (1998). A new definition of children with special health care needs. *Pediatrics*, *102*(1 Pt 1), 137–140. https://doi.org/10.1542/peds.102.1.137
McQuaid, E. L. (2018). Barriers to medication adherence in asthma: The importance of culture and context. *Annals of Allergy, Asthma & Immunology*, *121*(1), 37–42. https://doi.org/10.1016/j.anai.2018.03.024
McVicar, K. L., Ivanitskaya, L. V., Bradley, D. W., & Montero, J. T. (2019). Primary care and public health collaboration reports: A qualitative review of integration aims, participants, and success determinants. *Population Health Management*, *22*(5), 422–432. https://doi.org/10.1089/pop.2018.0160
McWilliams, J. M., Weinreb, G., Ding, L., Ndumele, C. D., & Wallace, J. (2023). Risk adjustment and promoting health equity in population-based payment: Concepts and evidence. *Health Affairs*, *42*(1), 105–114. https://doi.org/10.1377/hlthaff.2022.00916
Medalie, J. H., & Cole-Kelly, K. (2002). The clinical importance of defining family. *American Family Physician*, *65*(7), 1277–1279.

Medicaid and CHIP Payment and Access Commission (MACPAC). (n.d). *Overview of the Affordable Care Act and Medicaid.* https://www.macpac.gov/subtopic/overview-of-the-affordable-care-act-and-medicaid/

_______. (2015a). *Comparing CHIP benefits to Medicaid, exchange plans, and employer-sponsored insurance.* https://www.macpac.gov/wp-content/uploads/2015/03/Comparing-CHIP-Benefits-to-Medicaid-Exchange-Plans-and-Employer-Sponsored-Insurance.pdf

_______. (2015b). Provider networks and access: Issues for children's coverage. In *Report to Congress on Medicaid and CHIP* (pp. 59–71). https://www.macpac.gov/wp-content/uploads/2015/03/Provider-Networks-and-Access-Issues-for-Children%E2%80%99s-Coverage.pdf

_______. (2016). *Employer-sponsored insurance for low- and moderate-income children.* https://www.macpac.gov/wp-content/uploads/2016/01/Employer-Sponsored-Insurance-for-Low-and-Moderate-Income-Children.pdf

_______. (2017). *Medicaid hospital payment: A comparison across states and to Medicare.* https://www.macpac.gov/wp-content/uploads/2017/04/Medicaid-Hospital-Payment-A-Comparison-across-States-and-to-Medicare.pdf

_______. (2018a). *Federal requirements and state options: Premium assistance.* https://www.macpac.gov/wp-content/uploads/2017/11/Federal-Requirements-and-State-Options-Premium-Assistance.pdf

_______. (2018b). *School-based behavioral health services: Findings from stakeholder interviews.* https://www.macpac.gov/wp-content/uploads/2018/04/Medicaid-in-Schools.pdf

_______. (2019). *Medicaid payment initiatives to improve maternal and birth outcomes* (Issue Brief). https://www.macpac.gov/wp-content/uploads/2019/04/Medicaid-Payment-Initiatives-to-Improve-Maternal-and-Birth-Outcomes.pdf

_______. (2020). *MACStats: Medicaid and CHIP data book.* https://www.macpac.gov/wp-content/uploads/2020/12/MACStats-Medicaid-and-CHIP-Data-Book-December-2020.pdf

_______. (2021a). *Medicaid base and supplemental payments to hospitals* (Issue Brief). https://www.macpac.gov/wp-content/uploads/2020/03/Medicaid-Base-and-Supplemental-Payments-to-Hospitals.pdf

_______. (2021b). *Medicaid and CHIP in the territories.* https://www.macpac.gov/wp-content/uploads/2019/07/Medicaid-and-CHIP-in-the-Territories.pdf

_______. (2021c). *Upper payment limit supplemental payments.* https://www.macpac.gov/wp-content/uploads/2021/11/Upper-Payment-Limit-Supplemental-Payments.pdf

_______. (2022). *Directed payments in Medicaid managed care.* https://www.macpac.gov/wp-content/uploads/2022/06/June-2022-Directed-Payments-Issue-Brief-FINAL.pdf

_______. (2023a). *MACStats: Medicaid and CHIP data book.* https://www.macpac.gov/wp-content/uploads/2023/12/EXHIBIT-25.-Medicaid-Supplemental-Payments-to-Non-Hospital-Providers-by-State-FY-2022-millions.pdf

_______. (2023b). *Medicaid base and supplemental payments to hospitals.* https://www.macpac.gov/wp-content/uploads/2023/03/Medicaid-Base-and-Supplemental-Payments-to-Hospitals-Issue-Brief.pdf

_______. (2023c). *Percentage of Medicaid enrollees in managed care by state and eligibility group, FY 2021. Program enrollment and spending.* https://www.macpac.gov/wp-content/uploads/2023/12/EXHIBIT-30.-Percentage-of-Medicaid-Enrollees-in-Managed-Care-by-State-and-Eligibility-Group-FY-2021.pdf

_______. (2024a). *Annual analysis of Medicaid disproportionate share hospital allotments to states.* https://www.macpac.gov/wp-content/uploads/2024/03/Chapter-3-Annual-Analysis-of-Medicaid-Disproportionate-Share-Hospital-Allotments-to-States.pdf

_______. (2024b). *Issue brief: School-based services for students enrolled in Medicaid.* https://www.macpac.gov/wp-content/uploads/2024/04/School-Based-Services-for-Students-Enrolled-in-Medicaid.pdf

Medicaid Program; Ensuring Access to Medicaid Services, 89 F.R. 40542 (effective July 9, 2024) (codified at 42 CFR § 421, 438, 441, & 447). https://www.federalregister.gov/documents/2024/05/09/2024-08084/medicaid-program-ensuring-access-to-medicaid-serviceshttps://www.federalregister.gov/documents/2024/05/10/2024-08363/medicaid-program-ensuring-access-to-medicaid-services

Medicaid Program: Medicaid and Children's Health Insurance Program (CHIP) Managed Care Access, Finance, and Quality, 89 FR 41002 (effective July 9, 2024) (codified at 42 CFR § 431, 438, & 457). https://www.federalregister.gov/documents/2024/05/10/2024-08085/medicaid-program-medicaid-and-childrens-health-insurance-program-chip-managed-care-access-finance

Medicare Payment Advisory Commission (MedPAC). (2018). Chapter 8: Medicare payment strategies to improve price competition and value for Part B drugs. In MedPAC, *Report to the Congress: Medicare and the health care delivery system* (pp. 211–236). https://www.medpac.gov/wp-content/uploads/import_data/scrape_files/docs/default-source/reports/jun18_ch8_medpacreport_sec.pdf

________. (2023a). Medicare advantage. In *A data book: Health care spending and the Medicare program* (pp. 119–132). https://www.medpac.gov/wp-content/uploads/2023/07/July2023_MedPAC_DataBook_Sec9_SEC.pdf

________. (2023b). The Medicare advantage program: Status report. In *Report to the Congress: Medicare Payment Policy* (pp. 319–379). https://www.medpac.gov/wp-content/uploads/2023/03/Ch11_Mar23_MedPAC_Report_To_Congress_SEC.pdf

________. (2023c). Standardized benefits in Medicare Advantage plans. In *Report to the Congress: Medicare and the Health Care Delivery System* (pp. 107–150). https://www.medpac.gov/wp-content/uploads/2023/06/Jun23_Ch3_MedPAC_Report_To_Congress_SEC.pdf

Meert, K. L., Clark, J., & Eggly, S. (2013). Family-centered care in the pediatric intensive care unit. *Pediatric Clinics of North America*, *60*(3), 761–772. https://doi.org/10.1016/j.pcl.2013.02.011

Mehrotra, A., Wang, M. C., Lave, J. R., Adams, J. L., & McGlynn, E. A. (2008). Retail clinics, primary care physicians, and emergency departments: A comparison of patients' visits. *Health Affairs (Project Hope)*, *27*(5), 1272–1282. https://doi.org/10.1377/hlthaff.27.5.1272

Mehta, L. S., Sharma, G., Creanga, A., Hameed, A., Hollier, L., Johnson, J., Leffert, L., McCullough, L., Mujahid, M., Watson, K., White, C., & American Heart Association Advocacy Coordinating Committee. (2021). Call to action: Maternal health and saving mothers: A policy statement from the American Heart Association. *Circulation*, *144*(15). https://doi.org/10.1161/CIR.0000000000001000

Melnychuk, E., Sallade, T. D., & Kraus, C. K. (2022). Hospitals as disaster victims: Lessons not learned? *Journal of the American College of Emergency Physicians Open, 3*(1), e12632. https://doi.org/10.1002/emp2.12632

Mendelsohn, A. L., Dreyer, B. P., Flynn, V., Tomopoulos, S., Rovira, I., Tineo, W., Pebenito, C., Torres, C., Torres, H., & Nixon, A. F. (2005). Use of videotaped interactions during pediatric well-child care to promote child development: A randomized, controlled trial. *Journal of Developmental & Behavioral Pediatrics*, *26*(1), 34–41.

Mendelsohn, A. L., Huberman, H. S., Berkule, S. B., Brockmeyer, C. A., Morrow, L. M., & Dreyer, B. P. (2011). Primary care strategies for promoting parent-child interactions and school readiness in at-risk families: The Bellevue Project for early language, literacy, and education success. *Archives of Pediatrics & Adolescent Medicine*, *165*(1), 33–41. https://doi.org/10.1001/archpediatrics.2010.254

Mennella, C., Maniscalco, U., De Pietro, G., & Esposito, M. (2024). Ethical and regulatory challenges of AI technologies in healthcare: A narrative review. *Heliyon*, *10*(4), e26297. https://doi.org/10.1016/j.heliyon.2024.e26297

Mental Health America. (2018). *The state of mental health in America 2018*. https://mhanational.org/issues/state-mental-health-america-2018

Merikangas, K. R., Calkins, M. E., Burstein, M., He, J. P., Chiavacci, R., Lateef, T., Ruparel, K., Gur, R. C., Lehner, T., Hakonarson, H., & Gur, R. E. (2015). Comorbidity of physical and mental disorders in the neurodevelopmental genomics cohort study. *Pediatrics*, *135*(4), e927–938. https://doi.org/10.1542/peds.2014-1444

Merrick, M. T., Ford, D. C., Ports, K. A., Guinn, A. S., Chen, J., Klevens, J., Metzler, M., Jones, C. M., Simon, T. R., Daniel, V. M., Ottley, P., & Mercy, J. A. (2019). *Vital Signs*: Estimated proportion of adult health problems attributable to adverse childhood experiences and implications for prevention–25 States, 2015–2017. *Morbidity and Mortality Weekly Report*, *68*(44), 999–1005. https://doi.org/10.15585/mmwr.mm6844e1

Mersky, J. P., Choi, C., Plummer Lee, C., & Janczewski, C. E. (2021). Disparities in adverse childhood experiences by race/ethnicity, gender, and economic status: Intersectional analysis of a nationally representative sample. *Child Abuse & Neglect*, *117*, 105066. https://doi.org/10.1016/j.chiabu.2021.105066

Mervosh, S., & Paris, F. (2024, March 29). Why school absences have 'exploded' almost everywhere. *The New York Times*. https://www.nytimes.com/interactive/2024/03/29/us/chronic-absences.html

Meyer, B. D., & Wherry, L. (2012). *Saving teens: Using a policy discontinuity to estimate the effects of Medicaid eligibility* (NBER Working Paper No. w18309). National Bureau of Economic Research. https://papers.ssrn.com/sol3/papers.cfm?abstract_id=2131681

Michaud, J., & Kates, J. (2017). *Public health in Puerto Rico after Hurricane Maria*. KFF. https://www.kff.org/mental-health/issue-brief/public-health-in-puerto-rico-after-hurricane-maria/

Michener, J. D. (2021). Politics, pandemic, and racial justice through the lens of Medicaid. *American Journal of Public Health*, *111*(4), 643–646. https://doi.org/10.2105/ajph.2020.306126

Midgett, A., Doumas, D. M., Peralta, C., Bond, L., & Flay, B. (2020). Impact of a brief, bystander bullying prevention program on depressive symptoms and passive suicidal ideation: A program evaluation model for school personnel. *Journal of Prevention and Health Promotion*, *1*(1), 80–103. https://doi.org/10.1177/2632077020942959

Miech, R. A., Johnston, L. D., Patrick, M. E., O'Malley, P. M., Bachman, J. G., & Schulenberg, J. E. (2023). *Monitoring the Future national survey results on drug use, 1975-2022: Overview, key findings on adolescent drug use*. Ann Arbor: Institute for Social Research, University of Michigan. https://monitoringthefuture.org/wp-content/uploads/2022/12/mtf2022.pdf

Mijakoski, D., Bislimovska, J., Milosevic, M., Mustajbegović, J., Stoleski, S., & Minov, J. (2015). Differences in burnout, work demands and team work between Croatian and Macedonian hospital nurses. *Cognition, Brain, Behavior. An Interdisciplinary Journal*, *XIX*, 179–200.

Miles, P. V. (2009). Maintenance of certification: The role of the American Board of Pediatrics in improving children's health care. *Pediatric Clinics of North America*, *56*(4), 987–994. https://doi.org/10.1016/j.pcl.2009.05.010

Miller, A. (2023). CDC to reduce funding for states' child vaccination programs. *KFF Health News*. https://kffhealthnews.org/news/article/cdc-childhood-vaccinations-programs-funding-cut-public-health/

Miller, D. S., and J. D. Rivera. (n.d.). Town and gown: Understanding the past to improve the future. *International Journal of the Humanities*, *3*(8), 215–224. https://www.researchgate.net/publication/325183850_Town_and_Gown_Understanding_the_Past_to_Improve_the_Future

Miller, E. B., Canfield, C. F., Roby, E., Wippick, H., Shaw, D. S., Mendelsohn, A. L., & Morris-Perez, P. A. (2023). Enhancing early language and literacy skills for racial/ethnic minority children with low incomes through a randomized clinical trial: The mediating role of cognitively stimulating parent–child interactions. *Child Development*, *95*(4), 1172–1185. https://doi.org/10.1111/cdev.14064

Miller, F., & Miller, P. (2021). Transgenerational trauma and trust restoration. *AMA Journal of Ethics*, *23*(6), E480–E486. https://doi.org/10.1001/amajethics.2021.480

Miller, S., & Wherry, L. R. (2019). The long-term effects of early life Medicaid coverage. *Journal of Human Resources*, *54*(3), 785–824. https://doi.org/10.3368/jhr.54.3.0816.8173R1

Milne Wenderlich, A., & Herendeen, N. (2021). Telehealth in pediatric primary care. *Current Problems in Pediatric and Adolescent Health Care*, 51(1), 100951. https://doi.org/10.1016/j.cppeds.2021.100951

Mimila, N. A., Chung, P. J., Elliott, M. N., Bethell, C. D., Chacon, S., Biely, C., Contreras, S., Chavis, T., Bruno, Y., Moss, T., & Coker, T. R. (2017). Well-child care redesign: A mixed methods analysis of parent experiences in the PARENT trial. *Academic Pediatrics*, *17*(7), 747–754. https://doi.org/10.1016/j.acap.2017.02.004

Minh, A., Muhajarine, N., Janus, M., Brownell, M., & Guhn, M. (2017). A review of neighborhood effects and early child development: How, where, and for whom, do neighborhoods matter? *Health & Place*, *46*, 155–174. https://doi.org/10.1016/j.healthplace.2017.04.012

Minkovitz, C. S., Hughart, N., Strobino, D., Scharfstein, D., Grason, H., Hou, W., Miller, T., Bishai, D., Augustyn, M., McLearn, K. T., & Guyer, B. (2003). A practice-based intervention to enhance quality of care in the first 3 years of life: The HealthySteps for Young Children Program. *Journal of the American Medical Association*, *290*(23), 3081–3091. https://doi.org/10.1001/jama.290.23.3081

Minkovitz, C. S., Strobino, D., Mistry, K. B., Scharfstein, D. O., Grason, H., Hou, W., Ialongo, N., & Guyer, B. (2007). HealthySteps for Young Children: Sustained results at 5.5 years. *Pediatrics*, *120*(3), e658–e668. https://doi.org/10.1542/peds.2006-1205

Miranda, M. L., Lilienfeld, A., Tootoo, J., & Bravo, M. A. (2023). Segregation and childhood blood lead levels in North Carolina. *Pediatrics, 152*(3), e2022058661. https://doi.org/10.1542/peds.2022-058661

Miranda-Mendizabal, A., Castellví, P., Parés-Badell, O., Alayo, I., Almenara, J., Alonso, I., Blasco, M. J., Cebrià, A., Gabilondo, A., Gili, M., Lagares, C., Piqueras, J. A., Rodríguez-Jiménez, T., Rodríguez-Marín, J., Roca, M., Soto-Sanz, V., Vilagut, G., & Alonso, J. (2019). Gender differences in suicidal behavior in adolescents and young adults: Systematic review and meta-analysis of longitudinal studies. *International Journal of Public Health*, *64*(2), 265–283. https://doi.org/10.1007/s00038-018-1196-1

Mistry, K. B., Minkovitz, C. S., Riley, A. W., Johnson, S. B., Grason, H. A., Dubay, L. C., & Guyer, B. (2012). A new framework for childhood health promotion: The role of policies and programs in building capacity and foundations of early childhood health. *American Journal of Public Health*, *102*(9), 1688–1696. https://doi.org/10.2105/AJPH.2012.300687

Mitchell, P., Wynia, M., Golden, R., McNellis, B., Okun, S., Webb, C.E., Rohrbach, V., & Von Kohorn, I. (2012). *Core principles & values of effective team-based health care* [Discussion Paper].

Mohammadifirouzeh, M., Oh, K. M., Basnyat, I., & Gimm, G. (2023). Factors associated with professional mental help-seeking among U.S. immigrants: A systematic review. *Journal of Immigrant and Minority Health*, *25*(5), 1118–1136. https://doi.org/10.1007/s10903-023-01475-4

Moheize, S., Hsu, M., Matiz, L. A., Peretz, P., Medina, K., Esteves, A., Meyer, D., Maletz, B., Pineda, L., & Berger-Jenkins, E. (2024). The role of an early childhood community health worker in addressing psycho-social needs in the perinatal and early childhood period. *Journal of Primary Care & Community Health*, *15*, 21501319241234478. https://doi.org/10.1177/21501319241234478

Molnár, Z., Bódai, V., Szakacs, G., Erdélyi, B., Fogarassy, Z., Sáfrán, G., Varga, T., Kónya, Z., Tóth-Szeles, E., Szücs, R., & Lagzi, I. (2018). Green synthesis of gold nanoparticles by thermophilic filamentous fungi. *Scientific Reports*, *8*, 3943. https://doi.org/10.1038/s41598-018-22112-3

Monahan, E., McCrae, J. S., & Arbour, M. (2024). Participation in pediatric primary care innovation, DULCE, increases caregiver agency and resilience and decreases impact of stress. *Prevention Science*, *25*, 685–698. https://doi.org/10.1007/s11121-023-01608-z

Mongelli, F., Georgakopoulos, P., & Pato, M. T. (2020). Challenges and opportunities to meet the mental health needs of underserved and disenfranchised populations in the United States. *Focus (American Psychiatric Publishing)*, *18*(1), 16–24. https://doi.org/10.1176/appi.focus.20190028

Montalbano, A., Rodean, J., Canares, T., Burns, R., Lee, B., Alpern, E. R., & Hall, M. (2017). Urgent care utilization in the pediatric Medicaid population. *Journal of Pediatrics*, *191*, 238–243.e231. https://doi.org/10.1016/j.jpeds.2017.08.035

Montez, J. K. (2021). Diversity and inclusion in pediatrics is essential for promoting health equity. *American Academy of Pediatrics*. https://www.aap.org/en/news-room/aap-voices/diversity-and-inclusion-inpediatrics-is-essential-for-promoting-health-equity/

Moore, S., Timpe, Z., Rasberry, C. N., Hertz, M., Verlenden, J., Spencer, P., Murray, C., Lee, S., Barrios, L. C., Tripathi, T., McConnell, L., Iachan, R., & Pampati, S. (2024). Disparities in the implementation of school-based mental health supports among K–12 public schools. *Psychiatric Services*, *75*(1), 17–24. https://doi.org/10.1176/appi.ps.20220558

Morgan Health & NORC at the University of Chicago. (2022). *Health disparities in employer-sponsored insurance*. JPMorgan Chase & Co. https://www.jpmorganchase.com/content/dam/jpmc/jpmorgan-chase-and-co/who-we-are/our-business/documents/jpmc-morgan-health-norc-report-ada.pdf

Morishita, M., Takahashi, Y., Nishikawa, M., Sano, K., Kato, K., Yamashita, T., Imai, T., Saji, H., & Takakura, Y. (2015). Quantitative analysis of tissue distribution of the B16BL6-derived exosomes using a streptavidin-lactadherin fusion protein and iodine-125-labeled biotin derivative after intravenous injection in mice. *Journal of Pharmaceutical Sciences*, *104*(2), 705–713. https://doi.org/10.1002/jps.24251

Morrel-Samuels, S., Rupp, L. A., Eisman, A. B., Miller, A. L., Stoddard, S. A., Franzen, S. P., Hutchison, P., & Zimmerman, M. A. (2017). Measuring the Implementation of Youth Empowerment Solutions. *Health Promotion Practice*. https://doi.org/10.1177/1524839917736511

Mosher, D. K., Hook, J. N., Captari, L. E., Davis, D. E., DeBlaere, C., & Owen, J. (2017). Cultural humility: A therapeutic framework for engaging diverse clients. *Practice Innovations*, *2*(4), 221–233. https://doi.org/10.1037/pri0000055

Mosquera, D., Gonzalez, A., & Leeds, A. M. (2014). Early experience, structural dissociation, and emotional dysregulation in borderline personality disorder: The role of insecure and disorganized attachment. *Borderline Personality Disorder and Emotion Dysregulation*, *1*, 15. https://doi.org/10.1186/2051-6673-1-15

Mossey, J. M. (2011). Defining racial and ethnic disparities in pain management. *Clinical Orthopaedics and Related Research*, *469*, 1859–1870. https://link.springer.com/article/10.1007/s11999-011-1770-9

Mostashari, F. (2016). The paradox of size: How small, independent practices can thrive in value-based care. *Annals of Family Medicine*, *14*(1), 5–7. https://doi.org/10.1370/afm.1899

Moudatsou, M., Stavropoulou, A., Philalithis, A., & Koukouli, S. (2020). The role of empathy in health and social care professionals. *Healthcare*, *8*(1). https://doi.org/10.3390/healthcare8010026

Muehlenkamp, J. J., & Quinn-Lee, L. (2023). Effectiveness of a peer-led gatekeeper program: A longitudinal mixed-method analysis. *Journal of American College Health*, *71*(1), 282–291. https://doi.org/10.1080/07448481.2021.1891080

Muennig, P. A., Reynolds, M., Fink, D. S., Zafari, Z., & Geronimus, A. T. (2018). America's declining well-being, health, and life expectancy: Not just a white problem. *American Journal of Public Health*, *108*(12), 1626–1631. https://doi.org/10.2105/ajph.2018.304585

Mulcrone, P. L., Herzog, R. W., & Xiao, W. (2022). Adding recombinant AAVs to the cancer therapeutics mix. *Molecular Therapy Oncolytics*, *27*, 73–88. https://doi.org/10.1016/j.omto.2022.09.009

Mullin, A. P., Gokhale, A., Moreno-De-Luca, A., Sanyal, S., Waddington, J. L., & Faundez, V. (2013). Neurodevelopmental disorders: Mechanisms and boundary definitions from genomes, interactomes and proteomes. *Translational Psychiatry*, *3*(12), e329. https://doi.org/10.1038/tp.2013.108

Mulraney, M., Coghill, D., Bishop, C., Mehmed, Y., Sciberras, E., Sawyer, M., Efron, D., & Hiscock, H. (2021). A systematic review of the persistence of childhood mental health problems into adulthood. *Neuroscience and Biobehavioral Reviews*, *129*, 182–205. https://doi.org/10.1016/j.neubiorev.2021.07.030

Muralidharan, V., Burgart, A., Daneshjour, R., & Rose, S. (2023). Recommendations for the use of pediatric data in artificial intelligence and machine learning ACCEPT-AI. *NCBI*. https://www.ncbi.nlm.nih.gov/pmc/articles/PMC10482936/

Murillo, S. N., Rosenthal, A., Fenick, A. M., & Keene, D. (2022). The impact of a pediatric medical-legal partnership on pediatric providers: A qualitative study. *Academic Pediatrics*, *22*(3), 447–453. https://doi.org/10.1016/j.acap.2021.06.015

Murosko, D., Passerella, M., & Lorch, S. (2020). Racial segregation and intraventricular hemorrhage in preterm infants. *Pediatrics*, *145*(6). https://doi.org/10.1542/peds.2019-1508

Murphy, N. A., Alvey, J., Valentine, K. J., Mann, K., Wilkes, J., & Clark, E. B. (2020). Children with medical complexity: The 10-year experience of a single center. *Hospital Pediatrics*, *10*(8), 702–708. https://doi.org/10.1542/hpeds.2020-0085

Murphy, S. L., Kochanek, K. D., Xu, J., & Arias, E. (2021). *Mortality in the United States, 2020*. https://www.cdc.gov/nchs/products/databriefs/db427.htm

Murthy, K. S. (2021). *Confronting health misinformation*. Office of the U.S. Surgeon General, U.S. Department of Health and Human Services. https://www.hhs.gov/surgeongeneral/priorities/health-misinformation/index.html

Musich, S., Wang, S., Hawkins, K., & Klemes, A. (2016). The impact of personalized preventive care on health care quality, utilization, and expenditures. *Population Health Management*, *19*(6), 389–397. https://doi.org/10.1089/pop.2015.0171

Musumeci, M., Watts, M. O. M., Ammula, M., & Burns, A. (2022). *Medicaid financial eligibility in pathways based on old age or disability in 2022: Findings from a 50-state survey*. KFF. https://www.kff.org/report-section/medicaid-financial-eligibility-in-pathways-based-on-old-age-or-disability-in-2022-findings-from-a-50-state-survey-appendix/

Myers, D. (2017). *The new importance of children in America*. The Lucile Packard Foundation for Children's Health & Children's Hospital Association (CHA). https://lpfch.org/resource/the-new-importance-of-children-in-america/

Myers, K., Vander Stoep, A., Zhou, C., McCarty, C. A., & Katon, W. (2015). Effectiveness of a telehealth service delivery model for treating attention-deficit/hyperactivity disorder: A community-based randomized controlled trial. *Journal of the American Academy of Child and Adolescent Psychiatry*, *54*(4), 263–274. https://doi.org/10.1016/j.jaac.2015.01.009

Mykyta, L., Keisler-Starkey, K., & Bunch, L. (2022). *More children were covered by Medicaid and CHIP in 2021*. U.S. Census Bureau. https://www.census.gov/library/stories/2022/09/uninsured-rate-of-children-declines.html

Nahum, A. S., Vongsachang, H., Friedman, D. S., & Collins, M. E. (2022). Parental trust in school-based health care: A systematic review. *Journal of School Health*, *92*(1), 79–91.

Nakamura, M. M., Harper, M. B., & Jha, A. K. (2013). Change in adoption of electronic health records by US children's hospitals. *Pediatrics*, *131*(5), e1563–e1575. https://doi.org/10.1542/peds.2012-2904

Nardone, A., Casey, J. A., Morello-Frosch, R., Mujahid, M., Balmes, J. R., & Thakur, N. (2020). Associations between historical residential redlining and current age-adjusted rates of emergency department visits due to asthma across eight cities in California: an ecological study. *Lancet Planet Health*, *4*(1), e24–e31. https://doi.org/10.1016/s2542-5196(19)30241-4

National Academies of Sciences, Engineering, and Medicine (National Academies). (2015). *Mental disorders and disabilities among low-income children*. The National Academies Press. https://doi.org/10.17226/21780

_______. (2016). *Ending discrimination against people with mental and substance use disorders: The evidence for stigma change*. The National Academies Press. https://doi.org/10.17226/23442

_______. (2017a). *Communities in action: Pathways to health equity*. The National Academies Press. https://doi.org/10.17226/24624

_______. (2017b). *Training the future child health care workforce to improve the behavioral health of children, youth, and families: Proceedings of a workshop*. The National Academies Press. https://doi.org/10.17226/24877

_______. (2017c). *Communicating science effectively: A research agenda*. The National Academies Press. https://doi.org/10.17226/23674.

_______. (2018). *Opportunities for improving programs and services for children with disabilities*. The National Academies Press. https://doi.org/10.17226/25028

_______. (2019a). *A roadmap to reducing child poverty*. The National Academies Press. https://doi.org/10.17226/25246

_______. (2019b). *Fostering healthy mental, emotional, and behavioral development in children and youth: A national agenda*. The National Academies Press. https://doi.org/10.17226/25201

_______. (2019c). *The promise of adolescence: Realizing opportunity for all youth*. The National Academies Press. https://doi.org/10.17226/25388

_______. (2019d). *Vibrant and healthy kids: Aligning science, practice, and policy to advance health equity*. The National Academies Press. https://doi.org/10.17226/25466

_______. (2019e). *Taking action against clinician burnout: A systems approach to professional well-being*. The National Academies Press. https://doi.org/10.17226/25521

_______. (2020a). *Addressing health misinformation with health literacy strategies: Proceedings of a workshop—in brief*. The National Academies Press.

_______. (2020b). *Children's mental health and the life course model: A virtual workshop series: Proceedings of a workshop*. The National Academies Press. https://doi.org/10.17226/25941

_______. (2020c). *Framework for equitable allocation of COVID-19 vaccine*. The National Academies Press.

_______. (2020d). *Promoting positive adolescent health behaviors and outcomes: Thriving in the 21st century*. The National Academies Press. https://doi.org/10.17226/25552

_______. (2021a). *Considerations for using telemental health services for children and youth: Proceedings of a workshop–in brief*. The National Academies Press. https://doi.org/10.17226/26442.

_______. (2021b). *Implementing high-quality primary care: Rebuilding the foundation of health care*. The National Academies Press. https://doi.org/10.17226/25983
_______. (2021c). *Reimagining a system of care to promote the well-being of children and families: Proceedings of a workshop*. The National Academies Press. https://doi.org/10.17226/26098
_______. (2021d). *Strategies for building confidence in the COVID-19 vaccines*. The National Academies Press.
_______. (2021e). *The future of nursing 2020–2030: Charting a path to achieve health equity*. The National Academies Press. https://doi.org/10.17226/25982
_______. (2021f). *Exploring the role of critical health literacy in addressing the social determinants of health: Proceedings of a workshop—in brief*. The National Academies Press. https://doi.org/10.17226/26214
_______. (2022a). *Global roadmap for healthy longevity*. The National Academies Press. https://doi.org/10.17226/26144
_______. (2022b). *Responding to the current youth mental health crisis and preventing the next one: Proceedings of a workshop—in brief*. The National Academies Press. https://doi.org/10.17226/26669
_______. (2022c). *Optimizing care systems for people with intellectual and developmental disabilities: Proceedings of a workshop*. The National Academies Press. https://doi.org/10.17226/26624
_______. (2023a). *Achieving whole health: A new approach for veterans and the nation*. The National Academies Press. https://doi.org/10.17226/26854
_______. (2023b). *Addressing the long-term effects of the COVID-19 pandemic on children and families*. The National Academies Press. https://doi.org/10.17226/26809
_______. (2023c). *Closing the opportunity gap for young children*. The National Academies Press. https://doi.org/10.17226/26743
_______. (2023d). *Federal policy to advance racial, ethnic, and tribal health equity*. The National Academies Press.
_______. (2023e). *The future pediatric subspecialty physician workforce: Meeting the needs of infants, children, and adolescents*. The National Academies Press. https://doi.org/10.17226/27207
_______. (2023f). *Low birth weight babies and disability*. The National Academies Press. https://doi.org/10.17226/27375
_______. (2023g). *Reducing intergenerational poverty*. The National Academies Press.
_______. (2023h). *Social media and adolescent health*. The National Academies Press.
_______. (2023i). *Toward equitable innovation in health and medicine: A framework*. The National Academies Press. https://doi.org/10.17226/27184
_______. (2024a). *Addressing the rising mental health needs of an aging population: Proceedings of a workshop*. The National Academies Press. https://doi.org/10.17226/27340
_______. (2024b). *Ending unequal treatment: Strategies to achieve equitable health care and optimal health for all*. The National Academies Press. https://doi.org/10.17226/27820
National Academy for State Health Policy (NASHP). (2019). *A snapshot of state efforts to reach and enroll children for state Medicaid and CHIP programs*. https://nashp.org/a-snapshot-of-state-efforts-to-reach-and-enroll-children-for-state-medicaid-and-chip-programs/
National Academy of Medicine (NAM). (2023). *Emerging stronger from COVID-19: Priorities for health system transformation*. The National Academies Press. https://doi.org/10.17226/26657
_______. (2024). *Valuing America's health: Aligning financing to reward better health and well-being*. The National Academies Press. https://doi.org/10.17226/27141

National Alliance on Mental Illness (NAMI). (2016). *Out-of-network, out-of-pocket, out-of-options: The unfulfilled promise of parity.* https://www.nami.org/Support-Education/Publications-Reports/Public-Policy-Reports/Out-of-Network-Out-of-Pocket-Out-of-Options-The/Mental_Health_Parity2016.pdf

_______. (2017). *The doctor is out: Continuing disparities in access to mental and physical health care.* https://www.nami.org/wp-content/uploads/2023/08/DoctorIsOut.pdf

National Association of Community Health Centers (NACHC). (2014). *A sketch of community health centers chart book.*

_______. (2020). *Community health center chartbook.* https://www.nachc.org/wp-content/uploads/2020/01/Chartbook-2020-Final.pdf

_______. (2022). *America's health centers: 2022 snapshot.* https://www.nachc.org/resource/americas-health-centers-2022-snapshot/

_______. (2023a). *Closing the primary care gap: How community health centers can address the nation's primary care crisis.* https://www.nachc.org/wp-content/uploads/2023/06/Closing-the-Primary-Care-Gap_Full-Report_2023_digital-final.pdf

_______. (2023b). *Community health center chartbook: 2023.* https://www.nachc.org/wp-content/uploads/2023/07/Community-Health-Center-Chartbook-2023–2021UDS.pdf

National Association of County and City Health Officials (NACCHO). (2020). *NACCHO's 2019 Profile study: Local health department capacity to prepare for and respond to public health threats.* https://www.naccho.org/uploads/downloadable-resources/2019-Profile-Preparedness-Capacity.pdf

National Association of School Nurses. (2022). *Survey finds 45% of school nurses report mental health conditions.* https://www.nasn.org/blogs/nasn-inc/2022/09/22/survey-finds-45-of-school-nurses-report-mental-hea

_______. (2024). A contemporary *Framework* update for today's school nursing landscape: Introducing the *School Nursing Practice Framework™. NASN School Nurse.* https://doi.org/10.1177/1942602X241241092

National Association of Social Workers (NASW). (2023a). *Children, adolescents and young adults (CAYA) specialty practice section.* https://www.socialworkers.org/careers/specialty-practice-sections/Children-adolescents-and-young-adults

_______. (2023b). *Child welfare specialty practice section.* https://www.socialworkers.org/careers/specialty-practice-sections/child-welfare

National Center on Birth Defects and Developmental Disabilities (NCBDDD). (2023). *Fiscal year 2023 budget.* Centers for Disease Control and Prevention. https://www.cdc.gov/ncbddd/aboutus/budget/index.html#:~:text=CDC's%20National%20Center%20on%20Birth,Health%20Approach%20to%20Blood%20Disorders

National Center for Health Statistics. (n.d.). *CDC Data Finder.* Centers for Disease Control and Prevention. https://www.cdc.gov/nchs/index.htm

National Center for Health Workforce Analysis. (2023). *Health workforce projections.* Health Resources and Services Administration, U.S. Department of Health and Human Services. https://bhw.hrsa.gov/data-research/projecting-health-workforce-supply-demand

National Center for School Mental Health. (2020). Early intervention & treatment services & supports (Tiers 2 & 3). https://www.schoolmentalhealth.org/media/som/microsites/ncsmh/documents/quality-guides/Tiers-2-&-3.pdf

National Commission on the Certification of Physician Assistants (NCCPA). (2020). *2019 statistical profile of recently certified physician assistants.* https://www.nccpa.net/wp-content/uploads/2020/11/2019-Recently-Certified-Report-final_compressed.pdf

_______. (2023). *Pediatrics certificate of added qualifications (CAQ).* https://www.nccpa.net/specialty-certificates/#pediatrics

National Committee for Quality Assurance. (n.d.). *HEDIS measures.* https://www.ncqa.org/hedis/

_______. (2023). *Health plan accreditation.* https://www.ncqa.org/programs/health-plans/health-plan-accreditation-hpa/
National Council of Urban Indian Health (NCUIH). (2023). *Policy priorities 2023.* https://ncuih.org/wp-content/uploads/Policy-Priorities-23_NCUIH_D330_V4-1.pdf
National Home Visiting Resource Center (NHVRC). (2018). *2018 home visiting yearbook.* https://nhvrc.org/yearbook/2018-home-visiting-yearbook/
_______. (2020). *2020 Home visiting yearbook.* James Bell Associates. https://www.jbassoc.com/resource/2020-home-visiting-yearbook/
_______. (2023). *2023 home visiting yearbook.* James Bell Associates and the Urban Institute.
National Health Law Program. (2021). *Finding and analyzing Medicaid quality measures.* https://healthlaw.org/wp-content/uploads/2021/01/NHeLP_AnalyzingCoreMeasures01202021_embeddedlinks.pdf
National Human Genome Research Institute (NHGRI). (2024a). *Epigenetics.* https://www.genome.gov/genetics-glossary/Epigenetic
_______. (2024b). *Gene.* https://www.genome.gov/genetics-glossary/Gene.pdf
National Indian Child Welfare Association (NICWA). (2014). *Peer support programs.* https://www.nicwa.org/wp-content/uploads/2016/11/2014_PeerSupportPrograms_Newsletter.pdf
National Initiative on Mixed-Income Communities. (2020). *What works to promote inclusive, equitable mixed-income communities.* https://case.edu/socialwork/nimc/sites/default/files/2021-12/What%20Works%20book%202020.pdf
National Institute for Health and Care Excellence. (2018). *Attention deficit hyperactivity disorder: Diagnosis and management (NG87).* https://www.nice.org.uk/guidance/ng87
National Institute of Child Health and Human Development (NICHD). (n.d.). *Intellectual and developmental disabilities (IDDs).* https://www.nichd.nih.gov/health/topics/factsheets/idds
_______. (2021). *Oral health in America: Advances and challenges.* U.S. Department of Health and Human Services, National Institute of Dental and Craniofacial Research. https://www.nidcr.nih.gov/sites/default/files/2021-12/Oral-Health-in-America-Advances-and-Challenges.pdf
The National Organization of Nurse Practitioner Faculties. (2022). *Nurse practitioner role core competencies.* https://cdn.ymaws.com/www.nonpf.org/resource/resmgr/competencies/nonpf_np_role_core_competenc.pdf
National Partnership for Women & Families. (2023). *Case study: Leveraging value-based payment to advance health equity.* https://nationalpartnership.org/report/making-care-primary/
National Quality Forum. (2017). *A roadmap for promoting health equity and eliminating disparities: The four I's for health equity.* https://www.qualityforum.org/Publications/2017/09/A_Roadmap_for_Promoting_Health_Equity_and_Eliminating_Disparities__The_Four_I_s_for_Health_Equity.aspx
National Research Council (NRC). (2011). *Improving health in the United States: The role of health impact assessment.* National Academies Press. https://www.ncbi.nlm.nih.gov/books/NBK83538/
National Research Council (NRC) & Institute of Medicine (IOM). (1998). *Protecting youth at work: Health, safety, and development of working children and adolescents in the United States.* The National Academies Press. https://doi.org/10.17226/6019
_______. (2000). *From neurons to neighborhoods: The science of early childhood development.* The National Academies Press. https://doi.org/10.17226/9824
_______. (2004). *The National Academies collection: Reports funded by National Institutes of Health.* In *Children's Health, The Nation's Wealth: Assessing and Improving Child Health.* The National Academies Press. https://doi.org/10.17226/10886
_______. (2009). *Preventing mental, emotional, and behavioral disorders among young people: Progress and possibilities.* The National Academies Press. https://doi.org/10.17226/12480

_______. (2013). *U.S. health in international perspective: Shorter lives, poorer health.* The National Academies Press. https://doi.org/10.17226/13497

_______. (2015). *Transforming the workforce for children birth through age 8: A unifying foundation.* The National Academies Press. https://doi.org/10.17226/19401

National Rural Health Association (NRHA). (2015). *The future of rural behavioral health.* https://www.ruralhealth.us/getmedia/01d32ac2-da4c-45a7-b4d8-368accbd6682/The-Future-of-Rural-Behavioral-Health_Feb-2015.pdf

National School Lunch Program (NSLP). (2024). *National level annual summary tables: FY 1969–2023.* https://www.fns.usda.gov/pd/child-nutrition-tables

National Scientific Council on the Developing Child. (2020). *Connecting the brain to the rest of the body: Early childhood development and lifelong health are deeply intertwined.* https://developingchild.harvard.edu/resources/connecting-the-brain-to-the-rest-of-the-body-early-childhood-development-and-lifelong-health-are-deeply-intertwined/

National Task Force on Anchor Institutions (NTFAI). (2010). Anchor institutions task force. http://www.margainc.com/files_images/general/anchor_task_force_statement.pdf

National Vaccine Advisory Committee. (2013). Protecting the public's health: Critical functions of the Section 317 Immunization Program—A report of the National Vaccine Advisory Committee. *Public Health Reports*, *128*(2), 78–95. https://doi.org/10.1177/003335491312800203

Nationwide Children's Hospital. (n.d.a). *Healthy neighborhoods healthy families.* https://www.nationwidechildrens.org/about-us/population-health-and-wellness/healthy-neighborhoods-healthy-families

_______. (n.d.b). *What is substance use disorder (SUD)?* Nationwide Children's Hospital. https://www.nationwidechildrens.org/conditions/substance-use-disorder

Nchako, C., & Cai, L. (2018). *A closer look at who benefits from SNAP: State-by-state fact sheets.* Center on Budget and Policy Priorities.

Ndugga, N., & Artiga, S. (2023). *Disparities in health and health care: 5 key questions and answers.* KFF. https://www.kff.org/racial-equity-and-health-policy/issue-brief/disparities-in-health-and-health-care-5-key-question-and-answers/

Needlman, R., Fried, L. E., Morley, D. S., Taylor, S., & Zuckerman, B. (1991). Clinic-based intervention to promote literacy. A pilot study. *American Journal of Diseases of Children*, *145*(8), 881–884. https://doi.org/10.1001/archpedi.1991.02160080059021

Neil, A. L., & Christensen, H. (2009). Efficacy and effectiveness of school-based prevention and early intervention programs for anxiety. *Clinical Psychology Review*, *29*(3), 208–215. https://doi.org/10.1016/j.cpr.2009.01.002

Neitzel, A. J., Wolf, B., Guo, X., Shakarchi, A. F., Madden, N. A., Repka, M. X., Friedman, D. S., & Collins, M. E. (2021). Effect of a randomized interventional school-based vision program on academic performance of students in grades 3 to 7: A cluster randomized clinical trial. *JAMA Ophthalmology*, *139*(10), 1104–1114.

NEJM Catalyst. (2018). What is care coordination? *NEJM Catalyst.* Massachusetts Medical Society. https://catalyst.nejm.org/doi/full/10.1056/CAT.18.0291

Nelson, E. E., Lau, J. Y., & Jarcho, J. M. (2014). Growing pains and pleasures: How emotional learning guides development. *Trends in Cognitive Sciences*, *18*(2), 99–108. https://doi.org/10.1016/j.tics.2013.11.003

Neuwirth, Z. E. (2019). *Reframing healthcare: A roadmap for creating disruptive change.* Advantage Publishers.

New American Economy. (n.d.). *Undocumented immigrants.* New American Economy. https://www.newamericaneconomy.org/issues/undocumented-immigrants/

New York University (NYU) Langone Health. (n.d.). *Developmental–behavioral pediatrics research.* https://med.nyu.edu/departments-institutes/pediatrics/divisions/developmental-behavioral-pediatrics/research

Newgard, C. D., Lin, A., Malveau, S., Cook, J. N. B., Smith, M., Kuppermann, N., Remick, K. E., Gausche-Hill, M., Goldhaber-Fiebert, J., Burd, R. S., Hewes, H. A., Salvi, A., Xin, H., Ames, S. G., Jenkins, P. C., Marin, J., Hansen, M., Glass, N. E., Nathens, A. B., McConnell, K. J., & Pediatric Readiness Study Group. (2023). Emergency department pediatric readiness and short-term and long-term mortality among children receiving emergency care. *JAMA Network Open*, *6*(1), e2250941. https://doi.org/10.1001/jamanetworkopen.2022.50941

Newhouse, J. P. (2021). An ounce of prevention. *Journal of Economic Perspectives*, *35*(2), 101–118. https://doi.org/10.1257/jep.35.2.101

Nguyen, T. M., Crowther, C. A., Wilkinson, D., & Bain, E. (2013). Magnesium sulphate for women at term for neuroprotection of the fetus. *The Cochrane Database of Systematic Reviews*, (2), cd009395. https://doi.org/10.1002/14651858.CD009395.pub2

Nichols, L. M., & Taylor, L. A. (2018). Social determinants as public goods: A new approach to financing key investments in healthy communities. *Health Affairs*, *37*(8), 1223–1230. https://doi.org/10.1377/hlthaff.2018.0039

Nigg, J. T., Sibley, M. H., Thapar, A., & Karalunas, S. L. (2020). Development of ADHD: Etiology, heterogeneity, and early life course. *Annual Review of Developmental Psychology*, *2*(1), 559–583. https://doi.org/10.1146/annurev-devpsych-060320-093413

Niksch, M., & Papanicolas, I. (2023). *The provision of preventative health care for children and young people in selected high-income countries*. The National Academies Press.

Nock, M. K., & Favazza, A. R. (2009). Nonsuicidal self-injury: Definition and classification. In M. K. Nock (Ed.), *Understanding nonsuicidal self-injury* (pp. 9–18). American Psychological Association. http://www.jstor.org/stable/j.ctv1chrr2g.6

Nong, P. (2023). *AI in medicine need to counter bias, and not entrench it more*. NPR. https://www.npr.org/sections/health-shots/2023/06/06/1180314219/artificial-intelligence-racial-bias-health-care

Noorihekmat, S., Rahimi, H., Mehrolhassani, M. H., Chashmyazdan, M., Haghdoost, A. A., Ahmadi Tabatabaei, S. V., & Dehnavieh, R. (2020). Frameworks of performance measurement in public health and primary care system: A scoping review and meta-synthesis. *International Journal of Preventive Medicine*, *11*, 165. https://doi.org/10.4103/ijpvm.IJPVM_34_19

Norris, L. (2023). *How immigrants can obtain health coverage*. https://www.healthinsurance.org/obamacare/how-immigrants-are-getting-health-coverage/

Norris, T., & Howard, T. (2015). Can hospitals heal America's communities? "All in for mission" is the emerging model for impact. *Democracy Collaborative*. http://democracy-collaborative.org/content/can-hospitals-heal-americas-communities-0

North, S. (2023). Expanding telehealth in adolescent care: Moving beyond the COVID-19 pandemic. *Pediatrics*, *151*(Suppl 1). https://doi.org/10.1542/peds.2022-057267J

Novak, N. L., Lira, N., O'Connor, K. E., Harlow, S. D., Kardia, S. L. R., & Stern, A. M. (2018). Disproportionate sterilization of Latinos under California's eugenic sterilization program, 1920–1945. *American Journal of Public Health*, *108*(5), 611–613. https://doi.org/10.2105/ajph.2018.304369

Nutbeam, D. (2000). Health literacy as a public health goal: A challenge for contemporary health education and communication strategies into the 21st century. *Health Promotion International*, *15*(3), 259–267. https://doi.org/10.1093/heapro/15.3.259

Nuwarda, R. F., Ramzan, I., Weekes, L., & Kayser, V. (2022). Vaccine hesitancy: Contemporary issues and historical background. *Vaccines*, *10*(10). https://doi.org/10.3390/vaccines10101595

Nweke, N., Isom, J., & Fashaw-Walters, S. (2022). Health equity tourism: Reckoning with medical mistrust. *Journal of Medical Systems*, *46*(5), 27. https://doi.org/10.1007/s10916-022-01812-4

NYC Health + Hospitals. (2020). *NYC Health + Hospitals launches 3-2-1 Impact, a program that provides early intervention services to support the health and well-being of young children and families.* https://www.nychealthandhospitals.org/pressrelease/system-launches-3-2-1-impact-program-provides-early-intervention-services-to-families/

O'Connor, E., O'Connor, M., Gray, S., & Goldfeld, S. (2018). Profiles of mental health competence and difficulties as predictors of children's early learning. *School Mental Health, 10*(3), 402–416. https://doi.org/10.1007/s12310-018-9252-9

Office of the Attorney General. (2018). *The Attorney General's community benefits guidelines for non-profit hospitals.* Commonwealth of Massachusetts. https://www.mass.gov/doc/updated-nonprofit-hospital-community-benefits-guidelines/download

Office of Disease Prevention and Health Promotion (ODPHP). (n.d.a). *Healthy people 2030.* U.S. Department of Health and Human Services. https://health.gov/healthypeople/objectives-and-data/social-determinants-health

________. (n.d.b). *Healthy people 2030, leading health indicators.* U.S. Department of Health and Human Services. https://health.gov/healthypeople/objectives-and-data/leading-health-indicators

Office of Juvenile Justice and Delinquency Prevention. (2022a). *Estimated number of youth arrests.* U.S. Department of Justice. https://ojjdp.ojp.gov/statistical-briefing-book/crime/faqs/qa05101

________. (2022b). *OJJDP statistical briefing book, poverty status of children by family structure.* U.S. Department of Justice. https://ojjdp.ojp.gov/statistical-briefing-book/population/faqs/qa01203

Office of Head Start. (2023a). *About the office of Head Start.* U.S. Department of Health & Human Services, Administration for Children & Families. https://www.acf.hhs.gov/ohs/about

________. (2023b). *Head Start programs.* U.S. Department of Health & Human Services, Administration for Children & Families. https://www.acf.hhs.gov/ohs/about/head-start

________. (2023c). *Services snapshot.* U.S. Department of Health & Human Services, Administration for Children & Families. https://www.acf.hhs.gov/ohs/about/services-snapshot

Office of Management and Budget (OMB). (n.d.). *Table 15.1—Total outlays for health programs: 1962–2029. Historical Tables.* https://www.whitehouse.gov/omb/budget/historical-tables

________. (2023). *Appendix, budget of the United States government, fiscal year 2024.* U.S. Government Printing Office.

Office of the National Coordinator for Health Information Technology (ONC). (n.d.). *What is a health information exchange?* https://www.healthit.gov/topic/health-it-and-health-information-exchange-basics/what-hie

________. (2020). *Pediatric health information technology: Pediatric healthcare provider informational resource.* https://www.healthit.gov/sites/default/files/page/2020-12/Pediatric_HealthIT_Provider_IR_Print_508.pdf

________. (2023). *Patient-generated health data.* https://www.healthit.gov/topic/scientific-initiatives/pcor/patient-generated-health-data-pghd

Office of Special Education Programs. (2022). *IDEA section 618 data products.* U.S. Department of Education. https://data.ed.gov/dataset/idea-section-618-data-products

Office of the State Superintendent of Education. (n.d.). *National School Lunch Program (NSLP).* D.C. Government. https://osse.dc.gov/service/national-school-lunch-program-nslp

Office of the Surgeon General (OSG). (2021). *Protecting youth mental health: The U.S. Surgeon General's advisory.* U.S. Department of Health and Human Services. https://www.hhs.gov/sites/default/files/surgeon-general-youth-mental-health-advisory.pdf

________. (2024). *Firearm violence: A public health crisis in America: The U.S. Surgeon General's advisory.* U.S. Department of Health and Human Services. https://www.hhs.gov/sites/default/files/firearm-violence-advisory.pdf

Office on Violence Against Women. (2023). *Domestic violence.* U.S. Department of Justice. https://www.justice.gov/ovw/domestic-violence

Ofri, D. (2020, February 20). Why are nonprofit hospitals so highly profitable? *The New York Times.* https://www.nytimes.com/2020/02/20/opinion/nonprofit-hospitals.html

Ogden, C. L., Fryar, C. D., Martin, C. B., Freedman, D. S., Carroll, M. D., Gu, Q., & Hales, C. M. (2020). Trends in obesity prevalence by race and Hispanic origin-1999–2000 to 2017–2018. *Journal of the American Medical Association, 324*(12), 1208–1210. https://doi.org/10.1001/jama.2020.14590

Oh, W. O. (2023). Digital healthcare for child health nursing. *Journal of Pediatric Nursing, 64,* 1–10. https://doi.org/10.1016/j.pedn.2023.04.001

O'Hare, W. (2001). *The child population: First data from the 2000 census. A KIDS COUNT/PRB report on Census 2000.* Population Reference Bureau.

O'Hare, W., & Mayol-Garcia, Y. H. (2023). *The changing child population of the United States.* Annie E. Casey Foundation. https://www.aecf.org/resources/the-changing-child-population-of-the-united-states

Ohio Department of Health. (2020). *DataOhio. Infant mortality phase I.* https://data.ohio.gov/wps/portal/gov/data/projects/06infant-mortality

O'Keefe, V. M., Fish, J., Maudrie, T. L., Hunter, A. M., Tai Rakena, H. G., Ullrich, J. S., Clifford, C., Crawford, A., Brockie, T., Walls, M., Haroz, E. E., Cwik, M., Whitesell, N. R., & Barlow, A. (2022). Centering Indigenous knowledges and worldviews: Applying the Indigenist ecological systems model to youth mental health and wellness research and programs. *International Journal of Environmental Research and Public Health, 19*(10), 6271. https://doi.org/10.3390/ijerph19106271

O'Keefe, V. M., Maudrie, T. L., Cole, A. B., Ullrich, J. S., Fish, J., Hill, K. X., White, L. A., Redvers, N., Jernigan, V. B. B., Lewis, J. P., West, A. E., Apok, C. A., White, E. J., Ivanich, J. D., Schultz, K., Lewis, M. E., Sarche, M. C., Gonzalez, M. B., Parker, M., . . . Walls, M. L. (2023). Conceptualizing Indigenous strengths-based health and wellness research using group concept mapping. *Archives of Public Health, 81*(1), 71. https://doi.org/10.1186/s13690-023-01066-7

O'Loughlin, K., Shadowen, H. M., Haley, A. D., Gilbert, J., Kashiri, P. L., Webel, B., Huebschmann, A. G., & Krist, A. H. (2022). Patient preferences for discussing and acting on health-related needs in primary care. *Journal of Primary Care & Community Health, 13.* https://doi.org/10.1177/21501319221115946

Olds, D., Henderson, C., Tatelbaum, R., & Chamberlin, R. (1986). Improving the delivery of prenatal care and outcomes of pregnancy: A randomized trial of nurse home visitation. *Pediatrics, 77,* 16–28. https://doi.org/10.1542/peds.77.1.16

Olshansky, S. J., Passaro, D. J., Hershow, R. C., Layden, J., Carnes, B. A., Brody, J., Hayflick, L., Butler, R. N., Allison, D. B., & Ludwig, D. S. (2005). A potential decline in life expectancy in the United States in the 21st century. *New England Journal of Medicine, 352*(11), 1138–1145. https://doi.org/10.1056/NEJMsr043743

O'Mara, M. (2012). Beyond town and gown: University economic engagement and the legacy of the urban crisis. *The Journal of Technology Transfer, 37*(2), 234–250. https://doi.org/10.1007/s10961-010-9185-4

Omoloja, A., & Vundavalli, S. (2021). Patient generated health data: Benefits and challenges. *Current Problems in Pediatric and Adolescent Health Care, 51*(11), 101103. https://doi.org/10.1016/j.cppeds.2021.101103

O'Neil, J., Louzon, M. L., Talty, J., Matthews, J. D., & Bull, M. J. (2013). Child car seat inspection stations: Who attends and what is the benefit? *Annals of Advances in Automotive Medicine, 57,* 363–364.

Ong, M. K., Romano, P. S., Edgington, S., Aronow, H. U., Auerbach, A. D., Black, J. T., De Marco, T., Escarce, J. J., Evangelista, L. S., Hanna, B., Ganiats, T. G., Greenberg, B. H., Greenfield, S., Kaplan, S. H., Kimchi, A., Liu, H., Lombardo, D., Mangione, C. M., Sadeghi, B., . . . Fonarow, G. C. (2016). Effectiveness of remote patient monitoring after discharge of hospitalized patients with heart failure: The better effectiveness after transition—Heart failure (BEAT-HF) randomized clinical trial. *JAMA Internal Medicine*, *176*(3), 310–318. https://doi.org/10.1001/jamainternmed.2015.7712

Opipari-Arrigan, L., Dykes, D. M. H., Saeed, S. A., Thakkar, S., Burns, L., Chini, B. A., McPhail, G. L., Eslick, I., Margolis, P. A., & Kaplan, H. C. (2020). Technology-enabled health care collaboration in pediatric chronic illness: Pre-post interventional study for feasibility, acceptability, and clinical impact of an electronic health record–linked platform for patient-clinician partnership. *JMIR Mhealth Uhealth*, *8*(11), e11968. https://doi.org/10.2196/11968

Orchinik, L. J., Taylor, H. G., Espy, K. A., Minich, N., Klein, N., Sheffield, T., & Hack, M. (2011). Cognitive outcomes for extremely preterm/extremely low birth weight children in kindergarten. *Journal of the International Neuropsychological Society*, *17*(6), 1067–1079. https://doi.org/10.1017/s135561771100107x

Oregon Health Authority. (n.d.). *Health aspects of kindergarten readiness*. https://www.oregon.gov/oha/hpa/analytics/pages/kr-health.aspx

________. (2021). *Maximizing coverage through the Oregon Health Plan*. https://sharedsystems.dhsoha.state.or.us/DHSForms/Served/he3786b_2.pdf

________. (2023). *Oregon Health Plan: 2022–2027 demonstration amendment*. https://www.oregon.gov/oha/HSD/Medicaid-Policy/Documents/2022-2027-Demonstration-Amendment.pdf

Orenstein, W. A. (2023). *Congress passes law to establish vaccines for children program*. https://www.nfid.org/the-lifesaving-impact-of-vaccines-for-children/

Organisation for Economic Co-operation and Development (OECD). (2020). *Early learning and child well-being in the United States*. OECD iLibrary. https://doi.org/10.1787/198d8c99-en

________. (2022). *OECD child and well-being dashboard*. OECD iLibrary. https://www.oecd.org/els/family/child-well-being/data/dashboard/

Orr, C. J., Leslie, L. K., Schaechter, J., Williams, X. J., Montez, K. G., Deen, J. F., Evans, Y. N., Russell, C. J., Webb, J., Gaona, A. R., & Mendoza, F. S. (2024). Diversity, equity, and inclusion, child health, and the pediatric subspecialty workforce. *Pediatrics*, *153*(Suppl 2), e2023063678S. https://doi.org/10.1542/peds.2023-063678S

Orr, S. T., & Miller, C. A. (1997). Unintended pregnancy and the psychosocial well-being of pregnant women. *Women's Health Issues*, *7*(1), 38–46. https://doi.org/10.1016/s1049-3867(96)00017-5

Ortman, J. M., Velkoff, V. A., & Hogan, H. (2014). *An aging nation: The older population in the United States, population estimates and projections* (Current Population Report No. P25-1140). U.S. Census Bureau. https://www.census.gov/content/dam/Census/library/publications/2014/demo/p25-1140.pdf

Osofsky, J. D. (1999). The impact of violence on children. *The Future of Children*, *9*(3), 33–49. https://doi.org/10.2307/1602780

Ostergaard, M., & Guzzetta, C. (2021). *A guide to implementing child passenger safety inspection stations* (Report No. DOT HS 812 692). National Highway Traffic Safety Administration. https://rosap.ntl.bts.gov/view/dot/55179

Osterman, M. J. K., Hamilton, B. E., Martin, J. A., Driscoll, A. K., & Valenzuela, C. P. (2023). Births: Final data for 2021. *National Vital Statistics Reports*. https://pubmed.ncbi.nlm.nih.gov/36723449/

Overhage, L. N., Benson, N. M., Flores, M. W., & Cook, B. L. (2024). Self-pay outpatient mental health care for children and adolescents, by socioeconomic status. *Psychiatric Services*, *75*(9). https://doi.org/10.1176/appi.ps.20230524

Owen, M. C., Wallace, S. B., Committee on Adolescence, Alderman, E. M., Chung, R., Grubb, L. K., Lee, J., Powers, M. E., Rahmandar, M. H., & Upadhya, K. K. (2020). Advocacy and collaborative health care for justice-involved youth. *Pediatrics*, *146*(1). https://doi.org/10.1542/peds.2020-1755

Owen, M. J., Wright, M. S., Batalov, S., Kwon, Y., Ding, Y., Chau, K. K., Chowdhury, S., Sweeney, N. M., Kiernan, E., Richardson, A., Batton, E., Baer, R. J., Bandoli, G., Gleeson, J. G., Bainbridge, M., Chambers, C. D., & Kingsmore, S. F. (2023). Reclassification of the etiology of infant mortality with whole-genome sequencing. *JAMA Network Open*, *6*(2), e2254069–e2254069. https://doi.org/10.1001/jamanetworkopen.2022.54069

Owsley, K. M., Hamer, M. K., & Mays, G. P. (2020). The growing divide in the composition of public health delivery systems in US rural and urban communities, 2014–2018. *American Journal of Public Health*, *110*(S2), S204–S210. https://doi.org/10.2105/ajph.2020.305801

Owusu-Ansah, S., Moore, B., Shah, M. I., Gross, T., Brown, K., Gausche-Hill, M., Remick, K., Adelgais, K., Rappaport, L., & Wright, J. (2015). Pediatric readiness in emergency medical services systems. *Annals of Emergency Medicine*, *66*(6), 619–629. https://doi.org/10.1111/1475-6773.12657

Ozeke, O., Ozeke, V., Coskun, O., & Budakoglu, I. I. (2019). Second victims in health care: Current perspectives. *Advances in Medical Education and Practice*, *10*, 593–603. https://doi.org/10.2147/amep.S185912

Ozer, E. J., Abraczinskas, M., Duarte, C., Mathur, R., Ballard, P. J., Gibbs, L., Olivas, E. T., Bewa, M. J., & Afifi, R. (2020). Youth participatory approaches and health equity: Conceptualization and integrative review. *American Journal of Community Psychology*, *66*(3-4), 267–278. https://doi.org/10.1002/ajcp.12451

Oztek Celebi, F. Z., & Senel, S. (2021). Patients with chronic conditions and their complex care needs in a tertiary care hospital. *Archives de Pédiatrie*, *28*(6), 470–474. https://doi.org/10.1016/j.arcped.2021.05.001

Pabayo, R., Ehntholt, A., Davis, K., Liu, S. Y., Muennig, P., & Cook, D. M. (2019). Structural racism and odds for infant mortality among infants born in the United States 2010. *Journal of Racial and Ethnic Health Disparities*, *6*(6), 1095–1106. https://doi.org/10.1007/s40615-019-00612-w

Pachter, L. M., & García Coll, C. (2009). Racism and child health: A review of the literature and future directions. *Journal of Developmental and Behavioral Pediatrics*, *30*(3), 255–263. https://doi.org/10.1097/DBP.0b013e3181a7ed5a

Palfrey, J. S., Sofis, L. A., Davidson, E. J., Liu, J., Freeman, L., & Ganz, M. L. (2004). The pediatric alliance for coordinated care: Evaluation of a medical home model. *Pediatrics*, *113*(Suppl 4), 1507–1516. https://doi.org/10.1542/peds.113.S4.1507

Pan American Health Organization. (n.d.). *Support kids with cancer—Early diagnosis of childhood cancer.* https://www.paho.org/en/campaigns/support-kids-cancer-early-diagnosis-childhood-cancer

_______. (2015). *Advancing the health in all policies approach in the Americas: What is the health sector's role? A brief guide and recommendations for promoting intersectoral collaboration.* PAHO. https://www3.paho.org/hq/dmdocuments/2015/hiap-Brief-Guide-and-Recomendations-ENG.pdf

Panchal, N. (2022). *The impact of gun violence on children and adolescents.* KFF. https://www.kff.org/mental-health/issue-brief/the-impact-of-gun-violence-on-children-and-adolescents/

Pandolfini, C., & Bonati, M. (2005). A literature review on off-label drug use in children. *European Journal of Pediatrics*, *164*(9), 552–558. https://doi.org/10.1007/s00431-005-1698-8

Pape, G. A., Hunt, J. S., Butler, K. L., Siemienczuk, J., LeBlanc, B. H., Gillanders, W., Rozenfeld, Y., & Bonin, K. (2011). Team-based care approach to cholesterol management in diabetes mellitus: Two-year cluster randomized controlled trial. *Archives of Internal Medicine, 171*(16), 1480–1486. https://doi.org/10.1001/archinternmed.2011.417

Paradies, Y., Ben, J., Denson, N., Elias, A., Priest, N., Pieterse, A., Gupta, A., Kelaher, M., & Gee, G. (2015). Racism as a determinant of health: A systematic review and meta-analysis. *PLoS One, 10*(9). https://doi.org/10.1371/journal.pone.0138511

Parish, S. L., Magaña, S., Swaine, J. G., & Son, E. (2013). Chapter five—Studying racial and ethnic health care disparities among children with intellectual and developmental disabilities using the national survey of children with special health care needs. In R. C. Urbano (Ed.), *International Review of Research in Developmental Disabilities* (Vol. 45, pp. 185–224). Academic Press. https://doi.org/10.1016/B978-0-12-407760-7.00005-0

Park, S. H., & Bao, G. (2021). CRISPR/Cas9 gene editing for curing sickle cell disease. *Transfusion and Apheresis Science, 60*(1), 103060–103060. https://doi.org/10.1016/j.transci.2021.103060

Parker, K., Menasce Horowits, J., Brown, A., Fry, R., Cohn, D., & Igielnik, R. (2018). *Demographic and economic trends in urban, suburban and rural communities.* Pew Research Center. https://www.pewresearch.org/social-trends/2018/05/22/demographic-and-economic-trends-in-urban-suburban-and-rural-communities/

Parker, M., Diamond, R., & Guercio, A. (2019). Care coordination of autism spectrum disorder: A solution-focused approach. *Issues in Mental Health Nursing, 41*, 1–8. https://doi.org/10.1080/01612840.2019.1624899

Parolin, Z., & Wimer, C. (2020). Forecasting estimates of poverty during the COVID-19 crisis. *Poverty and Social Policy*. https://ideas.repec.org/p/aji/briefs/2046.html

Paskett, E. D., Harrop, J. P., & Wells, K. J. (2011). Patient navigation: An update on the state of the science. *CA: A Cancer Journal for Clinicians, 61*(4), 237–249. https://doi.org/10.3322/caac.20111

Pathak, P. R., & Chou, A. (2019). Confidential care for adolescents in the U.S. health care system. *Journal of Patient-Centered Research and Reviews, 6*(1), 46–50. https://doi.org/10.17294/2330-0698.1656

Patient-Centered Outcomes Research Institute (PCORI). (2015). *Financial compensation of patients, caregivers, and patient/caregiver organizations engaged in PCORI-funded research as engaged research partners.* https://www.pcori.org/sites/default/files/PCORI-Compensation-Framework-for-Engaged-Research-Partners.pdf

Patient Protection and Affordable Care Act, 42 U.S.C. § 9007 (2010).

Patel, M., & Raphael, J. L. (2023). Pediatric subspecialty pipeline: Aligning care needs with a changing pediatric health care delivery environment. *Pediatric Research, 93*(7), 1791–1793. https://doi.org/10.1038/s41390-023-02599-x

Patel, N. (2020). Improving health outcomes through patient education and partnerships with patients. *Journal of Cardiology,* University of Florida College of Medicine. https://www.ncbi.nlm.nih.gov/pmc/articles/PMC5242136/

Patrick, S. W., Richards, M. R., Dupont, W. D., McNeer, E., Buntin, M. B., Martin, P. R., Davis, M. M., Davis, C. S., Hartmann, K. E., Leech, A. A., Lovell, K. S., Stein, B. D., & Cooper, W. O. (2020). Association of pregnancy and insurance status with treatment access for opioid use disorder. *JAMA Network Open, 3*(8), e2013456. https://doi.org/10.1001/jamanetworkopen.2020.13456

Payot, A., & Barrington, K. J. (2011). The quality of life of young children and infants with chronic medical problems: Review of the literature. *Current Problems in Pediatric and Adolescent Health Care, 41*(4), 91–101. https://doi.org/10.1016/j.cppeds.2010.10.008

Peahl, A. F., & Howell, J. D. (2021). The evolution of prenatal care delivery guidelines in the United States. *American Journal of Obstetrics and Gynecology*, *224*(4), 339–347. https://doi.org/10.1016/j.ajog.2020.12.016

Pediatric Nursing Certification Board (PNCB). (2021). *Position statement, optimizing the health and well-being of America's children: The value of PNCB pediatric nursing certification.* https://www.pncb.org/sites/default/files/resources/Value_of_PNCB_Certifications_to_Health_Care_Industry_2021_Final.pdf

_______. (2022). *Who provides nursing care for our kids? Pediatric nursing workforce report 2022.* https://www.pncb.org/sites/default/files/resources/PNCB_2022_Pediatric_Nursing_Workforce_Demographic_Report.pdf

Pediatric Research Equity Act, Pub. L. No. 108-155, 117 Stat. 1936 (2003).

Pediatrics Supporting Parents (PSP). (n.d). *Pediatrics supporting parents: Home.* https://www.pediatricssupportingparents.org/

PEDSnet. (n.d.). *A pediatric learning health system.* https://pedsnet.org/

Penmetsa, P., Wang, T., & Nambisan, S. (2017). *An assessment of child restraint system misuse in the United States* [Presentation]. Transportation Research Board 97th Annual Meeting, Washington, DC.

Perez, M. F., & Coutinho, M. T. (2021). An overview of health disparities in asthma. *Yale Journal of Biology and Medicine*, *94*(3), 497–507.

Permar, S. (2022). "When will kids under five get COVID vaccines?" and other questions [Interview]. *Scientific American.* https://www.scientificamerican.com/article/when-will-kids-under-five-get-covid-vaccines-and-other-questions/

Perrin, J. M., Anderson, L. E., & van Cleave, J. (2014). The rise in chronic conditions among infants, children, and youth can be met with continued health system innovations. *Health Affairs (Project Hope)*, *33*(12), 2099–2105. https://doi.org/10.1377/hlthaff.2014.0832

Perrin, J. M., Asarnow, J. R., Stancin, T., Melek, S. P., & Fritz, G. K. (2019). Mental health conditions and health care payments for children with chronic medical conditions. *Academic Pediatrics*, *19*(1), 44–50. https://doi.org/10.1016/j.acap.2018.10.001

Perrin, J. M., Bloom, S. R., & Gortmaker, S. L. (2007). The increase of childhood chronic conditions in the United States. *Journal of the American Medical Association*, *297*(24), 2755–2759. https://doi.org/10.1001/jama.297.24.2755

Perrin, J. M., Cheng, T. L., Stoll, B. J., Boat, T., & Fuentes-Afflick, E. (2023a). Children, youth, and the life course: IOM/NAM contributions and critical areas for the future. *NAM Perspectives, 2023.* https://doi.org/10.31478/202301a

Perrin, J. M., Duncan, G., Diaz, A., & Kelleher, K. (2020a). Principles and policies to strengthen child and adolescent health and well-being. *Health Affairs (Project Hope)*, *39*(10), 1677–1683. https://doi.org/10.1377/hlthaff.2020.00709

Perrin, J. M., Flanagan, P., Katkin, J., Barabell, G., & Price, J. (2023b). The unique value proposition of pediatric health care. *Pediatrics*, *151*(2). https://doi.org/10.1542/peds.2022-060681

Perrin, J. M., Greenspan, P., Bloom, S. R., Finkelstein, D., Yazdgerdi, S., Leventhal, J. M., Rodewald, L., Szilagyi, P., & Homer, C. J. (1996). Primary care involvement among hospitalized children. *Archives of Pediatrics & Adolescent Medicine*, *150*(5), 479–486.

Perrin, J. M., Kenney, G. M., & Rosenbaum, S. (2020b). Medicaid and child health equity. *New England Journal of Medicine*, *383*(27), 2595–2598. https://doi.org/10.1056/nejmp2030646

Perrin, J. M., Lu, M. C., Geller, A., & DeVoe, J. E. (2020c). Vibrant and healthy kids: Aligning science, practice, and policy to advance health equity. *Academic Pediatrics*, *20*(2), 160–162. https://doi.org/10.1016/j.acap.2019.11.019

Perrin, J. M., Valvona, J., & Sloan, F. A. (1986). Changing patterns of hospitalization for children requiring surgery. *Pediatrics*, *77*(4), 587–592.

Perrin, J. M., Zimmerman, E., Hertz, A., Johnson, T., Merrill, T., & Smith, D. (2017). Pediatric accountable care organizations: Insight from early adopters. *Pediatrics*, *139*(2). https://doi.org/10.1542/peds.2016-1840

Perry, D. F., Allen, M., Brennan, E. M., & Bradley, J. (2010). The evidence base for mental health consultation in early childhood settings: A research synthesis addressing children's behavioral outcomes. *Early Education and Development*, *21*(6), 795–824. https://doi.org/10.1080/10409280903475444

Perry, D. F., Dunne, M. C., McFadden, L., & Campbell, D. (2008). Reducing the risk for preschool expulsion: Mental health consultation for young children with challenging behaviors. *Journal of Child and Family Studies*, *17*(1), 44–54.

Peterson, C., Aslam, M. V., Niolon, P. H., Bacon, S., Bellis, M. A., Mercy, J. A., & Florence, C. (2023). Economic burden of health conditions associated with adverse childhood experiences among US adults. *JAMA Network Open*, *6*(12), e2346323. https://doi.org/10.1001/jamanetworkopen.2023.46323

Peterson-KFF Health System Tracker. (2022). Length of life: Life expectancy. https://www.healthsystemtracker.org/indicator/health-well-being/life-expectancy/#Life%20expectancy%20at%20birth,%20by%20state,%202020

Pethe, K., Baxterbeck, A., Rosenthal, S. L., & Stockwell, M. S. (2019). Why parents use the emergency department despite having a medical home. *Clinical Pediatrics*, *58*(1), 95–99. https://doi.org/10.1177/0009922818809447

Petit-Steeghs, V., Lips, S. R., Schuitmaker-Warnaar, T. J., & Broerse, J. E. W. (2019). Client-centred maternity care from women's perspectives: Need for responsiveness. *Midwifery*, *74*, 76–83. https://doi.org/10.1016/j.midw.2019.03.016

Petiwala, A., Lanford, D., Landers, G., & Minyard, K. (2021). Community voice in cross-sector alignment: Concepts and strategies from a scoping review of the health collaboration literature. *BMC Public Health*, *21*(1), 712. https://doi.org/10.1186/s12889-021-10741-9

Petkovic, J., Barton, J. L., Flurey, C., Goel, N., Bartels, C. M., Barnabe, C., de Wit, M. P. T., Lyddiatt, A., Lacaille, D., Welch, V., Boonen, A., Shea, B., Christensen, R., Maxwell, L. J., Campbell, W., Jull, J., Toupin-April, K., Singh, J. A., Goldsmith, C. H., . . . Tugwell, P. S. (2017). Health equity considerations for developing and reporting patient-reported outcomes in clinical trials: A report from the OMERACT equity special interest group. *Journal of Rheumatology*, *44*(11), 1727–1733. https://doi.org/10.3899/jrheum.160975

The Pew Charitable Trusts. (2022). *The long-term decline in fertility—and what it means for state budgets*. https://www.pewtrusts.org/en/research-and-analysis/issue-briefs/2022/12/the-long-term-decline-in-fertility-and-what-it-means-for-state-budgets

Pew Research Center. (2015). *Modern immigration wave brings 59 million to U.S., driving population growth and change through 2065: Views of immigration's impact on U.S. society mixed*. https://search.issuelab.org/resources/23118/23118.pdf

Pham, S., Porta, G., Biernesser, C., Walker Payne, M., Iyengar, S., Melhem, N., & Brent, D. A. (2018). The burden of bereavement: Early-onset depression and impairment in youths bereaved by sudden parental death in a 7-year prospective study. *American Journal of Psychiatry*, *175*(9), 887–896. https://doi.org/10.1176/appi.ajp.2018.17070792

Phelan, S. M., Salinas, M., Pankey, T., Cummings, G., Allen, J. P., Waniger, A., Miller, N. E., Lebow, J., Dovidio, J. F., van Ryn, M., & Doubeni, C. A. (2023). Patient and health care professional perspectives on stigma in integrated behavioral health: Barriers and recommendations. *Annals of Family Medicine*, *21*(Suppl 2), S56–S60. https://doi.org/10.1370/afm.2924

Phibbs, C. S., Baker, L. C., Caughey, A. B., Danielsen, B., Schmitt, S. K., & Phibbs, R. H. (2007). Level and volume of neonatal intensive care and mortality in very-low-birth-weight infants. *New England Journal of Medicine*, *356*(21), 2165–2175. https://doi.org/10.1056/NEJMsa065029

Phillips, J. (2020). Pediatric vital signs: Measuring and improving the health of a population. *Pediatrics Nationwide*. https://pediatricsnationwide.org/2020/10/01/pediatric-vital-signs-measuring-and-improving-the-health-of-a-population/

Phillips, R. L., McCann, J. L., Bazemore, A., Fryer, G. E., Klein, L. S., & Weitzman, M. (2005). *Report to the task force on the care of children by family physicians*. https://www.graham-center.org/content/dam/rgc/documents/publications-reports/monographs-books/rgcmo-care-children.pdf

Pianta, R. C., & Hamre, B. K. (2009). Conceptualization, measurement, and improvement of classroom processes: Standardized observation can leverage capacity. *Educational Researcher*, *38*(2), 109–119.

Pica, N., & Bourgeois, F. (2016). Discontinuation and nonpublication of randomized clinical trials conducted in children. *Pediatrics*, *138*(3). https://doi.org/10.1542/peds.2016-0223

Piccolo, L. R., Roby, E., Canfield, C. F., Seery, A. M., Weisleder, A., Cates, C. B., Tutasig, L., Matalon, M., Custode, A., Rodriguez, L., & Mendelsohn, A. L. (2023). Supporting responsive parenting in real-world implementation: Minimal effective dose of the Video Interaction Project. *Pediatric Research*, *95*, 1295–1300. https://doi.org/10.1038/s41390-023-02916-4

Pillai, D., & Artiga, S. (2022). *2022 Changes to the public charge inadmissibility rule and the implications for health care*. KFF. https://www.kff.org/racial-equity-and-health-policy/issue-brief/2022-changes-to-the-public-charge-inadmissibility-rule-and-the-implications-for-health-care/

Pillai, D., Artiga, S., Hamel, L., Shumacher, S., Kirzinger, A., Presiado, M., & Kearney, A. (2023). *Health and health care experiences of immigrants: The 2023 KFF/LA Times survey of immigrants*. KFF. https://www.kff.org/racial-equity-and-health-policy/issue-brief/health-and-health-care-experiences-of-immigrants-the-2023-kff-la-times-survey-of-immigrants/

Pinedo, M., & Villatoro, A. P. (2020). The role of perceived treatment need in explaining racial/ethnic disparities in the use of substance abuse treatment services. *Journal of Substance Abuse Treatment*, *118*, 108105. https://doi.org/10.1016/j.jsat.2020.108105

Pinto-Coelho, L. (2023). How artificial intelligence is shaping medical imaging technology: A survey of innovations and applications. *Bioengineering*, *10*(12). https://doi.org/10.3390/bioengineering10121435

Piotrowski, C., Talavera, G., & Mayer, J. (2009). HealthySteps: A systematic review of a preventive practice-based model of pediatric care. *Journal of Developmental and Behavioral Pediatrics*, *30*, 91–103. https://doi.org/10.1097/DBP.0b013e3181976a95

Piper, K. N., Baxter, K. J., McCarthy, I., & Raval, M. V. (2020). Distinguishing children's hospitals from non-children's hospitals in large claims data. *Hospital Pediatrics*, *10*(2), 123–128. https://doi.org/10.1542/hpeds.2019-0218

Pires, S., McLean, J., & Allen, K. (2018). *Faces of Medicaid data series: Examining children's behavioral health service use and expenditures, 2005–2011*. Center for Health Care Strategies, Inc. https://www.chcs.org/media/Childrens-Faces-of-Medicaid-2018_072718-1.pdf

Platt, J. E., Jacobson, P. D., & Kardia, S. L. R. (2018). Public trust in health information sharing: A measure of system trust. *Health Services Research*, *53*(2), 824–845. https://doi.org/10.1111/1475-6773.12654

PlayReadVIP. (2024). *PlayReadVIP*. https://www.playreadvip.org/

Plummer, E., Letchuman, S., Fang, S., & Bai, G. (2023). Financial characteristics of nonprofit social welfare organizations in the US health care system. *JAMA Health Forum*, *4*(6), e231507. https://doi.org/10.1001/jamahealthforum.2023.1507

Pollack Porter, K. M., Rutkow, L., & McGinty, E. E. (2018). The importance of policy change for addressing public health problems. *Public Health Reports*, *133*(Suppl 1), 9S–14S. https://doi.org/10.1177/0033354918788880

Poowuttikul, P., Saini, S., & Seth, D. (2019). Inner-city asthma in children. *Clinical Reviews in Allergy & Immunology*, *56*(2), 248–268. https://doi.org/10.1007/s12016-019-08728-x

Poudel, A., & Gautam, S. (2017). Age of onset of substance use and psychosocial problems among individuals with substance use disorders. *BMC Psychiatry*, *17*(1), 10. https://doi.org/10.1186/s12888-016-1191-0

Pratt, R., Gyllstrom, B., Gearin, K., Lange, C., Hahn, D., Baldwin, L.-M., VanRaemdonck, L., Nease, D., & Zahner, S. (2018). Identifying barriers to collaboration between primary care and public health: Experiences at the local level. *Public Health Reports*, *133*(3), 311–317. https://doi.org/10.1177/0033354918764391

Prior, M., McManus, M., White, P., & Davidson, L. (2014). Measuring the "triple aim" in transition care: A systematic review. *Pediatrics*, *134*(6), e1648–e1661. https://doi.org/10.1542/peds.2014-1704

Project SEARCH. (2018). *Project SEARCH*. https://www.projectsearch.us/

Pronk, N., Kleinman, D. V., Goekler, S. F., Ochiai, E., Blakey, C., & Brewer, K. H. (2021). Promoting health and well-being in Healthy People 2030. *Journal of Public Health Management and Practice*, *27*(Suppl 6), S242–S248. https://doi.org/10.1097/PHH.0000000000001254

Pronovost, P., Johns, M. M. E., Palmer, S., Bono, R. C., Fridsma, D. B., Gettinger, A., Goldman, J., Johnson, W., Karney, M., Samitt, C., Sriram, R. D., Zenooz, A., & Wang, Y. C. (Eds.). (2018). *Procuring interoperability: Achieving high-quality, connected, and person-centered care*. National Academy of Medicine.

Pylypchuk, Y., & Selden, T. M. (2008). A discrete choice decomposition analysis of racial and ethnic differences in children's health insurance coverage. *Journal of Health Economics*, *27*(4), 1109–1128. https://doi.org/10.1016/j.jhealeco.2007.12.001

Pyone, D., Qureshi, N. K., Ha, L., Goldberg, V., McCune, E., Wojtowicz, J., Sullivan, K., Sigman, G., & O'Keefe, J. C. (2021). Social determinants of health screening at well child visits: A pilot program implemented during the COVID-19 pandemic. *Journal of Primary Care & Community Health*, *12*, 21501327211058912. https://doi.org/10.1177/21501327211058912

Qi, M., Santos, H., Pinheiro, P., McGuinness, D. L., & Bennett, K. P. (2023). Demographic and socioeconomic determinants of access to care: A subgroup disparity analysis using new equity-focused measurements. *PLoS One*, *18*(11). https://doi.org/10.1371/journal.pone.0290692

Qin, X., Zahran, H. S., Leon-Nguyen, M., Kilmer, G., Collins, P., Welch, P., & Malilay, J. (2022). Trends in asthma-related school health policies and practices in the US states. *The Journal of School Health*, *92*(3), 252–260. https://doi.org/10.1111/josh.13124

QPR Institute. (n.d.). *What is QPR? Our mission*. https://qprinstitute.com/about-qpr

Qureshi, J. A., & Gangopadhyaya, A. (2021). Childhood Medicaid eligibility and human capital. *Economics of Education Review*, *82*, 102103. https://doi.org/10.1016/j.econedurev.2021.102103

Rabbitt, M., Hales, L. J., Reed-Jones, M., & Coleman-Jensen, A. C. (2023b). *Survey tools*. United States Department of Agriculture, Economic Research Service. https://www.ers.usda.gov/topics/food-nutrition-assistance/food-security-in-the-u-s/survey-tools/

Rabbitt, M. P., Hales, L. J., Burke, M. P., & Coleman-Jensen, A. (2023a). *Household food security in the United States in 2022* (Report No. ERR-325). U.S. Department of Agriculture.

Raffington, L. (2024). Utilizing epigenetics to study the shared nature of development and biological aging across the lifespan. *NPJ Science of Learning*, *9*(1), 24. https://doi.org/10.1038/s41539-024-00239-5

Rahman, M. T., Sobur, M. A., Islam, M. S., Ievy, S., Hossain, M. J., El Zowalaty, M. E., Rahman, A. T., & Ashour, H. M. (2020). Zoonotic diseases: Etiology, impact, and control. *Microorganisms*, *8*(9), 1405. https://doi.org/10.3390/microorganisms8091405

Rakshit, S., McGough, M., & Amin, K. (2024). *How does U.S. life expectancy compare to other countries?* Peterson-KFF Health System Tracker. https://www.healthsystemtracker.org/chart-collection/u-s-life-expectancy-compare-countries/

Ralston, K. & Coleman-Jensen, A. (2017). *USDA's National School Lunch Program reduces food insecurity.* U.S. Department of Agriculture, Economic Research Service. https://www.ers.usda.gov/amber-waves/2017/august/usda-s-national-school-lunch-program-reduces-food-insecurity/

Ralston, K., Newman, C., Clauson, A., Guthrie, J., & Buzby, J. (2008). *The National School Lunch Program: Background, trends, and issues.* U.S. Department of Agriculture, Economic Research Service. https://www.ers.usda.gov/webdocs/publications/46043/12051_err61_1_.pdf?v=0

Ramadan, A. M. H., & Ataallah, A. G. (2021). Are climate change and mental health correlated? *General Psychiatry, 34*(6), e100648. https://doi.org/10.1136/gpsych-2021-100648

Ramos, M. C., Barreto, J. O. M., Shimizu, H. E., Moraes, A. P. G., & Silva, E. N. D. (2020). Regionalization for health improvement: A systematic review. *PLoS One*, *15*(12), e0244078. https://doi.org/10.1371/journal.pone.0244078

Ran, T., Chattopadhyay, S. K., & Hahn, R. A. (2016). Economic evaluation of school-based health centers: A community guide systematic review. *American Journal of Preventive Medicine*, *51*(1), 129–138. https://doi.org/10.1016/j.amepre.2016.01.017

Ranade-Kharkar, P., Narus, S. P., Anderson, G. L., Conway, T., & Del Fiol, G. (2018). Data standards for interoperability of care team information to support care coordination of complex pediatric patients. *Journal of Biomedical Informatics*, *85*, 1–9. https://doi.org/10.1016/j.jbi.2018.07.009

Randolph, C. (2021). Community health workers in home visits and asthma outcomes. *Pediatrics*, *148*(Suppl 3), S56–S57.

Rankin, K. A., Mosier-Mills, A., Hsiang, W., & Wiznia, D. H. (2022). Secret shopper studies: An unorthodox design that measures inequities in healthcare access. *Archives of Public Health*, *80*(1), 226. https://doi.org/10.1186/s13690-022-00979-z

Raphael, J. L., Beers, L. S., Perrin, J. M., & Garg, A. (2020). Public charge: An expanding challenge to child health care policy. *Academic Pediatrics*, *20*(1), 6–8. https://doi.org/10.1016/j.acap.2019.09.001

Raphael, J. L., & Oyeku, S. O. (2020). Implicit bias in pediatrics: An emerging focus in health equity research. *Pediatrics*, *145*(5), e20200512. https://doi.org/10.1542/peds.2020-0512

Rasberry, C. N., Lee, S. M., Robin, L., Laris, B. A., Russell, L. A., Coyle, K. K., & Nihiser, A. J. (2011). The association between school-based physical activity, including physical education, and academic performance: A systematic review of the literature. *Preventive Medicine*, *52*, S10–S20.

Rathore, B., & Kadin, M. E. (2010). Hodgkin's lymphoma therapy: Past, present, and future. *Expert Opinion on Pharmacotherapy*, *11*(17), 2891–2906. https://doi.org/10.1517/14656566.2010.515979

Rau, J. (2020a). Amid coronavirus distress, wealthy hospitals hoard millions. *The Washington Post.* https://www.washingtonpost.com/local/amid-coronavirus-distress-wealthy-hospitals-hoard-millions/2020/04/27/9c84ccc0-866b-11ea-878a-86477a724bdb_story.html

________. (2020b, May 13). *Wealthy hospitals rake in U.S. disaster aid for COVID-19 costs.* Kaiser Health News. https://khn.org/news/wealthy-hospitals-rake-in-u-s-disaster-aid-for-covid-19-costs/

Raval, M. V., Reiter, A. J., & McCarthy, I. M. (2022). Association of children's hospital status with value for common surgical conditions. *JAMA Network Open*, *5*(6), e2218348. https://doi.org/10.1001/jamanetworkopen.2022.18348

Ravi, N., Gitz, K. M., Burton, D. R., & Ray, K. N. (2021). Pediatric non-urgent emergency department visits and prior care-seeking at primary care. *BMC Health Services Research*, *21*(1), 466. https://doi.org/10.1186/s12913-021-06480-7

Ray, B. D. (2024). Homeschooling: The research. *NHERI*. https://www.nheri.org/research-facts-on-homeschooling/

Ray, K. N., Shi, Z., Ganguli, I., Rao, A., Orav, E. J., & Mehrotra, A. (2020). Trends in pediatric primary care visits among commercially insured US children, 2008–2016. *JAMA Pediatrics*, *174*(4), 350–357. https://doi.org/10.1001/jamapediatrics.2019.5509

Rebbe, R., Sattler, K. M., & Mienko, J. A. (2022). The association of race, ethnicity, and poverty with child maltreatment reporting. *Pediatrics*, *150*(2). https://doi.org/10.1542/peds.2021-053346

Rechel, B. (2020). Integrating primary care and public health. *Eurohealth*, *26*(1).

Redmond, C., Akinoso-Imran, A. Q., Heaney, L. G., Sheikh, A., Kee, F., & Busby, J. (2022). Socioeconomic disparities in asthma health care utilization, exacerbations, and mortality: A systematic review and meta-analysis. *Journal of Allergy and Clinical Immunology*, *149*(5), 1617–1627. https://doi.org/10.1016/j.jaci.2021.10.007

Reed, S. M., Arbet, J., & Staubli, L. (2021). Clinical nurse specialists in the United States registered with a national provider identifier. *Clinical Nurse Specialist*, *35*(3), 119–128. https://doi.org/10.1097/NUR.0000000000000592

Registered Nurses' Association of Ontario. (n.d.). *About RNAO*. https://rnao.ca

Rehabilitation Act of 1973, 29 U.S.C. § 794 (1973). https://www.govinfo.gov/content/pkg/USCODE-2016-title29/html/USCODE-2016-title29-chap16-subchapV-sec794.htm

Rehman, M. U., Shafique, A., Khalid, S., Driss, M., & Rubaiee, S. (2021). Future forecasting of COVID-19: A supervised learning approach. *Sensors*, *21*(10), 3322. https://doi.org/10.3390/s21103322

Rehner, T., Brazeal, M., & Doty, S. T. (2017). Embedding a social work-led behavioral health program in a primary care system: A 2012–2018 case study. *Journal of Public Health Management and Practice*, *23*(Suppl 6), S40–S46. https://doi.org/10.1097/PHH.0000000000000657

Reilly, J. J., Methven, E., McDowell, Z. C., Hacking, B., Alexander, D., Stewart, L., & Kelnar, C. J. (2003). Health consequences of obesity. *Archives of Disease in Childhood*, *88*(9), 748–752. https://doi.org/10.1136/adc.88.9.748

Reilly, P. R. (2015). Eugenics and involuntary sterilization: 1907–2015. *Annual Review of Genomics and Human Genetics*, *16*, 351–368. https://doi.org/10.1146/annurev-genom-090314-024930

Reiss-Brennan, B. (2014). Mental health integration: Normalizing team care. *Journal of Primary Care & Community Health*, *5*(1), 55–60. https://doi.org/10.1177/2150131913508983

Reiss-Brennan, B., Brunisholz, K. D., Dredge, C., Briot, P., Grazier, K., Wilcox, A., Marcz, L., & James, B. (2016). Association of integrated team-based care with health care quality, utilization, and cost. *Journal of the American Medical Association*, *316*(8), 826. https://doi.org/10.1001/jama.2016.11232

Reopell, L., Nolan, T. S., Gray II, D. M., Williams, A., Brewer, L. C., Bryant, A. L., Wilson, G., Williams, E., Jones, C., McKoy, A., Grever, J., Soliman, A., Baez, J., Nawaz, S., Walker, D. M., Metlock, F., Zappe, L., Gregory, J., & Joseph, J. J. (2023). Community engagement and clinical trial diversity: Navigating barriers and co-designing solutions—A report from the "Health Equity through Diversity" seminar series. *PLoS One*, *18*(2). https://doi.org/10.1371/journal.pone.0281940

Return2Learn Tracker. (2023). *Chronic absenteeism: 2017–2023*. https://www.returntolearn-tracker.net/

Reuben, A. (2018). Childhood lead exposure and adult neurodegenerative disease. *Journal of Alzheimer's Disease*, *64*(1), 17. https://doi.org/10.3233/JAD-180267

Reynolds, C. A., & Maughan, E. D. (2015). Telehealth in the school setting: An integrative review. *Journal of School Nursing*, *31*(1), 44–53. https://doi.org/10.1177/1059840514540534

Rice, C. E., Rosanoff, M., Dawson, G., Durkin, M. S., Croen, L. A., Singer, A., & Yeargin-Allsopp, M. (2012). Evaluating changes in the prevalence of the autism spectrum disorders (ASDs). *Public Health Review*, *34*(2), 1–22. https://doi.org/10.1007/bf03391685

Rieselbach, R., Epperly, T., McConnell, E., Noren, J., Nycz, G., & Shin, P. (2019). Community health centers: A key partner to achieve Medicaid expansion. *Journal of General Internal Medicine*, *34*(10), 2268–2272. https://doi.org/10.1007/s11606-019-05194-1

Riley, C. (2023, April 4). *All children thrive: Co-creating system transformation so that every child can thrive* [Presentation]. Committee on Improving the Health and Wellbeing of Children and Youth Through Health Care System Transformation, Washington, DC. https://www.nationalacademies.org/documents/embed/link/LF2255DA3DD1C41C0A42D3BEF0989ACAECE3053A6A9B/file/DC6861792530729124825704O7AC8E53D9F332A4DA49?noSaveAs=1

Riley, M., Morrison, L., & McEvoy, A. (2019). Health maintenance in school-aged children: Part I. History, physical examination, screening, and immunizations. *American Family Physician*, *100*(4), 213–218. https://www.aafp.org/pubs/afp/issues/2019/0815/p213.html

Riley, T., Clary, A., & Higgins, E. (2019). *Identifying gaps in federal oversight of hospitals' community benefit investments: Opportunities for state policy*. National Academy for State Health Policy. https://nashp.org/identifying-gaps-in-federal-oversight-of-hospitals-community-benefit-investments-opportunities-for-state-policy/

Rising Ground. (n.d.). *Rising ground*. https://www.risingground.org/

Rivara, F., Adhia, A., Lyons, V., Massey, A., Mills, B., Morgan, E., Simckes, M., & Rowhani-Rahbar, A. (2019). The effects of violence on health. *Health Affairs*, *38*(10), 1622–1629. https://doi.org/10.1377/hlthaff.2019.00480

Rivers, S. E., Brackett, M. A., Reyes, M. R., Elbertson, N. A., & Salovey, P. (2013). Improving the social and emotional climate of classrooms: A clustered randomized controlled trial testing the RULER approach. *Prevention Science*, *14*(1), 77–87.

The Robert Wood Johnson Foundation. (n.d.). *RWJF's approach: Align for health framework*. https://www.alignforhealth.org/framework/

Roberts, M. C., & R. G. Steele. (2017). *Handbook of pediatric psychology* (5th ed.). Guilford Press.

Roberts, M. S., Stokes, J. A., King, M. A., Lynne, T. A., Purdie, D. M., Glasziou, P. P., Wilson, D. A., McCarthy, S. T., Brooks, G. E., de Looze, F. J., & Del Mar, C. B. (2001). Outcomes of a randomized controlled trial of a clinical pharmacy intervention in 52 nursing homes. *British Journal of Clinical Pharmacology*, *51*(3), 257–265. https://doi.org/10.1046/j.1365-2125.2001.00347.x

Robertson, A. A., Newgard, C. D., Malveau, S. E., Lin, A., Caughey, A. B., & Schmitt, J. (2023). Emergency department pediatric readiness and mortality among children receiving emergency care. *JAMA Network Open*, *6*(1), e2249846. https://doi.org/10.1001/jamanetworkopen.2022.49846

Robinson, L. R., Bitsko, R. H., Thompson, R. A., Dworkin, P. H., McCabe, M. A., Peacock, G., & Thorpe, P. G. (2017). CDC grand rounds: Addressing health disparities in early childhood. *Morbidity and Mortality Weekly Report*, *66*, 769–772. https://doi.org/10.15585/mmwr.mm6629a1

Robinson, T., & McDonald, K. (2023, September 7). *Population health: Nationwide children's approach to health equity* [Presentation]. Committee on Improving the Health and Wellbeing of Children and Youth Through Health Care System Transformation, Washington, DC.

Robling, M., Bekkers, M. J., Bell, K., Butler, C. C., Cannings-John, R., Channon, S., Martin, B. C., Gregory, J. W., Hood, K., Kemp, A., Kenkre, J., Montgomery, A. A., Moody, G., Owen-Jones, E., Pickett, K., Richardson, G., Roberts, Z. E., Ronaldson, S., Sanders, J., ... Torgerson, D. (2016). Effectiveness of a nurse-led intensive home-visitation programme for first-time teenage mothers (Building Blocks): A pragmatic randomised controlled trial. *The Lancet*, *387*(10014), 146–155. https://doi.org/10.1016/s0140-6736(15)00392-x

Roby, E., Miller, E. B., Shaw, D. S., Morris, P., Gill, A., Bogen, D. L., Rosas, J., Canfield, C. F., Hails, K. A., Wippick, H., Honoroff, J., Cates, C. B., Weisleder, A., Chadwick, K. A., Raak, C. D., & Mendelsohn, A. L. (2021). Improving parent-child interactions in pediatric health care: A two-site randomized controlled trial. *Pediatrics*, *147*(3). https://doi.org/10.1542/peds.2020-1799

Roche, J., Bell, L., Galvão, C., Golumbic, Y. N., Kloetzer, L., Knoben, N., Laakso, M., Lorke, J., Mannion, G., Massetti, L., Mauchline, A., Pata, K., Ruck, A., Taraba, P., & Winter, S. (2020). Citizen science, education, and learning: Challenges and opportunities [Conceptual Analysis]. *Frontiers in Sociology*, *5*. https://doi.org/10.3389/fsoc.2020.613814

Rodgers, C. R. R., Flores, M. W., Bassey, O., Augenblick, J. M., & Cook, B. L. (2022). Racial/ethnic disparity trends in children's mental health care access and expenditures from 2010–2017: Disparities remain despite sweeping policy reform. *Journal of the American Academy of Child and Adolescent Psychiatry*, *61*(7), 915–925. https://doi.org/10.1016/j.jaac.2021.09.420

Rodriguez, D., & McGrath, K. (2021). Perspectives of immigrant families and persons with disabilities during COVID-19. *Developmental Disabilities Network Journal*, *1*(2). https://digitalcommons.usu.edu/cgi/viewcontent.cgi?article=1028&context=ddnj

Rodriguez-Quintana, N., Walker, M., & Lewis, C. (2021). In search of reliability: Expert-informed training methods for conducting observational coding of cognitive behavioral therapy fidelity. *Journal of Cognitive Psychotherapy*, *35*, 308–329. https://doi.org/10.1891/JCPSY-D-20-00045

Roehrig, C. (2016). Mental disorders top the list of the most costly conditions in the United States: $201 billion. *Health Affairs*, *35*(6), 1130–1135. https://doi.org/10.1377/hlthaff.2015.1659

Rogers, H., Hershey, J., Morone, J., Lipman, T., Wilson-Hall, L., Anderson, K., & Hawkes, C. (2023). Perspectives of pediatric community health workers: Roles, successes, and challenges. *Health Promotion Practice*, *24*, 1206–1214. https://doi.org/10.1177/15248399221112866

Ronen, T. (2021). *The role of coping skills for developing resilience among children and adolescents*. In MC. L. Kern & M. L. Wehmeyer (Eds.), *The Palgrave Handbook of Positive Education* (pp. 345–368). Springer International Publishing. https://doi.org/10.1007/978-3-030-64537-3_14

Ronis, S. D., McConnochie, K. M., Wang, H., & Wood, N. E. (2017). Urban telemedicine enables equity in access to acute illness care. *Telemedicine and e-Health*, *23*(2), 105–112. https://doi.org/10.1089/tmj.2016.0098

Rosen, D. S., Elster, A., Hedberg, V., & Paperny, D. (1997). Clinical preventive services for adolescents: position paper of the Society for Adolescent Medicine. *Journal of Adolescent Health*, *21*(3), 203–214. https://doi.org/10.1016/s1054-139x(97)00116-x

Rosenbaum, S. (2014). Medicaid payments and access to care. *New England Journal of Medicine*, *371*(25), 2345–2347. https://doi.org/10.1056/NEJMp1412488

Rosenbaum, S., & Johnson, K. (2023). *A twenty-first century Medicaid child health policy: Modernizing EPSDT.* The Milbank Quarterly, Milbank Memorial Fund. https://www.milbank.org/quarterly/opinions/a-twenty-first-century-medicaid-child-health-policy-modernizing-epsdt/

Rosenberg, J., Shabanova, V., McCollum, S., & Sharifi, M. (2022). Insurance and health care outcomes in regions where undocumented children are Medicaid-eligible. *Pediatrics, 150*(3). https://doi.org/10.1542/peds.2022-057034

Rosenblatt, A., Pederson, R., Davis-Sandfoss, T., Irwin, L., Mitsos, R., & Manworren, R. (2024). Child life specialist services, practice, and utilization across health care: A scoping review. *JBI Evidence Synthesis.* https://doi.org/10.11124/JBIES-23-00025

Rosenthal, E. L. (1998). *A summary of the national community health advisor study.* Annie E. Casey Foundation.

Rosenthal, E. L., Brownstein, J. N., Rush, C. H., Hirsch, G. R., Willaert, A. M., Scott, J. R., Holderby, L. R., & Fox, D. J. (2010). Community health workers: Part of the solution. *Health Affairs (Project Hope), 29*(7), 1338–1342. https://doi.org/10.1377/hlthaff.2010.0081

Rosino, M. L. (2016). Boundaries and barriers: Racialized dynamics of political power. *Sociology Compass, 10*(10), 939–951. https://doi.org/10.1111/soc4.12412

Ross, A., Arnold, J., Gormley, A., Locke, S., Shanske, S., & Tardiff, C. (2018). Care coordination in pediatric health care settings: The critical role of social work. *Social Work in Health Care, 58*(1), 1–13.

Ross, M., & Bateman, N. (2019). *Meet the low-wage workforce.* The Brookings Institution. https://www.brookings.edu/articles/meet-the-low-wage-workforce/

Rossati, A. (2017). Global warming and its health impact. *International Journal of Occupational and Environmental Medicine, 8*(1), 7–20. https://doi.org/10.15171/ijoem.2017.963

Rossin-Slater, M. (2022). *Surviving a school shooting: Impacts on the mental health, education, and earnings of American youth.* Stanford Institute for Economic Policy Research. https://siepr.stanford.edu/publications/health/surviving-school-shooting-impacts-mental-health-education-and-earnings-american

Rossin-Slater, M., & Wüst, M. (2020). What is the added value of preschool for poor children? Long-term and intergenerational impacts and interactions with an infant health intervention. *American Economic Journal: Applied Economics, 12*(3). https://www.aeaweb.org/articles?id=10.1257/app.20180698

Roter, D. L. (1983). Physician/patient communication: Transmission of information and patient effects. *Maryland State Medical Journal, 32*(4), 260–265.

Roth, K. B., Kahn, G., Storr, C. L., & Wilcox, H. C. (2024). Childhood factors associated with unnatural death through midadulthood. *JAMA Network Open, 7*(2), e240327. https://doi.org/10.1001/jamanetworkopen.2024.0327

Rouse, D. J., Hirtz, D. G., Thom, E., Varner, M. W., Spong, C. Y., Mercer, B. M., Iams, J. D., Wapner, R. J., Sorokin, Y., Alexander, J. M., Harper, M., Thorp, J. M., Jr., Ramin, S. M., Malone, F. D., Carpenter, M., Miodovnik, M., Moawad, A., O'Sullivan, M. J., Peaceman, A. M., & Roberts, J. M. (2008). A randomized, controlled trial of magnesium sulfate for the prevention of cerebral palsy. *New England Journal of Medicine, 359*(9), 895–905. https://doi.org/10.1056/NEJMoa0801187

Routledge, R. (2020). Integrating specialty care into primary care: The Nuka approach. *British Columbia Medical Journal, 62*(1), 26–28. https://bcmj.org/premise/integrating-specialty-care-primary-care-nuka-approach

Rowan-Legg, A. (2013). Oral health care for children—A call for action. *Paediatrics & Child Health, 18*(1), 37–43.

Rozier, M. D. (2020). Nonprofit hospital community benefit in the U.S.: A scoping review from 2010 to 2019. *Frontiers in Public Health, 8*, 72. https://doi.org/10.3389/fpubh.2020.00072

Rubin, V., & Rose, K. (2015). *Strategies for strengthening anchor institutions' community impact*. PolicyLink.

Ruggiero, K., Pratt, P., & Antonelli, R. (2019). Improving outcomes through care coordination: Measuring care coordination of nurse practitioners. *Journal of the American Association of Nurse Practitioners, 31*(8), 476–481. https://doi.org/10.1097/jxx.0000000000000276

Ryder, J. R. (2018). Fetal antecedents of cardiovascular disease. *Journal of the American Heart Association, 7*(19), e010507. https://doi.org/10.1161/jaha.118.010507

Sabin, J. A., & Greenwald, A. G. (2012). The influence of implicit bias on treatment recommendations for 4 common pediatric conditions: Pain, urinary tract infection, attention deficit hyperactivity disorder, and asthma. *American Journal of Public Health, 102*(5), 988–995. https://doi.org/10.2105/AJPH.2011.300621

Sacks, V., & Murphey, D. (2018). *The prevalence of adverse childhood experiences, nationally, by state, and by race/ethnicity*. Child Trends. https://childtrends.org/publications/prevalence-adverse-childhood-experiences-nationally-state-race-ethnicity

Sadler, L. S., & Daley, A. M. (2002). A model of teen-friendly care for young women with negative pregnancy test results. *Nursing Clinics of North America, 37*(3), 523–535. https://doi.org/10.1016/s0029-6465(02)00018-x

Sakran, J. V., & Bulger, E. M. (2023). Defining a roadmap to firearm injury prevention: In reply to Jones and colleagues. *Journal of the American College of Surgeons, 237*(2), 384–385. https://doi.org/10.1097/xcs.0000000000000731

Salari, N., Ghasemi, H., Abdoli, N., Rahmani, A., Shiri, M. H., Hashemian, A. H., Akbari, H., & Mohammadi, M. (2023). The global prevalence of ADHD in children and adolescents: A systematic review and meta-analysis. *Italian Journal of Pediatrics, 49*(1), 48. https://doi.org/10.1186/s13052-023-01456-1

Salinsky, E. (2017). *The Nuka system of care*. Grantmakers In Health. https://scfnuka.com/wp-content/uploads/2016/09/NUKA-CaseStudy.pdf

Salm, M., & Schunk, D. (2012). The relationship between child health, developmental gaps, and parental education: Evidence from administrative data. *Journal of the European Economic Association, 10*(6), 1425–1449.

Salston, M., & Figley, C. (2003). Secondary traumatic stress effects of working with survivors of criminal victimization. *Journal of Traumatic Stress, 16*, 167–174. https://doi.org/10.1023/A:1022899207206

Saluja, B., & Bryant, Z. (2021). How implicit bias contributes to racial disparities in maternal morbidity and mortality in the United States. *Journal of Women's Health, 30*(2), 270–273. https://doi.org/10.1089/jwh.2020.8874

Samuelson, K. (2024, January 17). Pediatric care for non-white children is universally worse across U.S. *Northwestern University*. https://news.northwestern.edu/stories/2024/01/pediatric-care-for-non-white-children-is-universally-worse-across-u-s/

Sandstrom, H. (2019). Early childhood home visiting programs and health. *Health Affairs*. https://doi.org/10.1377/hpb20190321.382895

Sanner, S., Baldwin, D., Cannella, K. A., Charles, J., & Parker, L. (2010). The impact of cultural diversity forum on students' openness to diversity. *Journal of Cultural Diversity, 17*(2), 56–61.

Santos, T. (2020). Non-profit hospital targeted health priorities and collaboration with local health departments in the first national descriptive study. *Frontiers in Public Health, 8*, 124. https://doi.org/10.3389/fpubh.2020.00124

Sartin, E., Bell, T. R., McDonald, C. C., & Mirman, J. H. (2019). Assessment of caregiver-targeted interventions for use of motor vehicle passenger safety systems for children: A systematic review and meta-analysis. *JAMA Network Open, 2*(10), e1914180. https://doi.org/10.1001/jamanetworkopen.2019.14180

Saulsberry, L., Seo, V., & Fung, V. (2019). The impact of changes in Medicaid provider fees on provider participation and enrollees' care: A systematic literature review. *Journal of General Internal Medicine*, *34*(10), 2200–2209. https://doi.org/10.1007/s11606-019-05160-x

Saunders, M. M. (2015). Clinical nurse specialists' perceptions of work patterns, outcomes, desires, and emerging trends. *Journal of Nursing Administration*, *45*(4), 212–217. https://doi.org/10.1097/nna.0000000000000187

Sawyer, S. M., Azzopardi, P. S., Wickremarathne, D., & Patton, G. C. (2018). The age of adolescence. *The Lancet Child & Adolescent Health*, 2(3), 223–228.

Schaaf, M., Warthin, C., Freedman, L., & Topp, S. M. (2020). The community health worker as service extender, cultural broker and social change agent: A critical interpretive synthesis of roles, intent and accountability. *BMJ Global Health*, *5*(6). https://doi.org/10.1136/bmjgh-2020-002296

Scharff, D. P., Mathews, K. J., Jackson, P., Hoffsuemmer, J., Martin, E., & Edwards, D. (2010). More than Tuskegee: Understanding mistrust about research participation. *Journal of Health Care for the Poor and Underserved*, *21*(3), 879–897. https://doi.org/10.1353/hpu.0.0323

Schering, S. (2024). *Pediatrics fill rate dips during 2024 Match; AAP leaders highlight workforce issues, need to recruit more to field.* AAP News. https://publications.aap.org/aapnews/news/28441/Pediatrics-fill-rate-dips-during-2024-Match-AAP?autologincheck=redirected

Schiff, J. S., Filice, C., & Chen, C. (2024). 15 years of Medicaid and CHIP quality measurement: Challenges, progress, and a path forward. *Health Affairs Forefront*. https://www.healthaffairs.org/do/10.1377/forefront.20230313.382895/full/

Schmidt, A., Ilango, S. M., McManus, M. A., Rogers, K. K., & White, P. H. (2020). Outcomes of pediatric to adult health care transition interventions: An updated systematic review. *Journal of Pediatric Nursing, 51*, 92–107. https://doi.org/10.1016/j.pedn.2020.01.002

Schneider, A., Klukoff, H., & Lehan, M. (2023). *An introduction to managed care in CHIP.* Georgetown University McCourt School of Public Policy Center for Children & Families. https://ccf.georgetown.edu/2023/01/01/an-introduction-to-managed-care-in-chip/

Schnierle, J., Christian-Brathwaite, N., & Louisias, M. (2019). Implicit bias: What every pediatrician should know about the effect of bias on health and future directions. *Current Problems in Pediatric and Adolescent Health Care*, *49*(2), 34–44. https://doi.org/10.1016/j.cppeds.2019.01.003

Schonert-Reichl, K. A., Oberle, E., Lawlor, M. S., Abbott, D., Thomson, K., Oberlander, T. F., & Diamond, A. (2015). Enhancing cognitive and social–emotional development through a simple-to-administer mindfulness-based school program for elementary school children: A randomized controlled trial. *Developmental Psychology*, *51*(1), 52.

School-Based Health Alliance (SBHA). (n.d.). *Medicaid policies that work for SBHCs*. https://www.sbh4all.org/federal-policy-and-advocacy/medicaid-policies-that-work-for-sbhcs/

________. (2014). *2013-14 digital census report*. http://censusreport.sbh4all.org/

________. (2023a). *Findings from the 2022 national census of school-based health centers.* https://sbh4all.org/wp-content/uploads/2023/10/findings-from-the-2022-national-census-of-school-based-health-centers-09.20.23.pdf

________. (2023b). *State policy maps*. https://www.sbh4all.org/federal-policy-and-advocacy/state-policy-maps/

Schor, E. L., & Bergman, D. (2021). Pediatric preventive care: Population health and individualized care. *Pediatrics*, *148*(3). https://doi.org/10.1542/peds.2020-049877

Schrott, R., Song, A., & Ladd-Acosta, C. (2022). Epigenetics as a biomarker for early-life environmental exposure. *Current Environmental Health Reports*, *9*(4), 604–624. https://doi.org/10.1007/s40572-022-00373-5

Schultz, D. J., Byker Shanks, C., & Houghtaling, B. (2015). The impact of the 2009 Special Supplemental Nutrition Program for Women, Infants, and Children (WIC) food package revisions on dietary intake: A systematic review. *Journal of the Academy of Nutrition and Dietetics*, *115*(11), 1832–1846. https://doi.org/10.1016/j.jand.2015.06.381

Schultz Family Foundation. (2024, May 15). Eleven states launch new initiative to address America's youth mental health crisis. *AmeriCorps*. https://americorps.gov/newsroom/press-release/eleven-states-launch-new-initiative-address-americas-youth-mental-health

Schwartz, G. L., Feldman, J. M., Wang, S. S., & Glied, S. A. (2022). Eviction, healthcare utilization, and disenrollment among New York City Medicaid patients. *American Journal of Preventive Medicine*, *62*(2), 157–164. https://doi.org/10.1016/j.amepre.2021.07.018

Schwartz, G. L., Leifheit, K. M., Berkman, L. F., Chen, J. T., & Arcaya, M. C. (2021). Health selection into eviction: Adverse birth outcomes and children's risk of eviction through age 5 years. *American Journal of Epidemiology*, *190*(7), 1260–1269. https://doi.org/10.1093/aje/kwab007

Schwartz, K., & Damico, A. (2020). *Distribution of CARES Act funding among hospitals*. KFF. https://www.kff.org/coronavirus-covid-19/issue-brief/distribution-of-cares-act-funding-among-hospitals/

Schwarzenberg, S. J., & Georgieff, M. K. (2018). Advocacy for improving nutrition in the first 1000 days to support childhood development and adult health. *Pediatrics*, *141*(2). https://doi.org/10.1542/peds.2017-3716

Scorza, P., Duarte, C. S., Hipwell, A. E., Posner, J., Ortin, A., Canino, G., Monk, C., & Program Collaborators for Environmental influences on Child Health Outcomes. (2019). Research review: Intergenerational transmission of disadvantage: Epigenetics and parents' childhoods as the first exposure. *Journal of Child Psychology and Psychiatry, and Allied Disciplines*, *60*(2), 119–132. https://doi.org/10.1111/jcpp.12877

Seervai, S. (2017). *How Hurricane Maria worsened Puerto Rico's health care crisis*. The Commonwealth Fund. https://www.commonwealthfund.org/publications/other-publication/2017/dec/how-hurricane-maria-worsened-puerto-ricos-health-care

Sege, R. D., & Harper Browne, C. (2017). Responding to ACEs with HOPE: Health outcomes from positive experiences. *Academic Pediatrics*, *17*(Suppl 7), S79–S85. https://doi.org/10.1016/j.acap.2017.03.007

Seiler, N., Malcarney, M.-B., Horton, K., & Dafflitto, S. (2014). Coverage of clinical preventive services under the Affordable Care Act: From law to access. *Public Health Reports*, *129*(6), 526–532. https://doi.org/10.1177/003335491412900611

Seither, R., Calhoun, K., Yusuf, O. B., Dramann, D., Mugerwa-Kasujja, A., Knighton, C. L., & Black, C. L. (2023a). Vaccination coverage with selected vaccines and exemption rates among children in kindergarten—United States, 2021–22 school year. *Morbidity and Mortality Weekly Report*. Centers for Disease Control and Prevention. https://www.cdc.gov/mmwr/volumes/72/wr/mm7202a2.htm?s_cid=mm7202a2_w

Seither, R., Yusuf., O., Dramann D., Calhoun, K., Mugerwa-Kasujja, A., & Knighton, C. L. (2023b). *Coverage with selected vaccines and exemption from school vaccine requirements among children in kindergarten—United States, 2022–23 school year*. http://dx.doi.org/10.15585/mmwr.mm7245a2

Sekmen, M., Grijalva, C. G., Zhu, Y., Williams, D. J., Feinstein, J. A., Stassun, J. C., Johnson, J. A., Tanguturi, Y. C., Gay, J. C., & Antoon, J. W. (2023). Characteristics associated with serious self-harm events in children and adolescents. *Pediatrics*, *151*(6), e2022059817. https://doi.org/10.1542/peds.2022-059817

Semanco, M., Wright, S., & Rich, R. L. (2022). Improving initial sepsis management through a nurse-driven rapid response team protocol. *Critical Care Nurse*, *42*(5), 51–57. https://doi.org/10.4037/ccn2022608

Seniwati, T., Rustina, Y., Nurhaeni, N., & Wanda, D. (2023). Patient and family-centered care for children: A concept analysis. *Belitung Nursing Journal*, *9*(1), 17–24. https://doi.org/10.33546/bnj.2350

Seow, H., Barbera, L. C., McGrail, K., Burge, F., Guthrie, D. M., Lawson, B., Chan, K. K. W., Peacock, S. J., & Sutradhar, R. (2022). Effect of early palliative care on end-of-life health care costs: A population-based, propensity score–matched cohort study. *JCO Oncology Practice*, *18*(1), e183. https://doi.org/10.1200/OP.21.00299

Serang, F., Thompson, J. P., & Howard, T. (2013). *The anchor mission: Leveraging the power of anchor institutions to build community wealth*. The Democracy Collaborative, University of Maryland. https://institute.coop/sites/default/files/resources/006%202013_Serang_The%20Anchor%20Mission%20Leveraging%20the%20Power%20of%20Anchor%20Institutions%20to%20Build%20Community%20Wealth.pdf

Shachar, C., Gruppuso, P. A., & Adashi, E. Y. (2023). Pediatric drug and other shortages in the age of supply chain disruption. *Journal of the American Medical Association*, *329*(24), 2127–2128. https://doi.org/10.1001/jama.2023.4755

Shafer, P. R. (2024). Does supporting children help their parents thrive? *JAMA Network Open*, *7*(2), e2356376.

Shafer, P. R., Gutiérrez, K. M., Ettinger de Cuba, S., Bovell-Ammon, A., & Raifman, J. (2022). Association of the implementation of Child Tax Credit advance payments with food insufficiency in US households. *JAMA Network Open*, *5*(1), e2143296–e2143296. https://doi.org/10.1001/jamanetworkopen.2021.43296

Shah, A. C., & Badawy, S. M. (2021). Telemedicine in pediatrics: Systematic review of randomized controlled trials. *JMIR Pediatrics and Parenting*, *4*(1), e22696. https://doi.org/10.2196/22696

Shain, B., Committee on Adolescence, Braverman, P. K., Adelman, W. P., Alderman, E. M., Breuner, C. C., Levine, D. A., Marcell, A. V., & O'Brien, R. F. (2016). Suicide and suicide attempts in adolescents. *Pediatrics*, *138*(1), e20161420. https://doi.org/10.1542/peds.2016-1420

Shalaby, R. H., & Agyapong, V. (2020). Peer support in mental health: Literature review. *JMIR Mental Health*, *7*(6), e15572. https://mental.jmir.org/2020/6/e15572

Sharkey, P. (2018). The long reach of violence: A broader perspective on data, theory, and evidence on the prevalence and consequences of exposure to violence. *Annual Review of Criminology*, *1*(1), 85–102. https://doi.org/10.1146/annurev-criminol-032317-092316

Sheldrick, R. C., Bair-Merritt, M. H., Durham, M. P., Rosenberg, J., Tamene, M., Bonacci, C., Daftary, G., Tang, M. H., Sengupta, N., Morris, A., & Feinberg, E. (2022). Integrating pediatric universal behavioral health care at federally qualified health centers. *Pediatrics*, *149*(4). https://doi.org/10.1542/peds.2021-051822

Sheridan, S. M., Knoche, L. L., Kupzyk, K. A., Edwards, C. P., & Marvin, C. A. (2011). A randomized trial examining the effects of parent engagement on early language and literacy: The Getting Ready intervention. *Journal of School Psychology*, *49*(3), 361–383. https://doi.org/10.1016/j.jsp.2011.03.001

Sherman, A. D. F., McDowell, A., Clark, K. D., Balthazar, M., Klepper, M., & Bower, K. (2021). Transgender and gender diverse health education for future nurses: Students' knowledge and attitudes. *Nurse Education Today*, *97*, 104690. https://doi.org/10.1016/j.nedt.2020.104690

Sherwood Valley Band of Pomo Indians. (n.d.). *Sherwood Valley band of Pomo Indians*. https://www.sherwoodvalleybandofpomo.com/tribal-youth-diversion-program.html

Shi, Y., Inoue, H., Wu, J. C., & Yamanaka, S. (2017). Induced pluripotent stem cell technology: A decade of progress. *Nature Reviews Drug Discovery*, *16*(2), 115–130. https://doi.org/10.1038/nrd.2016.245

Shim, R. S., & Compton, M. T. (2020). The social determinants of mental health: Psychiatrists' roles in addressing discrimination and food insecurity. *Focus*. https://doi.org/10.1176/appi.focus.20190035

Shimamoto, K. (2023). Advancing digital health equity. *Children's Hospital Association*. https://www.childrenshospitals.org/news/childrens-hospitals-today/2023/09/advancing-digital-health-equity

Shivers, E. M., Faragó, F., & Gal-Szabo, D. E. (2022). The role of infant and early childhood mental health consultation in reducing racial and gender relational and discipline disparities between Black and white preschoolers. *Psychology in the Schools*, *59*(10), 1965–1983. https://doi.org/10.1002/pits.22573

Shmerling, R. H. (2022). *Why life expectancy in the US is falling*. Harvard Health Publishing. https://www.health.harvard.edu/blog/why-life-expectancy-in-the-us-is-falling-202210202835

Shortell, S. M., Toussaint, J. S., Halvorson, G. C., Kingsdale, J. M., Scheffler, R. M., Schwartz, A. Y., Wadsworth, P. A., & Wilensky, G. (2023). The Better Care Plan: A blueprint for improving America's healthcare system. *Health Affairs Scholar*, *1*(1). https://doi.org/10.1093/haschl/qxad007

Shrider, E. A. & Creamer, J. (2023). *Poverty in the United States: 2022*. U.S. Census Bureau. https://www.census.gov/library/publications/2023/demo/p60-280.html.

Sia, C., Tonniges, T. F., Osterhus, E., & Taba, S. (2004). History of the medical home concept. *Pediatrics*, *113*(Suppl 5), 1473–1478.

Silliman, R., & Schleifer, D. (2020). *A two way street: Building trust between people with Medicaid and primary care doctors*. Public Agenda. https://www.publicagenda.org/reports/a-two-way-street-building-trust-between-people-with-medicaid-and-primary-care-doctors/

Silver, H. C., & Zinsser, K. M. (2020). The interplay among early childhood teachers' social and emotional well-being, mental health consultation, and preschool expulsion. *Early Education and Development*, *31*(7), 1133–1150. https://doi.org/10.1080/10409289.2020.1785267

Silvola, S., Restelli, U., Bonfanti, M., & Croce, D. (2023). Co-design as enabling factor for patient-centred healthcare: A bibliometric literature review. *ClinicoEconomics and Outcomes Research*, *15*, 333–347. https://doi.org/10.2147/ceor.S403243

Simmonds, M., Llewellyn, A., Owen, C. G., & Woolacott, N. (2016). Predicting adult obesity from childhood obesity: A systematic review and meta-analysis. *Obesity Reviews*, *17*(2), 95–107. https://doi.org/10.1111/obr.12334

Simmons-Duffin, S. (2022, August 27). *As states try to define when life begins, science, religion and politics clash*. NPR. https://www.npr.org/sections/health-shots/2022/08/27/1119684376/when-does-life-begin-as-state-laws-define-it-science-politics-and-religion-clash

Simon, A. E., Rossen, L. M., Schoendorf, K. C., Larson, K., & Olson, L. M. (2015). Location of usual source of care among children and adolescents in the United States, 1997–2013. *Journal of Pediatrics*, *167*(6), 1409–1414. https://doi.org/10.1016/j.jpeds.2015.09.026

Simon, M., Choudhry, N. K., Frankfort, J., Margolius, D., Murphy, J., Paita, L., Wang, T., & Milstein, A. (2017). Exploring attributes of high-value primary care. *Annals of Family Medicine*, *15*(6), 529–534. https://doi.org/10.1370/afm.2153

Simon, T. D., Berry, J., Feudtner, C., Stone, B. L., Sheng, X., Bratton, S. L., Dean, J. M., & Srivastava, R. (2010). Children with complex chronic conditions in inpatient hospital settings in the United States. *Pediatrics*, *126*(4), 647–655. https://doi.org/10.1542/peds.2009-3266

Simon, T. D., Haaland, W., Hawley, K., Lambka, K., & Mangione-Smith, R. (2018). Development and validation of the pediatric medical complexity algorithm (PMCA) version 3.0. *Academic Pediatrics*, *18*(5), 577–580. https://doi.org/10.1016/j.acap.2018.02.010

Sinclair, E. M., McCleery, E. J., Koepsell, L., Zuckerman, K. E., & Stevenson, E. B. (2019). Shared reading practices and early literacy promotion in the first year of life. *Journal of Developmental & Behavioral Pediatrics*, *40*(7), 538–546. https://doi.org/10.1097/DBP.0000000000000690

Singh, G. K., Yu, S. M., & Kogan, M. D. (2013). Health, chronic conditions, and behavioral risk disparities among U.S. immigrant children and adolescents. *Public Health Reports*, *128*(6), 463–479. https://doi.org/10.1177/003335491312800606

Sinha, S., Bedgood, M., Puttagunta, R., Kataria, A., Bourgeois, F., Lee, J. A., Vodzak, J., Hall, E., Levy, B., & Vawdrey, D. K. (2023). Variation in pediatric and adolescent electronic health data sharing practices under the 21st Century Cures Act. *Journal of the American Medical Informatics Association*, *30*(12), 2021–2027. https://doi.org/10.1093/jamia/ocad172

Sisk, B., & Baker, J. N. (2019). A model of interpersonal trust, credibility, and relationship maintenance. *Pediatrics*, *144*(6). https://doi.org/10.1542/peds.2019-1319

Sisodia, R. C., Rodriguez, J. A., & Sequist, T. D. (2021). Digital disparities: Lessons learned from a patient-reported outcomes program during the COVID-19 pandemic. *Journal of the American Medical Informatics Association*, *28*(10), 2265–2268. https://doi.org/10.1093/jamia/ocab138

Skolnick, A. A. (1997). A FACCT-filled agenda for public information. *Journal of the American Medical Association*, *278*(19), 1558–1558. https://doi.org/10.1001/jama.1997.03550190022011

Slabaugh, S. L., Shah, M., Zack, M., Happe, L., Cordier, T., Havens, E., Davidson, E., Miao, M., Prewitt, T., & Jia, H. (2017). Leveraging health-related quality of life in population health management: The case for healthy days. *Population Health Management*, *20*(1), 13–22. https://doi.org/10.1089/pop.2015.0162

Slopen, N., Chang, A. R., Johnson, T. J., Anderson, A. T., Bate, A. M., Clark, S., Cohen, A., Jindal, M., Karbeah, J., Pachter, L. M., Priest, N., Suglia, S. F., Bryce, N., Fawcett, A., & Heard-Garris, N. (2024). Racial and ethnic inequities in the quality of paediatric care in the USA: A review of quantitative evidence. *The Lancet Child & Adolescent Health*, *8*(2), 147–158. https://doi.org/10.1016/S2352-4642(23)00251-1

Smith, C. D., Balatbat, C., Corbridge, S., Dopp, A. L., Fried, J., Harter, R., Landefeld, S., Martin, C., Opelka, F., Sandy, L., Sato, L., & Sinsky, C. (2018). Implementing optimal team-based care to reduce clinician burnout. *NAM Perspectives*. https://doi.org/10.31478/201801b

Smith, J. D., Cruden, G. H., Rojas, L. M., Van Ryzin, M., Fu, E., Davis, M. M., Landsverk, J., & Brown, C. H. (2020). Parenting interventions in pediatric primary care: A systematic review. *Pediatrics*, *146*(1), e20193548. https://doi.org/10.1542/peds.2019-3548

Smith, S. N., Almirall, D., Choi, S. Y., Koschmann, E., Rusch, A., Bilek, E., Lane, A., Abelson, J. L., Eisenberg, D., Himle, J. A., Fitzgerald, K. D., Liebrecht, C., & Kilbourne, A. M. (2022). Primary aim results of a clustered SMART for developing a school-level, adaptive implementation strategy to support CBT delivery at high schools in Michigan. *Implementation Science, 17*, 42. https://doi.org/10.1186/s13012-022-01211-w

Smokowski, P. R., & Evans, C. B. R. (2019). *Bullying and victimization across the lifespan: Playground politics and power*. Springer Cham. https://doi.org/10.1007/978-3-030-20293-4

Snowden, L. R., & Graaf, G. (2023). States' racial resentment correlates with administrative distancing and lower rates of health plan selection in Affordable Care Act marketplaces: A cross-sectional analysis. *BMC Health Services Research*, *23*(1), 1191. https://doi.org/10.1186/s12913-023-10252-w

Social and Character Development Research Consortium. (2010). *Efficacy of schoolwide programs to promote social and character development and reduce problem behavior in elementary school children* (NCER 2011–2001). National Center for Education Research, Institute of Education Sciences, U.S. Department of Education. https://ies.ed.gov/ncer/pubs/20112001/pdf/20112001.pdf

Social Security Act of 1935, Pub. L. No. 74-271, § 501, 49 Stat. 620 (1935).

Social Security Act § 1902(a)(30)(A), 42 U.S.C. § 1396a(a)(30)(A) (2024).

Social Security Administration (SSA). (n.d.). *Compilation of the social security laws, definitions.* https://www.ssa.gov/OP_Home/ssact/title21/2110.htm#:~:text=(B)%20a%20child%20who%20is,public%20agency%20in%20the%20State.

Society for Adolescent Health and Medicine. (2021). Medication for adolescents and young adults with opioid use disorder. *Journal of Adolescent Health, 68*(3), 632–636. https://doi.org/10.1016/j.jadohealth.2020.12.129

Society of Pediatric Psychology. (2023). *Who we are.* https://pedpsych.org/about-us/

Sockalingam, S., Arena, A., Serhal, E., Mohri, L., Alloo, J., & Crawford, A. (2018). Building provincial mental health capacity in primary care: An evaluation of a Project ECHO mental health program. *Academic Psychiatry, 42*(4), 451–457. https://doi.org/10.1007/s40596-017-0735-z

Soleimanpour, S. (2020). School-based health centers: At the intersection of health and education. *Journal of Adolescent Health, 67*(3), 317–318. https://doi.org/10.1016/j.jadohealth.2020.05.009

Soleimanpour, S., Brindis, C., Geierstanger, S., Kandawalla, S., & Kurlaender, T. (2008). Incorporating youth-led community participatory research into school health center programs and policies. *Public Health Reports, 123*(6), 709–716. https://doi.org/10.1177/003335490812300607

Soleimanpour, S., Cushing, K., Christensen, J., Ng, S., Yang, J., Saphir, M., Geierstanger, S., Even, M., & Brey, L. (2023). *Findings from the 2022 National Census of School-Based Health Centers.* School-Based Health Alliance.

Soleimanpour, S., Geierstanger, S. P., Kaller, S., McCarter, V., & Brindis, C. D. (2010). The role of school health centers in health care access and client outcomes. *American Journal of Public Health, 100*(9), 1597–1603. https://doi.org/10.2105/AJPH.2009.186833

Sommers, B. D., & Oellerich, D. (2013). The poverty-reducing effect of Medicaid. *Journal of Health Economics, 32*(5), 816–832. https://doi.org/10.1016/j.jhealeco.2013.06.005

Song, Z., Zubizarreta, J. R., Giuriato, M., Koh, K. A., & Sacks, C. A. (2023). Firearm injuries in children and adolescents: Health and economic consequences among survivors and family members. *Health Affairs, 42*(11), 1541–1550. https://doi.org/10.1377/hlthaff.2023.00587

Soto, M., Sicotte, C., & Motulsky, A. (2019). Using health information exchange: Usability and usefulness evaluation. *Studies in Health Technology and Informatics, 264*, 1036–1040. https://doi.org/10.3233/SHTI190382

Soucy, N. L., Terrell, R. M., Chedid, R. A., & Phillips, K. P. (2023). Best practices in prenatal health promotion: Perceptions, experiences, and recommendations of Ottawa, Canada, prenatal key informants. *Women's Health, 19*. https://doi.org/10.1177/17455057231158223

Sousa, A. C., Ferrinho, S. N., & Travassos, B. (2023). The use of wearable technologies in the assessment of physical activity in preschool- and school-age youth: Systematic review. *International Journal of Environmental Research and Public Health, 20*(4). https://doi.org/10.3390/ijerph20043402

Southcentral Foundation Nuka System of Care. (n.d.). *About us: Southcentral Foundation* https://scfnuka.com/about-us/#what

________. (2019). *Southcentral Foundation's Nuka System of Care.* https://transform-integratedcommunitycare.com/wp-content/uploads/2019/09/overview-of-the-case-studies.pdf

Spencer, A., & Ohene-Ntow, A. (2022). *Engaging communities of color to promote health equity: Five lessons from New York-based health care organizations.* Center for Health Care Strategies. https://www.chcs.org/resource/engaging-communities-of-color-topromote-health-equity-five-lessons-from-new-york-based-health-care-organizations/

Spiegelman, M. (2020). School nurses in U.S. public schools. *Data Point. NCES 2020-086.* Institute of Education Sciences, National Center for Education Statistics. https://nces.ed.gov/pubs2020/2020086.pdf

Spiker, S. (2023). Medical-financial partnerships: An innovative approach to improving community health. *One Degree.* https://about.1degree.org/medical-financial-partnerships-an-innovative-approach-to-improving-community-health/

Splett, J. W., Fowler, J., Weist, M. D., McDaniel, H., & Dvorsky, M. (2013). The critical role of school psychology in the school mental health movement. *Psychology in the Schools, 50*(3), 245–258.

Stabile, M. (2023). *Approaches to address child mental health and well-being: An international perspective* [Paper Presentation]. Committee on Improving the Health and Wellbeing of Children and Youth through Health Care Transformation.

Stack, M. L., Ozawa, S., Bishai, D. M., Mirelman, A., Tam, Y., Niessen, L., Walker, D. G., & Levine, O. S. (2011). Estimated economic benefits during the 'decade of vaccines' include treatment savings, gains in labor productivity. *Health Affairs (Project Hope), 30*(6), 1021–1028. https://doi.org/10.1377/hlthaff.2011.0382

State Monitoring Requirements 42 CFR § 438.66 (2024).

State of Childhood Obesity. (n.d.). *The child and adult care food program (CACFP).* The Robert Wood Johnson Foundation. https://stateofchildhoodobesity.org/policy-topic/child-and-adult-care-food-program/

Statista. (n.d.). *Hospital supported employment as a percentage of total employment in 2016, by US region.* Statista. https://www.statista.com/statistics/285814/us-hospital-employment-as-a-percentage-of-total-regional-employment

Steel-Fisher, G. K., Findling, M. G., Caporello, H. L., Lubell, K. M., Vidoloff Melville, K. G., Lane, L., Boyea, A. A., Schafer, T. J., & Ben-Porath, E. N. (2023). Trust in US federal, state, and local public health agencies during COVID-19: Responses and policy implications. *Health Affairs (Project Hope), 42*(3), 328–337. https://doi.org/10.1377/hlthaff.2022.01204

Stein, R., Perrin, J., & Iezzoni, L. I. (2010). Access and medical support for youth and young adults with chronic health conditions and disabilities. In D. Lollar (Ed.), *Launching into adulthood: An integrated response to support transition of youth with chronic health conditions and disabilities* (pp. 77–102). https://www.researchgate.net/publication/288030028_Access_and_medical_support_for_youth_and_young_adults_with_chronic_health_conditions_and_disabilities

Stein, R. E., Gortmaker, S. L., Perrin, E. C., Perrin, J. M., Pless, I. B., Walker, D. K., & Weitzman, M. (1987). Severity of illness: Concepts and measurements. *The Lancet, 2*(8574), 1506–1509. https://doi.org/10.1016/s0140-6736(87)92633-x

Steiner, M. J., Hall, M., Sutton, A. G., Stephens, J. R., Keyenaar, J. K., Chase, L., & McDaniels, C. E. (2023). Pediatric hospitalization trends at children's and general hospitals, 2000–2019. *Journal of the American Medical Association, 330*(19), 1906–1908. https://doi.org/10.1001/jama.2023.19268

Stewart, L. A., Hernan, R. R., Mardy, C., Hahn, E., Chung, W. K., Bacha, E. A., Krishnamurthy, G., Duron, V. P., & Krishnan, U. S. (2023). Congenital heart disease with congenital diaphragmatic hernia: Surgical decision making and outcomes. *Journal of Pediatrics, 260*, 113530. https://doi.org/10.1016/j.jpeds.2023.113530

Stewart, S., & Svihovec, S. (2022). A delivery service model for genetics: The use of a genetic counselor and nurse practitioner team for diagnosis and care in specific condition populations. *Nursing Forum, 57*(5), 819–824. https://doi.org/10.1111/nuf.12769

Stille, C., Turchi, R. M., Antonelli, R., Cabana, M. D., Cheng, T. L., Laraque, D., & Perrin, J. (2010). The family-centered medical home: Specific considerations for child health research and policy. *Academic Pediatrics, 10*(4), 211–217. https://doi.org/10.1016/j.acap.2010.05.002

Straussner, S. L. A., & Fewell, C. H. (2018). A review of recent literature on the impact of parental substance use disorders on children and the provision of effective services. *Current Opinion in Psychiatry*, *31*(4), 363–367. https://doi.org/10.1097/yco.0000000000000421

Strianese, O., Rizzo, F., Ciccarelli, M., Galasso, G., D'Agostino, Y., Salvati, A., Del Giudice, C., Tesorio, P., & Rusciano, M. R. (2020). Precision and personalized medicine: How genomic approach improves the management of cardiovascular and neurodegenerative disease. *Genes*, *11*(7), 747. https://doi.org/10.3390/genes11070747

Strolin-Goltzman, J., Sisselman, A., Melekis, K., & Auerbach, C. (2014). Understanding the relationship between school-based health center use, school connection, and academic performance. *Health & Social Work*, *39*(2), 83–91.

Subcommittee of the President's Council on Fitness, Sports and Nutrition. (2012). *Physical activity guidelines for Americans—Midcourse report: Strategies to increase physical activity among youth*. U.S. Department of Health and Human Services.

Substance Abuse and Mental Health Services Administration (SAMHSA). (2014). *Expert convening on infant and early childhood mental health consultation*. U.S. Department of Health and Human Services. https://www.samhsa.gov/sites/default/files/programs_campaigns/IECMHC/iecmhc-expert-convening-summary.pdf

_______. (2015). *Racial/ethnic differences in mental health service use among adults* (HHS Publication No. SMA-15-4906). U.S. Department of Health and Human Services. https://www.samhsa.gov/data/sites/default/files/MHServicesUseAmongAdults/MHServicesUseAmongAdults.pdf

_______. (2017). *Family/parent/caregiver support for behavioral health*. U.S. Department of Health and Human Services. https://www.samhsa.gov/sites/default/files/programs_campaigns/brss_tacs/family-parent-caregiver-support-behavioral-health-2017.pdf

_______. (2019). *Ready, set, go, review: Screening for behavioral health risk in schools*. U.S. Department of Health and Human Services. https://www.samhsa.gov/resource/ebp/ready-set-go-review-screening-behavioral-health-risk-schools

_______. (2020). *Key substance use and mental health indicators in the United States: Results from the 2019 national survey on drug use and health*. U.S. Department of Health and Human Services.

_______. (2021). *Highlights for the 2021 national survey on drug use and health*. U.S. Department of Health and Human Services. https://www.samhsa.gov/data/sites/default/files/2022-12/2021NSDUHFFRHighlights092722.pdf

_______. (2022a). *2022 NSDUH detailed tables*. U.S. Department of Health and Human Services. https://www.samhsa.gov/data/report/2022-nsduh-detailed-tables

_______. (2022b). *FY 2022 infant and early childhood mental health program*. U.S. Department of Health and Human Services. https://www.samhsa.gov/sites/default/files/grants/pdf/fy-22-iecmh-nofo.pdf

_______. (2022c). *FY 2022 SAMHSA operating plan*. U.S. Department of Health and Human Services. https://www.samhsa.gov/sites/default/files/about_us/budget/fy-2022-samhsa-operating-plan.pdf

_______. (2022d). *Key substance use and mental health indicators in the United States: Results from the 2021 national survey on drug use and health* (HHS Publication No. PEP22-07-01-005, NSDUH Series H-57). U.S. Department of Health and Human Services. https://www.samhsa.gov/data/report/2021-nsduh-annual-national-report

_______. (2023a). Infant early childhood mental health (IECMH) grant program. U.S. Department of Health and Human Services. https://www.samhsa.gov/early-childhood-mental-health-programs/iecmh-grant-program

_______. (2023b). *Project linking actions for unmet needs in children's health (Project LAUNCH)*. U.S. Department of Health and Human Services. https://www.samhsa.gov/early-childhood-mental-health-programs/project-launch

_______. (2024). *About NCTSI.* U.S. Department of Health and Human Services. https://www.samhsa.gov/child-trauma/about-nctsi

Sullivan, E. E., & Ellner, A. (2015). Strong patient-provider relationships drive healthier outcomes. *Harvard Business Review.* https://hbr.org/2015/10/strong-patient-provider-relationships-drive-healthier-outcomes

Sullivan, J., Wilton, L., & Apfelbaum, E. P. (2020). Adults delay conversations about race because they underestimate children's processing of race. *Journal of Experimental Psychology: General.* https://doi.org/10.1037/xge0000851

Sun, S., Cao, W., Ge, Y., Siegel, M., & Wellenius, G. A. (2022). Analysis of firearm violence during the COVID-19 pandemic in the US. *JAMA Network Open, 5*(4), e229393. https://doi.org/10.1001/jamanetworkopen.2022.9393

Swedo, E. A., D'Angelo, D. V., Fasula, A. M., Clayton, H. B., & Ports, K. A. (2023). Associations of adverse childhood experiences with pregnancy and infant health. *American Journal of Preventive Medicine, 64*(4), 512–524. https://doi.org/10.1016/j.amepre.2022.10.01

Sykes, S., Wills, J., Rowlands, G., & Popple, K. (2013). Understanding critical health literacy: A concept analysis. *BMC Public Health, 13*, 150. https://doi.org/10.1186/1471-2458-13-150

Szarfman, A., Levine, J. G., Tonning, J. M., Weichold, F., Bloom, J. C., Soreth, J. M., Geanacopoulos, M., Callahan, L., Spotnitz, M., Ryan, Q., Pease-Fye, M., Brownstein, J. S., Hammond, W. E., Reich, C., & Altman, R. B. (2022). Recommendations for achieving interoperable and shareable medical data in the USA. *Communications Medicine, 2*, 86. https://doi.org/10.1038/s43856-022-00148-x

Takanishi, R. (1978). Childhood as a social issue: Historical roots of contemporary child advocacy movements. *Journal of Social Issues, 34*(2), 8–28. https://doi.org/10.1111/j.1540-4560.1978.tb01026.x

Takeshita, J., Wang, S., Loren, A. W., Mitra, N., Shults, J., Shin, D. B., & Sawinski, D. L. (2020). Association of racial/ethnic and gender concordance between patients and physicians with patient experience ratings. *JAMA Network Open, 3*(11), e2024583. https://doi.org/10.1001/jamanetworkopen.2020.24583

Talbert, A. (2017). *Youth-led programs.* Voinovich School of Leadership and Public Affairs at Ohio University. https://www.ohio.edu/voinovich-school/sites/ohio.edu.voinovich-school/files/sites/voinovich/files/Youth-Led-Programs_FINAL.pdf

Talbird, S. E., Carrico, J., La, E. M., Carias, C., Marshall, G. S., Roberts, C. S., Chen, Y. T., & Nyaku, M. K. (2022). Impact of routine childhood immunization in reducing vaccine-preventable diseases in the United States. *Pediatrics, 150*(3). https://doi.org/10.1542/peds.2021-056013

Talmi, A., Muther, E. F., Margolis, K., Buchholz, M., Asherin, R., & Bunik, M. (2016). The scope of behavioral health integration in a pediatric primary care setting. *Journal of Pediatric Psychology, 41*(10), 1120–1132. https://doi.org/10.1093/jpepsy/jsw065

Tan, J., Zhang, Z., Yan, L. L., & Xu, X. (2024). The developmental origins of health and disease and intergenerational inheritance: A scoping review of multigenerational cohort studies. *Journal of Developmental Origins of Health and Disease*, 1–12. https://doi.org/10.1017/s2040174424000035

Tang, S. S., Hudak, M. L., Cooley, D. M., Shenkin, B. N., & Racine, A. D. (2018). Increased Medicaid payment and participation by office-based primary care pediatricians. *Pediatrics, 141*(1). https://doi.org/10.1542/peds.2017-2570

Taras, H., Wright, S., Brennan, J., Campana, J., & Lofgren, R. (2004). Impact of school nurse case management on students with asthma. *The Journal of School Health, 74*(6), 213–219. https://doi.org/10.1111/j.1746-1561.2004.tb07935.x

Taylor, H. L., & G. Luter. (2013). *Anchor institutions: An interpretative review essay.* Anchor Institution Task Force. https://ubwp.buffalo.edu/aps-cus/wp-content/uploads/sites/16/2015/07/Literature_Review_2013.pdf

Taylor, S. (2020). Anxiety disorders, climate change, and the challenges ahead: Introduction to the special issue. *Journal of Anxiety Disorders*, *76*, 102313. https://doi.org/10.1016/j.janxdis.2020.102313

Temple, M. W., Sisk, B., Krams, L. A., Schneider, J. H., Kirkendall, E. S., & Lehmann, C. U. (2019). Trends in use of electronic health records in pediatric office settings. *Journal of Pediatrics*, *206*, 164–171.e2. https://doi.org/10.1016/j.jpeds.2018.10.039

Tennessee Department of Health. (2015). *2015 Edition of the State Health Plan*. https://www.tn.gov/content/dam/tn/health/documents/2015_Edition_of_the_State_Health_Plan.pdf

Terao, M., Hoffman, J.M., Brilli, R.J. Finch, A., Walsh, K. E., & Coffey, M. (2019). Accelerating improvement in children's healthcare through quality improvement collaboratives: A synthesis of recent efforts. *Current Treatment Options in Pediatrics*, *5*, 111–130.

Tessier, K. (2010). Effectiveness of hands-on education for correct child restraint use by parents. *Accident Analysis and Prevention*, *42*, 1041–1047. https://doi.org/10.1016/j.aap.2009.12.011

Tester, J. M., Leung, C. W., & Crawford, P. B. (2016). Revised WIC food package and children's diet quality. *Pediatrics*, *137*(5), e20153557. https://doi.org/10.1542/peds.2015-3557

Teye, S. O., Yanosky, J. D., Cuffee, Y., Weng, X., Luquis, R., Farace, E., & Wang, L. (2021). Exploring persistent racial/ethnic disparities in lead exposure among American children aged 1–5 years: Results from NHANES 1999–2016. *International Archives of Occupational and Environmental Health*, *94*(4), 723–730. https://doi.org/10.1007/s00420-020-01616-4

Thakrar, A. P., Forrest, A. D., Maltenfort, M. G., & Forrest, C. B. (2018). Child mortality in the US and 19 OECD comparator nations: A 50-year time-trend analysis. *Health Affairs*, *37*(1), 140–149.

Therriault, C., Ahmed, N., Zucker, S., Passarelli, M., Dudack, D., Sibley, S., Martini-Carvell, K., & Dworkin, P. H. (2021). *Help Me Grow building impact report*. Help Me Grow National Center. https://helpmegrownational.org/wp-content/uploads/2022/08/Help-Me-Grow-Building-Impact-Report_Full_-2021.pdf

Thiede, M., Akweongo, P., & McIntyre, D. (2007). Exploring the dimensions of access. In D. McIntyre & G. Mooney (Eds.), *The economics of health equity* (pp. 103–123). Cambridge University Press.

Thomas, L. T., Lee, C. M. Y., McClelland, K., Nunis, G., Robinson, S., & Norman, R. (2023). Health workforce perceptions on telehealth augmentation opportunities. *BMC Health Services Research*, *23*(1), 182. https://doi.org/10.1186/s12913-023-09174-4

Thomas, M., Miller, D., & Morrissey, T. (2019). Food insecurity and child health. *Pediatrics*, *144*, e20190397. https://doi.org/10.1542/peds.2019-0397

Thomasius, R., Paschke, K., & Arnaud, N. (2022). Substance-use disorders in children and adolescents. *Deutsches Ärzteblatt International*, *119*(25), 440–450. https://doi.org/10.3238/arztebl.m2022.0122

Thompson, O. (2017). The long-term health impacts of Medicaid and CHIP. *Journal of Health Economics*, *51*, 26–40. https://doi.org/10.1016/j.jhealeco.2016.10.003

Thornton, R. L. J., Glover, C. M., Cené, C. W., Glik, D. C., Henderson, J. A., & Williams, D. R. (2016). Evaluating strategies for reducing health disparities by addressing the social determinants of health. *Health Affairs (Project Hope)*, *35*(8), 1416–1423. https://doi.org/10.1377/hlthaff.2015.1357

Thyen, U., Kuhlthau, K., & Perrin, J. M. (1999). Employment, child care, and mental health of mothers caring for children assisted by technology. *Pediatrics*, *103*(6 Pt 1), 1235–1242. https://doi.org/10.1542/peds.103.6.1235

Tieder, J. S., Sisk, B., Hudak, M., Richerson, J. E., & Perrin, J. M. (2018). General pediatricians and value-based payments. *Pediatrics*, *142*(4). https://doi.org/10.1542/peds.2018-0502

Tiel Groenestege-Kreb, D., van Maarseveen, O., & Leenen, L. (2014). Trauma team. *British Journal of Anaesthesia*, *113*(2), 258–265. https://doi.org/10.1093/bja/aeu236

Tilala, M. H., Chenchala, P. K., Choppadandi, A., Kaur, J., Naguri, S., Saoji, R., & Devaguptapu, B. (2024). Ethical considerations in the use of artificial intelligence and machine learning in health care: A comprehensive review. *Cureus, 16*(6), e62443. https://doi.org/10.7759/cureus.62443

Toia, J., Murtagh, K., Heald, L., Leake, K., & Jhaveri, R. (2024). Advanced practice providers in pediatric infectious diseases. *Journal of the Pediatric Infectious Diseases Society*, *13*(3), 228–231. https://doi.org/10.1093/jpids/piae008

Tolbert, J., Drake, P., & Damico, A. (2023). *Key facts about the uninsured population.* KFF. https://www.kff.org/uninsured/issue-brief/key-facts-about-the-uninsured-population/

Topmiller, M., McCann, J., Hoang, H., Rankin, J., Grandmont, J., Pelzer, M., & Sripipatana, A. (2023). Health centres and social determinants of health: An analysis of enabling services provision and clinical quality. *Family Medicine and Community Health*, *11*(3). https://doi.org/10.1136/fmch-2023-002227

Toossi, S., & Jones, J. W. (2024). The food and nutrition assistance landscape: Fiscal year 2023 annual report. *Economic Research Service.* https://www.ers.usda.gov/webdocs/publications/109314/eib-274.pdf?v=4937.6

Totten, A. M., McDonagh, M. S., & Wagner, J. H. (2020). *The evidence base for telehealth: Reassurance in the face of rapid expansion during the COVID-19 pandemic.* Agency for Healthcare Research and Quality. https://www.ncbi.nlm.nih.gov/books/NBK557174/

Toure, D. M., Kumar, G., Walker, C., Turman, J. E., Jr., & Su, D. (2022). Barriers to pediatric mental healthcare access: Qualitative insights from caregivers. *Journal of Social Service Research*, *48*(4), 485–495. https://doi.org/10.1080/01488376.2022.2088949

Towe, V. L., Leviton, L., Chandra, A., Sloan, J. C., Tait, M., & Orleans, T. (2016). Cross-sector collaborations and partnerships: Essential ingredients to help shape health and well-being. *Health Affairs (Project Hope)*, *35*(11), 1964–1969. https://doi.org/10.1377/hlthaff.2016.0604

TRAILS to Wellness. (n.d.). *Our programs.* https://trailstowellness.org/our-programs

Transnational Forum on Integrated Community Care (TFICC). (2019). *Overview of case studies: Southcentral Foundation's Nuka System of Care.* https://transform-integratedcommunitycare.com/wp-content/uploads/2019/09/overview-of-the-case-studies.pdf

Trent, M., Dooley, D. G., & Dougé, J. (2019). The impact of racism on child and adolescent health. *Pediatrics*, *144*(2). https://doi.org/10.1542/peds.2019-1765

Tribal Budget Formulation Workgroup. (2022). *Advancing health equity through the federal trust responsibility: Full mandatory funding for the Indian Health Service and strengthening nation-to-nation relationships.* National Indian Health Board. https://www.nihb.org/docs/09072022/FY%202024%20Tribal%20Budget%20Formulation%20Workgroup%20Recommendations.pdf

Tripathi, S., McGarvey, J., Lee, K., Staubach, K., Gehring, E., Sisson, P., McCaskey, M., Mack, E., Hord, J., Pallotto, E. K., Lyren, A., & Coffey, M. (2023). Compliance with central line maintenance bundle and infection rates. *Pediatrics*, *152*(3), e2022059688. https://doi.org/10.1542/peds.2022-059688

Trost, S. L., Beauregard, J., Njie, F., Berry, J., Harvey, A., & Goodman, D. A. (2022). *Pregnancy-related deaths: Data from maternal mortality review committees in 36 US states, 2017–2019.* Centers for Disease Control and Prevention, U.S. Department of Health and Human Services. https://www.cdc.gov/reproductivehealth/maternal-mortality/erase-mm/data-mmrc.html

Trounson, A., Boyd, N. R., & Boyd, R. L. (2019). Toward a universal solution: Editing compatibility into pluripotent stem cells. *Cell Stem Cell*, *24*(4), 508–510. https://doi.org/10.1016/j.stem.2019.03.003

Trippe, C., Tadler, C., Johnson, P., Giannarelli, L., & Betson, D. (2019). *National- and state-level estimates of WIC eligibility and WIC program reach in 2016*. U.S. Department of Agriculture, Food and Nutrition Service, Office of Policy Support.

Trust for America's Health. (2022). *Racial and ethnic approaches to community health*. https://www.tfah.org/wp-content/uploads/2022/03/Final-FY23-Racial-and-Ethnic-Approaches-to-Community-Health.pdf

________. (2023). *The prevention and public health fund: Preventing disease and reducing long-term health costs*. https://www.tfah.org/wp-content/uploads/2023/09/PPHF_Backgrounder_September2023.pdf

Tsai, D. (2022). *Centers for Medicare & Medicaid Services informational bulletin: Information on school-based services in Medicaid: Funding, documentation and expanding services*. U.S. Department of Health and Human Services. https://www.medicaid.gov/federal-policy-guidance/downloads/sbscib081820222.pdf

Tschudy, M. M., Toomey, S. L., & Cheng, T. L. (2013). Merging systems: Integrating home visitation and the family-centered medical home. *Pediatrics*, *132*(Suppl 2), S74–S81. https://doi.org/10.1542/peds.2013-1021E

Tsimberidou, A. M., Fountzilas, E., Nikanjam, M., & Kurzrock, R. (2020). Review of precision cancer medicine: Evolution of the treatment paradigm. *Cancer Treatment Reviews*, *86*, 102019. https://doi.org/10.1016/j.ctrv.2020.102019

Tsoi, M. F., Li, H. L., Feng, Q., Cheung, C. L., Cheung, T. T., & Cheung, B. M. Y. (2022). Prevalence of childhood obesity in the United States in 1999–2018: A 20-year analysis. *Obesity Facts*, *15*(4), 560–569. https://doi.org/10.1159/000524261

Turner, A., Ricketts, T., & Leslie, L. K. (2020). Comparison of number and geographic distribution of pediatric subspecialists and patient proximity to specialized care in the US between 2003 and 2019. *JAMA Pediatrics*, *174*(9), 852–860. https://doi.org/10.1001/jamapediatrics.2020.1124

Turner, C., McClure, R., Nixon, J., & Spinks, A. (2005). Community-based programs to promote car seat restraints in children 0-16 years—A systematic review. *Accident Analysis and Prevention*, *37*, 77–83. https://doi.org/10.1016/j.aap.2003.12.004

Turner, S., Nunn, A. J., Fielding, K., & Choonara, I. (1999). Adverse drug reactions to unlicensed and off-label drugs on paediatric wards: A prospective study. *Acta Paediatrica*, *88*(9), 965–968. https://doi.org/10.1080/08035259950168469

Turner Lee, N., Resnick, P., & Barton, G. (2019). Algorithmic bias detection and mitigation: Best practices and policies to reduce consumer harms. *The Brookings Institution*. https://www.brookings.edu/articles/algorithmic-bias-detection-and-mitigation-best-practices-and-policies-to-reduce-consumer-harms/

Tylee, A., Haller, D. M., Graham, T., Churchill, R., & Sanci, L. A. (2007). Youth-friendly primary-care services: How are we doing and what more needs to be done? *The Lancet*, *369*(9572), 1565–1573. https://doi.org/10.1016/s0140-6736(07)60371-7

Tyler, E. T., Hulkower, R. L., & Kaminski, J. W. (2017). *Behavioral health integration in pediatric primary care: Considerations and opportunities for policymakers, planners, and providers*. Milbank Memorial Fund. https://www.milbank.org/wp-content/uploads/2017/03/MMF_BHI_REPORT_FINAL.pdf

Umberson, D., & Montez, J. K. (2010). Social relationships and health: A flashpoint for health policy. *Journal of Health and Social Behavior*, *51*(Suppl), S54. https://doi.org/10.1177/0022146510383501

United Kingdom Department of Health and Social Care. (2020). *Health in all policies*. https://www.health-ni.gov.uk/articles/health-all-policies

United Nations International Children's Emergency Fund (UNICEF). (n.d.). *How to improve primary healthcare to prepare for future pandemics*. https://www.unicef.org/stories/how-to-improve-primary-healthcare-to-prepare-for-pandemics

________. (1997). *The state of the world's children 1997*. https://www.unicef.org/reports/state-worlds-children-1997

________. (2005). *Report card no. 6: Child poverty in rich countries 2005*. UNICEF Innocenti Research Centre. https://www.unicef-irc.org/publications/pdf/repcard6e.pdf

________. (2020). *Worlds of influence: Understanding what shapes child well-being in rich countries*. (Innocenti Report Card No. 16). UNICEF Office of Research–Innocenti. https://www.unicef.org/innocenti/media/1816/file/UNICEF-Report-Card-16-Worlds-of-Influence-EN.pdf

United States Congress. (2020). *Consolidated Appropriations Act, 2022*, H.R. 2471, 117th Cong. (2022). https://www.congress.gov/bill/117th-congress/house-bill/2471

________. (2020). *Coronavirus Aid, Relief, and Economic Security Act*, Pub. L. No. 116-136, 134 Stat. 281. https://www.congress.gov/116/plaws/publ136/PLAW-116publ136.pdf

________. (2024). *Indian Self-Determination and Education Assistance: Congressional Statement of Findings*.

University of California, Los Angeles. (n.d.). *Introducing data informed futures*. https://healthychild.ucla.edu/news/introducing-data-informed-futures

University of Texas Rio Grande Valley School of Medicine. (n.d.). Texas Child Health Access Through Telemedicine (TCHATT). https://www.utrgv.edu/school-of-medicine/departments/psychiatry/tcmhcc/tchatt/index.htm

University of Vermont Medical Center. (2020). *Benefits & compensation*. https://www.uvmhealth.org/gme/about-gme/benefits-compensation

University of Wisconsin Population Health Institute. (2024). *County Health Rankings Program*. https://www.countyhealthrankings.org

Upadhya, K. K., Psoter, K. J., Connor, K. A., Mistry, K. B., Levy, D. J., & Cheng, T. L. (2020). Cluster randomized trial of a pre/interconception health intervention for mothers in pediatric visits. *Academic Pediatrics*, *20*(5), 660–669. https://doi.org/10.1016/j.acap.2019.10.003

Urban Institute. (2024). *The US population is aging*. https://www.urban.org/policy-centers/cross-center-initiatives/program-retirement-policy/projects/data-warehouse/what-future-holds/us-population-aging

USAFacts. (2023). How much money do doctors make in the US? https://usafacts.org/articles/how-much-money-do-doctors-make-in-the-us/

Vaks, Y., Bensen, R., Steidtmann, D., Wang, T. D., Platchek, T. S., Zulman, D. M., Malcolm, E., & Milstein, A. (2016). Better health, less spending: Redesigning the transition from pediatric to adult healthcare for youth with chronic illness. *Healthcare*, *4*(1), 57–68. https://doi.org/10.1016/j.hjdsi.2015.09.001

Valado, T., Tracey, J., Goldfinger, J., & Briggs, R. (2019). HealthySteps: Transforming the promise of pediatric care. *The Future of Children*, *29*(1). https://files.eric.ed.gov/fulltext/EJ1220075.pdf

Valaitis, R. K., Wong, S. T., MacDonald, M., Martin-Misener, R., O'Mara, L., Meagher-Stewart, D., Isaacs, S., Murray, N., Baumann, A., Burge, F., Green, M., Kaczorowski, J., & Savage, R. (2020). Addressing quadruple aims through primary care and public health collaboration: Ten Canadian case studies. *BMC Public Health*, *20*(1), 507. https://doi.org/10.1186/s12889-020-08610-y

Valdivia, H. R. (2022). The pediatric clinical nurse specialist: A children's hospital journey. *Journal of Pediatric Nursing*, *66*, 213–215. https://doi.org/10.1016/j.pedn.2022.07.019

Valido, A., Robinson, L. E., Woolweaver, A. B., Drescher, A., Espelage, D. L., Wright, A. A., Ishmeal, D., Dailey, M. M., Long, A. C. J., & LoMurray, S. (2023). Pilot evaluation of the elementary social-emotional learning program sources of strength. *School Mental Health, 15*(2), 528–539. https://doi.org/10.1007/s12310-023-09567-0

Validova, A., Strane, D., Matone, M., Wang, X., Rosenquist, R., Luan, X., & Rubin, D. (2023). Underinsurance among children with special health care needs in the United States. *JAMA Network Open*, *6*(12), e2348890. https://doi.org/10.1001/jamanetworkopen.2023.48890

van den Berg, M. J., van Loenen, T., & Westert, G. P. (2016). Accessible and continuous primary care may help reduce rates of emergency department use: An international survey in 34 countries. *Family Practice*, *33*(1), 42–50. https://doi.org/10.1093/fampra/cmv082

van Ryn, M., & Burke, J. (2000). The effect of patient race and socio-economic status on physicians' perceptions of patients. *Social Science & Medicine*, *50*(6), 813–828. https://doi.org/10.1016/s0277-9536(99)00338-x

Van Veen, B. (2014). *Patient and family advisory councils: Engaging patients in how care is designed, delivered and experienced: A literature review.* https://dspace.library.uvic.ca/handle/1828/5797

Vargas, E. D., & Pirog, M. A. (2016). Mixed-status families and WIC uptake: The effects of risk of deportation on program use. *Social Science Quarterly*, *97*(3), 555–572. https://doi.org/10.1111/ssqu.12286

Vargas, C., Whelan, J., Brimblecombe, J., & Allender, S. (2022). Co-creation, co-design, co-production for public health—A perspective on definition and distinctions. *Public Health Research & Practice*, *32*. https://doi.org/10.17061/phrp3222211

Varshney, K. (2022). Are federally qualified health centers accessible to pediatric populations in most need throughout Detroit? A visualization using proximity analysis. *Journal of Health Care for the Poor and Underserved*, *33*(1), 356–361. https://doi.org/10.1353/hpu.2022.0026

Vasan, A., Morgan, J. W., Mitra, N., Xu, C., Long, J. A., Asch, D. A., & Kangovi, S. (2020). Effects of a standardized community health worker intervention on hospitalization among disadvantaged patients with multiple chronic conditions: A pooled analysis of three clinical trials. *Health Services Research*, *55*(Suppl 2), 894–901. https://doi.org/10.1111/1475-6773.13321

Vela, M. B., Erondu, A. I., Smith, N. A., Peek, M. E., Woodruff, J. N., & Chin, M. H. (2022). Eliminating explicit and implicit biases in health care: Evidence and research needs. *Annual Review of Public Health*, *43*(1), 477–501. https://doi.org/10.1146/annurev-publhealth-052620-103528

Velázquez, N. (2022, May 3). *Testimony before the House Committee on Energy and Commerce, subcommittee on health.* U.S. House of Representatives. https://energycommerce.house.gov/sites/democrats.energycommerce.house.gov/files/documents/Witness%20Testimony_Velazquez_HE_2022.05.03.pdf

Venkataramani, M., Pollack, C. E., & Roberts, E. T. (2017). Spillover effects of adult Medicaid expansions on children's use of preventive services. *Pediatrics*, *140*(6). https://doi.org/10.1542/peds.2017-0953

Vespa, J., Medina, L., & Armstrong, D. M. (2020). *Demographic turning points for the United States: Population projections for 2020 to 2060.* U.S. Census Bureau. https://www.census.gov/content/dam/Census/library/publications/2020/demo/p25-1144.pdf

Vicetti Miguel, C. P., Dasgupta-Tsinikas, S., Lamb, G. S., Olarte, L., & Santos, R. P. (2022). Race, ethnicity, and health disparities in US children with COVID-19: A review of the evidence and recommendations for the future. *Journal of the Pediatric Infectious Diseases Society*, *11*(Suppl 4), S132–S140. https://doi.org/10.1093/jpids/piac099

Video Interaction Project. (n.d.). PlayReadVIP. *Video interaction project.* https://www.playreadvip.org/

Vinci, R. J. (2021). The pediatric workforce: Recent data trends, questions, and challenges for the future. *Pediatrics, 147*(6). https://doi.org/10.1542/peds.2020-013292

Viner, R. M., Ozer, E. M., Denny, S., Marmot, M., Resnick, M., Fatusi, A., & Currie, C. (2012). Adolescence and the social determinants of health. *Lancet, 379*(9826), 1641–1652. https://doi.org/10.1016/s0140-6736(12)60149-4

Vision to Learn. (2022). *A decade of progress.* https://visiontolearn.org/wp-content/uploads/VTL-A-Decade-of-Progress.pdf

_______. (2023). *2022–2023 annual report.* https://visiontolearn.org/wp-content/uploads/VTL_AnnualReport_2023_12_screen.pdf

Viswanathan, M., Kraschnewski, J. L., Nishikawa, B., Morgan, L. C., Honeycutt, A. A., Thieda, P., Lohr, K. N., & Jonas, D. E. (2010). Outcomes and costs of community health worker interventions: A systematic review. *Medical Care, 48*(9), 792–808. https://doi.org/10.1097/MLR.0b013e3181e35b51

Viswanathan, M., Wallace, I., Middleton, J. C., Kennedy, S.M., McKeeman, J., Hudson, K., Rains, C., Vander Schaaf, E. B., & Kahwati, L. (2022). Screening for depression, anxiety, and suicide risk in children and adolescents: An evidence review for the U.S. Preventive Services Task Force. *Agency for Healthcare Research and Quality (US).* https://www.ncbi.nlm.nih.gov/books/NBK585407/

Viswanathan, M., Urrutia, R. P., Hudson, K. N., Middleton, J. C., & Kahwati, L. C. (2023). Folic acid supplementation to prevent neural tube defects: Updated evidence report and systematic review for the US Preventive Services Task Force. *Journal of the American Medical Association, 330*(5), 460–466. https://doi.org/10.1001/jama.2023.9864

Viveiros, J., & Sturtevant, L. (2016). *The role of anchor institutions in restoring neighborhoods: Health institutions as a catalyst for affordable housing and community development.* National Housing Conference. https://nhc.org/wp-content/uploads/2017/03/The-Role-of-Anchor-Institutions-in-Restoring-Neighborhoods-Health-Institutions-as-a-Catalyst-for-Affordable-Housing-and-Community-Development-.pdf

Vogel, J. A., Rising, K. L., Jones, J., Bowden, M. L., Ginde, A. A., & Havranek, E. P. (2019). Reasons patients choose the emergency department over primary care: A qualitative metasynthesis. *Journal of General Internal Medicine, 34*(11), 2610–2619. https://doi.org/10.1007/s11606-019-05128-x

Voss, P. (2013). Sensitive and critical periods in visual sensory deprivation. *Frontiers in Psychology, 4*, 664. https://doi.org/10.3389/fpsyg.2013.00664

Wakefield, E. O., Pantaleao, A., Popp, J. M., Dale, L. P., Santanelli, J. P., Litt, M. D., & Zempsky, W. T. (2018). Describing perceived racial bias among youth with sickle cell disease. *Journal of Pediatric Psychology, 43*(7), 779–788. https://doi.org/10.1093/jpepsy/jsy015

Walford, H., Trinih, S., Winecrot, A., & Lu, M. (2011). *Role of prenatal care in reducing racial and ethnic disparities.* In A. Handler, J. Kennelly, & N. Peacock (Eds.), *Reducing racial/ethnic disparities in reproductive and perinatal outcomes: The evidence from population-based interventions.* Springer Science & Business Print Media.

Walker, A. T., Smith, P. J., Kolasa, M., & Centers for Disease Control and Prevention. (2014). Reduction of racial/ethnic disparities in vaccination coverage, 1995–2011. *MMWR Supplements, 63*(1), 7–12.

Walker, B. H., Brown, D. C., Walker, C. S., Stubbs-Richardson, M., Oliveros, A. D., & Buttross, S. (2022). Childhood adversity associated with poorer health: Evidence from the U.S. National Survey of Children's Health. *Child Abuse & Neglect, 134*, 105871. https://doi.org/10.1016/j.chiabu.2022.105871

Walker, S. C., Kerns, S. E., Lyon, A. R., Bruns, E. J., & Cosgrove, T. J. (2010). Impact of school-based health center use on academic outcomes. *Journal of Adolescent Health, 46*(3), 251–257.

Wallerich, L., Fillol, A., Rivadeneyra, A., Vandentorren, S., Wittwer, J., & Cambon, L. (2023). Environment and child well-being: A scoping review of reviews to guide policies. *Health Promotion Perspectives*, *13*(3), 168–182. https://doi.org/10.34172/hpp.2023.20

Walsh, E. E., Pérez Marc, G., Zareba, A. M., Falsey, A. R., Jiang, Q., Patton, M., Polack, F. P., Llapur, C., Doreski, P. A., Ilangovan, K., Rämet, M., Fukushima, Y., Hussen, N., Bont, L. J., Cardona, J., DeHaan, E., Castillo Villa, G., Ingilizova, M., Eiras, D., Mikati, T., . . . RENOIR Clinical Trial Group (2023). Efficacy and safety of a bivalent RSV prefusion F vaccine in older adults. *New England Journal of Medicine*, *388*(16), 1465–1477. https://doi.org/10.1056/NEJMoa2213836

Walter, H. J., Vernacchio, L., Trudell, E. K., Bromberg, J., Goodman, E., Barton, J., Young, G. J., DeMaso, D. R., & Focht, G. (2019). Five-year outcomes of behavioral health integration in pediatric primary care. *Pediatrics*, *144*(1), e20183243. https://doi.org/10.1542/peds.2018-3243

Wang, B., Frank, R., & Glied, S. (2023). Lasting scars: The impact of depression in early adulthood on subsequent labor market outcomes. *Health Economics*, *32*(12), 2694–2708. https://doi.org/10.1002/hec.4747

Wang, G., Schwartz, G. L., Kershaw, K. N., McGowan, C., Kim, M. H., & Hamad, R. (2022). The association of residential racial segregation with health among U.S. children: A nationwide longitudinal study. *SSM–Population Health*, 19. https://doi.org/10.1016/j.ssmph.2022.101250

Wang, L. Y., Vernon-Smiley, M., Gapinski, M. A., Desisto, M., Maughan, E., & Sheetz, A. (2014). Cost-benefit study of school nursing services. *JAMA Pediatrics*, *168*(7), 642–648. https://doi.org/10.1001/jamapediatrics.2013.5441

Ward, N., & Batalova, J. (2023). *Frequently requested statistics on immigrants and immigration in the United States*. Migration Policy Institute. https://www.migrationpolicy.org/sites/default/files/publications/frs-print-2023.pdf

Warren, M. D., & Kavanagh, L. D. (2023). Over a century of leadership for maternal and child health in the United States: An updated history of the maternal and child health bureau. *Maternal and Child Health Journal*, 1–15. https://doi.org/10.1007/s10995-023-03629-0

Wasserman, R. C., Varni, S. E., Hollander, M. C., & Harder, V. S. (2019). Change in site of children's primary care: A longitudinal population-based analysis. *Annals of Family Medicine*, *17*(5), 390–395. https://doi.org/10.1370/afm.2416

Watson, J. B., & Rayner, R. (1920). Conditioned emotional reactions. *Journal of Experimental Psychology*, *3*(1), 1–14.

Waxman, E., Gundersen, C., & Thompson, M. (2018). *How far do SNAP benefits fall short of covering the cost of a meal?* Urban Institute. https://www.urban.org/research/publication/how-far-do-snap-benefits-fall-short-covering-cost-meal

Weaver, C. A., Ball, M. J., Kim, G. R., & Kiel, J. M. (Eds.). (2013). *Healthcare information management systems: Cases, strategies, and solutions*. Springer. https://doi.org/10.1007/978-3-319-20765-0

Webber, M. P., Carpiniello, K. E., Oruwariye, T., Lo, Y., Burton, W. B., & Appel, D. K. (2003). Burden of asthma in inner-city elementary schoolchildren: Do school-based health centers make a difference? *Archives of Pediatrics & Adolescent Medicine*, *157*(2), 125–129.

Wehby, G. L. (2022). The impact of household health insurance coverage gains on children's academic achievement in Iowa: Evidence from the ACA. *Health Affairs*, *41*(1). https://doi.org/10.1377/hlthaff.2021.01222

Wehman, P., Schall, C., McDonough, J., Graham, C., Brooke, V., Riehle, J. E., Brooke, A., Ham, W., Lau, S., Allen, J., & Avellone, L. (2017). Effects of an employer-based intervention on employment outcomes for youth with significant support needs due to autism. *Autism*, *21*(3), 276–290. https://doi.org/10.1177/1362361316635826

Wehman, P., Schall, C., McDonough, J., Sima, A., Brooke, A., Ham, W., Whittenburg, H., Brooke, V., Avellone, L., & Riehle, E. (2020). Competitive employment for transition-aged youth with significant impact from autism: A multi-site randomized clinical trial. *Journal of Autism and Developmental Disorders*, *50*(6), 1882–1897. https://doi.org/10.1007/s10803-019-03940-2

Wehrle, F. M., Caflisch, J., Eichelberger, D. A., Haller, G., Latal, B., Largo, R. H., Kakebeeke, T. H., & Jenni, O. G. (2020). The importance of childhood for adult health and development—Study protocol of the Zurich longitudinal studies. *Frontiers in Human Neuroscience*, *14*. https://doi.org/10.3389/fnhum.2020.612453

Weinberg, S. T., Monsen, C., Lehmann, C. U., & Leu, M. G. (2021). Integrating web services/applications to improve pediatric functionalities in electronic health records. *Pediatrics*, *148*(1). https://doi.org/10.1542/peds.2021-052047

Weiss, A. J., Liang, L., & Martin, K. (2022). Overview of hospital stays among children and adolescents, 2019. *Agency for Healthcare Research and Quality*. www.hcup-us.ahrq.gov/reports/statbriefs/sb299-Hospital-Stays-Children-2019.pdf

Weitzman Institute. (2023). *Prescription for play*. https://www.weitzmaninstitute.org/prescription-for-play/

Welch, T. R., Olson, B. G., Nelsen, E., Beck Dallaghan, G. L., Kennedy, G. A., & Botash, A. (2017). United States medical licensing examination and American Board of Pediatrics certification examination results: Does the residency program contribute to trainee achievement. *Journal of Pediatrics*, *188*, 270–274.e3. https://doi.org/10.1016/j.jpeds.2017.05.057

Welp, A., & Manser, T. (2016). Integrating teamwork, clinician occupational well-being and patient safety—Development of a conceptual framework based on a systematic review. *BMC Health Services Research*, *16*, 281. https://doi.org/10.1186/s12913-016-1535-y

Wen, H., Hockenberry, J. M., & Cummings, J. R. (2017). The effect of Medicaid expansion on crime reduction: Evidence from HIFA-waiver expansions. *Journal of Public Economics*, *154*, 67–94. https://doi.org/10.1016/j.jpubeco.2017.09.001

Wen, H., Wilk, A. S., Druss, B. G., & Cummings, J. R. (2019). Medicaid acceptance by psychiatrists before and after Medicaid expansion. *JAMA Psychiatry*, *76*(9), 981–983. https://doi.org/10.1001/jamapsychiatry.2019.0958

Werner-Seidler, A., Spanos, S., Calear, A. L., Perry, Y., Torok, M., O'Dea, B., Christensen, H., & Newby, J. M. (2021). School-based depression and anxiety prevention programs: An updated systematic review and meta-analysis. *Clinical Psychology Review*, *89*, 102079. https://doi.org/10.1016/j.cpr.2021.102079

Wernham, A. (2011). Health impact assessments are needed in decision making about environmental and land-use policy. *Health Affairs*, *30*(5), 947–956. https://doi.org/10.1377/hlthaff.2011.0050

Wherry, L. R. (2018). State Medicaid expansions for parents led to increased coverage and prenatal care utilization among pregnant mothers. *Health Services Research*, *53*(5), 3569–3591. https://doi.org/10.1111/1475-6773.12820

Wherry, L. R., Kenney, G. M., & Sommers, B. D. (2016). The role of public health insurance in reducing child poverty. *Academic Pediatrics*, *16*(Suppl 3), S98–S104. https://doi.org/10.1016/j.acap.2015.12.011

Wherry, L. R., Miller, S., Kaestner, R., & Meyer, B. D. (2015). Child Medicaid coverage and later life health care utilization. *National Bureau of Economic Research*. https://www.nber.org/system/files/working_papers/w20929/w20929.pdf

White, A., Liburd, L. C., & Coronado, F. (2021). Addressing racial and ethnic disparities in COVID-19 among school-aged children: Are we doing enough? *Preventing Chronic Disease*, *18*, 210084. http://dx.doi.org/10.5888/pcd18.210084

White, K., & Belachew, B. (2022). Role of psychologists in pediatric subspecialties: Integrated psychological services overarching concepts across pediatric subspecialties. *Pediatric Clinics of North America*, *69*(5), 825–837.

White, P. H., Cooley, W. C., Transitions Clinical Report Authoring Group, American Academy of Pediatrics, American Academy of Family Physicians, & American College of Physicians. (2018). Supporting the health care transition from adolescence to adulthood in the medical home. *Pediatrics*, *142*(5), e20183610. https://doi.org/10.1542/peds.2018-2587

White House Council on Environmental Quality & Office of Science and Technology Policy. (2022). *Guidance for federal departments and agencies on indigenous knowledge*. https://www.whitehouse.gov/wp-content/uploads/2022/12/OSTP-CEQ-IK-Guidance.pdf

Whitehead, L., Robinson, S., Arabiat, D., Jenkins, M., & Morelius, E. (2024). The report of access and engagement with digital health interventions among children and young people: Systematic review. *JMIR Pediatrics and Parenting*, *7*, e44199. https://doi.org/10.2196/44199

Whitener, K. (2024). *New rule seeks to improve transparency of state Medicaid provider payment rates*. https://ccf.georgetown.edu/2024/05/22/new-rule-seeks-to-improve-transparency-of-state-medicaid-provider-payment-rates/

Whitlock, J., & Lloyd-Richardson, E. E. (2019). *Healing self-injury, a compassionate guide for parents and other loved ones*. Oxford University Press.

Whitney, C. G., Zhou, F., Singleton, J., & Schuchat, A. (2014). *Benefits from immunization during the vaccines for children program era—United States, 1994–2013*. Centers for Disease Control and Prevention. https://www.cdc.gov/mmwr/preview/mmwrhtml/mm631Sp6a4.htm

Whitney, D. G., & Peterson, M. D. (2019). US national and state-level prevalence of mental health disorders and disparities of mental health care use in children. *JAMA Pediatrics*, *173*(4), 389–391. https://doi.org/10.1001/jamapediatrics.2018.5399

Whole Child Health Alliance. (2023). *Key elements of whole child health models; Updated*. https://www.nemours.org/content/dam/nemours/nemoursorg/en/documents/whole-child-health-alliance-key-elements.pdf

Whyte, L. E., & Evans, M. (2023). Children are dying in ill-prepared emergency rooms across America. *The Wall Street Journal*. https://www.wsj.com/health/healthcare/hospitals-emergency-rooms-cost-childrens-lives-d6c9fc23

Wight, V., Kaushal, N., Waldfogel, J., & Garfinkel, I. (2014). Understanding the link between poverty and food insecurity among children: Does the definition of poverty matter? *Journal of Child Poverty*, *20*(1), 1–20. https://doi.org/10.1080/10796126.2014.891973

Wikle, S., & Wagner, J. (2023). Medicaid unwinding. *National Health Law Program*. https://healthlaw.org/unwinding/

Wilcox, H. C., Kellam, S. G., Brown, C. H., Poduska, J. M., Ialongo, N. S., Wang, W., & Anthony, J. C. (2008). The impact of two universal randomized first- and second-grade classroom interventions on young adult suicide ideation and attempts. *Drug and Alcohol Dependence*, *95*(Suppl 1), S60–S73. https://doi.org/10.1016/j.drugalcdep.2008.01.005

Wilens, T. E., & Spencer, T. J. (2010). Understanding attention-deficit/hyperactivity disorder from childhood to adulthood. *Postgraduate Medicine*, *122*(5), 97–109. https://doi.org/10.3810/pgm.2010.09.2206

Wiley, L. F. (2016). The struggle for the soul of public health. *Journal of Health Politics, Policy and Law*, *41*(6), 1083–1096. https://doi.org/10.1215/03616878-3665967

Wiley, L. F., & Matthews, G. W. (2017). Health care system transformation and integration: A call to action for public health. *Journal of Law, Medicine & Ethics*, *45*(Suppl 1), 94–97. https://doi.org/10.1177/1073110517703335

Wilkerson, I. (2020). *Caste: The origins of our discontents*. Allen Lane.

Wilkinson, A., Gabriel, A., Stratford, B., Carter, M., Rodriguez, Y., Okogbue, O., Somers, S., Young, D., & Harper, K. (2020). *Early evidence of Medicaid's important role in school-based health services*. Child Trends. https://www.childtrends.org/publications/early-evidence-medicaid-role-school-based-heath-services

Willgerodt, M. A., Brock, D., & Tanner, A. (2023). National school nurse workforce study 2.0. *National Association of Nurses*. https://www.nasn.org/research/school-nurse-workforce

Willgerodt, M. A., Brock, D. M., & Maughan, E. D. (2018). Public school nursing practice in the United States. *The Journal of School Nursing*, *34*(3), 232–244. https://doi.org/10.1177/1059840517752456

Willgerodt, M. A., Tanner, A., McCabe, E., Jameson, B., & Brock, D. (2024). Public school nurses in the United States: National school nurse workforce study 2.0. *The Journal of School Nursing*. https://doi.org/10.1177/10598405241253565

Williams, C., Mostashari, F., Mertz, K., Hogin, E., & Atwal, P. (2012). From the Office of the National Coordinator: The strategy for advancing the exchange of health information. *Health Affairs (Project Hope)*, *31*(3), 527–536. https://doi.org/10.1377/hlthaff.2011.1314

Williams, D. R. (2018). Stress and the mental health of populations of color: Advancing our understanding of race-related stressors. *Journal of Health and Social Behavior*, *59*(4), 466–485. https://doi.org/10.1177/0022146518814251

Williams, D. R., & Collins, C. (2001). Racial residential segregation: A fundamental cause of racial disparities in health. *Public Health Reports*, *116*(5), 404–416. https://doi.org/10.1093/phr/116.5.404

Williams, E., Burns, A., & Rudowitz, R. (2023). *Obesity rates among children: A closer look at implications for children covered by Medicaid*. https://www.kff.org/medicaid/issue-brief/obesity-rates-among-children-a-closer-look-at-implications-for-children-covered-by-medicaid/

Williams, E., & Musumeci, M. (2021). *Children with special health care needs: Coverage, affordability, and HCBS access*. KFF. https://www.kff.org/medicaid/issue-brief/children-with-special-health-care-needs-coverage-affordability-and-hcbs-access/

Willis, J. A. B., Bazemore, A., Jetty, A., Petterson, S., George, J., Rosario, B. L., Scheufele, E., Rajmane, A., Dankwa-Mullan, I., & Rhee, K. (2020). *The state of primary care in the United States: A chartbook of facts and statistics*. The Robert Graham Center. https://www.graham-center.org/content/dam/rgc/documents/publications-reports/reports/PrimaryCareChartbook2021.pdf

Willis, V. C., Thomas Craig, K. J., Jabbarpour, Y., Scheufele, E. L., Arriaga, Y. E., Ajinkya, M., Rhee, K. B., & Bazemore, A. (2022). Digital health interventions to enhance prevention in primary care: Scoping review. *JMIR Medical Informatics*, *10*(1), e33518. https://doi.org/10.2196/33518

Wilson, A., Hodgetts-Morton, V. A., Marson, E. J., Markland, A. D., Larkai, E., Papadopoulou, A., Coomarasamy, A., Tobias, A., Chou, D., Oladapo, O. T., Price, M. J., Morris, K., & Gallos, I. D. (2022). Tocolytics for delaying preterm birth: A network meta-analysis (0924). *The Cochrane Database of Systematic Reviews*, *8*(8), CD014978. https://doi.org/10.1002/14651858.CD014978.pub2

Wise, P. H. (2008). Transforming preconceptional, prenatal, and interconceptional care into a comprehensive commitment to women's health. *Women's Health Issues*, *18*(Suppl 6), S13–S18. https://doi.org/10.1016/j.whi.2008.07.014

Wissow, L. S., Platt, R., & Sarvet, B. (2021). Policy recommendations to promote integrated mental health care for children and youth. *Academic Pediatrics*, *21*(3), 401–407. https://doi.org/10.1016/j.acap.2020.08.014

Witt, R., Vatti, T., Lasko, L., & Witt, A. M. (2021). Team-based breastfeeding support at a federally qualified health center: Efficacy, utilization, and patient satisfaction. *Breastfeeding Medicine: The Official Journal of the Academy of Breastfeeding Medicine*, *16*(9), 741–749.

Wolraich, M. L., Hagan, J. F., Jr., Allan, C., Chan, E., Davison, D., Earls, M., Evans, S. W., Flinn, S. K., Froehlich, T., Frost, J., Holbrook, J. R., Lehmann, C. U., Lessin, H. R., Okechukwu, K., Pierce, K. L., Winner, J. D., & Zurhellen, W. (2019). Clinical practice guideline for the diagnosis, evaluation, and treatment of attention-deficit/hyperactivity disorder in children and adolescents. *Pediatrics*, *144*(4). https://doi.org/10.1542/peds.2019-2528

Wong, C. A., Bain, A., Polsky, D., Merchant, R. M., Antwi, Y. A., Slap, G., Rubin, D., & Ford, C. A. (2017). The use and out-of-pocket cost of urgent care clinics and retail-based clinics by adolescents and young adults compared with children. *Journal of Adolescent Health*, *60*(1), 107–112.

Wong, C. A., Houry, D., & Cohen, M. K. (2024). Integrating public health and health care—Protecting health as a team sport. *New England Journal of Medicine*, *390*(19), 1739–1742. https://doi.org/10.1056/NEJMp2403274

Wong, N. T., Zimmerman, M. A., & Parker, E. A. (2010). A typology of youth participation and empowerment for child and adolescent health promotion. *American Journal of Community Psychology*, *46*(1–2), 100–114. https://doi.org/10.1007/s10464-010-9330-0

Wood, L., & McDaniel, T. (2020). A preliminary investigation of universal mental health screening practices in schools. *Journal of Applied School Psychology*, *36*(4), 323–342.

Woodward, J., & Rice, E. (2015). Case management. *Nursing Clinics of North America*, *50*(1), 109–121. https://doi.org/10.1016/j.cnur.2014.10.009

Woolf, S. H., & Schoomaker, H. (2019). Life expectancy and mortality rates in the United States, 1959–2017. *Journal of the American Medical Association*, *322*(20), 1996–2016. https://doi.org/10.1001/jama.2019.16932

Woolf, S. H., Wolf, E. R., & Rivara, F. P. (2023). The new crisis of increasing all-cause mortality in US children and adolescents. *Journal of the American Medical Association*, *329*(12), 975. https://doi.org/10.1001/jama.2023.3517

World Health Organization (WHO). (n.d.a). *Health topics: Adolescent health*. https://www.who.int/health-topics/adolescent-health#tab=tab_1

_______. (n.d.b). *Maternal health*. https://www.who.int/health-topics/maternal-health#tab=tab_1

_______. (n.d.c). *Patient safety*. https://www.who.int/teams/integrated-health-services/patient-safety

_______. (1986, November 21). *The Ottawa charter for health promotion: First international conference on health promotion*. https://www.who.int/teams/health-promotion/enhanced-wellbeing/first-global-conference

_______. (2013). *How to use the ICF—A practical manual for using the international classification of functioning, disability and health*. https://www.who.int/publications/m/item/how-to-use-the-icf---a-practical-manual-for-using-the-international-classification-of-functioning-disability-and-health

_______. (2018). *Integrating health services*. https://www.who.int/docs/default-source/primary-health-care-conference/linkages.pdf

_______. (2019). *Accountability as a driver of health equity*. https://www.who.int/europe/publications/i/item/9789289054096

_______. (2021). *Cancer in children*. https://www.who.int/news-room/fact-sheets/detail/cancer-in-children

_______. (2023). *Asthma*. https://www.who.int/news-room/fact-sheets/detail/asthma

_______. (2024). *Disinformation and public health*. https://www.who.int/news-room/questions-and-answers/item/disinformation-and-public-health

World Health Organization & United Nations Children's Fund. (1978). *Primary health care: Report of the International Conference on Primary Health Care, Alma-Ata, USSR, 6–12 September 1978*. https://www.who.int/publications/i/item/9241800011

World Obesity Federation. (2023). *World obesity atlas 2023*. https://data.worldobesity.org/publications/?cat=19

Wright, C. F., Campbell, P., Eberhardt, R. Y., Aitken, S., Perrett, D., Brent, S., Danecek, P., Gardner, E. J., Chundru, V. K., Lindsay, S. J., Andrews, K., Hampstead, J., Kaplanis, J., Samocha, K. E., Middleton, A., Foreman, J., Hobson, R. J., Parker, M. J., Martin, H. C., . . . Firth, H. V. (2023). Genomic diagnosis of rare pediatric disease in the United Kingdom and Ireland. *New England Journal of Medicine*, *388*(17), 1559–1571. https://doi.org/10.1056/nejmoa2209046

Wright, J. L., Davis, W. S., Joseph, M. M., Ellison, A. M., Heard-Garris, N. J., & Johnson, T. L. (2022). Eliminating race-based medicine. *Pediatrics*, *150*(1). https://doi.org/10.1542/peds.2022-057998

Wu, A. G., Madhavan, G., Deakins, K., Evans, D., Hayward, A., Pugh, C., Carter Stutts, A., Mustin, L., Staubach, K. C., Sisson, P., Coffey, M., Lyren, A., Lee, G.M, Gupta, S., Pereira-Argenziano, L., & Priebe, G. P. (2023). Pediatric ventilator-associated events before and after a multicenter quality improvement initiative. *JAMA Network Open*, *6*(12), e2346545. https://doi.org/10.1001/jamanetworkopen.2023.46545

Wyman, P., Brown, C. H., LoMurray, M., Schmeelk-Cone, K., Petrova, M., Yu, Q., Walsh, E., Tu, X., & Wang, W. (2010). An outcome evaluation of the sources of strength suicide prevention program delivered by adolescent peer leaders in high schools. *American Journal of Public Health*, *100*(9), 1653–1661. https://doi.org/10.2105/ajph.2009.190025

Wyman, P., Cero, I., Brown, C. H., Espelage, D., Pisani, A., Kuehl, T., & Schmeelk-Cone, K. (2023). Impact of sources of strength on adolescent suicide deaths across three randomized trials. *Injury Prevention*, *29*(5), 442–445. https://doi.org/10.1136/ip-2023-044944

Xierali, I. M., Nivet, M. A., & Rayburn, W. F. (2021). Full-time faculty in clinical and basic science departments by sex and underrepresented in medicine status: A 40-year review. *Academic Medicine*, *96*(4), 568–575. https://doi.org/10.1097/ACM.0000000000003925

Xiong, X., Buekens, P., Fraser, W. D., Beck, J., & Offenbacher, S. (2006). Periodontal disease and adverse pregnancy outcomes: A systematic review. *BJOG: An International Journal of Obstetrics and Gynaecology*, *113*(2), 135–143. https://doi.org/10.1111/j.1471-0528.2005.00827.x

Yee, A. B., Fagnano, M., & Halterman, J. S. (2013). Preventive asthma care delivery in the primary care office: Missed opportunities for children with persistent asthma symptoms. *Academic Pediatrics*, *13*(2), 98–104. https://doi.org/10.1016/j.acap.2012.10.009

Yeung Thompson, R. S., & Leadbeater, B. J. (2013). Peer victimization and internalizing symptoms from adolescence into young adulthood: Building strength through emotional support. *Journal of Research on Adolescence*, *23*(2), 290–303. https://doi.org/10.1111/j.1532-7795.2012.00827.x

Yonek, J., Lee, C. M., Harrison, A., Mangurian, C., & Tolou-Shams, M. (2020). Key components of effective pediatric integrated mental health care models: A systematic review. *JAMA Pediatrics*, *174*(5), 487–498. https://doi.org/10.1001/jamapediatrics.2020.0023

Yoong, S. Y. C., Ang, P. H., Chong, S.-L., Ong, Y.-K. G., Zakaria, N. D. B., Lee, K. P., & Pek, J. H. (2021). Common diagnoses among pediatric attendances at emergency departments. *BMC Pediatrics*, *21*(1), 172. https://doi.org/10.1186/s12887-021-02646-8

Young, N. A. E. (2021). *Childhood disability in the United States: 2019* (ACSBR-006). U.S. Census Bureau. https://www.census.gov/library/publications/2021/acs/acsbr-006.html

Young, N. A. E., & Crankshaw, K. (2021). Disability rates highest among American Indian and Alaska Native children and children living in poverty. *United States Census Bureau*. https://www.census.gov/library/stories/2021/03/united-states-childhood-disability-rate-up-in-2019-from-2008.html

Young, S., Connolly Sollose, L., & Carey, J. P. (2020). Addressing chronic absenteeism in middle school: A cost-effective approach. *Children & Schools*, *42*(2), 131–138. https://doi.org/10.1093/cs/cdaa009

Youth.gov. (n.d.). *Involving youth in positive youth development.* https://youth.gov/youth-topics/involving-youth-positive-youth-development

YouthPower Learning & YouthPower Action. (n.d.). *YouthPower action.* https://www.youthpower.org/youthpower-action

Yu, H., Kolko, D. J., & Torres, E. (2017). Collaborative mental health care for pediatric behavior disorders in primary care: Does it reduce mental health care costs? *Families, Systems, & Health*, *35*(1), 46–57. https://doi.org/10.1037/fsh0000251

Yu, J., Perrin, J. M., Hagerman, T., & Houtrow, A. J. (2022). Underinsurance among children in the United States. *Pediatrics*, *149*(1), e2021050353. https://doi.org/10.1542/peds.2021-050353

Yun, J., & Yun, Y. H. (2023). Health-promoting behavior to enhance perceived meaning and control of life in chronic disease patients with role limitations and depressive symptoms: A network approach. *Scientific Reports, 13*(1), 1–15. https://doi.org/10.1038/s41598-023-31867-3

Zablotsky, B., & Ng, A. E. (2023). *Mental health treatment among children aged 5–17 years: United States, 2021.* U.S. Department of Health and Human Services. https://www.cdc.gov/nchs//data/databriefs/db472.pdf

Zablotsky, B., Ng, A. E., Black, L. I., & Blumberg, S. J. (2023). *Diagnosed developmental disabilities in children aged 3–17 years: United States, 2019–2021.* Centers for Disease Control and Prevention, National Center for Health Statistics. https://www.cdc.gov/nchs/products/databriefs/db473.htm#Key_finding

Zacarian, D., Alvarez-Ortiz, L., & Haynes, J. (2017). *Teaching to strengths: Supporting students living with trauma, violence, and chronic stress* (1st ed.). ASCD.

Zare, H., Eisenberg, M. D., & Anderson, G. (2022). Comparing the value of community benefit and tax-exemption in non-profit hospitals. *Health Services Research*, *57*(2), 270–284. https://doi.org/10.1111/1475-6773.13668

Zaza, S., Sleet, D. A., Thompson, R. S., Sosin, D.M, Bolen, J. C., & Task Force on Community Preventive Services. (2001). Reviews of evidence regarding interventions to increase use of child safety seats. *American Journal of Preventive Medicine*, *21*(Suppl 4), 31–47.

Zeanah, C. H., & Fox, N. A. (2019). How early experience shapes human development: The case of psychosocial deprivation. *Neural Plasticity*. https://doi.org/10.1155/2019/1676285

Zerhouni, E. A. (2006). Research funding. NIH in the post-doubling era: Realities and strategies. *Science*, *314*(5802), 1088–1090. https://doi.org/10.1126/science.1136931

Zhang, Y., Ding, Z., Perentesis, J. P., Khuntia, D., Pfister, S. X., & Sharma, R. A. (2021). Can rational combination of ultra-high dose rate FLASH radiotherapy with immunotherapy provide a novel approach to cancer treatment? *Clinical Oncology (Royal College of Radiologists)*, *33*(11), 713–722. https://doi.org/10.1016/j.clon.2021.09.003

Zhang, X., Perez-Stable, E. J., Bourne, P. E., Peprah, E., & Boulware, L. E. (2023). Telehealth usage among low-income racial and ethnic minority groups during the COVID-19 pandemic. *Journal of Medical Internet Research*, *25*, e43604. https://doi.org/10.2196/43604

Zhou, C., Crawford, A., Serhal, E., Kurdyak, P., & Sockalingam, S. (2016). The impact of Project ECHO on participant and patient outcomes: A systematic review. *Academic Medicine*, *91*(10), 1439–1461. https://doi.org/10.1097/acm.0000000000001328

Zhou, F., Shefer, A., Wenger, J., Messonnier, M., Wang, L. Y., Lopez, A., Moore, M., Murphy, T. V., Cortese, M., & Rodewald, L. (2014). Economic evaluation of the routine childhood immunization program in the United States, 2009. *Pediatrics*, *133*(4), 577–585. https://doi.org/10.1542/peds.2013-0698

Zimmerman, S., & Lieberman, M. (2020). *The Safe Routes to School Program Census Project: 2019 national program assessment report.* Safe Routes Partnership. https://saferoutespartnership.org/sites/default/files/resource_files/national_srts_census_report_final.pdf

Zipursky, A. R., Olson, K. L., Bode, L., Geva, A., Jones, J., Mandl, K. D., & McMurry, A. (2023). Emergency department visits and boarding for pediatric patients with suicidality before and during the COVID-19 pandemic. *PLoS One*, *18*(11), e0286035. https://doi.org/10.1371/journal.pone.0286035

Zuckerman, B., Amaro, H., Bauchner, H., & Cabral, H. (1989). Depressive symptoms during pregnancy: Relationship to poor health behaviors. *American Journal of Obstetrics & Gynecology*, *160*(5 Pt 1), 1107–1111. https://doi.org/10.1016/0002-9378(89)90170-1

Zuckerman, S., Skopec, L., & Aarons, J. (2021). Medicaid physician fees remained substantially below fees paid by Medicare in 2019. *Health Affairs*, *40*(2), 343–348. https://doi.org/10.1377/hlthaff.2020.00611

Zuckerman, S., Williams, A. F., & Stockley, K. E. (2009). Trends in Medicaid physician fees, 2003–2008. *Health Affairs (Project Hope)*, *28*(3), w510–w519. https://doi.org/10.1377/hlthaff.28.3.w510

Zupkovich, D. (2022). *Success in our state.* CliniSync. https://clinisync.org/wp-content/uploads/2022/03/ISBH-Success-Story.pdf

Appendix A

Biosketches of Committee Members and Staff

COMMITTEE MEMBERS

Tina L. Cheng (*Co-Chair*, she/her) is the B.K. Rachford Professor and Chair of Pediatrics at the University of Cincinnati College of Medicine, director of the Cincinnati Children's Research Foundation, and chief medical officer at Cincinnati Children's Hospital Medical Center. She was previously chair of pediatrics and pediatrician-in-chief at Johns Hopkins University. Her clinical work, teaching, and research focus on child, adolescent, and family perspectives on improving health; community-integrated models to interrupt the intergenerational cycle of disadvantage; as well as innovation and transformation for excellent and equitable health outcomes. Cheng completed Brown University's 7-year program in medicine. She also completed her pediatrics residency and chief residency at the University of California, San Francisco, and San Francisco General Hospital. At the University of California, Berkeley, she received an MPH in epidemiology and completed a preventive medicine residency, followed by a fellowship in academic general pediatrics at the University of Massachusetts. She is a member of the National Academy of Medicine and has served on National Academies Committees and the Forum for Children's Well-Being. Cheng currently is consulting editor for *Pediatric Clinics of North America* and past president of the Academic Pediatric Association and holds leadership roles in the American Academy of Pediatrics and the Association of Medical School Pediatric Department Chairs.

James M. Perrin (*Co-Chair,* he/him) is professor of pediatrics at Harvard Medical School and formerly directed the Division of General Pediatrics at the MassGeneral Hospital for Children and its Center for Child and Adolescent Health Policy. Perrin currently holds the MGH John C. Robinson Distinguished Chair in Pediatrics. He has been on faculty at the University of Rochester as well as Vanderbilt University. His work has recently addressed how to improve Medicaid for younger people in Massachusetts and nationally, with an emphasis on children and youth with chronic conditions. Perrin is a graduate of Harvard College and Case Western Reserve School of Medicine, and did his residency and fellowship at the University of Rochester. He developed a rural community health center between Rochester and Buffalo. He has served on the boards of Family Voices, the Frank Porter Graham Child Development Institute (University of North Carolina), and the Institute for Exceptional Care. A member of the National Academy of Medicine, he has been on several National Academies committees. He is past president of the Academic Pediatric Association (APA) and the American Academy of Pediatrics (AAP), and he currently chairs the AAP Committee on Child Health Financing. He was founding editor of the APA journal *Academic Pediatrics*.

Louis P. Appel (he/him) serves as director of pediatrics at People's Community Clinic (PCC), a federally qualified health center in Austin, Texas. He previously served as chief medical officer of PCC. At PCC, Appel has championed the promotion of early relational health and projects on group pediatric well-child checks, postpartum depression screening, lactation support, and childhood obesity prevention focused on the prenatal and immediate postpartum periods. He is a fellow of the American Academy of Pediatrics (AAP), a member of the American Public Health Association, and a member of the Harvard Center on the Developing Child's Pediatric Innovation Initiative. Appel received an MD from Harvard Medical School and obtained an MPH at the Harvard School of Public Health, with a concentration in public management and community health. He completed his pediatric residency at the University of Washington in Seattle. Appel serves on a Medicaid advisory committee for BlueCross BlueShield of Texas and is immediate past president of the Texas Pediatric Society, the Texas chapter of the AAP.

Christina Bethell (she/her) is professor at Johns Hopkins University in the Bloomberg School of Public Health. Her research focuses on building and translating the science of healthy development to promote early and lifelong health of children, youth, families, and communities. Her roots are in national and state health care policy, financing reform, and delivery system redesign to promote whole child and family health and integrated services.

Bethell is founding director of the Child and Adolescent Health Measurement Initiative as well as the Data Resource Center for Child and Adolescent Health. She led the design and national use of adult-, child-, and family-centered quality and outcomes measures in common use today, including measures of medical homes, children with special health care needs, promoting healthy development, adverse childhood experiences, positive childhood experiences, family resilience, and child flourishing, as well as the Integrated Child Risk Index. Her research has shaped policies regarding adverse childhood experiences and relational health promotion, including providing testimony to the U.S. House Committee on Oversight and Reform on identifying, preventing, and treating childhood trauma. She earned an MBA and MPH from the University of California, Berkeley, and a PhD in public policy and health services research from The University of Chicago.

Ashleigh F. Bowman (she/her) is assistant professor of maternal child health nursing in the College of Nursing at the University of South Alabama. She maintains an active practice as a pediatric nurse practitioner in the Pediatric Emergency Center at USA Health Children's & Women's Hospital in Mobile, Alabama, with a particular interest in caring for critically ill and medically complex children. Bowman's professional expertise in pediatric emergency medicine has recently focused on caring for children who have been physically and/or sexually abused. Her research interest is focused on health care policy, particularly how policy intersects with advanced nursing practice and how policy impacts child health outcomes. She is a member of the National Association of Pediatric Nurse Practitioners where she serves on the Health Policy Committee and the International Association of Forensic Nurses. She received a DNP from the University of South Alabama and is a board-certified pediatric acute care nurse practitioner.

Nathan T. Chomilo (he/him) is medical director for the State of Minnesota's Medicaid and MinnesotaCare programs, adjunct assistant professor of pediatrics at the University of Minnesota Medical School, and general pediatrician with Park Nicollet Health Services/HealthPartners. He served as the State of Minnesota's COVID-19 vaccine equity director and as senior advisor on equity to the Minnesota Commissioner of Health. Chomilo received an MD from the University of Minnesota Medical School, where he also completed his combined residency in internal medicine and pediatrics and was a pediatric chief resident. Chomilo is a member of the American Academy of Pediatrics (AAP) and currently serves in an uncompensated advisory role for some of the organization's expert committees, including the Medicaid and CHIP Expert Advisory Panel, the Section on Minority Health Equity and Inclusion, and the Council on Early Childhood. He is a board member of the AAP chapter in Minnesota that operates independently from AAP.

Ashleigh D. Coser (she/her) is a health service psychologist with the Cherokee Nation. She oversees and provides integrated behavioral health services across multiple clinics and serves as an internship and practicum supervisor. Coser currently serves as a board member with the Oklahoma Psychological Association and recently served as chair for the Native American Special Interest Group with the Association for Behavioral and Cognitive Therapies. She is a member of the Choctaw Nation and a descendant of the Creek and Chickasaw nations. Her research interests include examining the parent–child relationship among American Indian families and maternal mental health. Her recent publications have focused on conducting behavioral research in American Indian communities and examining psychometric properties of measures used widely with that population. Coser earned her PhD in clinical psychology from Oklahoma State University and completed her internship at the Indian Health Care Resource Center in Tulsa, Oklahoma. She completed her postdoctoral training at University of Oklahoma Health Sciences Center.

Alison E. Cuellar (she/her) is professor of health administration and policy at George Mason University and research associate with the National Bureau of Economic Research. She serves as chair of the Community Preventive Services Task Force, an independent, nonfederal panel of public health and prevention experts that provides evidence-based findings and recommendations about community preventive services, programs, and other interventions aimed at improving population health; she is also an elected member of the National Academy of Social Insurance. Cuellar has extensive research experience in evaluation, including the impact of new organizational forms, such as hospital systems and physician alliances and their effects on quality, efficiency, costs, prices, and equity. She also studies Medicaid and private payer initiatives, payment and coverage policy related to primary care and behavioral health, and the intersection with the legal–carceral systems. She received a PhD at the University of California, Berkeley. Cuellar published the article "Value-based Payment, the Safety Net, and Rethinking Risk" in the *American Journal of Managed Care*.

Hala H. Durrah (she/her) is an independent patient family engagement consultant. Her passion for patient family engagement work stems from her experience as a mother of a chronically ill child who has undergone two liver transplants and a bone marrow transplant. As a subject matter expert and policy analyst in patient partnership and engagement, Durrah serves as a consultant on projects focused on patient-centered measurement, quality improvement, patient safety, health equity, child health, health care transformation, medical education and board certification, patient-partnered research, and patient experience. In 2020, she was elected to the

American Board of Emergency Medicine as their first public member director and recently selected to serve as the public member on the Committee for Certification to the American Board of Medical Specialties. Durrah has advised and provided her expertise to many organizations—including, but not limited to, the American Institutes for Research, National Association of Community Health Centers, Centers for Medicare & Medicaid Services, Agency for Healthcare Research and Quality, Community Catalyst, National Quality Forum, American Hospital Association, MedStar Health, and Anne Arundel Medical Center. She received a BA in international affairs and an MA in tourism administration, both from The George Washington University. Durrah currently serves as core faculty and family advisory lead for the Accelerating Child Health Transformation initiative led by the Center for Health Care Strategies with support from the Robert Wood Johnson Foundation. She has also published the article "My Child Is Sick; Don't Call Her A 'Consumer'" in *Health Affairs*.

Carole Roan Gresenz (she/her) is professor of public policy and health at Georgetown University and currently holds the Bette Jacobs endowed professorship. Previously, she was interim dean of the School of Nursing & Health Studies and senior advisor for Strategic Health Initiatives at Georgetown and served in various roles at the RAND Corporation, including as senior economist; director of the Economics, Sociology and Statistics Department; and director of the Health Economics, Finance, and Organization program. Her research background is broad-based and includes work on children's health insurance, access to health care among uninsured children, children's behavioral health care, gun violence, provider payment policies, and local health care policy making. She received an MA and PhD in economics from Brown University and a bachelor's degree in economics from Loyola University Maryland. Gresenz serves on the MedStar Healthcare Delivery Research advisory board and previously served on the scientific council for Georgetown/MedStar Health.

Kelly J. Kelleher (he/him) is the inaugural ADS chair of innovation and vice president for community health at Nationwide Children's Hospital (NCH) and distinguished professor of pediatrics, psychiatry and public health at The Ohio State University. He is founding director of the Center for Child Health Equity and Outcomes Research at NCH and developer of the Healthy Neighborhood/Healthy Family program in Columbus, Ohio, where his research and leadership focus on population health for children and young families, financing mechanisms that facilitate population health, and public–private collaborations for local community development on behalf of children. Kelleher received the national Hearst Population Health Prize and is steering committee chair for the national PEDSnet research consortium.

He received his BS and MD from The Ohio State University, his pediatric residency training from Northwestern University, his MPH from Johns Hopkins, and his fellowship training through the Epidemiology Training Program at the National Institute of Mental Health. He has also served on three previous consensus committees of the National Academies and the Forum for Children's Well-Being and was a founding participant in the pediatric Digital Learning subcommittee of the National Academy of Medicine Leadership Consortium for a Value and Science-Driven Health System, which led to the formation of PEDSnet. Kelleher is a member of the American Academy of Pediatrics. He published the article "Promoting Children's Mental, Emotional, and Behavioral (MEB) Health in All Public Systems, Post-COVID-19" in *Administration and Policy in Mental Health*.

William Martinez (he/him) is associate professor of psychiatry and behavioral sciences at the University of California, San Francisco (UCSF), and director of the Child and Adolescent Services clinic in the Division of Infant, Child, and Adolescent Psychiatry at Zuckerberg San Francisco General Hospital. He is currently director of pediatric mental health for the UCSF Health and Human Rights Initiative, a multidisciplinary group across several departments and hospitals focused on improving the health of asylees and their families. Martinez is also principal investigator of the Fuerte program, a school-based group prevention program targeting newcomer immigrant youth at risk for behavioral health concerns. His overall clinical and research aims are concentrated on reducing behavioral health disparities among ethnic minority youth, with a specific focus on Latinx and immigrant populations. He takes a socioecological approach to understanding these concerns across three areas of inquiry: (1) the impact of social determinants on behavioral health disparities; (2) implementation and dissemination of evidence-based prevention and intervention programming for traumatic stress; and (3) informed policy focused on improving conditions for asylee youth. Martinez received a PhD in clinical child psychology from DePaul University. He is board certified through the American Board of Professional Psychology in clinical child and adolescent psychology and has a certificate in implementation science through UCSF. He is retained by Psychological Assessment Resources, Inc., as a compensated member of an expert panel on a revision of the Trauma Symptom Checklist for Children.

Philip O. Ozuah (he/him) is president and CEO of Montefiore Einstein Medicine, the umbrella organization for Montefiore Health System and Albert Einstein College of Medicine. He previously served as president and chief operating officer of Montefiore Health System and professor and university chairman of pediatrics and physician-in-chief of the Children's Hospital at Montefiore. In these roles, Ozuah expanded access for underserved communities, advanced programs of excellence, fostered innovations, and improved financial and operational performance. His research focuses on addressing disparities in pediatric asthma and obesity. Ozuah is a member of the National Institutes of Health study sections; a member of the American Academy of Pediatrics, Academic Pediatric Association, Society for Pediatric Research, and American Pediatric Society. Most recently he was elected chair of the Health Systems Committee of the American Hospital Association. Ozuah earned an MD from the University of Ibadan, Nigeria; an MSc, with a specialization in medical education, from the University of Southern California, Los Angeles; and a PhD in educational leadership and administration from the University of Nebraska–Lincoln. During the COVID-19 pandemic, he published articles in *The New York Times* and in the *U.S. News & World Report* Best Hospitals issue on health inequities.

Sarah A. Stoddard (she/her) is associate professor of nursing and health behavior health education at the University of Michigan. Her career has focused on promoting the health and wellbeing of youth living in communities characterized by substantial health and social disparities. Stoddard has served as a public health nurse focused on maternal–child health and a nurse practitioner in community- and school-based clinics; she was also state adolescent health coordinator for the Minnesota Department of Health. Her research aims to improve understanding of youth development within adverse contexts and apply strengths-based approaches to prevention in school and community settings. Stoddard serves on the U.S. Department of Health and Human Services Community Preventive Services Task Force. She has held leadership positions for the Interdisciplinary Association for Population Health Science and the Society for Adolescent Health and Medicine, and served as a member of the executive committee for the National Network of State Adolescent Health Coordinators. She is a fellow of the Society of Adolescent Health and Medicine and the American Academy of Nursing. Stoddard received her undergraduate degree in nursing from Minnesota State University at Mankato, and an MS and PhD from the University of Minnesota.

Lequisha S. Turner (she/her) is a predoctoral psychology intern with the University of Nebraska Medical Center Munroe Meyer Institute. She is also a licensed mental health professional and faculty member in the University of Nebraska Omaha Grace Abbott School of Social Work. Turner works with children, adolescents, and families from historically underserved communities. She has provided behavioral health care in a federally qualified health center, a school-based health clinic, and multiple integrated primary care locations. She is also a member of American Psychological Association's Division 17 Society of Counseling Psychology and Division 45 Society for the Psychological Study of Culture, Ethnicity, and Race. Turner obtained both her BA and MSW from the University of Nebraska Omaha and is currently completing her PhD in educational psychology at the University of Nebraska–Lincoln.

Jennifer R. Walton (she/her) is section chief of developmental behavioral pediatrics at the University of Miami Miller School of Medicine's Department of Pediatrics and is part of the leadership of the university's Mailman Center for Child Development. She is a champion of health equity, diversity, inclusion, and intersectionality. Walton has served on the board of directors for the Society for Developmental Behavioral Pediatrics and on the executive committee of the Pediatric Section of the National Medical Association. She now serves on the professional advisory board for the Williams Syndrome Association. Walton received an MD from the Northeastern Ohio Universities College of Medicine (now called NEOMED) and an MPH from the University of Pennsylvania Perelman School of Medicine. She is a member and fellow of the American Academy of Pediatrics and volunteers on the executive committee for the member section on developmental behavioral pediatrics. She has been interviewed and contributed to articles on priorities for developmental and behavioral pediatrics and racism in pediatric health.

NATIONAL ACADEMY OF MEDICINE FELLOW

Kai N. Cheong is associate consultant pediatric specialist at the Hong Kong Children's Hospital at Kai Tak. As a specialist in pediatric immunology, infectious diseases, and rheumatology, she is responsible for translocating the hospital's existing tertiary service from Queen Mary Hospital at The University of Hong Kong, in addition to setting up and consolidating their entirely new quaternary regional service model in these specialties. Within just a few months, Cheong has led a small team to successfully implement a cost-efficient, innovative, one-stop, integrated, holistic, multidisciplinary service model in a Public Hospital Authority hospital within the framework of a public health care system heavily subsidized by the Hong Kong government. This service is the first of its kind in the region that is truly able to provide a comprehensive and personalized service for a large group of patients with complex diseases—at no extra cost to the patients and thus easily accessible to Hong Kong residents across all socioeconomic strata.

STAFF

Abigail Allen is an associate program officer with the National Academies of Sciences, Engineering, and Medicine's Committee on Law and Justice. Previously, she worked for the Animal Legal Defense Fund as a criminal defense law clerk and legislative affairs intern. Her research and writing centered on projects related to COVID-19's impact on the factory farming industry and aquatic animal law. Allen also worked as a criminal defense law clerk for a private firm in Fairfax, Virginia. She received both a BA in criminology, law, and society and a JD from George Mason University, after obtaining an associate degree from Northern Virginia Community College.

Emma Moore is senior program assistant with the Board on Children, Youth, and Families. She is a recent graduate of the University of Maryland, where she earned a BA in criminology and criminal justice and family science. Her interests include juvenile justice and the reciprocal relationship of the criminal justice system on families and youth. Prior to working at the National Academies of Sciences, Engineering, and Medicine, Moore held an internship at the Maryland Governor's Office of Crime Prevention, Youth, and Victim Services. She anticipates attending graduate school in the future to obtain an MSW.

Shaakira Parker is associate program officer with the Division of Behavioral and Social Sciences and Education. Before joining the National Academies of Sciences, Engineering, and Medicine, she was policy associate in the Child Health Advocacy Institute and the Early Childhood Innovation Network at Children's National Hospital, where she focused on policy, advocacy, and systems change to improve the public behavioral health system for children and families in the District of Columbia. Parker has a bachelor's degree in child development from Vanderbilt University and a master's in public health from The George Washington University Milken Institute School of Public Health. She is interested in how research can be used to develop evidence-based policies and prevention programs to address social and health disparities.

Julie Anne Schuck is senior program officer at the National Academies of Sciences, Engineering, and Medicine. In this role, Schuck regularly manages projects and staff teams; provides analytical, administrative, and editorial support for studies and convening activities; and serves as a technical writer. Projects have covered a wide range of subjects, including the health and wellbeing of children and youth, law and justice issues, incarceration and health, national security, STEM (science, technology, engineering, and mathematics) education, the science of human-system integration, workforce development, and the evaluations of several federal research and assistance programs. Schuck received a BS in engineering physics from the University of California, San Diego, and an MS in education from Cornell University.

Sunia Young is research associate with the National Academies of Sciences, Engineering, and Medicine's Board on Children, Youth, and Families. She previously worked as case manager at a Washington, DC–based behavioral health organization and as contact tracer for the State of Utah during the COVID-19 pandemic. Young also interned at the Carter Center's Mental Health Program and with a DC-based organization that supports Asian women who have experienced domestic violence and sexual assault. Additionally, she has studied the Persian language extensively and spent the summer of 2018 in Tajikistan studying the Iranian and Tajik dialects of Persian through the U.S. Department of State. Young graduated from Davidson College with a BS in psychology and a minor in Arab studies. Sunia is currently pursuing her master's in public health at Johns Hopkins University Bloomberg School of Public Health.

Appendix B

Previous National Academies Reports on Child and Adolescent Health and Health Care Reform

Despite remarkable advancements in medical science and developmental understanding, pediatric health care in the United States has yet to fully evolve to meet the complex challenges facing children and adolescents today. While strides have been made in treating acute illnesses and managing chronic conditions, this report reveals that the landscape of child and adolescent health care includes persistent gaps and disparities that demand urgent attention. There have been myriad calls across agencies and organizations looking to address critical shortcomings and ensure that all children and youth have access to the high-quality care they need and deserve.

Previous consensus reports by the National Academies of Sciences, Engineering, and Medicine have also provided insights into promising mechanisms and levers for innovation that can be implemented to improve the health and wellbeing of children and youth. Concerted collaborative, cross-sector efforts are still needed to translate these recommendations into actionable reforms that result in meaningful change.

Area of Focus	Report Title (Year)
Access to Care	• *Implementing High-Quality Primary Care: Rebuilding the Foundation of Health Care* (2021) • *Children's Health, the Nation's Wealth: Assessing and Improving Child Health* (2004) • *Crossing the Quality Chasm: A New Health System for the 21st Century* (2001) • *America's Children: Health Insurance and Access to Care* (1998)
Adolescent and Young Adult Health	• *Promoting Positive Adolescent Health Behaviors and Outcomes: Thriving in the 21st Century* (2020) • *The Promise of Adolescence: Realizing Opportunity for All Youth* (2019) • *Investing in the Health and Well-Being of Young Adults* (2015) • *Adolescent Health Services: Missing Opportunities* (2009) • *Adolescent Risk and Vulnerability: Concepts and Measurement* (2001)
Cancer	• *Childhood Cancer and Functional Impacts Across the Care Continuum* (2021) • *Childhood Cancer Survivorship: Improving Care and Quality of Life* (2003)
Community and Social Care	• *Integrating Social Care into the Delivery of Health Care: Moving Upstream to Improve the Nation's Health* (2019) • *Communities in Action: Pathways to Health Equity* (2017) • *Community-Oriented Primary Care: New Directions for Health Services Delivery* (1983)
Early Childhood	• *Transforming the Workforce for Children Birth Through Age 8: A Unifying Foundation* (2015) • *Depression in Parents, Parenting, and Children: Opportunities to Improve Identification, Treatment, and Prevention* (2009) • *From Neurons to Neighborhoods: The Science of Early Child Development* (2000)
Health Care Professionals and Workforce	• *The Future Pediatric Subspecialty Physician Workforce: Meeting the Needs of Infants, Children, and Adolescents* (2023) • *Graduate Medical Education That Meets the Nation's Health Needs* (2014)
Health Disparities	• *Closing the Opportunity Gap for Young Children* (2023) • *Federal Policy to Advance Racial, Ethnic, and Tribal Health Equity* (2023) • *Reducing Intergenerational Poverty* (2023) • *Vibrant and Healthy Kids: Aligning Science, Practice, and Policy to Advance Health Equity* (2019) • *A Roadmap to Reducing Child Poverty* (2019) • *The Health of Lesbian, Gay, Bisexual, and Transgender People: Building a Foundation for Better Understanding* (2011)

Immunizations	• *The Childhood Immunization Schedule and Safety: Stakeholder Concerns, Scientific Evidence, and Future Studies* (2013) • *Immunization Safety Review: Vaccines and Autism* (2004)
Injury Prevention	• *Preventing Bullying Through Science, Policy, and Practice* (2016) • *New Directions in Child Abuse and Neglect Research* (2014) • *Reducing the Burden of Injury: Advancing Prevention and Treatment* (1999) • *Injury in America: A Continuing Public Health Problem* (1985)
Mental and Behavioral Health	• *Fostering Healthy Mental, Emotional, and Behavioral Development in Children and Youth: A National Agenda* (2019) • *Preventing Mental, Emotional, and Behavioral Disorders Among Young People: Progress and Possibilities* (2009) • *Reducing Risks for Mental Disorders: Frontiers for Preventive Intervention Research* (1994)
National Children's Study	• *The National Children's Study 2014: An Assessment* (2014)
Obesity Prevention	• *Local Government Actions to Prevent Childhood Obesity* (2009) • *Preventing Childhood Obesity: Health in the Balance* (2005)
Parenting, Children, and Families	• *Addressing the Long-Term Effects of the COVID-19 Pandemic on Children and Families* (2023) • *Birth Settings in America: Outcomes, Quality, Access, and Choice* (2020) • *Parenting Matters: Supporting Parents of Children Ages 0–8* (2016)

SOURCE: Adapted from Perrin, Cheng, et al., 2023. All reports available at nap.edu.

Appendix C

Public Meeting Agendas

COMMITTEE ON IMPROVING THE HEALTH AND WELLBEING OF CHILDREN AND YOUTH THROUGH HEALTH CARE SYSTEM TRANSFORMATION

The Keck Center, 500 Fifth Street, NW
Washington, DC 20001

February 27, 2023

PUBLIC SESSION

11:30–11:45 Welcome and Introductions
Carlotta Arthur, Executive Director, DBASSE, National Academies
Natacha Blain, Senior Board Director, Board on Children, Youth, and Families
Tina Cheng, Committee Co-Chair, University of Cincinnati, Cincinnati Children's Hospital
James Perrin, Committee Co-Chair, Harvard Medical School, MassGeneral Hospital for Children

11:45–12:45 Discussion of the Statement of Task with Study Sponsors
Katherine Beckmann, The David & Lucile Packard Foundation (virtual)
Sandy Chung, American Academy of Pediatrics (virtual)

Ira Hillman, Einhorn Collaborative, Pediatrics Supporting Parents Collaborative (virtual)
Sara Kinsman, Health Resources and Services Administration
Amy Knight, Children's Hospital Association
Laurel K. Leslie, American Board of Pediatrics
Kamila Mistry, Agency for Healthcare Research and Quality

Also Attending
Brenda Harding, Agency for Healthcare Research and Quality (virtual)
Barry Solomon, Academic Pediatric Association

12:45–1:30 Lunch

1:30–2:00 Additional time for Committee and Sponsor Q&A

2:00–3:30 Public Information-Gathering Session

- Why is it important to invest in the health and wellbeing of children and youth?
- What is the purpose of transformation? Desired outcomes?
- What have been identified as key levers of change to guide innovation and transformation within health care systems?

Speakers:
Janet Currie, Princeton University (virtual)
Rachel Thornton, Nemours Children's Health (virtual)
Joshua Sharfstein, John Hopkins University (virtual)

February 28, 2023

PUBLIC SESSION

10:45–12:15 Welcome
Tina Cheng, Committee Co-Chair, University of Cincinnati, Cincinnati Children's Hospital
James Perrin, Committee Co-Chair, Harvard Medical School, MassGeneral Hospital for Children

Public Information-Gathering Session
- What are the desired outcomes of appropriate health care treatments and interventions for all children, youth, and families?
- Why is a life course perspective important for improving health and wellbeing?
- What are the special populations the study should consider?
- How does the rise in diversity among the U.S. population affect the administration of health care?

Speakers:
Michael Lu, University of California, Berkeley
Rahil Briggs, Zero to Three
Claire Brindis, University of California, San Francisco
Megie Okumura, University of California, San Francisco

The Keck Center, 500 Fifth Street, NW
Washington, DC 20001

March 29, 2023

PUBLIC SESSION

1:00–2:00 Understanding Health Care System Transformation
- Why is it important to invest in the health and wellbeing of children and youth?
- What is the future of pediatric health care delivery?
- What have been identified as key levers of change to guide innovation and transformation within health care systems?

Speakers
Neal Halfon, University of California, Los Angeles (invited)
Kay Johnson, Johnson Group Consulting, Inc. (virtual)
Edward Schor, Health Care System Consultant (virtual)

2:00–3:30 Lived Experience
- How should health care providers or health care systems be engaging families and communities in their care?

- What changes are needed in the child and adolescent health care system?
- What are patient and family expectations of high-quality care, evidence-based care, and health equity? How should these terms be defined to promote health care system change?
- What are promising policies and practices that incorporate the lived experiences of underserved children, adolescents, parents, and caregivers, and build the needed trust, partnerships, and long-term relationships to promote family-centered engagement, promote protective factors, and help address systemic inequities and disparities in access to and use of high-quality child and adolescent health care?

Speakers
Renee Boynton-Jarrett, Boston University, Vital Village Community Engagement Network
Tamela Milan-Alexander, EverThrive
Nikki Montgomery, Family Voices (virtual)

March 30, 2023

PUBLIC SESSION

1:00–2:00 Medicaid, Children's Health Insurance Program, and Alternative Payment Models

- What are the gaps and barriers in current payment models, for both public and commercial insurance, and what are potential solutions to overcome them?
- What are new strategies and/or models that should be considered for improving care for children and youth?
- What goals should be considered if financing health care is transformed and how should such transformation be advanced?

Speakers
Jacey Cooper, California Department of Health Care Services (virtual)
Sherry Glied, New York University (virtual)

The Keck Center, 500 Fifth Street, NW
Washington, DC 20001

June 15, 2023

PUBLIC SESSION

9:00–9:10	Welcome and Introductions *Tina Cheng, Committee Co-Chair* *James Perrin, Committee Co-Chair*
9:10–11:00	Collaborative Programs to Support Children's Health and Wellbeing Speakers (Virtual) *Elizabeth Koschmann, TRAILS to Wellness* *Carley Riley, Cincinnati Children's Hospital, All Children Thrive* *Christopher Greeley, Texas Children's Hospital, Baylor College of Medicine* *Doug Eby, Southcentral Foundation* Q&A Discussion with Committee Facilitator: *Christina Bethell, Committee Member*
11:00–11:15	Break
11:15–12:40	Importance of Investing in the Health and Wellbeing of Children and Adolescents Quality Health Care and Long-Term Social Benefit *David Erikson, Federal Reserve Bank of New York (virtual)* Quality Health Care for Young Adults Living with Chronic and Rare Conditions *Sneha Dave, Generation Patient* Quality Health Care for the Mental Health of Adolescents and Young Adults *Prameela Boorada, Mental Health America, Youth Mental Health Leadership Council* Q&A Discussion with Committee Facilitator: *Laquisha Turner, Committee Member*

12:40–1:30 Lunch

1:30–3:00 Scientific Advancements and the Future of Health Care Delivery

Biomedical Informatics and Artificial Intelligence
Eneida Mendonca, Cincinnati Children's Hospital
Genomic Medicine
Stephen Kingsmore, Rady Children's Hospital (virtual)
Medical Innovations and the Future of Children's Health
Paul Wise, Stanford University (virtual)

Q&A Discussion with Committee and Speakers
Facilitator: *Kelly Kelleher, Committee Member*

The Keck Center, 500 Fifth Street, NW
Washington, DC 20001

September 7, 2023

PUBLIC SESSION

9:00–9:05 Welcome
Tina Cheng, Committee Co-Chair
James Perrin, Committee Co-Chair

9:05–10:30 Policy and Financing Levers for Transforming the Child Health Care System

Speakers (Virtual)
Sara Rosenbaum, The George Washington University
Cindy Mann, Manatt Health
Mary Applegate, Ohio Department of Medicaid
Dana Hargunani, Oregon Health Authority

Q&A Discussion with Committee
Facilitator: *James Perrin, Committee Member*

10:30–10:45 Break

10:45–12:00	Messaging the Importance of Investing in Children's Health and Wellbeing Speakers *Bruce Lesley, First Focus on Children* *Sara Watson, Watson Strategies, LLC* *Nat Kendall-Taylor, Frameworks* *Tim Robinson, Nationwide Children's & Kenny McDonald, The Columbus Partnership (virtual)* Q&A Discussion with Committee and Speakers Facilitator: *Kelly Kelleher, Committee Member*
12:00–12:45	Lunch
12:45–1:30	Scientific Advancements and the Future of Health Care Delivery Speakers (Virtual) *Jim Taylor, Google* *Daniel Kraft, NextMed Health* Q&A Discussion with Committee and Speakers Facilitator: *Ashleigh Coser, Committee Member*
1:30–2:00	Findings from the Newly Released National Academies Report *The Future Pediatric Subspeciality Physician Workforce: Meeting the Needs of Infants, Children, and Adolescents* (Released September 7, 2023) Speakers (virtual) *Christopher Stille, University of Colorado, Children's Hospital Colorado* *Rachel Garfield, Vermont Child Health Improvement Program, University of Vermont*
2:00	Open Session Ends

Appendix D

Summary of Performance Measurement Topics Used across Seven Child Health Programs Involving Federal Funding

The seven child health programs involving federal funding include

1. Child Welfare [Administration for Children and Families] (CW)
2. Early Intervention [U.S. Department of Education] (EI)
3. Federally Qualified Health Centers [Health Resources and Services Administration] (FQHC)
4. Healthcare Effectiveness Data and Information Set (managed care organization measures) [National Committee for Quality Assurance] (HEDIS)
5. Maternal, Infant, and Early Childhood Home Visiting [Health Resources and Services Administration] (HV)
6. Medicaid and Children's Health Insurance Program (CHIP) [Centers for Medicare & Medicaid Services] (MCD)
7. Title V [Health Resources and Services Administration] (TV).

For each measurement topic, the number of measures used and names of agencies by code above with measures on this topic used as of 2022 are included in parentheses. This analysis was conducted by the Child and Adolescent Health Measurement Initiative (CAHMI) using information from the CAHMI Maternal and Child Health Measurement Compendium database.[1] This analysis was conducted to inform the formulation of the Engagement In Action Framework (EnAct!) for integrated child health systems (Bethell et al., 2023b).

[1] See https://www.cahmi.org/our-work-in-action/measurement-in-action/compendium

Measurement topics that address insurance, access, and utilization include 12 topics with a total of 38 measures. Six of 12 topics (50%) are used for two or more programs/measurement sets.

1. Adolescent well visits (4/TV, MCD, HEDIS)
2. Infants and toddlers with an individualized family services plan (IFSP) (2/EI)
3. Services were delivered in a home or community setting (1/EI)
4. Child and adolescent health insurance coverage, continuity and/or adequacy (3/TV, HV)
5. Outpatient visits, including telehealth (1/HEDIS)
6. Timely receipt of services for infants and toddler with an IFSP (2/EI)
7. Children and adolescents who are uninsured (1/TV)
8. Prenatal and postpartum care (6/TV, MCD, FQHC, HV, HEDIS)
9. Well-child visits (7/TV, HV, MCD, HEDIS)
10. Children and adolescents who did not receive needed health care (1/TV)
11. Receipt of dental care services (8/MCD, TV, FQHC, HEDIS)
12. Well-woman visits (3/TV, MCD, HEDIS)

Measurement topics that address quality of care, including screenings, referrals, and follow-ups include 17 topics with a total of 70 measures. Nine of 17 topics (52.9%) topics are used for two or more agencies.

1. Behavioral concerns of children (1/HV)
2. Early childhood developmental screening (6/TV, MCD, HV)
3. Parent–child interactions assessment (1/HV)
4. Cervical cancer screening (4/HEDIS)
5. Follow-up after hospitalization for mental illness (12/MCD, HEDIS)
6. Social needs follow-up (e.g., food security, housing) (3/HEDIS)
7. Chlamydia screening (2/MCD, HEDIS)
8. Follow-up care for prescribed medication for attention deficit hyperactivity disorder (ADHD) (6/MCD, HEDIS)
9. Social needs screening (e.g., food security, housing) (3/HEDIS)
10. Completed depression referrals (5/HEDIS, HV, FQHC)
11. Intimate partner violence referrals (1/HV)
12. Tobacco, alcohol, or other drug cessation referrals/treatments for adults and/or caregivers (7/FQHC, MCD, HEDIS)

13. Completed developmental status referrals (1/HV)
14. Intimate partner violence screening (1/HV)
15. Tobacco, alcohol, or other drug screening (2/FQHC, HV)
16. Depression screening (13/FQHC, TV, MCD, HV, HEDIS)
17. Lead screening (2, MCD, HEDIS)

Measurement topics that address quality of care, including the care process, education, and counseling include 11 topics with a total of 52 measures. Six of 11 topics (54.5%) are used for two or more measurement sets.

1. Antibiotic treatment (4/HEDIS)
2. Contraceptive care (6/HEDIS)
3. Transition of care (adolescents, early intervention) (2/TV, EI)
4. Asthma medication (2/MCD, HEDIS)
5. Labor and delivery care (4/TV, MCD)
6. Use of first-line psychosocial care for children and adolescents (2/MCD, HEDIS)
7. Children and adolescents receiving care in a setting that meets multipart medical home measure (2/TV)
8. Mediated dispute resolution (2/EI)
9. Weight assessment, counseling for nutrition, physical activity (9/FQHC, MCD, HEDIS)
10. Consumer assessment of health care providers and systems health plan—includes several experience-of-care measures (4/MCD, HEDIS)
11. Monitoring of children and adolescents on antipsychotics (15/MCD, HEDIS)

Measurement topics that address health-related and intermediate outcomes include 31 topics with 148 measures. Seven of 31 (22.6%) topics are used for two or more measurement sets.

1. Bullying (victimization or perpetration) (3/TV)
2. Children and adolescents with a mental or behavioral condition who receive treatment or counseling (1/TV)
3. Low birth weight (4/TV, HV, MCD)
4. Child and adolescent immunization status (60/FQHC, TV, MCD, HEDIS)
5. Children and adolescents with special health care needs (CSHCN) (1/TV)
6. Maternal mortality rate (1/TV)

7. Child and adolescent mortality rates, including suicide, motor vehicle accidents (4/TV)
8. Children and adolescents with special health care needs who receive care in a well-functioning system (1//TV)
9. Mental health disorder diagnosis (5/HEDIS)
10. Child and adolescent physical activity (3/TV)
11. Early/infant death mortality rates (6/TV)
12. Mothers breastfeeding (3/TV, HV)
13. Child maltreatment (3/HV, CW)
14. Early language and literacy activities or caregivers (e.g., daily reading) (1/HV)
15. Prenatal immunization status (3/HEDIS)
16. Child socioemotional knowledge, skills, and behavior (1/EI)
17. Emergency department visits and injury hospitalizations (4/TV, MCD, HV)
18. Preterm birth (2/TV, HV)
19. Children and adolescents diagnosed with attention deficit disorder or ADHD (1/TV)
20. Families using infant safe-sleep methods (4/TV, HV)
21. Primary caregiver education (1/HV)
22. Children and adolescents diagnosed with an autism spectrum disorder (1/TV)
23. Family knowledge of rights, communicating child's needs, and supporting development (1/EI)
24. Severe maternal morbidity (1/TV)
25. Children and adolescents in excellent or very good health (1/TV)
26. Foster-care related outcomes (e.g., timely placement) (23/CW)
27. Smoking/tobacco use (2/TV)
28. Children and adolescents who are obese (3/TV)
29. Infants born with alcohol or substance exposure (neonatal abstinence) (2/TV)
30. Teen birth rate (1/TV)
31. Children and adolescents who have decayed teeth or cavities (1/TV)

NOTE: New Title V national outcomes measures starting in 2024 will include school readiness, child flourishing, two or more adverse childhood experiences, housing instability, food insecurity, and more.